PRINCIPLES OF
DENTAL PUBLIC HEALTH

Principles of
Dental Public Health

Fourth Edition

James Morse Dunning, D.D.S., M.P.H., S.D.
Professor of Ecological Dentistry, Emeritus
Harvard University

HARVARD UNIVERSITY PRESS
Cambridge, Massachusetts, and London, England
1986

Library of Congress Cataloging-in-Publication Data

Dunning, James Morse, 1904–
    Principles of dental public health.

    Includes bibliographies and index.
    1. Dental public health. I. Title. [DNLM:
1. Public Health Dentistry. WU 113 D924p]
RK52.D8 1986   362.1'9'7600973   86–4632
ISBN 0–674–70550–5

To
Mae, Cornelia, and Rose

Preface

THIS BOOK is designed both for the student and for the general practitioner of dentistry. It gives an introduction to the broad field of public health and also detailed, specific material on the development of dental public health programs. Previous textbooks on dental public health have dealt almost exclusively with the dental aspects. This is a good method of approach if the text is to be used for teaching purposes in a situation where lecturers on the broader aspects of public health can fill in the background material. Practicing dentists, however, suddenly finding themselves so placed that they must design or participate in a community dental health program, need to know more than mere dentistry. They need to know the frame of reference in which their efforts will fit. They can read basic texts on public health but will find them designed for the physician and filled with much detail that appears irrelevant to them as dentists. They need a simplified approach to public health practice, and they need, particularly, an elementary knowledge of those tools of public health that will help them design and operate their own program. By tools I mean those basic sciences such as biostatistics and epidemiology which are essential to all study of mass disease, whether it be systemic or dental. The problems of dental disease are primarily those of chronic disease, the field toward which medicine is turning its sharpest attention these days and where epidemiology and biostatistics are indispensable aids.

This book is, in a very real sense, the crystallization of a course in dental public health which has been presented since 1947 to upperclass undergraduates at the Harvard School of Dental Medicine and, since 1955, in more or less the same form as an evening course for graduate dentists. Both student groups have been very rewarding, though in different ways. The undergraduates are closer to their period of basic science training in the Medical School. They give evidence of better background and of greater interest in the material grouped under the heading "Tools of Dental Public Health." The graduate group, with practical experience back of them, are more specifically interested in dental program planning. For the members of this group, the course has been their first contact with the broad field of public health, and they show great eagerness to understand the framework of public health administration within which they are operating. Both groups appear interested in continued education in dental public health because they find themselves, chiefly as a result of the advent of fluoridation, for the first time in history possessed of preventive techniques which can be applied at the community level. From these experiences and from others, I see clear evidence of the need for a textbook on dental public health that will reach all practitioners of dentistry and which will stand on its own feet as reading material for those practitioners unable to obtain formal teaching in the subject.

A book of this sort can serve only as an introduction to the larger field of public health. Biostatistics, for instance, is an extremely hard subject to learn by oneself. The chapters on biostatistics here are designed merely to present the statistical point of view, including the concept of variability and a few of the simpler tests commonly needed in the dental field. Students going more deeply into this field will need not only more advanced textbooks but also good teachers. The material on public health administration and personnel management is merely an introduction to a large field in which practical experience counts heavily. Dentists who suddenly find themselves in charge of a large working force will need additional help. This they can obtain from some of the textbooks referred to in the list of references and also by seeking aid from their public health colleagues. In the field of preventive dentistry, this book treats dental caries, periodontal disease, oral cancer, and the like in such a way as to give a basic understanding of their earlier signs and of those mass phenomena which are of interest from a public health point of view. The refinements of oral pathology can be learned from textbooks specifically devoted to the subject.

To the teacher of dental public health, this book should have value as a teaching outline, either for undergraduate dental students or for postgraduate students. Around it can be built a course which will have both breadth and detail, the detail often supplied by specialists from areas outside dentistry, where these are available. Where the teachers must do most of the work themselves, it is hoped that by reading as far as they can in the reference material presented here, they will be able to do a reasonably good job. It is hoped they will enjoy their teaching work as much as has the author over the past decades.

Since the third edition of this book went to press in 1978, the sharp drop in the incidence of dental caries in children in developed countries all over the world, coming at a time of high inflation and economic recession, has profoundly altered dental practice in the United States. No longer do children up through the teenage period require massive restorative dentistry. Fluoridation can claim a major share of the credit for this change, but epidemiologically the drop is a complex matter requiring further study.

The immediate result of this drop has been less work for dentists to do among children. Inflation has then urged dentists to raise their fees in such a way as to price many of them out of their market. This situation has forced a number of changes on the profession—some constructive, others destructive. Constructive changes have occurred in the marketing of private practices and in the greater attention paid to periodontal disease and to the care of adult and elderly patients. A destructive change has taken place in the opposition of the profession to the use of extended function auxiliaries at just the time when increases in the public delivery system for dental care are needed to reach low-income citizens and people in underserved areas.

The re-election of a conservative administration has made restoration of the recent drastic cuts in federal health programs unlikely. The gap between the "haves" and the "have-nots" in our society has widened, so that more and better public health programs are needed—not fewer programs. Dental care delivery systems, as a consequence, need careful study.

For all these reasons, dentists now appear to have greater opportunities for future public health action than formerly, even though the success of their preventive measures for caries has resulted in a lessening of the need for care for children. It is my hope that this textbook may continue to inspire and to facilitate the careful planning of programs and political actions for the future.

Even the English language has changed, in response to a lowering of sex barriers. A dentist can no longer be referred to uniformly as "he," nor an auxiliary as "she." Where this may still occur in the book, no sex preference is implied.

I am deeply indebted not only to a number of publishers and authors whose specific contributions are noted at appropriate points, but to many other workers and teachers in the fields of public health and of dentistry whose points of view and phraseology have influenced the writing of this text. Certain well-turned phrases and basic concepts become the vocabulary of any specialized field, and it is often impossible to credit their originators. More particularly, I wish to express gratitude to colleagues who read the original manuscript of this book and offered constructive criticism. Among these are Louis J. P. Calisti, Robert L. Glass, John E. Gordon, Demetrios M. Hadjimarkos, Leon B. Leach, Hugh R. Leavell, Benjamin F. Paul, Robert B. Reed, James H. Shaw, Reidar F. Sognnaes, William D. Wellock, and Marjorie A. C. Young. Within my immediate family, my first wife, Mae, and daughter Cornelia have given particularly helpful advice. I am also indebted to Laurence B. Brown for the preparation of most of the illustrations. To my father, the late William B. Dunning, I am indebted for leadership both in dentistry and in writing. Dr. Dunning saw the first chapter of the book in time to lend it his encouragement.

Help in this revision has come from a number of quarters, but particular acknowledgments are due to Robin M. Lawrence (for the comprehensive revision of Chapter 23), Theodore Rebich, Jr. (for the New York material), David E. Barmes, Gregory N. Connolly, Chester W. Douglass, and Jonathan Director. My wife, Nora Dunning, has provided valuable editorial assistance, as well as doing the word-processing and the heavy cut-and-paste work in the preparation of the revised manuscript.

Contents

PART I. Background

1. Public Health in Theory   3
2. Public Health in Practice   18
3. Milestones in Dental Public Health   43

PART II. The Tools of Dental Public Health

4. Biostatistics: Selection of Data   59
5. Biostatistics: Appraisal of Variability   74
6. Biostatistics: Correlation and Other Tests   93
7. Epidemiology: General Principles   112
8. Epidemiology: Dental Caries   131
9. Epidemiology: Periodontal and Other Diseases   167
10. The Social Sciences   185

11. *Principles of Administration*   208
12. *Preventive Dentistry*   230

Part III.   Dental Health Programs

13. *Dental Needs and Resources*   269
14. *Surveying*   310
15. *Dental Health Education*   363
16. *Water Fluoridation*   393
17. *Delivery of Dental Care*   433
18. *Payment for Dental Care*   476
19. *Evaluating the Quality of Dental Care*   501
20. *Community Dental Health Programs*   526
21. *Special Dental Health Programs*   552
22. *State Dental Health Programs*   578
23. *United States Federal Programs*   595
24. *Foreign and International Programs*   613

Part IV.   The Future

25. *Conquest or Equilibrium?*   629

References   641
Index   679

PART I

Background

CHAPTER 1

Public Health in Theory

FOR DENTISTS, whose profession over the past century has been built upon the high-quality restorative treatment performed by private practitioners, public health is a relatively new subject. It is a subject, however, to which dentists turned inevitably, once the almost universal prevalence of dental disease became an established fact. In a country where the principle of equal rights among men was taken seriously, it was impossible that any profession could concentrate its entire attention on elaborate care for a privileged group to the exclusion of the needs of the great masses of the population.

The problem of providing dental care for entire populations involves methods and concepts which are new and challenging to the average dentist. Prevention takes on a new meaning where manpower is obviously insufficient to render all needed restorative care. Teamwork becomes a necessity in extending the scope of care to the largest population and at the lowest cost per unit of care consistent with work of good quality. Group financing must be undertaken to aid the individual patient in the lower income brackets. The test of any public health measure now becomes, "How much will it do for the person who can't afford private care?" This is a fruitful new field for the dentist to enter. It makes him one with the social planners and the health officials who are prime movers in making his community a good place to live in.

The enlargement of the private practice point of view to embrace the public health point of view can become easy if a few important similarities are borne in mind. There is still an operator; not one person in a white coat, but a public health team variously attired and with various skills. There is still a patient: not one person with a complaint to treat, but a community composed of many persons, some with complaints, some with undiscovered disease, and some entirely healthy. Surveying and evaluation are the community equivalents of diagnosis. Actual methods of health education and of treatment differ only slightly from those of the private office, and the basic principles are unchanged. Society is composed of individuals.

Public health, as an organized effort to protect the well-being of the human race, is a development of many centuries' standing, perhaps almost as old as its parent discipline, medicine. Among the earliest recorded health codes are those of the Mosaic law of the Hebrews, in the first books of the Bible. Isolation of cases of infectious disease is provided for there: dietary rules are laid down, some of them arbitrary to a modern viewer but most of them recognizably useful in controlling infectious disease. Here was a strong society acting for its own protection.

The late Charles-Edward A. Winslow of Yale has given us an excellent definition of public health as "the art and science of preventing disease, prolonging life, and promoting physical and mental efficiency through organized community effort."[1] The important concept in this sentence is contained in the last words, *through organized community effort*. No longer is the individual patient the sole object of study; now the entire community is the focus. This includes not only the sufferers from disease in all degrees of severity, from the subclinical to the fatal, and those persons who have been left disabled in the wake of disease, but also well people, both resistant and susceptible to disease. The positive nature of the modern concept of health is well stated by the World Health Organization in its constitution: "Health is a state of complete physical, mental, and social well-being, and not merely the absence of disease or infirmity."

Historically, many public health programs have evolved as the result of the inability of some group within the population to receive adequate prevention of or treatment for existing disease. Thus the first activity of the United States Public Health Service beyond quarantine, upon its organization in 1798, was a medical care plan; later a chain of hospitals was established for seamen unable to obtain medical care through other means. This was essentially an extension of private medical care, but a group was at the giving end and a group at the receiving end. As group techniques evolved, they were applied to the well in addition to the sick, until now the preventive services of the U.S. Public Health Service constitute a far more important endeavor than its medical care services.

In dentistry there has been a somewhat similar transition. A century ago dentistry consisted mainly of careful restorative work for those individuals afflicted with dental disease and able to pay for treatment in private offices. About 1910 the first large institutions were formed to give dental care to indigent groups: the Forsyth Dental Infirmary for Children in Boston, and the Eastman Dental Dispensary in Rochester, New York. Even this was not public health as we know it today. Practical preventive methods for dental disease did not exist of a type to justify community dental health programs. Today the story is different. Oral hygiene, diet, water fluoridation, and fluoride rinses are all practical enough now to form good bases for communitywide programs to prevent dental caries. Water fluoridation presents a problem which precipitates the dentist into civic affairs alongside other public health workers who have taken a deep interest in this measure. These matters, and the health education to get them across, are the real core of dental public health.

The Council on Dental Education of the American Dental Association has given an apt definition which will also serve to indicate the scope of this book: "Dental public health is the science and art of preventing and controlling dental diseases and promoting dental health through organized community efforts. It is that form of dental practice which serves the community as a patient rather than the individual. It is concerned with dental health education of the public, applied dental research, and the administration of group dental care programs, as well as the prevention and control of dental diseases on a community basis."[2]

THE PUBLIC HEALTH METHOD

Public health work exhibits a certain number of characteristics that are different from individual practice in the same field. Most important perhaps is the fact that public health work must be done in areas where *group responsibility* is recognized. For this reason contagious diseases received some of the earliest attention, since it was obviously a group responsibility that a man be made safe from his neighbor. This concept led first to quarantine and isolation procedures, later to the mass preventive measures that loom so large today. Acute communicable diseases were the earliest to demand attention. Success in controlling many of these, as the science of bacteriology gave the means for doing so, led to a shift of attention, in the more developed countries, to chronic disease. This is the focus today. It is due in part to the fact that people live long enough now to fall victim to degenerative diseases they seldom had a chance to contract a century ago.

Another characteristic of the public health method is its reliance upon *teamwork*. This is due partly to the necessity of efficient handling of large groups of people and partly to the fact that many processes which are involved in prevention lend themselves particularly well to teamwork. Physical examination of schoolchildren for gross defects is a good example here. The same work could be done by private physicians in their own offices, but it is far easier to handle large groups of children in institutional surroundings, with systematic delegation of many procedures to properly supervised auxiliary personnel.

Prevention is in itself a major objective of public health programs. There are really three reasons for this. The first is ethical: that prevention of disease is an even greater good in life than the cure of disease. The second is the advantage of teamwork, as has just been mentioned. The third is cost efficiency, since prevention is far cheaper than cure in a program where there is responsibility for both approaches.

Group responsibility has also been recognized from the start in the area of the indigent. The completely indigent have been the easiest to recognize, as in the case of the destitute merchant seamen. Later on came the concept of *medical indigence:* an inability to pay large bills for medical care. This situation is found chiefly in the area of chronic disease, where the life savings of otherwise independent people are easily wiped out. Thus cancer has become a public health problem in recent years. The processes involved in screening for cancer are expensive in themselves, and the disease, once contracted, is extremely expensive to treat. As an outgrowth of aid to the medically indigent, the concept has arisen in the United States that health care is a *right* of citizenship and hence to be provided by government to the extent available. Public health agencies are inevitably affected by this new philosophy. The implications of the change are discussed in Chapters 22 and 23.

A further characteristic of public health work lies in its ability to deal with all sorts of problems involving the host population and the environment, beyond the range of the individual physician or dentist. No longer need a disease be considered a phenomenon caused by one "agent" within the individual patient. The disease can be studied on a communitywide basis and can be recognized for what it really is: a *multifactorial* problem. This introduces a new complexity into the search for causes of disease, and has given rise to the science of *epidemiology,* which has been called "the diagnostic procedure in mass disease."[3] Even in a disease as clearcut as measles, the epidemiologist will look for host factors and environmental factors and try to control them. These factors are often seen much more clearly when a group is studied, rather than an individual. Every disease can be thought of in terms of a chain or web of causation, to be broken either at the easiest spot, if such can be found, or at various spots. In a disease where no one preventive measure is highly effective or where exact causative factors are not known, a shotgun approach to various factors may possibly prove the most effective. This is often true of dental caries, as will be seen later. The science of epidemiology has been built up around the concept of multifactorial disease and the medical detective work needed to uncover various factors. Originally dealing only with epidemics of contagious disease, the epidemiologist now deals with all sorts of problems where his methods will apply, even automobile accidents. Time, place, and person are the best factors to study here.

The necessities of epidemiologic work have given rise to another characteristic of public health work which differentiates it from private practice: dependence on the *biostatistical method.* The existence of a disease in an individual patient can usually be described on a yes-or-no basis. This same disease would probably be present at all times in a large population group, its frequency affected by a multiplicity of factors. The time factor becomes important, since changes in the prevalence of disease can be measured only by observations over a number of years. These problems require accurate measurement of rates and lead us to the question whether differences between rates are real or are merely chance phenomena. Mathematical measurement of probability becomes necessary. The aim of biostatistics is not to erect complicated mathematical pyramids upon possibly shaky foundations, but to appraise the variability and the errors to be found in almost all arithmetic measurements of disease in large populations.

In recent years, *computer science* has vastly increased the ease of data analysis, even with small samples. The public health worker finds himself in more frequent contact with computers and with the computer center, to his great advantage. One new danger faces him, however. Computer analysis is now so easy that the temptation is strong to measure any situation even if the parameters are poor and then give undue importance to the computer print-outs.

Another characteristic of public health is that, through his efforts to attain prevention of disease, the public health worker deals with *healthy* or *apparently healthy people* as well as with the sick, and the first two categories are by far the largest. This brings a cheerful, hopeful atmosphere to the work, but also brings with it certain problems. The worker must go looking for minimal disease instead of waiting for frank disease to come to him. He must adapt himself to those testing methods which can be used effectively on large populations. He must learn to take more satisfaction from the recognition and interception of early disease than from the control of advanced disease.

From the public's point of view, it requires a stretch of the imagination to realize the need for periodic health examination and to accept preventive measures, except for those diseases which are most dramatic in their disabling or fatal effects. The *education of the public*, therefore, becomes a prime objective of public health work; so also, we now realize, does the *adaptation of public health programs to community culture*. The social sciences such as cultural anthropology and social psychology help us understand why people react in an apparently strange manner when health measures are introduced contrary to accepted cultural patterns.

Public health agencies have become increasingly involved in the delivery of care to people in disadvantaged or isolated locations, such as the inner cities or the outer rural areas. *Logistics* requires attention here, with attention to the location of and transportation to health care facilities. In general, care should be brought as close as possible to where the people are normally concentrated: hence the advantage of neighborhood health centers, or of school-based dental care facilities for school children.

Another mechanism, coming into increasing use in the payment for health care, is the *insurance* principle. Rare, catastrophic occurrences such as prolonged hospitalization and major surgery are fairly easy to insure, as the load can be borne in large part by those who never need the service. More common occurrences such as the need for restorative dentistry are much harder to handle, but the budgeting of payment in regular installments provides an aid which closely resembles insurance and is usually called that.

The occasional social failures of public health have much to teach us. Benjamin D. Paul, an anthropologist, has assembled a large and instructive volume dealing almost exclusively with such failures.[4] They occur with equal frequency in primitive communities, where witch doctors are getting their first competition, and in civilized societies, where people will not recognize the existence of such (to them) distasteful problems as mental disease. The rebuffs which have been dealt to water fluoridation in certain areas are the most obvious examples of social reaction in the dental field. In dentistry there is the additional difficulty that the common dental diseases are not thought to be contagious. Their relation to systemic disease is difficult enough to trace so that they are seldom considered causes of disability or death. With proper social planning, followed by education of the public, these problems may usually be put in their proper perspective.

ETHICS IN PUBLIC HEALTH

Much can be learned of the nature of public health by a consideration of the ethical problems it creates and a comparison of those problems with the more familiar ones of medical and dental practice. Ethics, here, may be defined as the science of the ideal human character and behavior in situations where distinction must be made between right and wrong, duty must be followed, and good interpersonal relations maintained.

One of the sharpest ethical distinctions we are called upon to make is that between the welfare of an individual and the welfare of society. Does society exist for the benefit of the individual or the individual for the benefit of society? The individualistic philosophy is well stated by Ralph Barton Perry: "The goodness of anything consists in its relation to feeling, desire, emotion, will or some similar attitude—this much having been assumed, there would then remain the further question as to where such attitudes of favor and disfavor are to be found. The answer of social democracy is that they are found, and found only, in individuals."[5]

Respect for the individual finds its way into the Golden Rule and is one of the most important teachings of Jesus. Western civilization has emphasized respect for the individual. This concept underlies our Bill of Rights. We do compile vital statistics, but are pretty careful to remember that vital statistics are "people with the tears wiped away," as someone has aptly said. In a negative sense, we show our respect for the individual by an unwillingness to dabble in compulsory eugenics or euthanasia.

Present-day principles of medical ethics also emphasize service to the individual. The American Medical Association postulates "full respect for the dignity of man" and the obligation of a physician not to reveal confidences entrusted to him. Only at the very end of the American Medical Association's *Principles of Medical Ethics* is there mention of society, in a section which reads: "The honored ideals of the medical profession imply that the responsibilities of the physician extend not only to the individual but also to society."[6] There is certainly no hint that society is more important than the individual.

The opposite philosophy is that which places greatest value on the welfare of the group. This is more than a recognition of the obvious fact that, when people are crowded together, one person's freedom ends "where the other person's nose begins." A social group is more than a mere aggregate, an arithmetical sum of its parts. The mark of an aggregate is that its parts can be joined or separated without essential change in their internal characteristics. No genuine social group is such an aggregate—its members are too interdependent. Every group has an esprit de corps, a common interest, a collective will, a kind of group mind.[6] Totalitarian governments are designed to recognize this philosophy; so also to a lesser extent are democratic governments, for the welfare of a majority of the people and the welfare of the state are often synonymous. This concept inevitably finds its way into public health. An example will illustrate the problems which may arise from conflict between this group-welfare philosophy and that of the welfare of the individual.

The American Typhus Commission in the Middle East during World War II had the assignment of working with local health authorities in the face of a major outbreak of typhus, the worst in the recorded history of the area, and accompanied by a high mortality rate. The Commission was exceptionally well prepared to be of help. They had discovered a new drug which sharply reduced the clinical severity of the disease and, if given early in adequate dosage, reduced the mortality almost to zero. They also had a recently discovered vaccine which was both safe and highly effective in preventing new cases of typhus. Finally, they were armed with DDT, which had just been found to be of value in controlling the human body lice which transmitted typhus. "Several physicians from the Middle East," says Dr. John C. Snyder, a member of this Commission,

were assigned by their government to collaborate with us in the studies. They regarded our intensive efforts, conducted without respect for days of the week or hours of the day, as rather difficult to explain or justify. We had long discussions with them of a friendly and philosophical sort. They stressed the disturbances which mass application of the newly devised epidemic-control measures would cause to the whole country in due course. Interference with the events of nature would result in a more crowded population, more wide-spread hunger, more intense misery. Death from hunger rather than typhus was the prospect. Therefore, they said, by what right did we presume to intervene when in their view the consequences to the people involved were worse than the disease we were seeking to prevent.[7]

Here was a peculiarly frustrating situation, but one faced by health organizations constantly these days in underdeveloped countries where populations are increasing rapidly. It was essentially a conflict between the immediate welfare of the individual and the long-range welfare of society. It forces a consideration of birth control, improvement of agriculture, and other socioeconomic problems not ordinarily thought of as matters of public health. Answers to these questions are often possible but not easy.

Fortunately, few of the ethical decisions in the realm of public health are as difficult as that which faced the Typhus Commission. Students of the population problem in the United States see little reason in the near future to fear either a declining population and cultural suicide or a runaway population that the country will be unable to support adequately. Birth control efforts here are gaining importance, but chiefly to the end that efforts to extend the life span will not result in overpopulation, and that unwanted pregnancies may be prevented. Public health workers here can usually feel that they are benefiting both the individual and society through their acts. By eliminating the pain of disease, by preventing or rehabilitating physical disability, and by extending the life of the population, they will assist in their cultural and physical growth of the country. In the words of Max Lerner, "The extension of life expectancy gives the individual a chance to fulfill his promise; it gives the culture a larger proportion of people who can spend their productive years in work."[8]

Ethical problems of a different nature confront the medical and dental professions in the United States today. A conservative federal administration, cutting back on health programs to finance an immense military budget, has accentuated the gap that has always existed between the "haves" and the "have-nots" in our society.

We see environmental conditions deteriorating in favor of for-profit industry. We see public health services for mothers, children, and the elderly cut back, passing added responsibility to the private sector. At the same time we see private medical and dental fees rising more rapidly than inflation, just when low-income people can least afford them.[9] In dentistry, as in medicine, we see the "quality" cry leading to increased sophistication and cost for specialized operations. At the same time the equitable distribution of primary care to all segments of our population remains far worse than in many other countries.

We ought not to deny the provision of quality care to those who can afford it, any more than we should forbid the manufacture of luxury cars, but can we as true professionals allow the rich to monopolize our services without also providing primary care for all people? Research must go forward in basic areas and in areas of currently limited clinical usefulness. We applaud marketing programs which increase the availability of private practitioners to the public. The trouble comes when major dental organizations limit the accessibility to dental care for parts of our population by opposing the delegation to auxiliaries of operations they are known to be competent to perform. This opposition, all too common today in the United States, and the current disparagement of public health care programs constitute a serious lack of ethics in our health professions.

PREVENTIVE MEDICINE AND PUBLIC HEALTH

Since public health work so often deals with prevention, the question usually arises whether preventive medicine is a science by itself and, if so, who is responsible for it. The concept of "prevention," of course, can be applied at almost any stage of medical or dental treatment. Primary prevention covers those measures taken before any disease appears, as is discussed in Chapter 12, on preventive dentistry. Secondary prevention is synonymous with early disease control. Thus control of early dental caries is prevention of crown-bridge work. Full-denture prosthesis forestalls problems in nutrition. According to this, preventive medicine or dentistry is a point of view to be applied in all phases of treatment, both for the limitation of disability at that stage and for the interception of disease at the next later stage.

Applying this analogy to a dental school curriculum, one would expect to find the teaching of preventive dentistry dealt with most frequently in departments of operative dentistry, oral diagnosis, or pedodontics: in fact, pervading all phases of clinical dentistry. No one will deny that this represents a valuable point of view. If this were all there were to prevention, no separate personnel would be needed to teach it and the whole matter could be handled through dental school staff meetings and such other channels of communication as are used to transmit standards of teaching. As it is, this concept more commonly goes by the name of "control," for control of present disease is really the matter in hand. The preventive concept, by being everyone's business, might become no one's. Hence there is logic in combining it with the community setting where it is most easily practiced, and in creating the departments of "community and preventive dentistry" so commonly seen in dental schools today.

A somewhat more accurate use of the word "prevention" involves primary focus on those measures taken in the period before any sign of frank disease has appeared: primary prevention. Such a concept might imply handing all phases of the teaching of prevention over to the person who presents the public health methodology. This is the desired solution where teachers of public health are available and are in close enough contact with the teachers of the traditional phases of clinical dentistry. Not only does it place responsibility squarely on one person's shoulders—a situation conducive to better accomplishment—but it allows group preventive methods to be considered alongside methods applicable to the individual case.

The true value of prevention can often be appreciated only by seeing what happens in a population group. Thanks to heredity and other factors, one child may have beautiful teeth without ever brushing them and another child have rampant dental caries even with the best of brushing. A layman, or even a teacher of dentistry, may misinterpret this as evidence that tooth brushing has no value. Only when groups of people are studied by proper public health methods can the actual benefit of tooth brushing be made clear. These concepts are treated in more detail in Chapter 12.

"SOCIALIZED MEDICINE"

With increasing populations in many parts of the world, and with the ability of government to equalize distribution of care among differing economic groups, there have been many attempts to bring all health activities under government control. The term "socialized medicine" has come to be attached to these programs, particularly where it was thought that the health of each individual in the community was a matter for government financing and should be paid for through the use of tax funds. This usually came to involve first payment to and then control of the medical and dental professions through government agencies. It interjected a third party into the doctor-patient relation, with sometimes real, sometimes imagined, alteration of this relation. Since socialized medicine in this form involves questions of political theory and ultimately of legislation, it has become controversial. In the words of Winslow, it is now a term which "stimulates the endocrines and deadens the neurones."

In a society where the independence of the private practitioner of medicine or dentistry is considered to be important, the relation between the activities of these practitioners and those of the public health workers must be carefully studied and a logical division of labor worked out. Public health should not ordinarily concern itself, above the level of primary care, with the treatment of individuals who are able to pay for their own care. A sharp line must thus occasionally be drawn between community prevention of disease and the treatment of disease. Current philosophy in the United States indicates that where public health workers pick up the signs of early disease they should refer their patients to, and cooperate with, private practitioners rather than unnecessarily assume responsibility for treatment themselves. Such a division of labor protects the doctor-patient relation for a majority of the population in any community, keeps down the cost of government, and makes best use of a manpower resource already in existence. It thus helps forestall "socialized medicine," in the usually accepted sense of the term.

It is impossible, however, to ignore the fact that government-rendered health care has long been on the increase in the United States. In 1919 there were approximately 32,000 veterans in receipt of compensation or pension for service-incurred disabilities, and eligible to receive medical care regardless of economic status.[10] In 1956, this same group numbered 2,739,000. This is not only an enormous numerical increase, it is also an increase from less than 1 percent of the veteran population potentially eligible for care in 1919 to almost 20 percent in 1956. The enactment of Medicare (health insurance for the aged) in 1966 now carries the country a long step further in the delivery of health care at government expense.

These changes open the question as to whether health care, to the extent available, should be considered a basic human right. The "inalienable rights" set forth in the Declaration of Independence, and later spelled out in the Bill of Rights, are freedoms, not services. Education, of course, is now considered a "right" here, and expensive school systems are charged to the taxpayer regardless of whether he has children to utilize them or not. The enthusiasm of the American public for similarly financed health care is tempered by a consideration of the large new tax burden involved, and the fact that third-party administration of health care increases rather than reduces its cost.

It is a prime mistake to assume that any one pattern for society is right and all others wrong. Some countries, as for instance England, have yielded far more in the way of health activities to government control than we have in the United States and yet are apparently reasonably happy with the result. Even within the United States there are variations in the degree to which people seek out and are happy under group-controlled health services. In the field of ordinary medical and dental care, insurance and budgeting plans offer great attraction to those who, though economically independent in the ordinary sense, need aid for extraordinary expenses. The administration of insurance, especially where groups of patients must be formed, involves a certain (though usually small) degree of loss of individual freedom. The distinction between voluntary and compulsory insurance plans is often difficult to maintain. The old American concept that voluntary health insurance is to be equated with progress and compulsory health insurance with dictatorial bureaucracy seems to be undergoing modification.

Public health involves the efforts of man to better his health through organized community effort. Prevention of disease is a prime objective in public health work, and one where teamwork is most often of great advantage. Community responsibility may also include the treatment of disease for certain groups within the population, and the limitation of disability in the wake of disease.

Based solidly upon medical science, public health also has additional disciplines and characteristics of its own. Social anthropology, epidemiology, biostatistics, behavioral science, and education are among the disciplines. The unqiue characteristics of public health work stem chiefly from the need to work more with well people than with sick people, and from the recognition of most disease as a multifactorial problem. Not only are the agents of disease to be studied, but the group characteristics of the host population, and, above all, the environment in which the agent operates.

Public health work has ethical problems of its own. Chief among them is the conflict between the welfare of the individual and the welfare of the group, most obvious now in the less developed countries where prolonging of life without control of births can lead to population overgrowth. The United States at the moment does not face this problem.

Dentistry is a newcomer to the field of public health, because good preventive measures have been lacking until recently and because dental disease is only indirectly a killer. Yet the place of dentistry in a public health program is now well established, and new preventive measures have now resulted in a striking decrease of dental caries incidence among the children in developed countries. Dental care facilities are now less needed than formerly for these child populations, but needs heretofore unmet exist in dental care for adult and elderly populations and for economically underprivileged population groups both here and abroad. These challenges arouse our interest not only in the science of public health but in the art of public health practice.

CHAPTER 2

Public Health in Practice

Since dental public health programs will almost never be organized except as part of a comprehensive public health program, and since the basic problems in the dental field are much the same as those in other areas of health service, it becomes of interest to study public health practice as it is commonly found today. Public health programs present an almost infinite variety in size and content, from small local programs to great national ones such as that of the U.S. Public Health Service.

Certain basic activities are to be found in all of these programs, but the method of approach and degree of specialization will vary greatly with the size of the program, and detailed content will vary with the needs of the areas involved. Because specialized training is needed for public health officers and because the essence of public health is the handling of groups, there is a certain minimum population below which a structured health department cannot be well supported by available tax funds. This population is commonly thought to be from 35,000 to 50,000. Rural areas or small towns with populations below this range must combine on a county or district basis if they are to have efficient health service. Boards of health, rather than departments, are found in small towns, but are more correctly considered to be parts of the political structure than the service structure of their community. They are largely staffed and frequently chaired by laymen. Service activities commonly are arranged by groups of towns such as counties.

The local health departments, naturally, are concerned with direct service to the public. These are the departments that hire public health nurses to visit individuals and families, that organize well-baby clinics to teach mothers the principles of child hygiene, that send out sanitary inspectors to check the milk and the meat. These are the departments that supervise local water supplies and local sewage disposal, and that collect morbidity and mortality figures from local physicians and administer quarantine regulations. The education they do is usually directly to the public, through the individual, family, or small group. As local health departments grow larger they can add more and more specialists to their staff, both to provide special services and to supervise and educate the rank and file of the health workers. The small health departments must look to a larger unit such as the state for these specialists. The largest local health departments are those seen in our large cities, where one operating department may actually have charge of health for a population numbered in the millions. Much more common throughout the United States, however, are the medium-sized units serving counties, local health districts, or small cities.

The great number and variety of personnel employed by local health departments can be seen from Table 1, showing figures compiled by the Association of State and Territorial Health Officials' National Public Health Reporting System.[1] Both full- and part-time employees of state health agencies are included. Part-time physicians and dentists usually outnumber their full-time equivalents at the local level; less so at state level. Women employees are commonly full-time.

The specific functions of health organizations at all levels from local to international are discussed in later chapters. Suffice it at this point to say that the larger these departments and the more local organizations they have under them, the less contact they have with individual members of the public, the less responsibility they have for the direct operation of sanitary facilities, nursing services, and so forth, and the more advisory functions they have, chiefly education, supervision, financing, and research.

The public health profession has now grown to be a large one, characterized first by the variety of backgrounds of its members, and second by the fact that many of them have joined it some time after their original entry into professional life. Public health, involving as it does a community approach rather than a specialized focus on any one phase of health service, often fails to attract people until after they have had a few years of experience in medicine, dentistry, or the like.

Schools of public health in the United States commonly train for a variety of tasks and accept a large proportion of foreign students as well. Of a student body of 419 at the Harvard School of Public Health in 1984, 79 students were from outside the United States.

Table 1. Full-time equivalent staff of United States state health agencies, by position and program area, December 31, 1977.

Full-time staff	No.
All professional, administrative, technical employees	71,603
Physicians	3,937
Dentists	725
Veterinarians	117
Registered nurses	17,803
Licensed practical nurses	6,297
Nutritionists, dietitians	901
Social workers	2,280
Health educators	753
Other behavioral scientists	1,010
Professional and technical laboratory employees	6,235
Engineers, sanitarians, related employees	9,159
Planners, economists, statisticians, related employees	1,468
Legal and related employees	183
Other professional, administrative, technical employees	20,735

The school offers the degrees of Master of Public Health, Doctor of Public Health, Master of Science in Hygiene, Master of Industrial Health, and Doctor of Science in Hygiene, and assists in programs leading to degrees of Master of Science (as in engineering), Master of Engineering, and Doctor of Philosophy. The physicians and dentists attending this and other schools of public health are most commonly candidates for the degree of Master of Public Health.

The American Public Health Association, founded in 1872, unites the public health profession in this country and publishes a monthly journal. The Association holds large annual conventions at which much of the scientific material is presented through section meetings, one of them on dental health with a membership of over 600. The membership of the entire Association in 1984 was 50,000. Similar associations and societies exist in other countries. The World Health Organization, through World Health Assemblies and other mechanisms, is beginning to bring health workers together on a larger-scale basis internationally.

In the field of dentistry, dental public health is one of the eight dental specialties recognized by the Council on Dental Education of the American Dental Association. The American Association of Public Health Dentistry sponsors a certification board described in Chapter 11, which conforms to ADA standards.

BASIC PUBLIC HEALTH ACTIVITIES

In order to understand the subject material usually dealt with by public health services, it helps to consider their basic activities one by one. This can best be done by reference to the organization chart of a large and well-developed department of health, the State of New York Department of Health, shown in Fig. 1. The description of this chart that follows has been supplied by Theodore Rebich, Jr., Chief of the Dental Research and Treatment Center of the Department of Health. Comments on the administrative design of departments of this type, together with such concepts as the span of control, are found in Chapter 11.

The Health Department is headed by a Commissioner, who presides over an organization employing more than 5,400 people at 28 statewide locations, including a network of regional and district

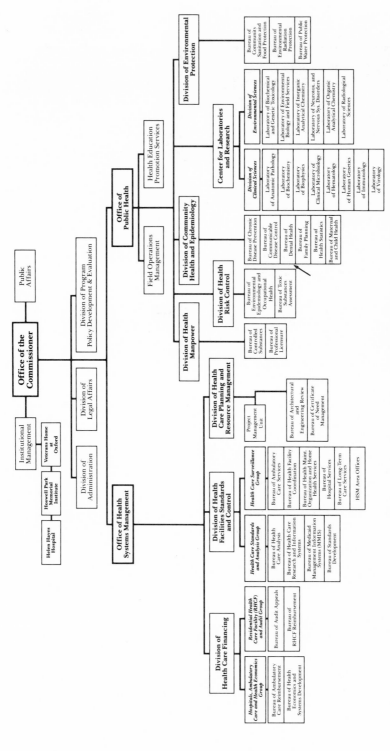

Figure 1. Organization chart of State of New York Department of Health, 1984. [Courtesy, State of New York Department of Health.]

offices and three research and patient treatment centers. These research and treatment centers are controlled by the Institutional Management Group, which reports directly to the Commissioner. Helen Hayes Hospital at West Haverstraw, N.Y., which is one of these three institutions, has recently initiated a Dental Research and Treatment Center with staff formerly of the Bureau of Dental Health, which is perhaps the first such state-funded dental center in the country.

The bulk of the Health Department is organized into two major program units: the Office of Public Health and the Office of Health Systems Management. The *Office of Health Systems Management* (OHSM) is responsible for ensuring that quality medical care is available to all New York residents regardless of where they live or their ability to pay. The department, through OHSM, has direct authority over all health care institutions in the state covered by the Public Health Law, including hospitals, nursing homes, diagnostic and treatment centers, and many home care providers. To protect the welfare of the patients, the state certifies all health care institutions and sets standards governing health facility operations. All health care institutions are inspected regularly to ensure that services meet state and federal requirements; complaints brought by patients, relatives, or employees are also investigated promptly.

Ensuring that limited health care dollars are prudently spent and administering programs to keep the cost of health care services within affordable limits are other primary goals of the department. In carrying out these mandates, OHSM develops reimbursement methods and sets the rate each health facility will be paid for services to patients covered by Medicaid. Those rates form the basis for Medicare, Blue Cross, Workers' Compensation, and No-Fault Insurance rates. OHSM also audits health facility costs and charges and reviews the financial implications of health facility construction and expansion.

Finally, OHSM is responsible for statewide planning to ensure that state health care resources are efficiently allocated to meet the population's needs. A major initiative is being undertaken to encourage innovative, cost-effective alternatives to institutional care, such as home health services, hospice, ambulatory surgery, and health maintenance organizations.

The *Office of Public Health* (OPH) is devoted to preserving the health of New York residents through education, research, and prevention of accidents and disease.

Many of the programs administered by OPH are aimed at enhancing child growth and development through early prenatal care, newborn screening, supplemental foods for pregnant women and children, immunization, prevention of dental disease, school health programs, and teen counseling. Other activities focus on occupation health hazards and the potential health threat of toxic contaminants in the environment. Still others are geared toward combating communicable diseases through continued monitoring of drinking water purity and restaurant sanitation and through follow-up investigation of hospital infections and sexually transmitted disease cases.

Research is one of the most important functions of the OPH. Hundreds of scientists, physicians, and technologists are exploring new ways to prevent and treat disease. Clinical, laboratory, and epidemiological studies are focused on such public health problems as birth defects, kidney disease, toxic effects of chemical substances and radiation, sexually transmitted diseases, and cancer. Other research efforts aim to improve laboratory testing methods, expand understanding of the body's basic biosystems, and reverse deterioration of lakes and streams.

OPH monitors the need for skilled health professionals throughout the state and identifies underserved areas for training support programs. It also oversees the medical conduct of physicians and takes disciplinary action against violators of the Public Health Law.

Finally, OPH is responsible for maintaining records of every birth, death, marriage, and divorce that occurs in the state and for protecting the confidentiality of those records. Using one of the most sophisticated computerized record-keeping systems in the nation, the department can quickly provide general trends or more detailed information on births and deaths for certain geographic areas or for the entire state.

The *Bureau of Dental Health* falls within the Division of Community Health and Epidemiology in OPH. In addition to its role in developing and implementing preventive dental programs, such as sealants, community water fluoridation, fluoride rinsing, and tablets, and in conducting dental health education, the Bureau of Dental Health has a long history of making significant contributions to dental public health research. Starting with the classic Newburgh-Kingston studies on community water fluoridation by Ast et al. in the 1940s, the bureau has conducted an active research program encompassing diverse areas.

The recent creation of the *Dental Research and Treatment Center* within the Department of Health, located at Helen Hayes Hospital, has resulted in a slight restructuring of the Bureau of Dental Health with the bulk of the research staff and programs now emanating from the center. The bureau's efforts are now largely concentrated on program development and administration, and the research efforts remaining in the bureau are program-related, such as the epidemiology of oral diseases among school children and the research related to identifying high-risk populations for the targeting of resources.

Education

In a democratic country, the field for governmental authority is far smaller than it is elsewhere, and there is need for much greater emphasis on education of the public. People must understand why health measures are valuable if they are to undertake them or support them of their own volition. To this extent, education permeates every activity within a health department.

Even a small health department can usually afford a health educator. This individual spends a great deal of time acting as a "resource" in the transmittal of health educational material to community agencies and to the public, and acts as an interpreter of the health department to the public. At the state level, divisions of health education usually appear, with specialized staff. The preparation of pamphlets and other material specially designed for use within the state now becomes a possibility. Specially trained health educators can be of great service as advisers to local programs. Professional training to the Master's level now reaches a growing number of persons in this field. More detailed consideration of health education, and its application in the dental field, is given in Chapter 15.

Vital Statistics

Another public health function of ancient origin is the compilation of vital statistics. The first task within this area has traditionally been census taking, and governments since the dawn of civilization have been taking censuses if for no other reason than to give an accurate base for taxation and for the recruiting of military manpower.

The next function in the field of vital statistics is registration of births, morbidity, and deaths for administrative purposes. Registration involves a complex system administered by departments of health. At the local level the health officer must see that physicians report these facts accurately, and he must then pass on to higher levels the facts that come to him. The interpretation of these figures is usually a state or national function and involves, among other things, international cooperation on terminology. The International Statistical Classification of Diseases, Injuries and Causes of Death is a guide to physicians all over the world, without which variations in terminology would make mortality comparisons between different countries impossible.[2] A classification of diseases of the buccal cavity is included.

The registration of morbidity is a far more difficult matter than the reporting of mortality. Disease is vastly more frequent than death, and only with the more serious communicable diseases is the need for morbidity registration sufficient to justify a state in resorting to compulsory rules. Governments, however, have certain functions to perform for the public which give them an opportunity to compile morbidity statistics beyond the field of reportable disease. One such opportunity comes through school health services, where periodic health appraisals of children give an opportunity for the collection of material relevant to health.

A division of vital statistics has an important function to perform in the standardization and analysis of the information which comes to it on frequency of disease. Sometimes the division is in a position to interpret these data; more often the function is performed by those in charge of epidemiology or some other specific program through which the information will be applied. The division of vital statistics should prepare frequency distributions, graphs, spot maps, and so forth, which may be of use to other divisions or to individuals or organizations other than governmental.

One of the big problems in the field of public health statistics is that of standardization and completeness of reporting. Not until 1933 were all of the states in the United States members of both the birth and the death registration areas. Membership in this instance was based upon two criteria: satisfactory state registration laws and 90 percent completeness in reporting. Even as recently as 1950 an analysis by the Bureau of the Census indicated that about 80,000 births, many of them illegitimate, went unregistered annually in the United States.[3]

Adult Health

Chronic disease and geriatric care are problems of increasing importance because control of acute infectious diseases has allowed the population to grow older and into the age bracket where chronic disease takes over. Two of the biggest endeavors here are the control of cancer through early detection and the control of heart disease through sensible living. Cancer work is a newcomer in the field of public health because of the recent rise in the incidence of this disease. Cancer detection is very difficult, comparatively speaking, and needs the cooperation of many medical specialists, important among them the dentist. Heart disease, again a newcomer because of recent high incidence, involves rehabilitation work as well as prevention in a public health program, because so much heart disease lies beyond our present preventive powers. The rehabilitation of the cardiac patient is a rewarding endeavor. Years of life and much happiness can be given to those who can be taught to live sensibly with their disabilities.

Aside from disease control, adult health programs deal with standards for nursing-home care and other environmental problems of the aging patient.

Dental Health

Almost all health departments in the United States now devote some attention to dental public health. An increasing number of larger ones have divisions of dental health with properly trained full-time personnel. This matter will receive detailed consideration in later chapters.

Hospitals

Hospitals are sometimes a responsibility of the large health department, sometimes not. Historically, the hospitals for certain wards of government (seamen, members of the armed forces, and others) and for patients with certain catastrophic diseases (such as tuberculosis) have grown up within the health department framework. Beyond this, state-level or even city-level standardization of hospital care is occasionally assumed by the health department. Separate departments of hospitals often assume these duties, but combined departments of health and hospitals with a single director are becoming more and more common.

Maternal and Child Health

One of the greatest periods of stress in human life is that of childbirth. Maternal mortality and mortality of newborn infants have always been higher than mortality among the population at large. Prevention of disease, disability, and death at this period has always been a peculiarly appealing public health problem, as well as one where teamwork has been very effective. Statistics show what striking advances have occurred in this field in the past 40 years. In 1915 almost 61 mothers died in connection with every 10,000 live births throughout the United States registration area.[4] In 1974 less than 2 died per 10,000 live births. In 1915 almost 100 (99.9) infants under 1 year of age died per 1,000 live births in the same area. In 1974 only 16.7 were dying per 1,000 births. Medicine and public health can share the honors for this improvement.

The public health endeavor centered upon childbirth has four important phases: prenatal care of the mother, medical care at the time of delivery, infant and preschool care for the child, and school health service. Only in occasional situations, usually where midwives are employed, does the department of public health have much to do with the actual delivery of babies. The other three phases of the maternal and child health effort, however, are standard responsibilities for a health department. *Prenatal and well-baby clinics* are constantly needed as outpatient facilities, or this work must be done in the home by public health nurses where the mother cannot attend the clinic. Health education is the prime objective at both periods. In addition to the basic facts that a mother must know about medical care, nutrition and dental care are very important secondary objectives.

The community services, according to Smillie, required to promote the health of the young child are:

1. Instruction of the parent in the techniques of child care and in the principles of nutrition and methods of protection against illness.

2. Facilities for periodic examination for the detection of defects, incipient disease, and the consequences of faulty care and training.

3. Medical and dental facilities for securing necessary correction and treatment of defects that are found.

4. Immunization against specific infectious diseases such as diphtheria and poliomyelitis.[5]

School health constitutes a major endeavor for any department of public health, unless, as sometimes occurs, the department of education assumes this responsibility. The gathering of children in a school not only imposes upon government a peculiar responsibility for the prevention of communicable disease, but gives government an unusual opportunity for health appraisal and the prevention of disease. In a quantitative sense, dental health is one of the large components of any school health program and will be discussed in Chapter 20. In fact, so largely was the public health dental program in any area concentrated upon schoolchildren that most of the early dental programs at the state level grew up as parts of divisions of maternal and child health.

Nursing

The public health nurse is to the bedside nurse as the health officer is to the private physician. This means that the public health nurse is most of the time engaged in promoting teamwork. She sees more patients than a private nurse would, doing less for each. Her primary function involves nursing care and health guidance to individuals and families at home, at school, at work, and at medical and health centers.[6] She does not do bedside nursing unless it is absolutely necessary. Her function rather is to demonstrate, teach, and supervise the nursing care that families, practical nurses, or other workers may assume safely in her absence. She does, however, perform diagnostic tests and preventive immunizations under the direction of a physician and interprets the findings of tests to individuals and families. When she enters a home in which there is illness, it is her job to "get the family organized" and see, if possible, that the illness found there does not spread beyond that one home. Aside from her work in homes, she has large responsibilities in collaborating with other professional and citizen groups to study, plan, and put into action a community health program. In order to undertake these various functions she should have special public health training in addition to her hospital course in nursing.

The public health nurse is needed on many different "task forces" within a health department. The division of communicable diseases needs her to find cases of latent disease and to trace down contacts. The school health service needs her for health screening and health education work among children. In this capacity she is often a permanent staff member in a school, knowing the health history and family background of the children better than anyone else in that school. On occasion, she can supervise a fluoride rinse program. She is essential in handling chronic illness among the indigent and aged in a community. She is needed in industry, though here it is usually the industry and not the health department that employs her.

It is the consensus of various groups who have studied the problem that there should be one public health nurse for each 5,000 population, where the functions of the nurse are those which have just been outlined. Where the nurse has any great amount of bedside care to perform, a better ratio is one to each 2,000 population. It can easily be seen, therefore, that even small health departments need a fair number of public health nurses. These women, with their supervisor or director, constitute an important division in all health departments. The cost of maintenance of a public health nursing program is one of the largest expenditures in most health department budgets.

Home bedside nursing care for low-income families usually falls outside the scope of health department activities. In the United States, this work has traditionally been performed by a voluntary visiting nurses' organization. The visiting nurse and the public health nurse, however, must often go to the same homes. Coordination between the two groups is of great importance in order to avoid duplication of effort and inefficient treatment through conflicting advice or failure to pool all available information upon a case. Thus, in some health departments, the visiting nurses and the public health nurses have their headquarters under one roof, and are integrated at the administrative level.

Disease Control

The control of specific diseases is one of the largest areas of activity in the field of public health and one of the oldest. Government has been concerned with controlling the spread of communicable disease ever since the days of the Mosaic law among the ancient Hebrews. Chronic-disease service is a more recent development, except for the programs that have arisen around tuberculosis and venereal disease. Most large health departments give separate bureau status to the services centered on these diseases. This may possibly be due to the historical development of the services but is undoubtedly perpetuated because of the magnitude of the problems involved. Both disease groups are endemic rather than epidemic most of the time; both necessitate an energetic search of unsuspected cases not only through contacts of known patients, but throughout the community at large. Both disease groups depend to a considerable extent upon environment factors for their frequency and both involve an extensive use of health education as a preventive measure. The high degree of hospitalization required for tuberculosis, however, and the careful social maneuvering needed in the handling of venereal disease, set each disease group apart from the other and both from the common run of other communicable diseases.

The control of acute communicable disease requires two types of effort not seen to a similar degree in other phases of health work: the science of epidemiology and the use of law.

For all the broad use that can be made of the epidemiological method, as will be discussed in Chapter 7, the fact remains that epidemiology started as the science of epidemics. The bulk of the work in the area is centered upon the tracing and appraising of acute communicable disease. The epidemiologist (whether or not he is actually so titled) must look at all parts of the chain of causation for the disease he is studying and appraise not only agent factors but host factors and environmental factors as well. Table 2 gives examples of some of the sources and modes of transmission of disease which must constantly be borne in mind. This is the "action phase" of the disease process, when the agent is on the move. There must also be background knowledge concerning susceptible hosts for diseases and favorable environments for their development. Some of the principles of the science of epidemiology are set forth in Chapter 7.

In the field of law, it is the group responsible for disease control that makes the rules for the reporting of infectious disease, secures legislation when needed, and shares with the division of vital statistics the responsibility for collecting and analyzing information. The division of disease control maintains case registers and administers quarantine and isolation procedure. It also arranges immunization programs, both compulsory and voluntary, for measles, polio, diphtheria, tetanus, and the like. On occasion, physical examinations may be required. An example of this is found in the premarital-examination laws which, in 1977, existed in 44 states. These laws usually require examination for both bride and groom and serological testing for syphilis before the issuance of the marriage license.

The success of communicable disease control in the United States is shown in Table 3 in terms of mortality. Morbidity, of course, is the large-scale problem. Immunizations are involved, as is reporting of actual disease. Then come problems of isolation, quarantine, and control of personal contacts, the premises of the cases, and the environment. Hanlon lists 49 communicable diseases commonly considered reportable in the United States in

Table 2. Some factors in the transmission of infectious disease.

Mechanism	Example
Source	
Human patients	Patients with active tuberculosis or syphilis
Human carriers	Occasional patients recovered from typhoid fever
Animal reservoirs	Ticks, carrying Rocky Mountain spotted fever
Inanimate reservoirs	Grain, carrying actinomycosis
Mode of transmission	
Direct contact	Syphilis
Droplet infection	Common cold
Inanimate transmitter	Soiled articles: staphylococcal infection Water: typhoid fever
Vector (animate)	Mosquitoes, carrying malaria or yellow fever

1974.[7] A constant watch must be kept upon these diseases, including those where mortality has dropped to zero. Smallpox is still on this list, though for the moment its occurrence has been eliminated worldwide.

Environmental Sanitation

Some of the earliest public health efforts come under the heading of environmental sanitation, since the theory of the miasmatic origin of disease preceded by centuries the discovery of bacteria. This theory placed an emphasis upon bad odors from decaying animal or vegetable proteins (miasmas) as causes of disease and suggested cleanliness of the environment as the best possible, if not the only, way to control disease. The initial phases of sanitation activities, to use Mark D. Hollis's phrase, center on keeping human excreta out of the diet. This emphasis continues today, with well over half the time and money of a sanitation department devoted to the purification of water and the disposal of sewage. Other activities include the inspection of food and milk, the maintenance of healthy conditions in industrial establishments, and the control of animate vectors of disease, such as mosquitoes. Removal of garbage and refuse may or may not be a function of a health department, but the sanitary inspectors will undoubtedly be interested in the efficiency of such removal. Control of air pollution and the maintenance of adequate housing standards are also mat-

Table 3. Decline in deaths from selected communicable diseases, United States, 1900–1971.

Cause of death	Deaths per 100,000 population per year	
	1900–1904	1971
Diphtheria	32.7	0.0
Pertussis	10.7	0.0
Measles	10.0	0.0
Typhoid fever	26.7	0.0
Diarrhea and enteritis	115.3	1.1
Syphilis	12.9	0.2
Tuberculosis	184.7	2.1

ters closely related to environmental sanitation, though requiring cooperative efforts beyond the normal duties of the health department.

The volume of work performed by health departments in the field of environmental sanitation is shown in a survey by the U.S. Public Health Service. By 1947 the following accomplishments were reported throughout the United States:

More than 14,000 systems provide water to about 85 million people and the quality of the water furnished is generally excellent.

More than 70 million people are served by sewerage systems and more than 5500 treatment plants have been installed which serve about 42 million people.

More than 70 percent of our market milk supply is pasteurized.

Practically all of our larger cities, and a constantly increasing number of the smaller ones, provide regular collection service of garbage and refuse, and disposal methods have been improved.[8]

By 1976 the number of water systems had increased, and they were serving 177 million people. By contrast, in 1973 there were still 65 small communities without public water supply in the thickly settled state of Massachusetts.

An interesting contrast exists between the activities of a sanitation department in a rural area and a similar department in a city. In rural areas, where communal water and sewerage facilities are for the most part impossible, it is necessary to educate individuals regarding standards of purity for water, the proper construction and use of privies, and other similar matters. Sanitation is a "do-it-yourself" affair. In large cities, where communal water and sewerage systems are the rule and where municipal codes govern the plumbing connections of these systems to homes, the homeowner needs almost no education. He needs only to turn a tap or flush a toilet. The engineering problem of the sanitation department, however, is infinitely larger and more complex.

Water fluoridation has brought dental public health into the field of environmental sanitation, and has given the dental profession as colleagues the more than 15,000 professional sanitarians in the country now employed in local health programs. Fifty-one percent of the total United States population now uses fluoridated water. Water-works engineers find the mechanism of fluoridation well within their range of chemical knowledge and well suited to the machinery they are accustomed to operate.

Laboratories

The rise of the science of bacteriology gave new tools to the public health worker, and also imposed upon him the responsibility for analyzing great numbers of specimens submitted to him from the field. The first known public health laboratory in the United States was established in 1892 in New York City following a severe outbreak of cholera. Since that time laboratories have become almost universal among large local health departments and state health departments. The U.S. Public Health Service and many industrial and university laboratories are also contributing both service and research in the field of public health. An offshoot of the analytical work performed by these laboratories has been the manufacture of sera, antitoxins, vaccines, and other biological materials for diagnosis, prevention, and treatment of disease. Manufacture is usually performed by state public health laboratories or by commercial laboratories operating under state or federal license.

A great variety of specimens are submitted to a health department for analysis. The water-works engineers need periodic analyses of water samples for both chemical and bacterial content. Physicians and hospitals need analyses of smears and blood in order to confirm a diagnosis of communicable disease. Local health officers or epidemiologists may be investigating a suspected outbreak of communicable disease in connection with which a large number of specimens may require examination. Sanitary inspectors will be submitting samples of food, milk, and so forth. In industry one of the largest problems is that of air analysis to determine whether toxic levels exist of dust, gases, vaporized toxic solvents, and so on.

At the national level, the laboratories of the National Bureau of Standards, the U.S. Food and Drug Administration, and the Environmental Protection Agency and, in the private sector, the American Dental Association Council on Dental Therapeutics are all of particular interest to dentists. The effect that these and other national laboratory groups have had upon standardization and improvement of our materia medica is indeed great.

Mental Health

A number of specialized problems, the product of our increasingly complex civilization, now require the attention of public health specialists and are represented by their own divisions or bureaus in the larger health departments. Mental health is perhaps the largest of these areas, and is often handled by a separate department. It involves a very heavy load of hospital care, much of it beyond the economic range of the individual patient. Mental hospitals are becoming less and less mere custodial institutions. The length of stay of the individual patient is decreasing; the percentage of cures is increasing. Community mental health centers now keep the mentally ill nearer to their families and family physicians. These centers permit easier outpatient service, both for prevention and for rehabilitation. Among preventive services, child-guidance clinics are perhaps the most interesting of a number of approaches designed to reduce those anxieties and tensions in modern society which are at the root of so much mental disease.

Nutrition

Nutrition is another large endeavor in many health departments. It is linked very closely with health education since the utilization of available foods is usually a much more important problem than the introduction of new food products in these days of energetic private enterprise. Dental health programs, of course, will do well to take advantage of all nutritional services that may be found at hand. Much dental disease can be prevented through the educational work of the nutritionist.

Industrial Health

Industrial health is an important subject for health departments which serve highly industrialized areas. The responsibility for prevention and care of industrial illnesses and injuries rests primarily with industry itself, but government agencies have found an increasing amount they could do to aid industry, particularly among plants with smaller working forces. In many ways industrial health resembles school health because of the concentration of healthy people in one place of work for a long period of time. The growing role of dentistry in an industrial health program receives attention in Chapter 21.

CHARACTERISTIC PUBLIC HEALTH TECHNIQUES

A number of techniques are characteristic of the public health method and have been developed by it because of the peculiar nature of the teamwork necessary for the prevention of disease. The use of the *health center, case finding,* and the use of the *community health council* are among the more important of these techniques.

Health Center

Health centers are community buildings to house health administration and a number of outpatient or preventive services not easily housed in a hospital. The health center is usually a dignified building in a central part of the community and as such becomes a visible symbol of health activity, enhancing the prestige and efficiency of the health department. The health center need not be far removed from the community hospital—in fact, there are many reasons why it should be quite close—yet it should have its own distinct entrance if for no other reason than that a health center is primarily for well people and a hospital primarily for sick people. There is a great deal to be said for keeping the two groups apart.

Typical health-center activities include the offices of the health department and of the public health and visiting nurses, central dental clinic for the community, prenatal, well-baby, and immunization clinics, rehabilitation facilities for the handicapped, mental health facilities, chest x-ray facilities, and perhaps headquarters for the local tuberculosis association and other voluntary agencies. A small auditorium for public health meetings is a valuable addition. The atmosphere of the building is that of a community center designed to help well people stay well. Its function, however, can be expanded until comprehensive outpatient medical and dental care for an entire area results. This is becoming increasingly common in low-income areas where public financing is a large factor.

One health center might be expected to serve a community of some 50,000 to 100,000 people. Large cities therefore have several such centers. Cities of intermediate size may have one health center, with outlying health units in certain public schools. These health units, in addition to serving as useful local nuclei for the school health program, can also house maternal, well-baby, and other clinic services in order to save travel time for those local people who attend.

A variant on the health unit, seen occasionally in the United States and Canada, and predominantly in New Zealand and Australia, is the school-based dental clinic. Dental care for children is thus brought right to where the children are normally congregated, with great reduction of logistic problems and great increase in utilization of service. Such dental clinics are often shared with the school nurse or physician.

Case Finding

As health departments found their way more and more into the field of preventive medicine, it became important to search apparently healthy populations for cases of early disease. This procedure has become known as *case finding* or *screening* and is centered upon simple tests for the more serious or prevalent diseases. One of the most familiar examples of case finding is that of miniature chest x-ray work (photofluorography) to discover tuberculosis. School physical examinations, as commonly performed, are also predominantly case finding. The object, of course, is to cover as large a population as possible with as simple a test as will yield helpful results. The most important danger lies in false negatives: cases of early disease missed because of inadequate detail in the method. This danger, however, is less than the danger the population will face if only a small proportion receive careful examination and the rest remain unexamined. Case finding or screening must be taken for what it is and must be supplemented wherever necessary by a more detailed method. Often case finding will point the way toward those stress groups where more detailed analysis becomes of great importance. Thus, forty years ago we saw great citywide chest x-ray surveys for tuberculosis. The findings of these surveys showed us where stress groups could be found. Such an analysis performed upon survey figures from Philadelphia is shown in Table 4.[9]

The current trend is not to survey entire populations by chest x-ray, but to concentrate upon those stress groups such as hos-

Table 4. Percentage of persons in different population groups showing possible tuberculosis upon mass chest x-ray survey, Philadelphia, 1946–1948.

Group	Percent
4,059 schoolchildren	0.3
32,535 food handlers	2.3
20,903 industrial workers	2.5
Admissions to Philadelphia General Hospital	6.4
3,106 diabetic patients	8.4

pital admissions and diabetic patients where the greatest findings are likely, and to use skin testing wherever possible. Radiation hazards aside, no public health program could afford periodic detailed x-ray examination of the entire population for tuberculosis, or more currently, lung cancer. Case finding or screening activities represent a compromise for this reason.

An interesting elaboration of case-finding procedure is that of *multiphasic screening.* This implies the taking of several tests at once for different diseases, thereby economizing upon time both for the operators and for the patients. Goldmann cites an example of such screening in San Francisco where the tests comprised height and weight, vision and hearing examinations, miniature (70-mm) photofluorograph of the chest, electrocardiogram, blood pressure, serological test for syphilis, tests for hemoglobin and blood sugar, and urine examination for sugar and albumin.[10]

Case-finding procedures in dentistry are at times a matter of controversy. There are some public health officials who feel that, because dental disease is almost universal, all schoolchildren should be routinely referred to sources of dental treatment. This attitude, however, neglects the health educational aspects of dental case-finding procedures and the stimulation they afford toward the seeking out of actual treatment. There are always a few caries-free children in every school class, and every child is likely to think himself one of these lucky few until it has been proved that he is not. The recent decrease in childhood dental caries throughout developed countries has reduced the need for routine school dental examination programs, except in underserved or known high-caries areas.

Voluntary versus Government Programs

The public health field is an extremely good one in which to observe the interaction of voluntary and government programming. The extent to which one or the other predominates will depend very largely on the culture of the country under observation, but any country is likely to exhibit both forms. The flexibility of the voluntary organizations gives them the opportunity to start new ideas, run pilot programs, and handle many problems of a fluctuating nature. Government programs, on the other hand, care more efficiently for the continuing community responsibilities and the heavy load of routine work, whether it be health education or medical care. As the scene shifts over the years, it is quite common to see voluntary activities become government supported as their need in the community becomes well established.

An interesting example of this, although not directly in the health field, is shown in the activities of CARE, the organization formed in the United States after World War II for the sending of food packages to foreign countries. Fig. 2 shows the financing of this organization over an 11-year period.[11] Note that it was supported entirely by voluntary contributions at the beginning, that its activities reached a peak after 3 years, after which the novelty of the work wore off and contributions dropped. The need for the service, however, continued, and government aid appeared at about the sixth year of the enterprise. Like many health activities, CARE has continued with a combination of voluntary and government support, the government support now forming the main bulk, but the voluntary support continuing steadily and carrying with it a broad public interest which is hard to maintain where financing is through tax channels alone.

A typical example of the interaction of government and voluntary work in the health field is the handling of health education, case finding, and rehabilitation for tuberculosis. Health departments and voluntary associations are often found sharing these tasks in a single community. The heavier service work in the area, and, of course, the hospitalization of patients, is taken on by the health department, but continued public interest in the program is maintained through community health planning in the voluntary tuberculosis association. The annual sale of Christmas seals has carried with it a large amount of health education and finances much of the preventive and rehabilitation work. As tuberculosis incidence has declined, these associations have often renamed themselves "lung" associations and taken on a wider spectrum of diseases and disabilities. The March of Dimes, originally formed to deal with poliomyelitis, thus now concerns itself largely with birth defects, since vaccination has sharply reduced the incidence of polio.

Community Health Councils

An essential feature of good public health practice is a broad desire on the part of people in all walks of life to see the health program a good one and to understand it. Such aims are best attained through councils of various sorts representing key people in the community from both voluntary and government agencies and the

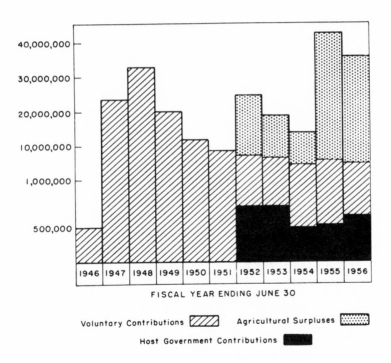

Figure 2. Value of volunteer and government contributions to CARE overseas distributions, 1946–1956 (not drawn to scale). [Courtesy, Cooperative for American Relief Everywhere, Inc.]

community at large. These councils are often associated with community fund-raising efforts under such banners as that of the Red Feather. The councils provide a forum for the exchange of information between various health agencies and the public and for the development of new ideas. In the larger communities, there may be a subdivision of council activities, often into such areas as health and hospitals, youth and leisure time, rehabilitation, child welfare, and so forth. Key people from government agencies, on the one hand, and from voluntary agencies and civilian organizations such as the service clubs, on the other hand, make a well-rounded membership for these community councils. Parent-teacher organizations are playing an increasing role in the area. Through council activity, large lay volunteer groups can be formed, informed, and active in public health matters. These volunteers not only perform a very useful service in a democratic society, but also serve as a recruiting ground for professional personnel.

In 1966, consumer participation in health planning became required by federal law, with consumers forming over one half of each board in a system of state and local health councils. In 1974, the National Health Planning and Resources Development Act (P.L. 93-641) redefined this system to include more than 200 area Health Systems Agencies (HSAs), and, in addition, Statewide Health Coordinating Councils. These agencies and councils not only serve as media for communication but also have approval or disapproval power over both new and existing institutional health services in their areas.

The manifestations of public health teamwork just described are characteristic of the United States today. Variations in pattern may be expected in other societies and other periods. All represent attempts to translate into community action procedures which were evolved by scientists or others as a result of study and planning. The adoption of these procedures must be motivated, must occasionally be clothed with authority, and must be communicated. The largest single task of public health agencies is to arrange their programs so that good health measures are understood, are consistent with community purposes and with the interests of citizens as individuals, and represent attainable goals. Unless these conditions apply, the best-laid plans cannot be translated into action.

CHAPTER 3

Milestones in Dental Public Health

RECORDS of dental treatment can be found in Egypt more than 1500 years before the birth of Christ, and efforts toward the prevention of dental disease date back to the time of Hippocrates. Dental health in terms of organized community effort, however, is a development of the past 100 years or so. It is interesting to trace through the centuries the steps that led to the widening of the field of treatment from the individual to the group, and to discover that even while the Dark Ages engulfed Europe a number of our present preventive techniques were finding their way into folk practice.

Some of the earliest references to mouth hygiene as a means of controlling dental disease are found in accounts of Arabian civilization in southern Europe about the ninth century A.D. The Arabs were leaders in medicine. They were also interested in care of the teeth rather than in their extraction and replacement, and mouth hygiene was a well-established technique. The instrument they used was called a *siwak*, and consisted of a small wooden stick, the end of which was often chewed, the wood fibers being used as a brush.[1]

During the Middle Ages in Europe a fairly definite set of rules for oral hygiene evolved, based on Arab writings. They appear in the fourteenth century, recorded by Guy de Chauliac, and again in the fifteenth century, recorded by Giovanni of Arcoli.[2] These rules involve a number of dietary prohibitions, including "viscous food such as figs and confectionery made with honey," and also directions for cleansing the teeth with dentifrice. Peter Foreest, a Dutch physician of the sixteenth century, concentrated upon the harmful effects of "sugar and all sweet things."

The first recognition of the removal of calcareous deposit as an important factor in the control of periodontal disease is credited to Abulcasis, an Arab in Spain in the late tenth century.[2] Other references to this procedure appear during the Middle Ages. In France in the eighteenth century Pierre Fauchard's book, *Le chirurgien dentiste,* emphasized the need to keep the teeth clean if disease were to be prevented. Several other writers soon afterward stressed preventive measures in the dental field, including the importance of diet. No health program, however, educational or otherwise, seems to have been devised during this entire period for the aid of large population groups.

THE NINETEENTH CENTURY

In the United States, the profession of dentistry grew to important stature through the medium of restorative procedures carried out in private practice. Dentists were essentially craftsmen who made beautiful gold restorations for the teeth of those who could afford their fees. There were a few early efforts, however, to aid the indigent. The first dispensary for the treatment of the poor was established by Skinner in 1791 in New York City. Dental service was offered there. In 1849, the Society of Dental Surgeons of the State of New York founded its own dental infirmary. In 1861, a dental service became part of the Charity Hospital of Philadelphia. In 1867, a small dental clinic for low-income people was opened in Boston. Nevertheless, there were no large-scale efforts made in the direction of dental treatment for low-income groups until the twentieth century.

Organized interest in dental health appears to have arisen in the United States about the year 1870. The American Dental Association, meeting that year in Nashville, Tennessee, passed a resolution calling for "a committee to correspond with the publishers of American school books and ascertain if some plan can be devised to have short, plain statements inserted of the number, name, form, and arrangement of the several teeth."[3] This should be done, it was felt, because "ignorance is one of the main causes of the loss of many teeth." The resolution, however, seems only to deal with dental anatomy. No prophylactic measures are mentioned.

Another step toward prevention of dental disease was taken by M. L. Rhein of New York City in 1884. This effort became better known, perhaps because the public was more nearly ready for it and because Rhein coined the term "oral hygiene," which proved popular.[4] Rhein urged dentists to teach their patients proper methods of tooth brushing. The efforts of the dental profession in the wake of this suggestion constitute the only true campaign to prevent caries put on before World War I. Even so, progress was slow. Another idea introduced about the turn of the century by the well-known dental histologist J. Leon Williams, became the slogan of the oral-hygiene campaign of the following two decades: "A clean tooth never decays." As Salzmann puts it, "While the truthfulness of this assertion is still being debated, there is no doubt but that it has been the inspiration and 'battle cry' which has led to higher standards of mouth hygiene."[1] Williams, following Miller and the chemicoparasitic theory of dental caries, emphasized the importance of gelatinous plaques as a shield beneath which destructive concentrations of acid could be generated, but thought the best way to render them harmless was through the use of germicides.[5,6]

In Europe, this same period saw the beginnings of public health dentistry for children through the establishment of dental clinics. In Strasbourg, Germany, the first children's dental clinic was established in 1865. Hanover followed suit in 1885, Offenbach and Würzburg in 1898. In England, through the stimulation of W. MacPherson Fisher of Dundee, the British Dental Association appointed a committee to carry on oral-hygiene work in the schools of that country. The committee was formed in 1890 and within the succeeding two decades influenced the appointment of dentists to many elementary schools.

THE EARLY TWENTIETH CENTURY

The opening of the twentieth century saw the various groups within the United States ready to approach the problem of dental public health along the lines of dental treatment for indigent children, and the education of all children on the subject of mouth hygiene, chiefly tooth brushing. The year 1910 stands as an impressive milestone in both endeavors. W. G. Ebersole of Cleveland, Ohio, was then in his second year as chairman of the Oral Hygiene Committee of the National (now American) Dental Association. In that year Ebersole wrote, "Tomorrow will show every dental organization in the world working in the oral hygiene field from an educational standpoint. Our government—municipal, state, and national—will be as insistent on healthy mouths in school children as they are upon vaccination."[7]

To implement this prophecy, the Oral Hygiene Committee was recommending the dental examination of all children, referral of reports to parents in order that correction of defects might be initiated, the establishment of dental clinics not only for treatment but for research into the problem of child dental hygiene, and a campaign for the education of the lay public largely through the medium of newspapers and lecturers. Dr. Ebersole did a great deal toward the fulfillment of the plans he had helped to sponsor. In July 1911 he organized a large oral-hygiene meeting in Cleveland, Ohio, at which he exhibited the mental and physical improvement of a group of 27 children, each of whom had been brought from a state of great dental neglect to a state of full dental health by a service he had sponsored in one of the Cleveland public schools.[8] This oral-hygiene meeting was attended by 3,200 persons, including the largest group of dentists ever assembled up to that time. In the wake of this meeting an oral-hygiene conference occurred out of which grew the National Mouth Hygiene Association. Ebersole had a clear vision of the importance of broad community backing for any program such as this to educate the public. As a result, leaders in public health, education, children's dentistry, women's clubs, and other lay groups were included among the officers.

The year 1910 also saw the establishment of the Rochester Dental Clinic, later endowed by George Eastman, and the incorporation of the Forsyth Dental Infirmary for Children in Boston. These two clinics constituted by a long margin the largest efforts the world had seen to bring dental care to the public without regard to its ability to pay. Chief emphasis at the time was upon restorative dentistry, but oral-hygiene instruction was an important part of the program and both institutions later added schools for dental hygienists. The clinics were opened in 1915 and have been in continuous operation ever since. A number of other children's clinics have been established since that time along similar lines, perhaps the most notable of which was the Murry and Leone Guggenheim Clinic in New York City.

Closely allied to the trend toward public dental care for civilians came the establishment in 1911 of the Dental Corps of the U.S. Army and in 1912 of that of the U.S. Navy. Though these services had small beginnings, each represented a decision on the part of government to assume full dental care for military personnel. The volume of care rendered through these services has steadily increased and has been matched by similar services in the Air Force, in the Public Health Service, and in the Veterans Administration, till the sum total of dental care now provided by the federal government is indeed impressive.

The first two decades of the twentieth century saw the introduction of the dentist's first professionally trained auxiliary: the *dental hygienist*. The original idea that dentists could delegate to supervised helpers some of their simpler duties in the care of the mouth seems to have come from C. M. Wright, who suggested in 1902 the formation of a subspecialty of the dental profession:

1. The practitioners of this separate and yet most important part of dentistry are to be women—women of education and refinement—who are seeking a field for work of an honorable and useful kind among people of culture.

2. The dental colleges are to offer opportunities for this partial and separate training; the course to consist of lectures on the anatomy of the teeth and gums, special pathology and physiology, and special clinical training in prophylactic therapeutics.

3. Upon the completion of this special course which shall require

one session, or one year of study, and practice under instruction in the college infirmary, and after presenting satisfactory evidence of proficiency in the polishing of teeth and caring for the mouth, the college shall grant a certificate of competence to the graduate of this course.

4. With this training and the dental college certificate, these ladies may be employed by dentists for this special work.[9]

Although Wright never carried out his suggestion, it is obvious that he was the first to visualize the dental hygienist and her course of training much as we know them today.

The man who put such ideas into practice was Dr. Alfred C. Fones of Bridgeport, Connecticut, and it was his activity with the Connecticut Dental Association that permitted him to do so. In 1905 Fones trained Mrs. Irene Newman in the procedures of dental prophylaxis. In 1906 Mrs. Newman was actually at work in Dr. Fones's office, and thus became the first dental hygienist. She had no legal status that year, however, and might soon have been forced to give up her work, for in 1907 a bill was introduced into the Connecticut State Legislature prohibiting dentists from employing unlicensed assistants in their operative work. Fortunately, Fones was at that time chairman of the Legislative Committee of the Connecticut Dental Association, and was able to insert a clause in the bill which would permit trained assistants to perform dental prophylaxis "in the immediate presence of and under the direct supervision of registered or licensed dentists." A potential legal obstacle was thus turned into the first legislative permission for the profession of dental hygiene.

It is of great interest to note that within 3 years Dr. Fones was urging a step which was still considered somewhat new and radical half a century later: the introduction of dental hygienists into a public school system. Between 1909 and 1913 Fones made several attempts to interest city officials in Bridgeport in a plan to establish a clinic to demonstrate the value of educational and preventive dental service for schoolchildren. He was ultimately successful in obtaining an initial $5,000 appropriation for this purpose and found himself at the same time faced with the responsibility of training young women to fill the posts he had created. Thus the first training school for dental hygienists came into being. Thirty-three women enrolled in the first class in November 1913, many of them with a background of dental assisting or school teaching. In June 1914, 27 of this group were graduated as dental hygienists. Ten started work in the Bridgeport school system the following autumn.[1]

Another public health milestone in the early twentieth century was the visit of Dr. G. V. Black to a meeting of the Colorado State Dental Association in 1908. This was the first occasion on which any group of professional people had ever discussed the dental phenomena we now associate with fluorine. The initiative had been taken by Dr. Frederic S. McKay, a practitioner in Colorado Springs, Colorado, who as early as 1905 had begun to assemble facts upon a brown discoloration then known as "Colorado stain." Until Black accepted McKay's invitation to come to Denver, McKay had been unable to excite interest in the subject of Colorado stain. After that meeting, study of the condition became widespread. Black named it "mottled enamel." A long series of epidemiological investigations culminated more than 20 years later in the discovery of fluorine as the causative agent of the stain. The term *fluorosis* was then coined to cover not only actual mottling but white enamel opacities of similar origin.

THE NINETEEN-TWENTIES

The period from 1919 to 1933—the period of prosperity and subsequent depression which succeeded World War I—was marked by few striking advances in the field of public health dentistry in the United States. Two important programs were established, however, which were to have a continuing influence over the programs and planning for the years to come. The first of these was the Dental Department of the U.S. Public Health Service, founded in 1919. The second was the dental clinic for home-office employees of the Metropolitan Life Insurance Company, organized by Thaddeus P. Hyatt in that same year. These events and their sequelae will be dealt with in more detail in Chapters 23 and 21 respectively.

By and large, the period following World War I was characterized by a broadening of the scientific basis for preventive dentistry and the identification of many of the factors we now consider predisposing to dental caries. The nutritional background for caries was really studied and stressed for the first time. The Mellanbys in England emphasized the importance of vitamin D in the diet; Hanke in Chicago discovered the role of vitamin C, but overstressed it beyond reason. Impressive evidence was assembled in support of both of these hypotheses, but the result at the time was controversy, not harmony. Researchers still felt they should be looking for *one* cause for caries. The chemico-parasitic theory for caries was very much in favor, and its firmer supporters, claiming that caries came from the outside of a tooth, not the inside, were frankly skeptical of the role of nutrition in any form. A climax, perhaps, to this controversy occurred in the 1920s when two well-known New York dentists held a formal debate on the question whether it is true that "A clean tooth never decays." The debate ended in a deadlock, largely because it became impossible to give an accurate definition of a "clean" tooth.

The decade following World War I also saw increasing recognition of the problem of dental health at the federal level. Two White House conferences on child health and protection were held in Washington, D.C., one in 1929 and the other in 1930. Both considered the problem of dental care. The latter conference, particularly, had a section on dentistry and oral hygiene at which Dr. Percy R. Howe, then director of the Forsyth Dental Infirmary for Children in Boston, proposed a program for continuing periodic dental supervision and cleaning of children's teeth, in addition to nutritional instruction to prevent dental disease. In 1927 the federal government formed a Committee on the Costs of Medical Care which launched an exhaustive 5-year study into economic and educational factors underlying the rendering of all phases of medical care throughout the United States. Among the many reports of this committee there is frequent reference to dentistry.[10] National attention was focused upon such problems as the inadequate supply of dentists in relation to the need for dental care throughout the country. In the meanwhile dental education was taking a long step forward in moving from proprietary schools run chiefly for profit to university schools with higher standards. Gies's report for the Carnegie Foundation in 1926 triggered this advance.[11] By 1929 the proprietary schools were virtually gone.

During the 1920s a surge of interest took place in public dental care programs at schools, private industrial plants, hospitals, and remote locations. Primary dental care (no gold work) was usually rendered. The total of such clinics has been roughly estimated at 3000. Among remote locations, Dr. Grenfell's hospitals in Labrador attracted volunteer summer dentists every year from half a dozen dental schools—Pennsylvania, Tufts, Columbia, and Harvard most frequently.

On the other side of the world another event of the 1920s rates as a milestone: the opening of the training school for dental nurses in Wellington, New Zealand, in 1921. This school came into being at the urging of T. A. Hunter, a founder of the New Zealand Dental Association and a pioneer in the establishment of a dental school in New Zealand. Hunter knew of the success of dental hygienists in the United States and saw in these women a means of correcting the deplorable defects he saw in the teeth of New Zealand children. In 1923, 29 dental nurses were graduated from the Wellington school. They were sent out into the government school system to provide dental care. These women and their successors have written a new chapter in the use of auxiliary dental personnel. Received with much skepticism at first, the New Zealand School Dental Service is now firmly established and is serving as an example for similar dental nurse plans in other parts of the world. The impact of this plan in various parts of the world, and its changes as childhood dental caries declined in so many developed countries, are discussed in Chapter 17.

THE NINETEEN-THIRTIES AND AFTER

In a very real sense the modern era in dental public health was ushered in as a result of the Great Depression. Events at this time made it clear that government could and should do much more for the people in a time of economic breakdown than had been thought either necessary or advisable in the United States in previous years. The need for health care increased rather than decreased as business activities stagnated. The public became unable to pay for private medical and dental service, and physicians and dentists were soon joining the ranks of the unemployed. One of the first activities of the Federal Emergency Relief Administration, therefore, was the establishment of large clinics in which relief clients could receive proper care. In the period between 1933 and

1935 an increase of more than 5 million occurred in the number of relief clients in the United States. Many physicians and dentists with dwindling practices were glad to be employed in these FERA clinics.

Another development stemming from the Depression was the Social Security Act passed by Congress in 1935. This law not only brought into being a form of unemployment compensation and old-age benefits with associated taxation, but provided for extensive federal aid to states for various health and welfare activities. Title V of the Social Security Act authorized federal grants for maternal and child health services, services for crippled children, and child welfare services. This, in the succeeding years, stimulated a tremendous growth in state dental services. The services often started as part of the divisions of maternal and child health in state health departments, but increasingly they became divisions of dental health in their own right. In 1934, only 14 states had administrative units responsible for dental health activities and these states employed only 8 full-time dentists. In 1941, only 6 years later, 38 states had dental health units of one sort or another, employing a total of 154 full-time dentists.[12]

What of the war years during both World War I and World War II? These periods saw vast expansions in dental service for armed forces all over the world. Young dentists were taken from their practices or from dental school and made parts of health teams in a way which was valuable to the men themselves, but so abnormal, in regard to both the organization of dental care and the type of care rendered, that the lessons of these periods for peacetime dental public health are of limited value. Many lessons were learned in the rapid rendering of restorative dental treatment, however, and these lessons are valuable today. Best of all, perhaps, in World War II the armed services became conscious of their role in graduate dental education, and through internship and fellowship programs and through their own dental schools have offered much valuable training to young men. Through travel, the armed services have lifted young dentists above provincialism and given them a broad point of view toward the care of populations, so valuable in public health work. Through the teamwork necessary in big clinics, the armed services have broken down some of the isolation of the individual dentists and prepared them for the group programs of the present and future.

Since World War II the growth of public health has proceeded along so many fronts that the identification of significant milestones becomes difficult. Surely a very important one occurred in 1945, with the initiation of water fluoridation on a trial basis in the two cities of Grand Rapids, Michigan, and Newburgh, New York. Each project was accompanied by intensive medical and dental appraisal for a period of 10 years, and each has provided statistical data of high quality on the dental benefits and safety of water fluoridation. The later fluoridation of major United States city water supplies are also milestones: Philadelphia in 1954, Chicago in 1956, and New York in 1965.

Another major development in the 1940s was a pioneering start in the field of voluntary prepaid comprehensive dental care. In 1945, Local 688 of the Teamsters' Union established a clinic in St. Louis to give comprehensive care to its members. This clinic became a leader in prepaid group practice. In 1948, Bissell B. Palmer of New York founded Group Health Dental Insurance, an open panel, professionally controlled insurance program which has contributed pioneer, though small-scale, experience in prepayment. In 1949, Group Health Association, a consumers' cooperative in Washington, D.C., established a clinic dental service which soon changed from a fee-for-service basis to prepayment. All these organizations attempted maintenance dental care on a periodic recall basis.

Another postwar development which is of historic importance was the establishment in England in the year 1948 of a national insurance scheme including comprehensive dental service. This daring attempt to provide an entire nation with dental service through the medium of compulsory health insurance and taxation has taught valuable lessons in what happens to a professional service when economic barriers to its utilization are suddenly swept away. Nevertheless, thousands of people in England who never received more than emergency dentistry before are now receiving fairly comprehensive dental care. Three decades after its establishment, the program is firmly in operation. The final verdict upon it is still to be made, but the beginning of the service in 1948 is an event of unquestionable importance.

The 1950s saw important advances in the financing of dental care in the United States. In 1954 the Washington State Dental Society organized the Washington State Dental Service Corporation to help administer the prepayment dental care plan for children of the International Longshoremen's and Warehousemen's Union-Pacific Maritime Association. This mechanism soon became recognized as the best means for the dental profession to maintain a responsible connection with group payment plans for dental care. The idea spread, and by 1984 a combination of commercial insurance companies, Delta Dental Plans, and other agencies were serving approximately 107 million beneficiaries.

MEDICARE, MEDICAID, AND HEALTH PLANNING

A milestone in the delivery of health care was reached on July 1, 1966, when Medicare (Title XVIII of the Social Security Act) brought medical care to the aged of the United States without regard to income. This legislation, opposed by many groups during the half century of debate which led up to it, did not include dental care. Title XIX, however, enacted at the same time and called Medicaid, did include dentistry, along with many other health services designed not merely for the recipients of general relief, but also for the entire lower middle class of the country. This legislation has opened problems of political theory, of taxation, of dental manpower, and of methodology in the rendering of dental care which are far from solution.

That same year, the "Partnership for Health" Act (P.L. 89-749) created a nationwide network of Comprehensive Health Planning agencies with the mandate that over one half of the governing boards be made up of consumers of health care. This network was renamed Health Systems Agencies in 1974, but the emphasis on consumer input was carried forward from 1966.

Another advance in the delivery of health care was the Health Maintenance Organization Act of 1973. This provided government support for organizations providing standardized comprehensive care to individuals in enrolled groups. Though dental care has seldom been included, the way is open for it, particularly for preventive and emergency services.

On the world scene, the dental service of the World Health Organization has taken on added stature. It has collaborated with other international groups in studies of dental care delivery in as many as 12 developed countries.[13] It has also established the WHO

Oral Epidemiological Data Bank, which is accumulating information on dental health and dental needs in many countries around the globe.

CHANGES IN DENTAL CARIES INCIDENCE

The major event so far in the 1980s has been the marked reduction in dental caries among children in many developed countries. Occurring in both fluoridated and unfluoridated areas, this reduction has been called a secular change, though there are also a number of specific causes, the chief one being water fluoridation. The reduction has produced an important change in dental needs by age in the United States, which are discussed in Chapters 8, 17, 20, and 21. The milestone best identified with the change has been the First International Conference on the Declining Prevalence of Dental Caries, held at Forsyth Dental Center, Boston, in June 1982.

Over the years there have been many more events which might be considered milestones in dental public health but are not mentioned here. Some of these will appear in later chapters, in connection with the specific subjects to which they relate.

PART II

The Tools of Dental Public Health

CHAPTER 4

Biostatistics: Selection of Data

THE WORKER with human material will find the statistical method of great value and will have even more need for it than will the laboratory worker. The laboratory worker, dealing with quick re-actions in a test tube and the somewhat slower though still marked reactions that follow surgical or environmental changes in a litter of experimental animals, will often find that he does not need the statistical method. By producing drastic changes over a relatively brief period of time and in a carefully controlled environment he will have little doubt whether his results could have occurred by chance. Claude Bernard, a French physiologist of the nineteenth century and a pioneer in laboratory research, writes: "We compile statistics only when we cannot possibly help it. Statistics yield prob-ability, never certainty—and can bring forth only conjectural sci-ences."[1]

The worker with human material, however, can seldom control environment, nor can he bring about drastic changes in his subjects quickly, particularly if he is studying chronic disease. The variability of human material, plus the fact that time allows the introduction of many additional factors which may contribute to a disease process, leaves the worker with quantitative data affected ·by a multiplicity of causes. Statistical methods become necessary, probability becomes of great interest, and conjecture based upon statistical probability may show a way to break the chain of causation of a disease even before all factors entering into the production of the disease are clearly understood. Yule has defined statistics as "methods specially adapted to the elucidation of quantitative data affected by a multiplicity of causes."[2]

The advent of possible methods to reduce dental caries in large groups of people has given importance to the accurate determination of dental-caries experience in such groups and the evaluation of differences observed between groups. The definite recognizability of most caries lesions and the number and accessibility of the teeth make the quantitative measurement of dental caries an easy procedure compared with the measurement of many other diseases. Counts of decayed, missing and filled (DMF) teeth and other dental findings are constantly reported in the literature as average values. The reliability of these averages, however, will depend upon the sizes of the samples from which they were drawn and upon many other factors. Comparisons between averages, therefore, may result in misleading statements that the prevalence or incidence of dental caries has been changed by a named percentage, when actually it was only a chance difference that was observed. Interpretation of the public health importance of such measures as fluoride rinse programs depends upon the validity of the data collected and of the statistical comparisons of results that are made. Good statistical procedure aims to eliminate errors so far as possible and measure those errors which cannot be eliminated.

Fully half the work in biostatistics involves common sense in the selection and interpretation of data. The magic of numbers is no substitute. Bernard points with derision at a German author who measured the salivary output of one submaxillary and one parotid gland in a dog for one hour.[1] This author then proceeded to deduce (1) the output of all salivary glands, right and left, (2) the total salivary output of a dog per kilogram per day, and finally

(3) the total output of saliva of a man per kilogram per day. The result, of course, was a very top-heavy structure built upon a set of observations entirely too small for the purpose. Work of this sort explains the jibes which so often ricochet upon better statisticians. Such mistakes can be avoided. Statisticians also suffer because they are so often content merely to collect and analyze data as an end in itself without the purpose or hope of producing new knowledge or a new concept. Conant, in his book *On Understanding Science,* makes it very clear that new concepts must alternate with the collection of data if an advance in our knowledge is to occur.[3]

PRELIMINARY GENERAL QUESTIONS

It is difficult to reduce common sense to rules, and for that reason I shall attempt to bring out through a series of examples certain questions which the statistician should answer for himself before he gets out his calculating machine.

First Example. A few years ago the Committee on Dentistry of the National Research Council received an inquiry from a research organization within the armed forces as to the propriety of authorizing a grant of $15,000 for raising rats under germ-free conditions. A smaller grant, made the year previously, had resulted in the development of techniques whereby only 5 out of hundreds of rats had survived in a germ-free state. The second grant was designed to assist the further development of techniques and also to permit the measurement of caries in caries-susceptible rats raised under germ-free conditions. Was such an expenditure of government funds, quite large by the standards of those days, justified where so few rats had survived?

After due consideration the National Research Council approved the grant. The Council agreed with the applicants for the money that an opportunity was presented here for the first time to test whether dental caries was actually an infectious disease to the extent that bacteria were necessary for its occurrence. It is a matter of history that the Notre Dame group in Indiana did succeed in raising many more rats under germ-free conditions, and could not produce dental caries in them even on a known cariogenic diet. The reintroduction of specific strains of bacteria into the germ-free environment again produced caries, and a series of important research reports has resulted.[4]

In this instance the National Research Council had to answer the question: *Would the proposed study produce new knowledge or possibly a new concept?* The answer was affirmative. A new concept of dental caries as an infectious disease might result.

Second Example. Shortly after World War I, the Metropolitan Life Insurance Company became interested in the teeth as foci of infection and wished to make a statistical study among their policyholders in order to determine whether certain specified impairments (cardiac diseases, circulatory disturbances, renal abnormalities, and so forth) could be associated with infected teeth. As a result they collected reports from over 17,000 physical examinations performed by physicians for the Company's ordinary policyholders.[5] Medical impairments were noted in these examinations, and the information that the policyholder was with or without "heavy dentistry." "Heavy dentistry" at that time implied large bridges constructed upon gold shell crowns, large fillings, and the like, many of which had been shown through the recently developed art of dental roentgenology to hide chronically infected teeth. The focal-infection theory was at its peak in those days, and patients with "heavy dentistry" were suspected of hiding more nonvital teeth than the rest of humanity. These examinations were not thorough ones made by dentists, but were actually quick inspections made by physicians. When percentages were computed and compared, no significant differences were found between the medical impairments of those with and without "heavy dentistry." Perhaps this is fortunate. Much "heavy dentistry" was good, and all of it indicated recourse to a dentist, with a reasonable probability that unsavable infected teeth had been removed. In reviewing this study today, it is quite obvious that no importance can be attached to the results. A more detailed, if smaller, study, based upon careful mouth examinations by dentists, would have been of far greater value. There was no reason to make use of poor data when better data could have been obtained.

The question to be answered, then, when undertaking a problem of this sort was: *Were the data of good enough quality for the purpose?* The answer here was "no."

Third Example. In 1927 a massive punched-card study was made of the dental records of over 12,000 employees of the Metropolitan Life Insurance Company.[6] These examinations were the work of dental hygienists, with dentists at hand for supervision and consultation. They were supported by a large number of x-rays, which were read by the dentists. Since careful work was involved, the resulting punched cards became a valuable source of information for further analyses in subsequent years. Some 10 years later a request was made that the cards be used for a study to show the correlation, if any, between occlusal and proximal caries, the theory being that a tooth with a pit or fissure on the occlusal would, by this fact, be made more susceptible to proximal caries. This study was not approved. It was the feeling of those in charge of the records that an unavoidable bias existed, since a large proportion of proximal cavities had been filled through the occlusal surface of the same tooth regardless of the existence of caries on the occlusal. It is very difficult to exclude bias of this sort in any study of adults where filled teeth must enter into the final appraisal.

The question to be answered in this instance was: *Were the data obviously biased?* They were. The inquirers were advised to seek new material among young patients for whom no filling work had been attempted.

Fourth Example. In 1948 the U.S. Public Health Service sent a dental officer along with an examining team whose mission it was to study all aspects of the health of workers in certain iron foundries in Illinois.[7] Careful dental-explorer examinations were made on more than 1,300 white workers in these foundries, and these examinations were compared with others made some years earlier of a group of mine and smelter workers. The statement was made that the foundry workers had "slightly more favorable caries experience" than the mine and smelter workers. Age, as a variable, was dealt with fairly well by division into 10-year age groups, but no mention was made of the geographical areas in which the different studies were performed, fluoride in the water supply, or possible examiner differences between the two studies. Was the comparison between the iron foundry workers and the mine and smelter workers justified, with the consequent inference that perhaps the mine and smelter workers were suffering from an occupational hazard of some sort? A negative reaction would seem indicated on this point until far more careful exclusion of remaining variables had been made.

The question to be answered, therefore, in evaluating this comparison between groups of workers, is: *Are the data comparable?* Probably they are not. Similar *exclusions of unnecessary variables* should be demonstrated in the two groups, and above all, *similar examination techniques.* The comparability of data from different studies cannot be taken for granted.

Fifth Example. Among the dental statistical studies which stand up well over the years may be mentioned an early work of H. Trendley Dean when he was attempting to correlate dental-caries prevalence with small amounts of fluoride in water supplies. This is the comparative study of the cities of Galesburg and Quincy, Illinois, one on the Mississippi River with no fluoride in the water, and the other inshore, using deep-well water which contained approximately 1.8 parts per million of fluoride.[8] Dean was careful with his explorer examinations, careful to use children of continuous residence in the two localities, and also careful with age and sex and all other variables within his control. Sample sizes were large enough so the unavoidable variability of human material could be ruled out as a probable cause of the impressive difference which was found between the two localities. Dean was wise enough, however, in the summary of his report, not to claim that this difference proved the inhibitory effect of fluoride in the water supply upon dental caries. After all, other trace elements unreported in either water supply might have coincided with fluoride and have been the true cause for the difference seen in dental-caries experience. Not until caries was reduced by the introduction of fluoride and fluoride alone into a fluoride-deficient water supply was conclusive proof possible.

The question which Dean, therefore, had both to ask and to answer was: *Does coincidence mean causation?* His frank acceptance of a possible negative answer led to other and more conclusive studies. A similar pitfall exists in the thought that because one event follows another time, the first is the cause of the second. This cannot be assumed.

Sixth Example. Studies on the prevalence of periodontal disease have been rare because of the difficulties involved in finding a good measure for this condition. Nevertheless, reasonably careful dental studies have been made of stress groups where increased periodontal disease was suspected. One such group was in daily contact with lead in a factory that manufactured storage batteries.[9]

Another group involved adult diabetic patients in a large diabetic clinic.[10] The desirability of control groups for both of these studies was clearly recognized by the authors, but such groups were not actually obtained owing to the difficulty of assembling population samples that would match the experimental groups in all matters such as age and sex, and the lack of the special desire to receive dental care that brings patients to the dental office. The chief requirement of a good control group is that it must match the experimental group as closely as possible in every relevant respect *except* the one under study: in this instance, exposure to an industrial hazard or existence of chronic disease.

The question which both authors had to answer, in this instance, unfortunately, in the negative, was: *Can an adequate control group be obtained?* As a result, both studies lack conclusive value.

EXAMINER VARIABILITY

Some of the foregoing examples hint at the attention one must pay to examiner variability in designing statistical studies or assembling data. Determination of what actually constitutes an early carious lesion or incipient periodontal damage is a difficult matter at best. Where a large number of examiners must be utilized, it is important that these persons be brought together for a brief indoctrination at the very least, so that interpretation of observations may be as uniform as possible. Better yet, the study should be confined to a small number of examiners either one person or a very small group whose members have worked together for some time. Beyond this, findings of dental disease may be expected to vary according to the type of examination (such as explorer alone, or explorer plus x-ray; see Chapter 14), time allotted for each examination, the quality of lighting at the time of examination, and so on.

One of the early efforts of the U.S. Public Health Service to obtain nationwide information by the questionnaire method sheds light on the size of the errors which may accumulate. A tremendous volume of data on the occurrence of dental disease and on the need for dental treatment all over the United States was collected from private dentists, school dentists, and occasionally dental hygienists and school nurses. These data were pub-

Table 5. Decayed, missing, and filled permanent teeth per person among children aged 12–14 from 5 cities by questionnaire in 1933–1934 and by oral examination in 1942.

City	1933–1934	1942	Difference (%)
Pueblo, Colo.	1.94	4.12	112
Colorado Springs, Colo.	1.65	2.46	49
Elkhart, Ind.	2.20	8.23	274
Michigan City, Ind.	5.25	10.37	98
Lima, Ohio	2.80	6.52	133

lished in U.S. Public Health Bulletin No. 226 in the year 1936.[11] Details of the examination methods used are not known and the methods probably differed a good deal. The Bulletin has a certain amount of value for internal comparisons. The best of these comparisons can be made between different age groups in the same area, or between similar age groups in fairly closely adjacent areas. Table 5, however, shows the exceedingly wide divergence of the findings reported in Bulletin 226 (1933–1934), both when compared internally with themselves and when compared externally with the explorer examination findings of Dean, Arnold, and Elvove (1942) in the same areas.[12] This material was assembled by a trained examining team working under uniform operating conditions and with uniform interpretation so far as possible.

ETHICAL CONSIDERATIONS

When proceedings other than routine dental examinations are involved, including the use of x-rays, informed consent may be needed from the subjects, their parents, or their school officials. The effect of such consent may be to spoil efforts at randomization of the sample and to introduce "placebo effects" in either the treated group or the control group, or both. The safety of any treatments or operations must usually be cleared with institutional committees on the protection of human subjects. Further consideration of these matters is found in Chapter 14.

QUESTIONNAIRES

Surveys conducted by questionnaire are those most liable to examiner error. Questionnaires have great value in the recording of subjective material, such as people's opinions upon various matters, and of facts that are available only through report, as for instance the income of dentists. In the recording of objective facts, however, questionnaires are most dangerous. Observations are actually reported by as many different observers, all unindoctrinated, as there are returned questionnaires. Semantic difficulties constantly arise: a given word will mean different things to different people. Matters of prestige may bias the answers to questions. A bias can exist even in the identity of those who do return questionnaires. Certain people are more deeply interested in certain questions than are other people, and there are some who actually enjoy filling out forms. All who return questionnaires are in a sense volunteers, and one must make up one's mind whether these volunteers are the people from whom one wishes to hear. The value of a questionnaire survey can be increased if trained interviewers, lay or professional, talk to the respondents personally and fill out the form according to semantically uniform techniques.

THE DOUBLE-BLIND TRIAL

Two of the problems attending clinical trials of disease-prevention methods are those of biased behavior on the part of the subject and wishful thinking on the part of the examiner. The patient may brush his teeth particularly well because he knows he is a test subject, or may "recover" from some disease symptom simply because he knows he is under treatment (the "placebo effect"). The examiner may see fewer new cavities in a study subject than a control subject simply because subconsciously he wants it that way. Both difficulties can be avoided by the double-blind trial method. The control subjects are given actual placebos or are given inert treatment in such a way that they do not know they are controls. The examiner, too, does not know whether he is examining a study subject or a control subject. Only through a coding process in the record system can the true outcome of the trial be known—afterward.

STATISTICAL TERMS DEFINED

At this point it will be useful to define certain of the terms that are used commonly by statisticians.

Universe, to the statistician, implies the sum total of all the persons or objects with the characteristics he is studying. Thus he may wish to study all cases of diabetes in the United States, or all cases of diabetes in New York State, or perhaps all children 12 to 14 years of age in the state of Illinois. In most cases he will be unable to survey the entire group he wishes to consider. He must, therefore, approximate the characteristics of his universe by studying a sample large enough to be typical of the universe in all relevant respects and to permit the evening out of those individual variations which usually remain after the most careful efforts have been made to eliminate unnecessary variables and bias.

It is a matter for common sense to decide whether the sample chosen from the universe shall be a *selected sample,* carefully chosen from individuals with special characteristics, or an *unselected sample,* chosen by a *random* method which very carefully excludes any possible choice between individuals on any other basis than chance. If one is trying to study the condition of a whole population, one wishes an unselected sample which will avoid bias and yet match the population in all major characteristics such as age and sex distribution. It is possible that a completely accidental method may be devised for doing this. More often a random sample must be planned in advance to avoid bias. If a pollster is making a random sampling of public opinion by interviewing people as he meets them in the street, he must remember that his sample will not contain an adequate representation of the invalids and the aged. If he is using the names at the head of each column in the telephone book, he must remember that he will miss the people not able to afford telephones. If he wishes to record the dental-caries experience of a community, he must not confine his attentions to dental patients, else he will find himself left with a sample biased on two counts which differentiate them from the public at large: first, they have dental defects which are obvious to them or they suspect such defects, and second, they have the education and the economic resources to seek dental care. In a similar sense a sample made up of hospital patients is a selected sample because it involves the more serious cases of systemic disease, and represents those patients both educated and able to secure hospital treatment.

Sample size is a matter of concern to be dealt with later in connection with analytical techniques. Public health work deals most frequently with large samples since the variables in human life are so many that no sampling method will reduce them beyond a certain point and large numbers of cases are needed so that unknown variables will even out. *Small samples,* so-called, are usually ones with less than 30 cases. Special small-sample formulas are needed for the analysis of these—a matter of more concern to the laboratory worker than the public health worker.

Sometimes, in order to get an unbiased sample from a heterogeneous population, it is necessary to resort to what is called *stratified sampling.* This is sampling where the population is first divided into more or less homogeneous subgroups or strata, then random samples are taken from these subgroups. The Statistics Section of the American Public Health Association lists two requirements where stratified sampling is to be undertaken:

1) It must be possible to divide the population into strata such that the mean of the measure that we are investigating, or the proportion having the particular characteristic, differs widely from one stratum to another; and

2) The number of members of the population in each stratum must be known.[13]

The second of these requirements permits samples to be taken from each stratum in proper proportion so that the final composite sample will have the same composition (in age, race, economic level, or whatever) as the entire population. This is necessary only where it is not planned to analyze each stratum (as, for instance, an age group) separately.

Special segments of the population can be used in the construction of *random samples* where the reason for the gathering of the group has nothing to do with a disease or other question under investigation. An example is the use of school populations for studies of disease prevalence in the child population. Children are not gathered in schools because of the presence or absence of most minor or acute disease processes. One must be careful, of course, to recognize that chronic invalids will be excluded. Industry likewise provides an excellent grouping of the adult population, when diseases that do not prevent employment are under study.

Though unselected samples from a broad universe are ordinarily sought where disease conditions are being described in a population, highly specified universes often prove best for the study of specific causative factors of a disease. Thus Dean made no attempt at all to obtain a broad universe in Galesburg or Quincy, Illinois, but confined himself to the most selected group he could find: boys of continuous residence, within a very restricted age span just large enough to supply him with numbers which would even out the individual variability between the boys. He avoided any selection directly dependent on caries status, such as a history of previous visits to a dental office. Having found what he was looking for in such a group, he proceeded to the study of wider age spans.

Every sample is to a certain extent random, to a certain extent selected. The very act of selecting a universe other than all mankind is selection in the statistical sense. At the other end of the scale, a highly focused sample must be protected from unconscious bias by certain rules which produce randomization. An examiner in Dean's position would have to take all available children in his selected category, or, let us say 100 by some random method in each school in town, if he wished to avoid the economic bias that might be introduced by examining children from only one school in town. Tables of *random numbers* are available and special methods of randomization described in many texts on statistics.

Age is the most common source of bias since so many conditions, caries included, vary with it. Two samples of broad age range (as 10 or more years) may be weighted, one with younger individuals, the other with older individuals. It is best to pinpoint age as closely as possible without sacrificing the sample size necessary to overcome unavoidable variables such as familial heredity. In working in school systems, children should be recorded by age, not by the grade they are in. In exact studies of children's teeth it is sometimes necessary for the researcher to go even further, measuring the posteruptive age of the teeth under actual study, since teeth do not always erupt at the same age.

Disease experience is another important variable to be considered where possible. Dental-caries experience, as noted at the time of initiation of a cohort study, will permit *pairing of cases,* so that the study group and the control group start off with equal caries susceptibility. If pairing is not easy, it will suffice to have the two samples more or less equal as to mean and standard deviation of disease experience.

Unknowns, to the statistician, are individual observations which were originally expected in their plan of action but which did not materialize. As an example, a statistician constructs a questionnaire survey through a system of carefully planned stratified sampling. The questionnaires are sent out, but he cannot control which questionnaires will be returned and which will not. How is he to evaluate conditions among the group that do not return their questionnaires? The simplest method, of course, is to assume a distribution of the unknowns according to the distribution to answers that did come back. Thus if the survey were to deal with income, it might be assumed that the incomes of those who did not return questionnaires were distributed in the same fashion as the incomes of those who did return questionnaires, and the former could therefore be ignored as not likely to alter the final result of the study. Such an assumption might easily be erroneous, since embarrassment could easily lead those with either extremely large or extremely small incomes not to reply as frequently as those with average incomes. Any study where there is a substantial proportion of unknown answers should contain a statement of the size of the unknown group and careful appraisal of its probable status.

Controls. Most studies involve comparisons within a population, not with some obvious "zero" situation (such as complete absence of dental caries), but with a level of the measured characteristic taken to be normal or endemic in the neighboring area. This requires use of a *control group,* which should ideally be similar to the experimental group in all respects except the one under analysis. Great care should be taken to select the control group in exactly the same manner as the experimental group. Matching of controls and experimentals may be done at any level from paired individuals to paired cities. If exact pairing of individuals cannot be done without reducing sample size too much, then study and control groups should be *balanced* so as to contain equal numbers of persons in such different categories as may be recognized (sex, economic status, and so forth). One good method for topical studies is the use of one half of the mouth of the subject as a control for the other. Thus many tests of topical fluoride therapy have been performed on one side only of the mouths of a group of children, the other side being treated with an inert solution. If any of the active solution crosses the midline, it minimizes rather than exaggerates the differences found. Another good control mechanism for topical treatment studies is the pairing of individuals according to previous caries (or other disease) experience. This improves the likelihood that subsequent incidence of disease, barring treatment, will be comparable.

Base-line data from previous years in the same population may be used for control purposes, if of comparable quality. This has been a common method in evaluation of water-supply fluoridation.

Rate, in its commonest form, applies to a series of observations made over a period of time: so many deaths per 100,000 persons per year, or so many new carious surfaces per child per year. The minimum number of observations by which a time rate can be determined is two. Average values for such characteristics as DMF teeth, when expressed per person or per a given number of persons, are also sometimes called rates. This is not a preferred use of the word. It is better to speak of a DMF *count,* when the observations which were averaged occurred at one point in time.

Mortality and *fatality* apply not only to people but to teeth. *Mortality* among people means deaths divided by population, a decimal fraction until it is multiplied by a power of 10 (1,000 or 100,000 is usually used). *Tooth mortality* means lost teeth divided by the total number of teeth possible in the group. Since the total number of teeth possible in the group is the number of persons times a constant, either 28 or 32, the constant is frequently omitted. Thus tooth mortality is often expressed as missing teeth per person, and is often a figure larger than 1.0. *Fatality* among persons means deaths divided by cases of a disease, then multiplied by a power of 10. *Tooth fatality* means missing teeth divided by DMF teeth (decayed plus missing plus filled). Since the count of DMF teeth is not a constant from individual to individual, it cannot be eliminated, and the tooth fatality is thus always a fraction less than 1 unless multiplied by a power of 10. Mortality and fatality *rates* usually refer to occurrences within a given interval of time, ordinarily one year, though it is not incorrect to use such terms in connection with a single event such as a disaster.

Experience, incidence, and prevalence are frequently confused, as they apply to dental caries or to any other condition. *Experience* refers to the cumulative effect of disease, past and present, up to the time of examination. It may be measured for caries in terms of cases or in terms of decayed, missing, and filled teeth, surfaces, or some other measure per person. *Incidence* is a rate, involving at least two measurements spaced apart by a definite interval of time, usually 1 year. It can be applied to new cases of disease, or to new teeth affected, and so on. Because of the nature of the measurement, caries incidence can be decreasing at a time when caries experience, since cumulative, is still increasing.

Prevalence is usually taken to refer to the proportion of a population affected by a disease or other condition at a given time. With caries, prevalence usually means the proportion of the population showing any evidence (experience) of caries, past or present. As an alternate meaning, caries prevalence may be used to designate the amount of untreated caries per person or the proportion of persons with untreated caries in the population at a given time, but *severity* is a better word for this. If the proportion is measured at one time, it is called *point prevalence.* When two measurements of point prevalence are separated by a period of time, the difference is called *period prevalence.*

This chapter has presented very briefly some of the commonsense factors to be considered when undertaking a statistical study. Some general statistical terms have been defined; more detailed dental terminology appears in Chapter 14. Chapter 5 takes up actual methods of statistical analysis.

Biostatistics: Appraisal of Variability

THERE COMES a time in the design of a study when data best suited to the study have been chosen, when bias and examiner error have been reduced to a minimum, perhaps to zero, and when the variability remaining in the sample will be that inherent in the sample itself: variability due to the diverse heredity, environment, and previous medical history found even in the most carefully selected groups of human beings. Such errors usually tend to even out if a large enough sample is studied. They scatter fairly evenly about the average or mean value for the sample. At this time the work of collecting data should proceed.

This chapter is not concerned with specific survey objectives, since suggestions of this nature are found in Chapter 14, nor is it concerned with such simple matters as tally sheets and the computing of averages or means. The construction of certain basic statistical tests, however, needs to be understood by the public health dentist, even if the actual completion of the test is done by computer. Various textbooks on statistics give this material in readable yet thorough form. Perhaps the best of these texts for the worker in the field of dental public health are Colton's *Statistics in Medicine* and Weintraub, Douglass, and Gillings's *Biostats*. The latter is a self-instructional book with problems, the solutions of which appear at the end of each chapter. Both volumes are written in such a way as to be valuable to the health worker without mathematical background. Certain basic principles in the presentation of statistical data, however, are worth including here; they are quoted in somewhat abbreviated form from Bradford Hill:

(i) The contents of a table as a whole and the items in each separate column should be clearly and fully defined. The unit of measurement must be included.

(ii) If the table includes rates, the basis upon which they are measured must be clearly stated—death rate per cent, or per thousand, or per million as the case may be.

(iii) Whenever possible the frequency distributions should be given in full. These are basic data from which conclusions are being drawn, and their presentation allows the reader to check the validity of the author's arguments. [A *frequency distribution* results whenever data are grouped into a number of different categories, as for instance DMF tooth counts, and it is wished to show how many examples of each category were found in the sample which was studied. A good example appears in Table 8.]

(iv) Rates or proportions should not be given alone without any information as to the numbers of observations upon which they are based. By giving only rates of observations and omitting the actual number of observations or frequency distributions, we are excluding the basic data.

(v) Where percentages are used it must be clearly indicated that these are not absolute numbers. Rather than combine too many types of figure in one table, it is often best to divide the material into two or three small tables.

(vi) Full particulars of any exclusion of observations from a collected series must be given. The reasons for and the criteria of exclusions must be clearly defined. [A good example of this in the dental field is the exclusion of third molars from DMF counts: a common practice, since so many third molars are either unerupted or impacted, yet a practice which must be recorded every time, since it is not universal.][1]

These rules for the presentation of tabular material make it plain that a table should stand on its own feet, and be reasonably understandable even without a reading of the accompanying text. Graphs, however, are a somewhat different proposition. A graph is a simplified presentation of material designed to make certain relations exceedingly clear. Exclusions and simplifications are the rule in graph work, as is also the selection of a scale which will make the graph easy to read. Careful titling of graphs is important, as is also a proper notation of the scale. Tabular material is the real meat of any scientific report; graphs are "propaganda." The textbooks already named and many others give directions for the preparation of the more important varieties of graphs.

MEASURES OF CENTRAL TENDENCY

Data, once recorded, must be summarized to be understood. Some one measurement must be taken as characteristic of all the observations in the sample, in order that comparison may be made with a similar characteristic measurement in another sample or samples. The central point of the frequency distribution is usually of most interest. The greatest number of observations is likely to be found here, with extreme values, high and low, fairly well distributed on either side. There are three measures of central tendency in common use: the mean, the median, and the mode.

The *mean,* or average, of a series of measurements is by far the most useful term for statistical analysis, as well as the most common. It is found by dividing the sum of all observations by the number of observations. It recognizes the arithmetic values of all the observations in the series, and is well suited to further work, such as the appraisal of variability soon to be discussed.

The *median* of a series of measurements is that value which represents the case at the exact center of the series when all observations have been arranged in order of magnitude. It is typical of a number of testing mechanisms which apply to rank lists and other collections of data where true number scales are misleading or impossible. This field is called *nonparametric statistics,* and it receives attention in Chapter 6.

There are times when the median is a better centering constant than the mean. This occurs when some isolated, very large observations a long way from the center will unduly influence the mean. Such observations, of course, have no distorting effect upon the

Table 6. Average net income of dentists according to certain types of practice organization or employment, United States, 1970.

	Net income (dollars)		
Type of employment	Mean	Standard deviation	Median
Independent practice without partners and without sharing of costs	28,798	15,545	26,700
Independent practice without partners but sharing costs of offices or assistants, etc.	31,515	17,090	29,100
All types of employment	29,487	16,095	26,900

median whatever. Table 6, abbreviated from an income survey of the American Dental Association Bureau of Economic Research and Statistics, may be used to illustrate this point.[2] It will be noted that the mean net income of dentists was in all instances larger than the median net income, a result of the distortion caused by certain very high and very infrequent incomes; 5.6 percent of the dentists reporting had annual incomes of $60,000 or more, each representing more than twice the median income. In a previous survey, 0.8 percent of the dentists were reported making more than five times the median income. Situations of this sort are generally typical of skewed curves, where the peak is asymmetrically placed.

The arrangement of measurements in order of magnitude also gives opportunity for dividing the sample according to *percentiles.* These are proportions named according to their location in the scale. The median is the 50th percentile. That point above which 25 percent of the observations are found and below which 74 percent of the observations are found is the 75th percentile, and so forth.

The *mode* is the observation occurring most frequently, or, in theory, the value at which the ideal frequency curve of the observations reaches its peak. The curve may on occasion have more than one peak, hence more than one mode.

Of the three central values, the mean is the easiest one to use for further mathematical analysis, particularly the testing of differences between populations to see whether such differences could have occurred by chance.

VARIABILITY

A statistician wishing to test the significance of a difference between two mean values must first determine the reliability of each mean. He has two chief criteria: the width of dispersal, or scatter, of individual scores about the mean, and the number of individuals in the sample. The first of these criteria is of prime importance as a measure of reliability, for it tells him in effect whether he is dealing with a "rifle" or a "shotgun." If all scores in a sample fall fairly close together, not many will be needed in order to establish a reliable central value. The more widely the scores scatter, the more scores will be needed in order to be sure that the apparent central value is a reasonable approximation of the true value for the universe under consideration.

Among possible measures of scatter, the most useful and best accepted is called the *standard deviation of the observations;* it is usually assigned the symbol s or the Greek equivalent σ (sigma). It is found by the following formula:

$$s = \sqrt{\frac{\text{The sum of the squares of all deviations from the mean}}{\text{The number of observations composing the mean}}}$$

$$= \sqrt{\frac{\Sigma(x - \bar{x})^2}{n}}$$

Table 7 deals with a hypothetical example of standard deviation and should make clear why statisticians value the term as an exceedingly descriptive one. The two samples in Table 7 are obviously alike in that they have a mean m of 7 DMF (decayed, missing, and filled) teeth per person. They are unlike in the way individual cases scatter around this mean. The first sample has twice the scatter of the second sample. There are various ways in which this scatter might be described. First to occur to one, perhaps, would be the *range* between the highest and the lowest observation. In the first sample this would be 8 (3 to 11), and in the second sample 4 (5 to 9). Range would do well enough in these two samples but would mean very little in the frequency distributions so often found, where the highest and lowest scores are very infrequent and are removed a long and an unpredictable distance from the main cluster of observations near the mean. The sum of all deviations is obviously of no help at all, for if the mean is properly located the deviations above and below it should add to zero, as indeed they do in these instances. Elimination of the minus signs on the deviations below the mean would help somewhat, but is arithmetically incorrect. Squaring the deviations, averaging them, and then extracting the square root effectively eliminates the minus signs and gives a value which, for reasons that need not be explained here, relates the deviations to the bell-shaped "normal" curve so often seen for the chance scatter of observations above and below a mean. The result of this process is termed the *standard deviation of the observations*. The square of the standard deviation (s^2), an easy figure to use in further calculations, is called the *variance*.

Fig. 3 shows such a normal curve drawn from its theoretical formula, and the relation to this curve of various multiples of the standard deviation. The term *confidence interval* is often applied to the distance which will enclose a given proportion of observations above and below the mean. Thus the "95 percent" confidence interval is between two standard deviations above and below the mean, while the "99 percent" interval is between three standard deviations above and below the mean. The end points of the interval are called *confidence limits*.

Table 7. Calculation of standard deviation: decayed, missing, and filled teeth per person in two hypothetical samples of five cases each.

First sample			Second sample		
DMF teeth	Deviation	(Deviation)^2	DMF teeth	Deviation	(Deviation)^2
3	−4	16	5	−2	4
5	−2	4	6	−1	1
7	0	0	7	0	0
9	2	4	8	1	1
11	4	16	9	2	4
5)35	0	5)40	5)35	0	5)10
$m = 7$		$s^2 = 8.0$	$m = 7$		$s^2 = 2.0$
		$s = 2.8$			$s = 1.4$

Fig. 4 shows actual curves for two groups of young men studied for their DMF teeth and showing the frequencies for various tooth scores found in Table 8.[3] In Fig. 4, the curve for Middle Atlantic midshipmen is strikingly like the theoretical curve except for two points which are rather out of line. The one for Southwestern midshipmen would be similar also if the zero values for DMF teeth could be translated into minus values such as must actually have existed in some of the men with very high (rather than just barely adequate) resistance to dental caries. The "resistant" mean would then have tapered off in decreasing frequency below zero just as the highly "susceptible" men do at the other end of the curve.

Referring once more to the theoretical curve in Fig. 3, we can see that a line drawn upward from the score scale one standard deviation either above or below the mean reaches the frequency

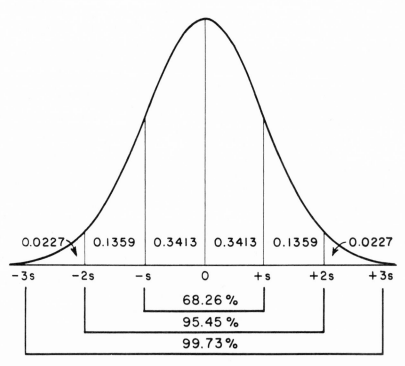

Figure 3. Normal frequency curve.

curve at its point of inflection: the point at which it changes from being convex to concave or vice versa. The area between plus and minus one standard deviation under the curve theoretically encloses in the typical case 68.26 percent of all observations; 31.74 percent of the observations fall outside. The area from plus to minus two standard deviations theoretically encloses 95.45 percent of all observations, and the area between plus and minus three standard deviations theoretically encloses 99.73 percent of the observations. Thus it can be seen that there is a real relation between the figure mathematically obtained for a standard deviation and the number of points in the series of observations which are likely to fall between various multiples of that standard deviation and the mean. Since the high frequencies of points are found near the mean in any series approaching typical proportions, the likelihood of a point arising distant from the mean can be computed in terms of the number of standard deviations it is removed from the mean.

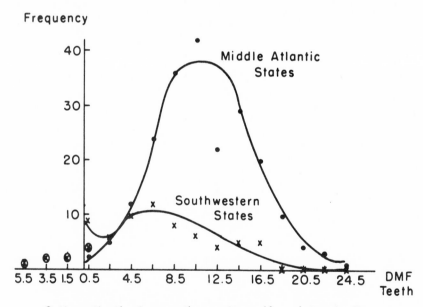

Figure 4. Actual frequency curves for DMF teeth for 275 U.S.N.R.M.S. midshipmen from two geographic regions, 1944.

This will be useful in the testing of differences between means, as we shall see later.

In each hypothetical sample in Table 7, the standard deviation *is that of the original observations.* There is only one case in each score category, but, even if each sample contained a large number of cases for each score group instead of one, the standard deviation of the observations would be the same provided that the cases were equally distributed among the score groups. The standard deviation, therefore, measures a fundamental characteristic of the sample regardless of its size: its variability.

Two graphic illustrations will help at this point to understand standard deviation. These are shown in Figs. 5 and 6. The first shows changes in the number of circulating leukocytes in the blood of experimental subjects who had received a drug designed to simulate stress.[4] An easily measured blood characteristic was desired which could be expected to change reliably under stress conditions. The graph shows a scatter diagram for each of three types of white blood cells: eosinophils, lymphocytes, and neutrophils. Each point represents one observation, and the hori-

Table 8. Frequency of DMF teeth, third molars excluded, among 275 midshipmen, aged approximately 21, selected because of birth in one of two selected areas, U.S.N.R.M.S., New York, 1944.

DMF teeth	Middle Atlantic states	Southwestern states
0–1	2	9
2–3	5	6
4–5	12	10
6–7	24	12
8–9	36	8
10–11	42	6
12–13	22	4
14–15	29	5
16–17	20	5
18–19	10	0
20–21	4	0
22–23	3	0
24–25	1	0
Total	210	65
Mean no. of teeth	11.21	7.36

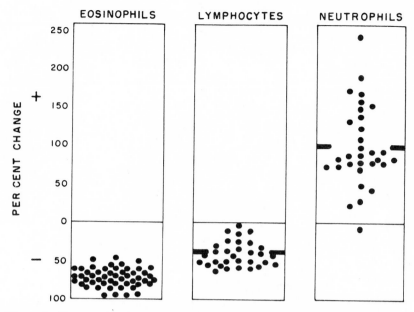

Figure 5. Changes in circulating leukocytes in non-Addisonians following 25 mg ACTH. [From P. H. Forsham, "Clinical Studies with Pituitary Adrenocorticotropin," *Journal of Clinical Endocrinology 8,* 22 (1948). Courtesy, Charles C Thomas, Publisher.]

zontal lines at either side of each box represent the mean value for change in the entire group of observations. It can be seen at a glance that the eosinophils have altered in a very regular fashion, clustering closely about their mean; that is, the standard deviation is small. The lymphocytes do not concentrate quite so well, and there is an added disadvantage that some of the observations show almost no change from zero, the original value. Neutrophils show the widest scatter of all: a very large standard deviation. Mere inspection makes it obvious that the eosinophils are the best measure of stress in this instance because of their small standard deviation.

Fig. 6 shows ascending mean values for dental-caries experience in terms of DMF teeth among a sample of 14,002 children together with the values for one and for two standard deviations plotted above and below the means.[5] The standard deviations had to be computed from the actual sample, but give us the most

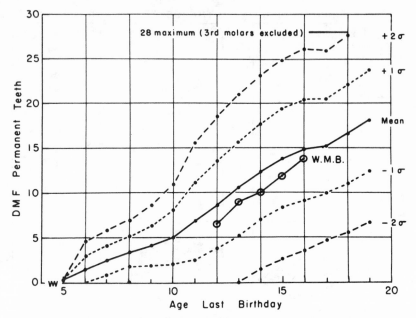

Figure 6. Dental caries experience in 14,002 children examined by explorer in 1951 in 28 representative Massachusetts communities, showing one and two standard deviations above and below the mean and a sample case plotted for a 5-year period.

probable scatter of observations among future samples taken from the same universe (Massachusetts in 1951). One would expect 68 percent of the children in any sample to have DMF counts within one standard deviation of the mean at a given age, and 95 percent of the children to have DMF counts within two standard deviations of the mean. Where either of these limits falls below zero, one would expect an accumulation of cases at zero, as in Fig. 4. Individual cases can be plotted upon Fig. 6, as has been done for the patient W.M.B. over a period of 4 years. Such plotting shows quickly and easily the relation of the individual not only to the mean but to the apparent frequency distribution of cases within the universe of which he is part.

Standard deviations can be computed for any frequency distribution by means of the formula used for Table 7. Where data are more numerous, however, or are grouped, with more than one case for each score, as in the data in Table 8, this method becomes cumbersome. Simpler mathematical formulas are available, the algebraic equivalents of the original one. They are:

for ungrouped data: $\quad s_x = \sqrt{\dfrac{\Sigma x^2}{n} - \bar{x}^2}$

for grouped data: $\quad s_x = \sqrt{\dfrac{\Sigma f x^2}{n} - \bar{x}^2}$

In these formulas, Σx^2 means the sum of the squares of the scores themselves; f means frequency, where more than one example of a given score occurs and data have been grouped; n means the number of cases in the sample; and $\bar{x}$ means the mean of all scores of variable x.

In referring to Table 7 it is quite obvious that the means shown there are far less reliable than they would be if there were 10 or 100 cases for each score instead of only one. The larger the sample is, the more nearly it approximates the full size of the universe and the more nearly the sample mean approximates the mean of the universe. The relation appeals to common sense, it can be tested experimentally as with the tossing of coins, and it can also be demonstrated mathematically. The reliability of a mean therefore depends not only upon the scatter of observations on either side of it, but also upon the number of cases—the sample size—upon which it is based. We want one figure which will recognize both of these criteria of reliability. This figure is known as the *standard error of the mean* and is obtained by dividing the standard deviation of the observations by the square root of the number of cases constituting the sample, thus:

$$S.E._{\cdot x} = \frac{s_x}{\sqrt{n}}$$

By this formula, the standard error of the first mean in Table 7 would be 2.8 divided by the square root of 5, the number of cases. The result is 1.25. Similarly the standard error of the second mean is 1.4 divided by the square root of 5, or 0.63. These values are often appended to the mean in the familiar form, 7 ± 1.25, or 7 ± 0.63. It is obvious that the larger the sample becomes the more the standard deviation of the observations is reduced by division and the smaller the standard error of the mean becomes. Thus the mean becomes more and more reliable statistically.

Means for samples tend to scatter around the mean for the universe according to the normal curve. The standard error of the mean gives an estimate of this scatter, and can be used for predicting what proportion of a series of sample means (of similar size) will fall a given distance from the mean of the universe. The mean for the universe is unknown, of course, but the mean of the sample at hand is taken as the best possible estimate of it.

SIGNIFICANCE OF DIFFERENCES BETWEEN MEANS

One of the prime reasons for estimating the standard error of a mean is to find out whether the difference between this mean and another mean could have arisen by chance or, instead, is likely to be a reliable finding indicating that the two samples were actually drawn from two different universes. The two frequency distributions shown in Figure 4 and recorded in detail in Table 8 will illustrate this point. They were part of a study of geographical variation in dental-caries experience, and it was desired to know from a testing of those two samples whether the midshipmen from the Middle Atlantic states and those from the Southwestern states actually came from one universe or from two. If the mean values for DMF teeth in these two groups were separated from each other by a difference that was small in proportion to the errors of each mean, one might assume that, if a large number of samples of 210 midshipmen of one sort and 65 of another sort were taken, the means would vary by chance, and small differences between the means would appear by chance, even if the men were all from the same universe. The wide scatter of individual cases in both groups emphasizes the need for further analysis.

In the end, therefore, the chief value of a mean lies in our ability to compare it with other means. We must test differences between means for their significance, and to do so we must find some measure for the *standard error of a difference* between means. Such a standard error ought to recognize the reliability of each of the means involved in the difference. This can be done by an algebraic manipulation of the standard errors of the two means. The formula is:

$$S.E._{Difference} = \sqrt{(S.E._{\bar{x}_1})^2 + (S.E._{\bar{x}_2})^2}$$

We are now ready for the final step in a significance test upon differences between means: the computation of a so-called t value, which is actually the difference divided by its own standard error. The formula for samples of more than 30 cases is:

$$t = \frac{\bar{x}_1 - \bar{x}_2}{S.E._{Difference}}$$

The reason for use of such a value can be understood if one imagines that both the samples being tested come from one universe (an assumption called the *null hypothesis,* since differences are "null"). If this were the case, we should expect the differences between samples to scatter according to the normal curve, and more or less evenly about a value of zero. If repeated tests were performed, zero itself would be the commonest difference. Moreover, if samples were made larger and larger until they approximated the size of the universe itself, differences between samples would again become smaller and smaller until they reached zero. A difference between samples, therefore, becomes significant only when it differs from zero more than might be expected under chance conditions.

The formula just stated allows us to compute a standard deviation for the difference based upon actual material, giving us at the same time probabilities which can be related to the normal curve just as were the standard deviations of the observations and the standard errors of the means. If a difference is equal to its own standard error, there will be approximately a 32 percent chance that this or a larger difference could have occurred accidentally in repeated tests. Obviously such a difference is meaningless. If the t value is 2, however, with the difference equal to twice its own standard error, reference to the normal curve tells us that only 5 percent of the time would a difference of this magnitude occur by chance. If the difference is three times its own standard error,

Table 9. Significance of a *t* value.

t value	Probability of chance occurrence, *P*	Interpretation
1.0	0.3174	Insignificant
2.0	.0456	Significant at 5% level ("borderline")
3.0	.0027	Significant at 1% level
4.0	.00006	Highly significant
5.0	.0000006	Highly significant

reference to the normal curve tells us that such a difference would occur by chance only 0.3 percent of the time. Therefore *t* values of 2 are taken to be of borderline significance by the statistician, and *t* values of 3 or more are taken to be of real significance. The mathematical probabilities for these and other values are shown in Table 9.

Table 10 shows full details of a significance test performed between the two frequency distributions shown in Table 8. Notice how nearly alike are the first measurements of variability, the standard deviations of the observations (4.55 and 4.81). Notice next that the standard error of the first mean is far smaller than the standard error of the second mean because the first is based upon a much larger number of cases. Notice finally that the standard error of the difference between the two means is somewhat greater than the standard error of either mean alone, but not as great as the two standard errors added together. The ultimate *t* value shows the difference to be almost six times its own standard error, which can be translated into a probability of less than one in 1 million for the accidental occurrence of a difference this size. The difference would therefore be termed highly significant. The arithmetic involved in this test may look formidable, but anyone with access to a modern calculating machine can run through the figures in a very short period of time. A properly programmed computer, of course, will do the job in no time at all.

Where human material must be used, statistical-significance tests should be performed and reported. If this is not done, frequency distributions of the DMF or other scores should be published so that the reader may perform his own tests.

Table 10. Calculation of significance of frequency distribution shown in Table 8.

DMF Teeth		Middle Atlantic States			Southwestern States		
Score	x	f	fx	fx^2	f	fx	fx^2
0–1	0.5	2	1.0	0.5	9	4.5	2.25
2–3	2.5	5	12.5	31.25	6	15.0	37.50
4–5	4.5	12	54.0	243.00	10	45.0	202.50
6–7	6.5	24	156.0	1014.00	12	78.0	507.00
8–9	8.5	36	306.0	2601.00	8	68.0	578.00
10–11	10.5	42	441.0	4630.50	6	63.0	661.50
12–13	12.5	22	275.0	3437.50	4	50.0	625.00
14–15	14.5	29	420.5	6097.25	5	72.5	1051.25
16–17	16.5	20	330.0	5445.00	5	82.5	1361.25
18–19	18.5	10	185.0	3422.50	0	0	0
20–21	20.5	4	82.0	1681.00	0	0	0
22–23	22.5	3	67.5	1518.75	0	0	0
24–25	24.5	1	24.5	600.25	0	0	0
		210	2355.0	30722.50	65	478.5	5026.25

$$s_{\text{M.A.}} = \sqrt{\frac{30{,}722}{210} - (11.21)^2} = \sqrt{146.30 - 125.66} = 4.55$$

$$s_{\text{S.W.}} = \sqrt{\frac{5{,}026}{65} - (7.36)^2} = \sqrt{77.33 - 54.20} = 4.81$$

$$\text{S.E.}_{\bar{x}_{\text{M.A.}}} = \frac{s_{\text{M.A.}}}{\sqrt{n}} = \frac{4.55}{\sqrt{210}} = 0.316$$

$$\text{S.E.}_{\bar{x}_{\text{S.W}}} = \frac{4.81}{\sqrt{65}} = 0.596$$

$$\text{S.E.}_{\text{Diff.}} = \sqrt{(\text{S.E.}_{\bar{x}_{\text{M.A.}}})^2 + (\text{S.E.}_{\bar{x}_{\text{S.W.}}})^2} = \sqrt{(0.316)^2 + (0.596)^2} = 0.674$$

$$t = \frac{\text{Difference}}{\text{S.E.}_{\text{Diff.}}} = \frac{11.21 - 7.36}{0.674} = \frac{3.85}{0.674} = 5.71$$

MORE ELABORATE TESTS

I shall not attempt here to describe more than one method of significance testing upon means. A common variation upon the test just given involves the use of the "null hypothesis," where an initial assumption is made that both samples came from the same universe and should therefore be described by the same "grand" standard deviation involving all observations from both samples. The result of this type of test is almost always quite close to results found by the method actually described. For use in small-sample work, the "t test" has been elaborated by Fisher.[6] The quantity t is again interpreted in terms of probability, but a further concept, *degree of freedom*, is added, a related form of which will be discussed in the next chapter.

Where more than two variables are to be related a method called *analysis of variance* is of value, making use of the squared deviations (variances) of the various observations from their means.[7] The objective of the method is to compare deviations between groups with the deviations within groups. An *F ratio* is determined, and the significance of this ratio appraised in accord with the number of comparisons and the sizes of the various samples. The basic question to be answered is whether deviations between groups exceed deviations within groups to such an extent that the groups should be considered to be drawn from different universes. Work of this degree of complexity will usually require the advice of an expert or, at the very least, further reading beyond the scope of this text.

CALCULATION OF SAMPLE SIZE

What is the implication of high variability of observations in the design of experiments to test methods of caries control? Fortunately, the apparent tendency for standard deviations to reach more or less predictable values among young adults gives us a hint. The formulas leading to a t value can be reversed and solved for the number of cases necessary in each sample, if fixed values are assumed for the difference between means and for the standard deviation. The formula thus becomes:

$$n = \frac{13.27s^2}{\text{Difference}^2}$$

The constant 13.27 implies a t value of 2.576, or a 1 percent chance that the difference between means will have occurred by chance. A less conservative approach would make use of a t value

Table 11. Minimum sample sizes, experimental or control, necessary to reduce chance occurrence of a stated difference between means to below 1%, if experimental and control groups are equal in size.[a]

Expected difference between means	Standard deviation(s)			
	3.0	4.0	5.0	6.0
1.0	119	212	332	478
2.0	30[b]	53	83	119
3.0	13[b]	23[b]	37	53
4.0	8[b]	13[b]	21[b]	30[b]

a. A *t* value of 2.6 is assumed, giving a probability of 1.0% that the difference between means might have occurred by chance.

b. Small-sample methods needed for analysis.

of 1.960, with a 5 percent probability of a chance difference. The constant in the numerator of the formula would then be 7.68. The quantity n is the number of cases in each sample, experimental, or control, and these samples are presumed to be equal in size.

A convenient table for size of sample (Table 11) can be constructed from this formula. No investigator will know in advance the exact means and standard deviations that his experiment will produce—otherwise he would not need to perform it. The general ranges of mean and standard-deviation values are often predictable, however, and permit some rough estimate of the sample sizes needed. The inference is obvious that where small differences in mean values are expected, particularly when accompanied by large standard deviations, large samples must be used. By making the samples a great deal larger than the minimum, additional accuracy can be obtained and unforeseen errors allowed for, provided of course that in making the increase in numbers one does not unduly impair the quality of the sample or of the examination method. Large samples also protect the investigator against the discovery of unsuitable or incompletely recorded cases, or, in longitudinal studies, against dropouts.

COVARIANCE ADJUSTMENT

The ideal statistical test involves comparison of two or more samples where all variables except those under study have been so controlled that biased results are unlikely. Unfortunately, circumstances occur where the groups are not equivalent in respect to certain important variables extraneous to the study. When this happens, covariance analysis permits adjustment of the main values of the groups to eliminate the effect of those extraneous variables that can be measured. The method for analysis involves a combination of the principles of regression analysis (correlation) and analysis of variance. The result not only gives figures by which means may be adjusted to eliminate the effects of the extraneous variables (covariates), but also an *F ratio* by which the significance of the differences between the adjusted means may be appraised. The figuring is so involved that it is very time-consuming to perform by hand, but modern computer programs make covariance analysis so easy that studies which might formerly have been discarded as involving too laborious analysis may now be brought quite quickly into a satisfactory degree of adjustment.

An example will illustrate the use of covariance analysis. Recent investigation of some potentially cariogenic food products was attempted in two state institutions in Massachusetts where a uniformly planned diet gave important advantages, but where the inmates of whole dormitories had to be assigned either to an experimental or to a control group—with no opportunity to assign individuals to groups at random. The study was a longitudinal one, covering a 2-year period. At the beginning of the study it was difficult enough to obtain dormitory groupings which provided samples of similar age distribution. It proved impossible to provide groups of similar past caries experience—a desirable procedure in order to secure equal levels of caries susceptibility. By the end of the 2-year period a number of dropouts had occurred from all study groups owing to discharge, transfer, or death. As a result, the groups no longer presented comparable mean ages. Covariance analysis was therefore used to adjust mean caries increments for group differences in age, past caries experience, and sound teeth at risk. Only after such adjustments could observed mean differences be compared with confidence.

CHAPTER 6

Biostatistics: Correlation and Other Tests

THE SCIENCE of statistics has given us a very large number of tests which can be applied to public health data. Only a very few of these belong in this volume: those which will illustrate principles of value in guiding the public health dentist in collection of the commoner types of data, and those which he will find himself using so frequently that recourse to a specialist in statistics will often be unnecessary. The significance test upon differences between means is certainly such a test; so also are the test for significance of difference between proportions, the X^2 (chi square) test, and the calculation of coefficient of correlation using parametric and nonparametric methods. Each is best adapted to data of a certain type, and an understanding of the tests will often guide a public health dentist toward the efficient collection of data which will fit one test particularly well.

DIFFERENCES BETWEEN PROPORTIONS

A test upon differences between means implies the existence of mean values expressed in numbers per person or some other baseline unit. Such is the case in many measures of physical characteristics and of disease. In dental public health, it is the case in the surveys of DMF teeth so necessary where caries prevalence is high. Where the prevalence of dental caries is low, however, DMF tooth counts vary less than they do under other conditions, and the proportion of the population showing one or more DMF teeth, conversely, becomes a more variable and a more interesting figure than the DMF count. It is also far easier to collect.

Such a survey procedure of course fails to disclose a great deal of the individual variability of human material, since instead of a long scale of numerical measurements we use only two categories: one negative and one positive. Because we want as much information upon variability as possible to guide us in estimating the significance of our findings, mean values per case should be assembled wherever there is an approximately even choice between this method and a yes-or-no method. There are many instances, however, where the estimation of dental disease on a yes-or-no basis is the most informative, others where it is the most reliable under adverse circumstances, and others yet where it is the only method possible (as in dealing with surveys expressed in affected teeth or tooth surfaces per 100 erupted teeth or surfaces, rather than per individual). For such surveys we need a significance test to be used upon differences between proportions. This test is actually simpler to perform than a test upon differences between means.

Several elementary textbooks on statistics develop in very clear style the application of the *binomial theorem* to the probability of error in a proportion. As material for an example Bradford Hill uses fatality rate in cases of a specific disease, showing how important it is to have a sample of adequate size if one is testing cures for this disease against a previously experienced fatality rate which for purposes of argument he assumes to have been 20 percent.[1] The fatality rate in a sample of one case will be either 100 percent or 0 percent, depending upon whether or not the patient dies. Both figures vary so widely from the previously experienced 20 percent fatality that comparison is impossible. When a sample of two patients is chosen, it is possible for both to recover, for one patient to recover and one to die (there are two ways for this to happen), or for both patients to die. These events, however, permit only three possible fatality rates: 0 percent, 50 percent, and 100 percent. Testing for any cure for the disease still remains, on the basis of chance alone, a highly inaccurate proceeding with such a small sample. Larger and larger samples are then discussed, until finally the general situation with n cases is developed, from which arises the formula for the *standard error of a proportion*. This formula is:

$$\text{S.E.} = \sqrt{\frac{pq}{n}}$$

where p represents the chance of an event occurring, q represents the chance of the event not occurring, n represents the number of cases in the sample.

The standard error of a proportion is a measure of the probable scatter, on the basis of chance alone, of many sampling proportions about the true value of this proportion in the universe. This scatter assumes a normal frequency curve, to which one turns for interpretation just as with the standard deviations and errors described in the previous chapter. The standard error of a proportion is a value parallel to the standard error of a mean, and fits into our significance-testing procedure at exactly the same point. It varies, obviously, with the number of cases in the sample.

The standard error of a proportion may be expressed in terms of percentage, without any decimal point, or as a decimal fraction. The latter method makes the arithmetic more difficult. The symbol q (the chance of an event not occurring) is in all instances 100 $- p$, or, if decimal fractions are used, $1.0 - p$. In the first instance, p is a whole number; in the second, it is less than one. Thus in Bradford Hill's example $p \times q$ is 20×80. The standard error is used exactly as one uses the standard error of a mean: it is combined with another value for another proportion in order to calculate a standard error for the difference between the two proportions. The formula for this, as in the previous chapter, is:

$$\text{S.E.}_{\text{Difference}} = \sqrt{\text{S.E.}_{\cdot p_1}{}^2 + \text{S.E.}_{\cdot p_2}{}^2}$$

The two separate steps, however, are unnecessary, as the two formulas given so far can be combined and the standard error of the difference computed directly from the original data:

$$S.E._{Difference} = \sqrt{\frac{p_1 q_1}{n_1} + \frac{p_2 q_2}{n_2}}$$

If the null hypothesis is used, with one overall probability for occurrence and nonoccurrence computed for both samples taken as one, then the formula becomes:

$$S.E._{Difference} = \sqrt{\frac{pq}{n_1} + \frac{pq}{n_2}}$$

Here n_1 and n_2, of course, are the sizes of the two samples involved in the test. The t value, as before, is the difference between proportions divided by its own standard error. This is interpreted as before, a value of 2 being of borderline (5 percent) significance and a value of 3 or more being clearly significant.

A typical example for testing is found in Knutson and Armstrong's second-year study of the effect of topically applied sodium fluoride solution upon caries incidence.[2] They report 97 carious teeth in 1944 from a group of 929 erupted but unattacked upper left teeth treated with sodium fluoride in 1942. The untreated upper right teeth showed 173 carious in 1944 out of 940 erupted but unattacked in 1942. The proportion of new caries on the experimental side is 10.4 percent; on the control side, 18.4 percent. Expressing the difference as a percent of a percent (a complicated but necessary step), the first figure is about 56 percent of the second, giving about 43 percent reduction in dental caries. A significance test may be made as follows:

$$t = \frac{18.4 - 10.4}{\sqrt{\dfrac{18.4 \times 81.6}{940} + \dfrac{10.4 \times 89.6}{929}}} = \frac{8.0}{1.6} = 5.0$$

A t value of this size implies a probability of the general magnitude of one in 1 million that such a difference would have occurred by chance.

The reader will note that p_1 and p_2 in this problem are the attacked teeth on the experimental side and on the control side respectively. If, however, the data from both sides are combined, an overall proportion of attacked teeth can be computed: 14.4 percent. With this proportion we can use the null hypotheses as follows:

$$t = \frac{18.4 - 10.4}{\sqrt{\dfrac{14.4 \times 85.6}{929} + \dfrac{14.4 \times 85.6}{940}}} = \frac{8.0}{1.6} = 5.0$$

If the arithmetic had been carried to one or two additional decimal places, small differences would have appeared between the two solutions to this problem, but these differences would have been quite unimportant in terms of probability.

All the tests described so far have been upon one pair of samples, from which were derived either one pair of means or one pair of proportions to be compared. It is often true that more than one pair of samples is available under circumstances where it is neither possible nor desirable to pool these samples into two groups for direct comparison. Several significant differences are to be sought all in one test, or perhaps a trend among certain progressive characteristics of a series of samples. Where the number of samples is small and perhaps related one to another in only a nominal way, the χ^2 *test* will show whether or not the differences we find are chance ones. Where we have a large number of observations to be compared, each related to the other on an interval scale (so in effect is a pair of observations), the calculation of a *correlation coefficient* gives us not only the probability of accidental occurrence for the relation we have observed, but also a numerical measure of the relation in terms of a coefficient from $+1.0$ to -1.0.

The χ^2 test is set up in such a way that the original number of cases entering into each sample becomes part of the calculation and affects interpretation of the answer. The test for correlation, on the other hand, allows merely a comparison of single figures, without any way to work into the calculations the size or variability of the sample from which it was drawn, if indeed a sample larger than one was involved. With such simplified pairs of observations, it is obvious that a larger number of pairs must be tested in order to establish a relation. Confidence can seldom be reposed in a correlation coefficient built upon less than a dozen pairs of observations, as will be seen later, unless the correlation is almost perfect, that is, where the coefficient approximates either $+1.0$ or -1.0.

THE x^2 TEST

The x^2 test is based upon a comparison between the observed measurement of a given characteristic in a sample and the measurement which ought to have been observed if the sample differed in no way from the universe upon which the test is based. The actual figure for x^2 is obtained by adding together all values of:

$$\frac{(\text{Observed number} - \text{expected number})^2}{\text{Expected number}}$$

It is important to note that all observations must be included in the test, whether positive or negative. Thus, in a caries problem, the cases showing no caries are just as important a part of the figuring as the cases of caries.

It is obvious that x^2 will equal zero if no sample involved in the test shows any difference between observed and expected values. It is also obvious that the more samples there are in the test, the larger x^2 will be. This latter fact needs to be recognized in the interpretation of x^2, and recognition is made of it by the computation of a figure called the number of *degrees of freedom*. This represents the number of compartments within a table which can be filled independently without the totals for the problem as a whole being incorrect. It is found by subtracting one from the number of columns in the table, subtracting one from the number of rows in the table, and multiplying these two figures together, except for the fact that the product is never less than 1.

After the calculation of x^2 and the determination of the number of degrees of freedom, the next step is to enter a master table, such as that prepared by Fisher (Table 12), and find the numbers closest to the value computed for x^2 in the line of the table which represents our figure for degrees of freedom (DF). Having located the number, one then follows to the head of the column and reads there the probability of chance occurrence of such a value of x^2, interpolating between column heads if necessary.

A good example for testing by x^2 can be found in an article describing the dental-caries status of children in several British

Table 12. Values for χ^2 for DF degrees of freedom and for different probabilities P that the given value will not be exceeded by chance alone.

DF			P		
	0.20	0.10	0.05	0.02	0.01
1	1.64	2.71	3.84	5.41	6.64
2	3.22	4.60	5.99	7.82	9.21
3	4.64	6.25	7.82	9.84	11.34
4	5.99	7.78	9.49	11.67	13.28
5	7.29	9.24	11.07	13.39	15.09
6	8.56	10.64	12.59	15.03	16.81
7	9.80	12.02	14.07	16.62	18.48
8	11.03	13.36	15.51	18.17	20.09
9	12.24	14.68	16.92	19.68	21.67
10	13.44	15.99	18.31	21.16	23.21

communities with varying degrees of fluoride in the water supply.[3] Table 13 gives the pertinent figures. Since we are testing not only the proportions of children involved but the sizes of the samples from which they are drawn, it becomes necessary to use the original numbers of children with or without caries from which the caries-free percentages were computed. This is done and the various steps of the χ^2 test are carried out in Table 14. Note that there are five columns and two rows in the test as it is finally set up. A study of the ten boxes in the table will clarify the reason for the formula for degrees of freedom. Let us concentrate on the observed figures for numbers of children, assuming that the total numbers in each locality sample and the total number without caries cannot be changed. If 16 of the 259 children studied in fluoride-free areas are caries-free, then 243 must show caries. Again in the next column, if 36 of the 119 children examined in Slough were caries-free, then 83 must show caries. The row for caries, therefore, is dependent upon the caries-free row, or vice versa. If we add the rows across horizontally, it becomes obvious that four numbers can be filled in independently, but the fifth cannot be if the row totals are to be 127 caries-free children and 456 with caries, respectively. The formula for degrees of freedom thus give us a figure of 4.

The expected numbers are found by applying to the total figure for each column the percentage figure for freedom from caries, and then for caries found for the entire study. Thus, for Essex and Surrey $259 \times 0.218 = 56$, in round numbers. In the caries row $259 \times 0.782 = 203$. To avoid the errors associated with samples smaller than those for which the test was designed, it is conventional to limit X^2 testing to situations where expected numbers are 5 or more.

The value of X^2, in this instance, is computed by adding the ten figures at the bottom of each box. The sum is 77.72. Since the largest figure on the line for four degrees of freedom in the X^2 table is 13.28, we realize the probability for chance occurrence of variations such as are seen in these five communities is a great deal less than 1 percent. We might get the same result by comparing the proportion of caries-free children in the two fluoride communities with the similar proportion for any one of the four nonfluoride communities mentioned, but we are much better off with a test which will give us the accumulated significance of all five communities at once. Note, however, that the test does not depend on an exact relation between the fluoride contents of the water supplies in the several communities. These figures do not appear in the calculation.

CORRELATION

When we were testing differences between means or differences between proportions we were essentially dealing with one variable

Table 13. Caries experience among children aged 12–14 in several British communities.

Area	Number of children examined	Percent of children caries-free
Essex and Surrey	259	6
Slough	119	30
Harwich	92	35
Burnham-on-Crouch	62	50
West Mersea	51	24
	583	

and measuring its occurrence in two sample situations. With χ^2 we were again dealing with one variable, but testing its occurrence in, say, two to six different situations, this being the type of problem for which χ^2 is best suited. In a sense, therefore, we are really dealing with two variables, although values for the second variable (fluoride content of water, in the example just cited for different British communities) need not be related one to another in any recognizable pattern.

Another type of problem quite commonly found is that where there are two variables, each susceptible of measurement according to a scale of its own. Each unit in the series we are testing consists of a pair of measurements, one for the first variable and one for the second variable. The number of pairs may be very large indeed, and in fact, the larger the number the more reliable

Table 14. Calculation of χ^2 from data of study described in Table 13.

Quantity	Essex and Surrey	Slough	Harwich	Burnham-on-Crouch	West Mersea	Total
		Caries-free				
No. observed	16	36	32	31	12	127
No. expected	56	26	20	14	11	127
Difference	-40	10	12	17	1	
Difference^2	1600	100	144	289	1	
$\dfrac{\text{Difference}^2}{\text{Expected}}$	28.57	3.85	7.20	20.64	0.09	
		With caries				
No. observed	243	83	60	31	39	456
No. expected	203	93	72	48	40	456
Difference	40	-10	-12	-17	-1	
Difference^2	1600	100	144	289	1	
$\dfrac{\text{Difference}^2}{\text{Expected}}$	7.88	1.08	2.00	6.02	0.03	
Total:						
Observed	259	119	92	62	51	583
Expected	259	119	92	62	51	583
Fraction caries-free	0.06	0.30	0.35	0.50	0.24	0.218

Degrees of freedom: DF $= (c - 1) \times (r - 1) = 4 \times 1 = 4$
$\chi^2 = 77.36$; $P \langle 0.01$
($P = 0.01$ for DF $= 4$ when χ^2 is 13.28 (Table 12); larger values of χ^2 mean *lower* probability of chance occurrence.)

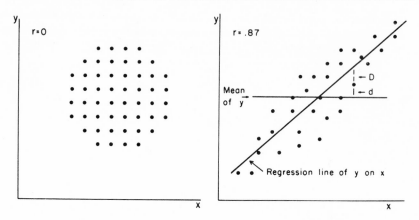

Figure 7–8. Hypothetical scatter diagrams showing correlation coefficients of 0 (*left*) and +0.87 (*right*).

the testing process. Such a situation is easiest to grasp in a so-called scatter diagram. Figs. 7 and 8 give such diagrams. If we are to attempt graphic analysis of the material in these two diagrams, we should try to draw some sort of line or curve which will typify the relation of one variable to the other. In Fig. 7 no line or curve of any sort can be drawn. There seems no way whatever to predict the value of *y* from a value of *x*. In Fig. 8, however, a relation becomes apparent, not perfect to be sure, yet recognizable. The diagonally ascending straight line is so drawn that the sum of the squares of the differences between the *y* values of the various points and the straight line will be as small as possible. The line itself is known as the *regression line* of *y* on *x*. The formula by which it is drawn is known as the *regression equation,* determined by the method of least squares. Another line not very different in slope and known as the regression line of *x* on *y* could be drawn in such a way as to minimize *x* variations. The measure of the distances of the various points from the line is summarized in *r,* the *correlation coefficient.* Fig. 7 has a correlation coefficient of 0; Fig. 8 has a correlation coefficient of +0.87. A correlation coefficient of +1.0 would mean that all points in Fig. 8 were located exactly on the ascending diagonal line. Values for *x* would thus increase as values for *y* increased (though the ratio need not be one to one), and for every possible value of *x* it would be possible to predict exactly the corresponding value for y. Inverse or negative correlation would imply a descending line, with values for x decreasing as values for y increased. If the correlation coefficient were -1.0, then all points would be located exactly on this descending straight line.

It is obvious that any given point can be tested for its scatter (or distance) from one of the two straight lines in Fig. 8. The first is the line representing the mean value for all observations of y and the second is the regression line of y on x. In Fig. 8, D and d are the distances between a given point and, respectively, the regression line and the mean for y. The symbol Σ means "sum of." The theoretical formula from which the correlation coefficient is computed is:

$$r = \sqrt{1 - \frac{\Sigma D^2}{\Sigma d^2}}$$

Where all points fall exactly on the regression line (and in this event, the two regression lines are the same), ΣD^2 becomes zero and r becomes 1.0. Where ΣD^2 and Σd^2 are equal, as they would be for any line we might draw upon Fig. 7, $\Sigma D^2 / \Sigma d^2$ becomes 1.0 and r becomes zero. For practical computation of r, either of the following formulas can be used:

$$r = \frac{\Sigma(x - \bar{x})(y - \bar{y})}{n s_x s_y} \qquad (a)$$

or

$$r = \frac{\dfrac{\Sigma xy}{n} - \bar{x}\bar{y}}{s_x s_y} \qquad (b)$$

Formula (a) makes use of the sum of all products of the deviations of one point from the mean of x and the deviations of the same point from the mean of y. This sum is divided by n, the number of pairs in the problem, times the product of the two standard deviations. Formula (b) is a simpler one to use in practice, since the original scores are multiplied together and not their differences from any mean. The two formulas are, of course, mathematically the same, and each is for ungrouped data. Where so many pairs of observations are to be tested that a frequency distribution must be constructed, the sum of the frequencies of the various products

Table 15. Approximate latitude of states on U.S. Atlantic coast compared with their mean ranks in three large studies of dental status.

State	Rank	Latitude
Florida	17	28
Georgia	19	33
South Carolina	18	34
North Carolina	15	36
Virginia	17	38
Maryland	34	39
Delaware	42	39
New Jersey	43	40
New York	44	42
Connecticut	41	41
Rhode Island	45	42
Massachusetts	44	42
New Hampshire	45	43
Maine	44	44

(fxy) is used in formula (b) instead of the sum of the products themselves (xy).

For those wishing to draw an exact line upon a graph, the *regression equation* for x on y is:

$$(x - \bar{x}) = r \left(\frac{s_x}{s_y}\right)(y - \bar{y})$$

An attempt to solve this equation for a specific value of y will soon demonstrate that it is merely an elaboration of the simple formula for a straight line, $x = a + by$, where a and b are constants. In the equation for the regression of y on x, the values of x and y are interchanged.

CALCULATION OF CORRELATION COEFFICIENT

A clear, though not ideal, example for simple correlation work is found in an ungrouped series of observations relating the rank in dental disease of the various states along the Atlantic seaboard of the United States to the approximate latitude of each state. Table 15 gives the figures. Details of the study appear in Chapter 8. The purpose of the test upon this particular group of states is to check the common impression that Northerners have more dental caries than Southerners. In this instance it was desired to exclude various factors seen in states away from the seacoast, notably the natural high fluoride in the water supply. The test therefore included only those states actually abutting on the Atlantic coast. With fourteen pairs of obvservations, we have data enough to develop a real regression line, and would find the X^2 test a clumsy one to use under the circumstances. Formula (b) is used, making use of the actual values for x and y rather than their differences from the mean of x and the mean of y.

The actual calculation of the correlation coefficient by the formula that has been given is so easily accomplished by computer software—and is so difficult by hand—that it is not given here. The coefficient proves to be 0.844, a high one. The regression coefficient for x on y becomes 2.4.

Fig. 9 is a graphic representation of the data, with the regression line drawn in. The regression line has been located by calculating two points and drawing a straight line between them. To obtain the first point, y was assumed to be 15, and the regression equation was solved for x by substituting 15 for y in the formula. For the second point, y was assumed to be 45, and again this value was substituted for y in the equation. Quite obviously there are limits to the usefulness of such a line. Several points fall some distance from it. In this instance, too, as in all others where a regression line is computed, it must not be unduly extended beyond the range of observed material.

As with differences between means and proportions, we cannot assume that a given correlation coefficient is the only one which would arise by chance if an indefinite number of samples were taken from the two universes of variables before us. The coefficients after repeated tests, however, should cluster more and more closely about a value away from zero if we are dealing with two related variables and about zero if we are dealing with unrelated variables. There is more than one way to deal with this situation, but the simplest for large samples involves a *standard error for a correlation coefficient* computed by the formula:

$$\text{S.E.}_{\cdot r} = \frac{1}{\sqrt{n - 1}}$$

where *n* is the number of paired observations on which the correlation coefficient is based. The correlation coefficient is then to be compared with its own standard error to see whether it differs significantly from zero. To do this it should be more than twice, and preferably more than three times, its own standard error. A t value is therefore computed as we have seen in former tests.

The very formula for standard error of the correlation coefficient makes it plain why small numbers of pairs cannot be tested reliably. If ten pairs are being tested, the standard error will be 1 divided by the square root of 9, which gives 0.333. Three times this

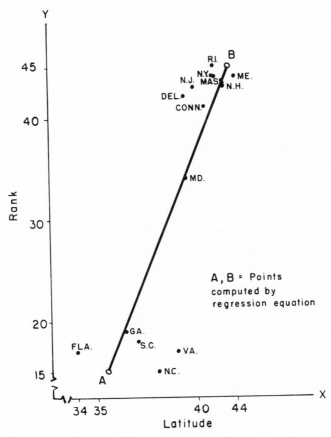

Figure 9. Approximate latitude of states on the Atlantic coast compared with their mean rank in three large studies of dental status.

figure is, of course, 1.0 or perfect correlation—an almost unheard-of finding. As the number of pairs in the test increases, the standard error diminishes, and first the very high correlation coefficients and later the medium-sized ones attain statistical significance. The t value for a correlation coefficient of 0.844 found from 14 pairs of observations is 3.047, which implies a probability between 1 in 100 and 1 in 1,000 of chance occurrence.

NONPARAMETRIC STATISTICS

Most of the statistical problems cited up to this point have involved normally distributed populations with somewhat similar variances and with good, clearly defined parameters, that is, characteristics which can be measured, preferably on an interval scale. However, a situation was mentioned in Chapter 5 where a skewed distribution was described, involving the income of dentists. Here a median value rather than a mean was seen to be the best measure of central tendency. The median bears no necessary relation to the magnitude of the observations on either side of it, but merely a relation to their number. The median often provides a meaningful description of a skewed frequency distribution. It is also useful in those situations where exact numbers cannot be used to describe intervals between observations and the best one can do is to compare the observations by their relative magnitude. When this procedure is carried out, an ordinal, or ranking, scale results. As an example, one might say that a sergeant ranks higher than a corporal, who in turn ranks higher than an Army private. There are even simpler situations where degrees of magnitude cannot be assigned and the scale is called nominal. Human eye color is a case in point. To deal with such situations, a series of relatively simple tests has been evolved, called nonparametric statistics.

The χ^2 test found in Tables 13 and 14 is an example of nonparametric statistics. The five communities tested there for differences in caries prevalence are not related by equal intervals of fluoride concentration in the water, and need not have been related to any measurable characteristic at all.

Another nonparametric test is found in Table 17, where climatological data from certain Australian cities have been arranged in rank order and the Spearman Rank Correlation Test applied. The formula for this test is as follows:

$$r_s = 1 - \frac{6\Sigma\Delta^2}{n(n^2 - 1)}$$

where Δ is the difference between ranks in a pair of observations and n the number of pairs in the series (Σ means "sum of"). The correlation coefficients noted at the foot of Table 17 are seen to resemble the coefficients for correlation described earlier in this chapter, in that they range from $+1.0$ to -1.0. The Spearman coefficients, however, are more simply calculated. They give less perspective on the variability of the data, and are therefore less efficient.

It is of interest to apply the Spearman Test to the data from the Atlantic states:

Parametric formula: $r = .844$ $SEr = .277$ $t = 3.05$
Spearman formula: $r = .903$ $SEr = .277$ $t = 3.26$

In terms of probability of chance occurrence, the two correlation coefficients are close together and both are significant.

In general, it may be stated that nonparametric tests are good for small samples; they are not dependent upon a normal distribution or an interval scale; they are quick and easy. The disadvantages of these tests lie in the fact that no mean or error can be computed, and they often neglect some of the information actually available in the original data. Nonparametric tests are being increasingly used, however. Siegel's text is a good one to consult where more detail is desired upon this subject.[4] His Chapter 3, on levels of measurement and choice of a statistical test, is particularly appropriate.

COMPUTER ANALYSIS

Within the past two decades computer services have become so easily available in urban centers that large-scale investigations hitherto considered impractical, and even small investigations not formerly considered worth transferring are now easily handled by a computer, with little if any increase in cost and a great gain in speed and accuracy. Chapter 14 takes up in some detail the types of dental recording most suitable for computer work. The main development in record technology has been through optical scanning. Original dental records can now be processed by a scanning machine in such a way that the data they contain are automatically transferred, or the data typed directly into the computer.

Much of the desirability of computer analysis depends upon the programs available at the specific computer centers. Programs for statistical tests and for the handling of certain unusual types of data are difficult and expensive to design. Once they have been prepared, however, and are available as software, they are very quickly used without additional cost. Computer programming, of course, is a special field in itself, making use of "languages" not easily learned by the beginner.

Some of the problems which come to mind as best suited for computer analysis involve complicated series of correlations, and covariance adjustment of means in studies where the groups are not equivalent in respect to certain underlying variables. Much simpler situations also lend themselves to computer analysis.

Among examples are the construction of study samples for research and the analysis of diet histories for clinical nutrition service. In the former category came the determination of average age and standard deviation of age in a group of state school dormitories where the residents in one entire dormitory were to receive one dietary supplement, the residents of another dormitory another supplement. In the diet analysis category, Chapter 12 describes a series of nutritional data banks where any public clinic or private dentist with as much as a personal computer and a modem can get detailed analysis of a one-day diet history for as little as three or four minutes of connected computer time.

INTERPRETATION

It is quite in order to close these chapters on biostatistics with some remarks on the interpretation of the tests which have been developed. Most important, perhaps, is to point out that neither differences nor correlations between sets of observations can prove causation unaided. It is very easy to translate strong positive or negative test results into an opinion that cause and effect can be found within the stated premises of the test. This temptation must be firmly avoided until it is known that all evidence is in and an unmistakable chain of reasoning exists. The results mean, of course, that something other than chance is operating. Perhaps the cause lies in factors, known or unknown, outside the scope of the test. The reader will recall Dean's hesitance at the time of his early epidemiological work on the caries-fluoride hypothesis. In spite of significant statistical results, his doubts as to the existence of unknown variables could be dispelled only by field trials in areas where the fluoride content of the water supply was the only major environmental factor to be altered.

One of the real dangers of the computer age is the temptation to measure irrelevant parameters simply because they are easy to measure. Thus a researcher, trying to assess the importance of predental college experience, once divided colleges into categories according to size of the student body. He totally neglected the unmeasurable criteria which differentiate good teaching from poor teaching.

If interpretation is difficult where test results have proved significant, it is all the more difficult where they are "not significant," that is, where the observed findings could have occurred so frequently by chance that we must discard them for the time being as a basis for further reasoning. At this point we must decide whether or not the findings are "suggestive." It is often true that our first glimpse of a real difference or a real correlation comes through the study of samples so small, so atypical, or so poorly examined that statistical significance cannot be attained. Under these circumstances it is a question for common sense whether the work should be done over under better conditions. If the work *is* worth doing over but there is no opportunity to do it, it may easily be worthwhile to publish the results with appropriate reservations, in the hope that someone else will carry the work on.

As for the possibility of technical errors along the way, one should not hesitate to ask for advice from the many available sources of statistical help—but one should think things through as far as possible first, and check the arithmetic. Remember the advice of a well-known yachtsman who said of navigation (another science based upon figures), "The *art* of navigation lies in the prompt recognition and correction of mistakes made in ascertaining a position at sea."

Significant biostatistical test findings, even when they accomplish nothing more, often serve as the basis upon which scientific theories can be constructed. A theory is to be judged not so much upon its ultimate truth as upon the aid it gives us in arranging our thoughts. This arrangement of thoughts, in turn, may lead to further scientific advances, or to practical measures of use in public health practice. Conant, in his book *On Understanding Science,* remarks wisely that "science emerges from the other progressive activities of man to the extent that new concepts arise from experiment and observation, and the new concepts in turn lead to further experiments and observations . . . The texture of modern science is the result of the interweaving of the fruitful concepts."[5]

Science can indeed be aided by results which are expressed in terms of probability, where statements in terms of certainty are impossible. The important thing in the field of biostatistics is to view the result of every test in the light of degree of its *probability.* This includes an estimate of the probable accuracy of the original data, the probable logic of the comparison which is to be made, and other commonsense considerations perhaps of greater importance than the probability of chance occurrence which is inherent in the figures themselves. The magic of numbers must not blind the investigator to these basic considerations.

CHAPTER 7

Epidemiology: General Principles

WHEN ATTEMPTS are made to understand the causes of diseases, there are two general approaches which may be taken. The first of these deals with the identification and tracing of the agent of the disease after it has entered or affected the individual host, and to this approach the name of *etiology* is usually given. This word is derived from the Greek *aitia*, cause, and *logos*, description or science. Here is a broad term for the "science of causes," which through common usage has come to be restricted for the most part to the study of the individual patient. The second approach looks further afield. The patient is seen set in his environment and as part of a group of similar patients, human or otherwise, all reacting to the same disease. This broader field of study involves consideration of many predisposing factors to disease as well as the apparent exciting cause and is thus concerned with the frequency of the disease in the group. To this approach to the study of disease the name *epidemiology* is commonly given. The term is derived from the Greek word *epi*, on or upon, then *demos*, the people, combined again with *logos* to denote description or science.

A good present-day definition of epidemiology is that of Clark, who calls it a science concerned with the study of factors that influence the occurrence and distribution of health, disease, defect, disability, or death in groups of individuals.[1] More practical is Gordon's concept that epidemiology is chiefly concerned with "the diagnostic procedure in mass disease."[2] Epidemiology, Gordon says, "is the counterpart of diagnosis with the same relationship to public health practice that clinical diagnosis has to treatment." As a science, epidemiology is closely related to ecology, that aspect of biology dealing with the mutual relations between organisms and their environment. Epidemiology, in fact, has been called medical ecology.

Practical epidemiology, of course, grew out of an effort to control epidemics of disease. An *epidemic* can be defined as the occurrence of a group of illnesses of similar nature clearly in excess of normal expectancy, and derived from a common or propagated source.[3] In contrast, *endemic* disease (*en,* in; *demos,* a people) has been taken to mean the usual low level of disease, chronic or acute, found within a population. Epidemics were originally considered to involve infectious disease only. In recent years the term has come to mean far more. The epidemiological approach is of great value in the study of noninfectious diseases, chronic diseases, mental and physical disabilities such as alcoholism, and even automobile accidents. Since the study of diseases in groups is peculiarly the responsibility of the public health worker, some description of the methods used in epidemiology, and of the terminology associated with it, will be of value at this point.

To understand the terms in which the epidemiologist must think, it will help to take a closer look at the science of *ecology* (another Greek word, from *oikos,* house, and *logos*). In its broadest, or holistic, sense, ecology views life in all its manifestations as a single system in process of interaction with the inorganic environment. Plant ecology, animal ecology, and human ecology are major sub-divisions of this system, but each must be viewed against the background of the whole. More practically, ecology aids the study of specific disturbances in ecological balance. A specific mass disease in man, or even a social phenomenon such as juvenile delinquency, may be studied in relation to all the animate things which either help to cause it or are affected by it or by its removal from the scene. Thus control of malaria in certain parts of India not only stimulates population growth (which is an undesirable phenomenon because it puts new strain upon an already inadequate food supply) but at the same time permits cultivation of land which previously could not be cultivated, thus in part perhaps restoring the balance. The ecological problem here is to determine the exact balance which will result, not only for human beings but for the other animal and plant inhabitants of the region.

The area of thought involved by ecology is extremely broad. Nevertheless, Gordon has developed with Adams five laws which they believe have general applicability.[4] These laws are:

1. All living things tend to produce more young than are needed to maintain the species. The resulting overpopulation, whether relative or absolute, brings into play a series of checks and counterchecks which dominates all biology.

2. A suitable food supply in adequate amount is the main factor in maintenance of a species. Species compete with each other and frequently rely upon each other for food supply. A balance thus occurs between species.

3. The physical environment of a species, including water, air, temperature, and similar natural forces, must be suited to its well-being.

4. Maintenance and survival depend on interspecies relations which permit survival from attack of natural enemies. This involves such cooperation between the species as is represented by parasitism.

5. Man, through his intelligence and by conscious effort, is able to control his environment to a remarkable extent. Culture, social structure of communities, species dominance, development of technologies, and social adaptation are important related concepts.

A director-general of the World Health Organization, speaking from an ecological point of view, has closely identified public health interests with the interests of conservationists:

The ecologist conceives the term "conservation" as the wise management and utilization of natural resources for the greatest good of the largest number. One may debate the position of man in such a universe, but only as to what level of hierarchy he may allocate himself. That he exists and affects his own kind and all else in the world is not debatable . . . man's history justifies the claim that he, like most other animal and plant life, is "an endangered species" . . . Man, in his struggle for survival, poses as many true ecological challenges as the more familiar lion, rhinoceros or whooping crane. The environment truly may be his friend or enemy.[5]

MULTIFACTORIAL DISEASE

The broad ecological view of man set in an environment which not only affects his resistance but also contains the agents of disease gives the epidemiologist a very practical approach to problems of mass disease. He soon finds that the conquest of most diseases depends upon many more factors than a mere knowledge of the biological mechanism which operates after the agent of the disease has entered the host. To the presence of the "main" cause of the disease must usually be added a list of contributing causes before the disease can affect large segments of a population. The result is a "chain" or "web" of causation which the public health worker may be able to break at various places. This multifactorial nature of disease is seen strikingly among the chronic diseases, where time permits the entry of a large number of factors, and is particularly apparent in those diseases such as diabetes where there is no obvious agent to trace. The epidemiologist studies the well people in addition to the sick in the community. He thus has more types of data at his disposal than has a physician treating an individual patient, and for this reason has more opportunity to consider disease as a multifactorial problem. The physician, to be sure, has the same need, but can do less about environmental factors than his public health colleague. The epidemiologist, because of this multiplicity of factors, finds himself constantly dependent upon biostatistics in the design of his studies and in the assembly and analysis of his data.

The broad look the epidemiologist must take at disease removes him somewhat from the actual treatment of individual cases. He can do much more about the prevention and control of future disease than about the cure of current disease. In this respect

Schneider has given us a good military analogy.[6] Epidemiology deals with the strategic aspect of the fight against disease, and medicine with the tactical. Epidemiology defines *when* and *where* action may be most effective against a disease rather than dealing with the *how* of treating it.

Both in the descriptive and in the planning phases of his work, the infectious-disease epidemiologist finds himself thinking of disease and health as "no more than selected instances among the many results of the total interaction between man and his environment."[2] To these two factors in the problem must usually be added a third: the agent of disease, if an agent exists. Thus the first step in epidemiologic (or ecologic) analysis involves a separation of the factors involved in a disease into three main groups: those pertaining to the *host* (namely, man), those pertaining to the *agent,* and those pertaining to the *environment.* The epidemiologist who deals more with noninfectious conditions is likely to refer to factors concerning *person, place,* and *time.* It will be useful for us to examine some of the common factors seen under each of these major headings, using for convenience the infectious-disease terminology.

HOST FACTORS

It is obvious that for a disease to obtain significant frequency in a population there must be a good reservoir of susceptible hosts. One would not expect as many cases of measles in a given community the following year if there had been a measles epidemic among the children the year before. So reliable and predictable is this phenomenon that it can be used in the absence of immunization programs to predict a cycle for such epidemics. This is the interval in which a new group of children grows up, sufficient in number to constitute a good chain for the communication of this highly infectious disease. Here, of course, we have an example of *active immunity* to disease acquired through infection.

Of equal interest is *natural resistance.* Thus tuberculosis is more common in the black race than in the white race for reasons perhaps genetic, perhaps associated with growth, development, physiology, specific immunity, or antibodies. The comparative natural resistance of the white race to tuberculosis is one of the constants of aid to a planner of an antituberculosis campaign. Natural resistance to disease will vary with the individual as well as with the race, and beyond a certain point such variation cannot be eliminated from the studies made by the epidemiologist.

Among variables affecting natural resistance there are a number which the epidemiologist can expect to find present in most of his studies. These are *age, sex, race,* and *family.* An example has already been given of racial variation in resistance to disease. *Race* is a difficult characteristic to assess, in part because so many of the divisions commonly thought of as racial in our society today are not that at all, but ethnic. The Jews, for instance, are an ethnic group, not a race. Another reason for difficulty in this area is that racial heredity, a legitimate host factor, is so closely linked in its effects to environmental factors such as social custom and cultural development that a clear distinction is very difficult. Custom has its effect upon diet, and diet in turn is usually dependent upon the availability of certain foods in the environment. Thus it is extremely hard to say whether the preference of Italians for leafy vegetables, oils, and wine is an ethnic (hence host) factor or an environmental factor in the causation or prevention of disease.

Age, on the contrary, is a very easy host factor with which to deal. Population statistics are easy to divide by age groups and it is almost automatic for the student of a disease to form a picture quite early of the age distribution of that disease. Age, of course, may operate through physiological changes, as for instance in dental caries, or through the mental growth and habits of the individual, the latter being the controlling factor in the high frequency of automobile accidents among teen-age boys. *Sex* is an equally easy characteristic to tabulate. Many diseases vary in their sex occurrence, but not nearly as many as vary in their occurrence with age. Some diseases show a sex variation merely because sex and occupation are linked. Thus tularemia is more common among Midwestern farmers than among their wives because of more frequent contact with ticks, rabbits, and other vectors of this disease.

Familial heredity is a very difficult characteristic to measure and will seldom prove an important factor in the epidemiological study of large groups. The dentist, however, has usually seen familial variations in occlusion, dental caries, and periodontal disease among his own patients. Familial inheritance of tooth form and face form is often seen and is easily recognized. Tooth structure, too, varies in different families, but whether this is truly the result of heredity or is the result of dietary and other habits within the family is a matter which can seldom be determined with accuracy. In medicine, familial tendencies in poliomyelitis and in hemophilia are among the many which are commonly known.

Inextricably associated with all of the host factors so far enumerated, one should look for *customs* and *habits*. Religious custom removes beef as a food in India. Social custom in Peru dictates that "sick" people should boil the water they drink and "well" people should use unboiled water.[7] Both these customs hinder the work of the public health official in one way or another. In this country, commercial sponsorship of certain products has developed habits of nationwide importance. The use of dentifrices and the use of soap are excellent examples of the results of such sponsorship. Both have induced good health habits. Cigarette advertising, on the other hand, is to be regretted by health workers.

The variable reaction of the host to the presence of a disease agent needs careful consideration. The spirochetes of Vincent's infection are present in practically all normal mouths yet do not cause disease. Not until lowered resistance or possibly an added dosage of spirochetes from outside occurs are the organisms in a position to multiply and cause trouble. The *resistance of the host* therefore is a cardinal factor to be looked for, not so much in terms of specific immunity as in terms of *general health* at a given time.

Closely akin to the subject of lowered resistance is that of *concomitant disease*. A diabetic is more susceptible to tuberculosis than a previously healthy individual, and tuberculosis conversely predisposes to diabetes. This opens up the interesting field of *synergism* and *antagonism*. Diseases occurring together may behave in three possible ways. First, there may be no reaction at all, each disease following its own course quite independently of the other. Second, the result may be greater than the sum of the independent effects of the two diseases; this is called synergism. Third, one disease may limit the effect of the other, a process which is called antagonism. Taylor and Gordon list many of these phenomena, both as they occur between pairs of infectious diseases and as they occur between infectious diseases and congenital anomalies or modifications of endocrine or metabolic functions.[8] The interaction of diabetes and tuberculosis, of course, is synergism. Diabetes, however, has been reported to be antagonistic to rheumatic fever, rheumatoid arthritis, and peptic ulcer. With congenital anomalies there are two excellent dental examples of synergism: cleft palate predisposes to sinusitis, and the mulberry molars of congenital syphilis (Hutchinson's teeth) are predisposed to dental caries. The epidemiologist may occasionally be able to turn synergism or antagonism to practical use. The antagonism between vaccinia (cow pox) and smallpox is the basis for smallpox vaccination. More important, he must constantly be on watch for the effects of *other* diseases on the one he is studying.

AGENT FACTORS

Many diseases have apparent agents, which may be either *biological, chemical,* or *physical.* Some well-understood diseases, however, have no apparent agent at all. Such a disease is diabetes. Obesity, to be sure, is so frequently associated with diabetes, and carbohydrates are so directly the cause of diabetic coma, that fats and carbohydrates might appear to be agents in this instance. Both, however, are essential nutrients and are of harm only when the human pancreas is unable to deal with them.

The best-known agents are *microbiological.* During the "Golden Age of Bacteriology" in the past century and early part of this century, an extraordinarily successful search was on for microbiological agents of disease, with consequent scant emphasis upon host and environmental factors. The search continues today, though with less of a single-track approach and with proportionally less attention to bacteria, more to viruses. Less space will be devoted here to these agents of disease than their importance would appear to warrant. The reason is that they can usually be isolated and first studied after they enter an experimental animal or an individual patient. In dental disease, streptococci have only recently been demonstrated to be causative agents—*streptococcus mutans* in particular. The concept of caries as an infectious disease is now leading to the concept that it is also contagious. This is one of the hypotheses that needs testing in connection with the recent decline in childhood caries in developed countries, discussed in Chapter 8. The trouble here is that human caries takes so long to develop that the sources of bacteria are virtually impossible to pinpoint.

Chemical agents are often hard to identify after they have done their work, hence are more often left to the epidemiologist to study. Fluoride, though it may be a nutrient under certain circumstances and a preventive of disease under other circumstances, can be the agent of disease if it is present in gross excess. The question of dosage here is all-important, as it is with chemical agents generally, so many of which are essential to the human body in small quantities. Heavy metals such as lead and mercury cause pathologic processes without the offsetting advantage of acting as recognized nutrients in small dosage. Poisonings of various sorts come under the heading of disease with a chemical agent. Many, of course, involve large enough dosages so that identification after ingestion is fairly easy.

Physical agents may vary all the way from radioactive fallout to the steering wheel of an automobile. Fallout is a "chronic" agent where accumulation is possible, and dosage must be figured not only in terms of the immediate amount but in terms of cumulative effect. Damaging effects may occur both to the individual exposed and also, through *mutagenesis,* to his or her offspring. The steering wheel of an automobile is an "acute" agent. Except at the moment of collision, it is a constructive, not a damaging, factor.

ENVIRONMENTAL FACTORS

The oldest field for mass study in the analysis of human diseases, and perhaps the most fruitful in terms of predisposing causes, is the environment. Before bacteria were known to exist, many diseases were explained solely in terms of terrestrial and meteorological influences. Thus the name "malaria" is merely a contraction of the Italian words for "bad air." The chief aspects of the environment which demand the attention of the epidemiologist are the physical environment, the biological environment, and the social environment. The sources, reservoirs, and carriers of disease are also important aspects of the environment. They may be either physical or biological.

The aspects of the *physical environment* which may appear to influence the occurrence of disease are almost innumerable.

Sometimes the factor may be a very specific one such as sunshine, with an easily recognizable connection to disease. Sunshine also acts to synthesize vitamin D and prevent rickets. Sometimes, however, the factor will be a vague one such as climate, where an interplay of many subfactors may operate in the causation of disease, giving the epidemiologist a very tangled skein to unravel. The many so-called tropical diseases may all be said to have a strong climatic factor, but each has a detailed epidemiology of its own. Dental caries occurs much more frequently in cold, moist climates, as we shall see later. Several subfactors undoubtedly contribute to this phenomenon.

The major climatological factors are obvious aspects of the physical environment to study: sunshine, temperature, rainfall, humidity and altitude. So also are the inanimate carriers of disease: air, water, soiled articles, and sewage. A water supply, by the way, may serve either as a vehicle for disease (as when it carries the typhoid bacillus with it), or as a protective agent (as when it carries an optimal quantity of fluoride for the prevention of dental caries). Untreated sewage is a major vehicle for disease. Air pollution is one of the big health problems of modern city life.

The *biologic environment* is a very important category for the epidemiologist. Food and nutrition fall within it, linking it to all forms of deficiency disease. Nutrition is also involved in many diseases on a basis other than that of deficiency manifestation. Thus lack of meat and dairy products affected the occurrence of tuberculosis in Denmark during World War I.[9] An increase in tuberculosis mortality followed the intensive export of meat and dairy products in an attempt to aid other countries at war, and later, when the submarine blockade made such export impossible, tuberculosis mortality returned quickly to prewar levels.

Another major problem in the biological environment is that of *animals hosts* and *vectors* of disease. Hogs may harbor *Trichinella spiralis,* transmitting trichinosis to humans who eat the meat insufficiently cooked. Various animals may be hosts for *Clostridium tetani,* their feces carrying tetanus to humans where wounds provide a portal of entry. Vectors are, by definition, arthropods.[3] Many insects are important vectors of disease: mosquitoes, fleas, lice, ticks, and flies. The classic example here is the control of yellow fever through the elimination of a certain type of mosquito (*Aëdes aegypti*) by Gorgas in the swamps of Central America. Until this was done, the Panama Canal could not be built.

The *social environment,* sometimes called socioeconomic environment, may actually influence disease through changing the physical environment of the host. It is more common, however, for social factors to exert an indirect influence through the educational status of the host population. Poor people with limited educational opportunities are less likely to understand the reasons for personal hygiene and for the avoidance of sources of infection than are people with better opportunities. This situation appears to explain the higher incidence of periodontal disease reported by Russell among low-income populations.[10] It is seldom, however, that an economic barrier alone is the deciding factor. The poorest segment of the population should receive welfare payments or other governmental aids sufficient to purchase minimum essential nutrients, and public medical care should be provided free of charge, but such is not often the case. Payments, commodity distributions, and food stamp programs fall far short of full coverage of the needy population, part of the trouble being these people's lack of ability to avail themselves of services which are actually offered.[11] Factors in the social and economic environment underlying such a situation can sometimes be measured with considerable clarity, sometimes not. An index for this purpose is described in Chapter 10.

INTERPLAY OF FACTORS

Various concepts will help in an understanding of the interplay of factors as they cause disease. Simplest of all is to consider the factors to be a *chain,* with disease occurring when the chain is complete and intact. Each link is as important as another in the chain, and the chain is no stronger than its weakest link. The chain can be broken by attack upon any link, whichever is most convenient. A variant of this concept is that of a *web,* where interconnections between factors are more numerous than in a chain. Webs can be broken, too.

Another helpful concept is that of the *seesaw,* with the host and the disease agent at opposite ends of the seesaw and the environment the fulcrum, as shown in Fig. 10. The greater the resistance

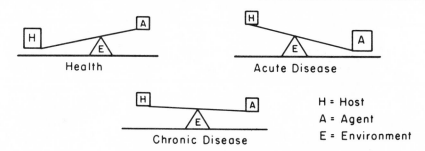

Figure 10. Balance of factors in disease.

of the host, the more he "weighs." If he outweighs the agent factor, he wins his health. A virulent disease agent, however, outweighs a susceptible host and disease is the result. The fulcrum, environment, can be shifted either toward the host or toward the agent, giving the one away from which it has been shifted additional leverage. An equilibrium, with the host and the disease agent weighing the same amount, represents symbiosis. If the weight or the placement of the fulcrum slightly favors the agent, the result is chronic disease, where both the host and the disease agent remain alive. It is only an unsuccessful agent of disease that kills its host and therefore, in the long run, itself as well.

MEASUREMENT OF MASS DISEASE

For the epidemiologist or the ecologist, the unit of observation is a group of living things within a natural environment. Three ecological groupings are commonly distinguished, according to increasing complexity: a *population,* a *community,* and an *ecosystem.*[4] A population is essentially a group of one kind of living thing. A community, or, as the ecologist would call it, a biotic community, is a more complex affair, embracing all populations in a rather small geographic area, both plant and animal, including man. This definition will not be used here, however, since it is too easily confused with the commoner use of the word community to imply a group of human beings living together in a local area with manmade limits. The ecosystem is the largest unit of all. Geographically it may include as large an area as can be found within which all animate and inanimate things can influence each other and blend into an organizational pattern. Dynamic behavior is an outstanding characteristic of an ecosystem, with an equilibrium existing between the various animate species, all of which react in a manner determined by the physical environment.

For practical purposes it is the population with which the epidemiologist has to deal most often. Populations have such traits as density, dispersion, intrinsic rates of natural increase, age distribution, morbidity, and mortality.[4] All these are characteristic of groups rather than of individuals. A population, therefore, must be considered a unit in itself, with many powers and potentialities not present in any of its components.

EPIDEMICS

One of the first tasks of an epidemiologist in dealing with a reported health hazard is to determine whether he is dealing with disease of significantly greater prevalence than normal (*epidemic* disease) or with a continuing problem involving normal disease prevalence (*endemic* disease). Unlike the physician, who can usually say "yes" or "no" to the presence of a given disease in an individual patient, the epidemiologist will almost never find his population without some prevalence of the commoner diseases. The large majority of the population may be healthy, but a fraction will show disease, either slight, moderate, or severe. Within this fraction will also be seen varying degrees of complication and death, and in the wake of certain diseases, varying degrees of disability. To this series of variations, the term *biologic gradient of disease* has been applied.[2] A large proportion of the population diseased and a steep rise of complication and death in this group as severity increases are the usual marks of an epidemic. Small prevalence and low gradient are characteristic of endemic disease. Fig. 11 shows two such gradients for diphtheria in Copenhagen, Denmark. Where vaccination produces the low gradient seen in group A of the clinical cases, the steeper gradient for group B (the unvaccinated) can justly be called an epidemic.

Morbidity and mortality rates are necessary to measure the biological gradient of disease. Morbidity is cases of disease divided by population, then multiplied by a convenient power of ten (usually 1,000 or 100,000). Mortality is deaths divided by population, and again multiplied by a convenient power of 10.

Improvement in diagnostic method may easily produce a steady upswing in the reported incidence of disease which has no basis in fact. The increasing use of x-rays in the dental field is a good example here, and marked changes in the total findings of surveys are seen when x-ray findings are added to explorer findings, as described in Chapter 14. An apparent increase in incidence of dental disease may in fact be due to improved diagnostic technique. Tuberculosis workers have found the same difficulty in analyzing statistics on the morbidity of that disease. Public awareness, too, has much to do with the reporting of disease. An epidemic of any sort sensitizes people to a disease, and more subacute cases are reported at the end than at the beginning.

Seasonal variations in disease are fairly common, both among infectious diseases and among accidents. We are all familiar with the fact that poliomyelitis epidemics occurred, if at all, in the late summer. Similarly measles appears to occur more frequently in the early spring. Accidents will vary with the conditions responsible for them. Automobile accidents in the New England area seem

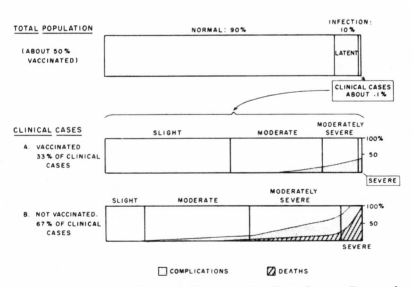

Figure 11. Biologic gradient of diphtheria in Copenhagen, Denmark, 1944. [Courtesy, Public Health Association of New York City.]

to be most prevalent in November and December, when ice and snow introduce hazards to which drivers have become unaccustomed.

Cyclic variations in disease may involve periods of anywhere from 2 to 15 years. An example has already been cited in the field of measles morbidity. The reasons for cycles of this sort are usually to be looked for in host-factor changes, where either the acquired immunity from the disease exhausts itself or a new susceptible population grows up in order to make possible another epidemic.

Slow changes in disease frequency which cannot be recognized as complete cycles and often cover centuries are termed *secular variations.* Usually they can be recognized only by a study of mortality rates, but every now and then a measure of morbidity can be found. In the field of dental disease we are fortunate, for ancient skulls often preserve evidence of tooth or bone damage. Dental caries thus is seen to have increased steadily over the centuries since earliest times in at least one country, as is discussed in the next chapter. Tuberculosis, on the other hand, as studied over the centuries through mortality, has been steadily on the downgrade, at least in the United States. Typical of the country as a whole are the death rates in Massachusetts.[12] In 1860, 444 persons per 100,000 died of this disease. In 1900, the figure was 253 per 100,000 and in 1940 only 36 per 100,000. Today the death rate is under 10 per 100,000. Tuberculosis morbidity of course continues, and at a much more slowly decreasing rate. The development of special antibacterial drugs like streptomycin and isoniazid has of course influenced both mortality and morbidity. Much of the change occurred, however, before the drugs were developed or even before sanatorium isolation became common.

In both caries and tuberculosis, the reasons for the swings are hard to identify. Gradual changes in dietary habit concomitant with our increase in civilization may possibly account for the increase in caries, and the gradual improvement of housing and sanitation may possibly account for the drop in tuberculosis, but many other factors must also be sought. Long-term changes in the virulence of the organisms are occasionally involved. The best example here is found in the long-term decline in mortality from scarlet fever in the United States, apparently from a change in the streptococci involved.

STRATEGY OF EPIDEMIOLOGY

In dealing with a multifactorial problem, especially in humans, where unwanted variables cannot be pushed aside as easily as with experimental animals, the epidemiological method becomes necessary. A strategy has arisen for epidemiological research which is well summarized by MacMahon and Pugh.[13] The methods they list are:

1. Descriptive epidemiology: description of the distribution of disease, with comparison of its frequency in different populations and in different segments of the same population.

2. Formulation of hypotheses: tentative theories designed to explain the observed distribution of the disease in terms of casual associations of the most direct nature possible.

3. Analytic epidemiology: observational studies designed specifically to examine the hypotheses developed as a result of the descriptive study.

4. Experimental epidemiology: experimental studies on human populations to test in a stringent manner those hypotheses that stand the test of observational and analytic studies.

Too often we are accustomed to focus attention only on the descriptive phase of epidemiology, to the neglect of the other three phases. Description, hypothesis formation, analysis, and testing are often so interwoven, however, that it is hard to tell where one begins and the other ends.

Water fluoridation provides excellent examples of these four processes, well known not only among dentists but among epidemiologists. The work of McKay, Dean, and others in mapping the occurrence of mottled enamel and later correlating these findings with fluoride content of water and finally with the occurrence of dental caries represented the descriptive stage. The formulation of the hypothesis that adjustment of the water supply to 1 part per million of fluoride would provide safe and acceptable caries control was the second stage. The studies of the caries-fluorine hypothesis in areas of natural fluoride water constituted the analytic phase. The construction of citywide field trials of water fluoridation, and the devising of better mechanical means for both fluoridation and de-fluoridation of water supplies, large and small, constituted the experimental phase of epidemiology. Few problems will present as complete a sequence of phases as does water fluoridation, yet this sequence must always be borne in mind. The epidemiological method will fall far short of its goal if the first phase, "descriptive epidemiology," is considered an end in itself.

METHODS OF EPIDEMIOLOGIC STUDY

There are various ways in which these methods can be used, ways which are common to all measurements of life processes and in particular to all dental diseases, not merely caries. A choice exists between cross-sectional and longitudinal studies. A *cross-sectional* study is a single effort made all at one time, either of necessity or because one is interested in the conditions seen at that particular time. It measures the effects of foregoing events, and is thus called *retrospective,* but its greater emphasis is upon the present. It is also called a case-history study. Thus one might perform a cross-sectional study of Eskimo children in Alaska merely because this was the only chance one had to get to Alaska, or perform a cross-sectional study of children in some nearby town in the current year because a new preventive measure was about to be introduced and it was desired to have data upon this particular year. In either case, the individuals making up the different age groups within the sample are *different* individuals. Human variability being what it is, the possibility exists that the children of age 12 in the sample, let us say, will show fewer DMF teeth per person than the children of age 11: a practical impossibility if one were studying progressive experience in the same persons. This trouble is most likely, of course, where samples are small. As samples increase in size, variability is controlled and a truer overall picture obtained in which such inconsistencies are infrequent.

The other kind is a *longitudinal* or *cohort* study. Here the *same* individuals are examined upon repeated occasions and the changes within the group recorded in terms of elapsed time between observations. This type of surveying does away with inter-age-group variability since the same persons are examined throughout. There is the added advantage, in the case of dental caries, that teeth can be followed as well as persons. This is particularly valuable in such studies as those which were made on the effect of topical fluoride treatment. Knutson in his work upon this subject wished to avoid the possible confusing influence of previous cavities and fillings in the teeth he was studying.[14] In his follow-up examinations, therefore, after topical application of sodium fluoride, he confined his attention to those teeth which were known to have been present and unattacked by caries at the pretreatment examination. His final results were expressed in percentages of teeth attacked, not of individuals. Longitudinal-survey work is ordinarily more accurate than cross-sectional work, but sources of variability still exist and samples must not be too small. The extreme difficulty in longitudinal work lies in getting repeated access to the same persons over long intervals of time. There is also the danger that time will introduce complicating factors other than the one under study.

THE EPIDEMIOLOGIST

If epidemiology is taken in its broadest sense, any researcher into the occurrence of disease or disability in groups of people is in fact an epidemiologist. Only large health departments, however, can usually afford specialists in this field. According to Smillie, an epidemiologist should have the five following qualifications:

1. He should be familiar with statistical techniques.
2. He should be well grounded in the diagnosis of disease.
3. He should be familiar with the history of medicine, particularly that portion of it that relates to epidemics of disease.
4. He should have a good knowledge of bacteriology and immunology and a thorough understanding of physiology, particularly in relation to the various environmental factors that may influence the health of individuals.
5. He must develop a point of view which will interrelate disease processes as they affect the community as a unit, rather than the individual. Thus he must have a real knowledge of the principles of preventive medicine.[15]

The epidemiologist is essentially a planner. Data come to him from many sources and his recommendations may be carried out by a great variety of different personnel, such as physicians, sanitarians, dentists, school nurses, government regulatory bodies, and the like. The epidemiologist, however, must keep close supervision over the collection of data and also serve as consultant to those in the field of public health administration. It is he who must determine when an epidemic of disease starts and when it has ceased to exist. He may not be able to do very much about the actual control of the epidemic once it has started, but if not, it is he who should apply the lessons learned to the design of measures which will prevent future epidemics.

EPIDEMIOLOGIC PROBLEMS IN THE DENTAL FIELD

The two following chapters of this book are devoted to the epidemiologic problems in dental caries and periodontal disease. Other challenging problems exist in the study of malocclusion, of genetics (including the effects of trauma during gestation), of posteruptive trauma to the teeth (the epidemiology of dental accidents), and finally of oral neoplasms and of radiation hazards to the oral structures. Dentists must educate themselves to make best use of these opportunities, and particularly to take a broader view of host factors. In rising to the challenge, they will find before them one of the most productive and fascinating new vistas in dental research.

CHAPTER 8

Epidemiology: Dental Caries

AT THE BEGINNING of the twentieth century, with Miller's chemico-parasitic theory newly propounded, there seemed little reason to look outside the human mouth for the causes of that almost universal disease, dental caries.[1] The oral environment, according to Miller, held the clue to the origin of this disease, and, if one could prevent the formation of bacterial plaques under which acid fermentation might occur, the whole problem of caries might be solved.

Dental research since that day has provided factor after factor which seemed to influence the occurrence of caries. Regardless of the validity of the Miller theory, the balance between dental health and dental caries was proving to be so delicate that a search for the predisposing factors of the disease became imperative. Detailed histological and chemical studies have shown the caries mechanism to be far more complicated than Miller dreamed it to be. Researchers for many years declared themselves to be in search of *"the* cause" of caries, but less and less have they really expected that one cause would lie at the end of their trail. The concept of multifactorial disease is now seen to fit dental caries as well as it does any other mass disease with which the epidemiologist has to deal. The public health dentist needs the tools of epidemiology in his fight against caries not only to develop a fuller understanding of the predisposing causes of the disease, but also to aid in planning the public programs which will control it and prevent it. Let us apply the epidemiological methods outlined in the last chapter to the subject of caries, reversing the order, however, and considering secular variations first, then host, agent, and environmental factors.

SECULAR VARIATIONS

The steady increase in proportion of the population affected by dental caries during most of recorded history has been touched upon in the previous chapter. Fig. 12 shows graphically the pace of this increase in Greece, from 3000 B.C. to the present time. The steady increase in percentage of teeth affected by caries, reaching its climax in modern times is matched by an equally striking increase in defective calcification.[2,3] Even at age 6, 73.6 percent of a recent sample of Greek children showed some degree of caries in their primary teeth.[4] Dental surveys in many parts of the world give the impression that similar increases have been the rule, with dental caries now almost universal among adults in civilized countries.

These changes all make dental caries look like a disease of civilization: a general hypothesis strengthened by observations upon present-day primitive tribes which have suddenly been overtaken by rampant dental caries coincidentally with the advent of modern prepared foods and the other appurtenances of a "civilized" environment. This is clearly suggested by Waugh in his studies of adjacent Eskimo settlements with and without imported white-man's food, and by Mellanby, who cites 17 primitive groups, only one showing as many as 28 percent of individuals with caries, and 23 recent European groups, most with over 80 percent caries and only one with as few as 46 percent.[5,6]

The introduction of water fluoridation and other preventive

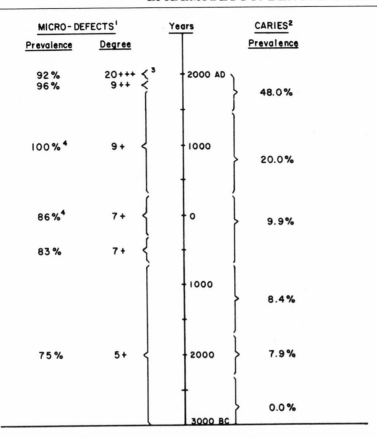

Figure 12. Prevalence of micro-defects (uncalcified interglobular spaces) and caries in teeth from Greek skulls, ancient and modern. From (1) Sognnaes, p. 547; (2) Krikos, p. 174. (3) The year 1948; (4) sample of fewer than 10 teeth.

measures in civilized areas were expected to make certain reversals in the upward trend of the disease, but suddenly during the late 1970s, reports of declining childhood caries began appearing from many developed countries, regardless of water fluoridation, and from nonfluoridated areas in the United States.[7] The developing countries, however, starting from severity levels below those of the developed countries, continued to show the familiar upward trend.[8]

Are these rapid changes in developed countries truly secular, as they are being called, or can specific causes be found for the decreases apart from elapsed time? A field for careful epidemiologic study lies ahead.

DENTAL CARIES AS A CHRONIC DISEASE

One of the outstanding features of dental caries is the long time it takes to develop. This is true not only of the individual lesion of caries, but the succession of lesions throughout the dentition as a whole, making caries a lifelong disease in most individuals who do not become edentulous at an early age.

What is a chronic disease? The time element of course must be present, but basically there are three types of chronic diseases and injuries. The first type is that which results from successful micro-biological symbiosis. The most successful disease from the point of view of the bacteria is that which allows the host to live longest, and therefore a successful infectious disease is a chronic disease. Tuberculosis is a good example. The second type results from a defect in or breakdown of metabolism or structure. Diabetes fits this pattern. The third is nutritional-deficiency disease. Over a period of time these types often blend, or one type leads to another. All three processes appear to be involved to some extent in dental caries.

All chronic diseases by their very nature are influenced by many factors, and these factors are often duplicated from one disease to another. We can therefore list to advantage the host, agent, and environment factors for other well-known diseases in order to compare those diseases with caries. This has been done in Table 16, with tuberculosis and diabetes taken as examples of their respective types. To this table might be added a nutritional-deficiency disease such as rickets, but when one has listed age and vitamin D in this instance all other factors seem to assume secondary importance. For this reason rickets has not been included.

A glance at Table 16 will show the great similarity between host and environmental factors in tuberculosis, diabetes, and caries. To which of the three classes of chronic disease does caries chiefly belong? Caries resembles tuberculosis in that so far it has been impossible to produce it experimentally without the introduction of microorganisms and microorganisms may even be able to transmit it.[9,10]

Table 16. Factors influencing occurrence of three chronic diseases.

Locus	Tuberculosis	Diabetes	Dental caries
Host	Race	Race	Race
	Familial heredity	Familial heredity	Familial heredity
	Age	Age	Age
	Sex	Sex (menopause)	Sex
			Developmental defects
	Concomitant disease	Concomitant disease	Emotional disturbances
		Obesity	
Agent	Tubercle bacillus	None known	Plaque-forming streptococci and suitable carbohydrate residue
	a. Strain (human vs. bovine)		
	b. Origin (endogenous vs. exogenous)		
Envi-ron-ment	Nutrition	Nutrition	Nutrition
	Occupation	Occupation (sedentary)	Fluoride
			Climate (sunshine, temperature, relative humidity)
	War	Urban life	War
	Social level	(Climate?)	Oral hygiene
	Housing		

Dental caries resembles diabetes in predisposing factors, since defective tooth structure has been shown to be somewhat more susceptible to dental carries than healthy tooth structure.[6] This simile cannot be carried too far, however, since the defective structure of any tissue of the body would be likely to increase the susceptibility of that tissue to the invasion of those diseases associated with it.

Is dental caries a deficiency disease which we can prevent with the assurance now felt in the field of rickets? To a certain extent, of course, it is; for a very large measure of prevention is possible through the ingestion of proper nutrients, including small quantities of fluoride ion, and the exclusion of excess in the way of refined carbohydrates. There is some evidence that vitamin C deficiency is associated with caries and more evidence that vitamin D deficiency is associated. Nevertheless, no nutrient or combination of nutrients seems the key to complete prevention of caries, and it falls far short of the facts to call caries a deficiency disease. All three major types of chronic disease, therefore, must be borne in mind, both in the collecting of data upon the epidemiology of dental caries and in planning public health programs for the control of caries.

HOST FACTORS

Race or Ethnic Group

Race or ethnic group has long been considered an important factor in the frequency of dental caries, yet little work has been done which would differentiate racial or ethnic heredity from environment. One of the best of the studies we do have is upon Army recruits during World War II.[11] A large study was made of draft rejection rates and a much smaller one of DMF tooth counts. Both gave similar results. The DMF material is reproduced in Fig. 13. The various racial and ethnic categories which are used are a little vague, yet considerable care was used in determining their limits. Environmental differences are probably at a minimum, since the recruits all resided in the same geographical area. The major contrasts which appear are not only in line with the clinical impression of most dentists, but are also corroborated at certain points by other studies. Specifically, both Chinese and black populations have been shown to have lower caries rates than corresponding white populations.[12] The U.S. Public Health Service National Dental Caries Prevalence Survey of 1979–80 confirms this as related to blacks.[13]

Age

It used to be generally believed that dental caries was "essentially a disease of childhood," and that its incidence among adults was very low compared with its pre- and postpubertal onslaught. This impression is borne out by the American Dental Association's 1965 survey of needs for dental care in the United States, where a very high peak in the number of teeth needing filling is seen to exist between the ages of 15 and 24.[14] This peak, however, represents accumulated needs and not necessarily current needs or dental-caries incidence. The impression that caries is a disease of youth is further borne out by a study at the Metropolitan Life Insurance Company, where affected teeth per person and, more particularly, affected surfaces per person (the equivalent of DMF teeth and DMF surfaces) are shown to accumulate far more rapidly at ages 17 to 19 and 20 to 24 than at older ages.[15] Other studies in terms of DMF teeth show more uniform incidence of caries.[16,17] On grounds of probability alone it seems much more likely that the incidence of lesions of dental caries should be lower immediately after the teeth have erupted than it would be a few years later, since time is needed for lesions of caries to develop to an obvious

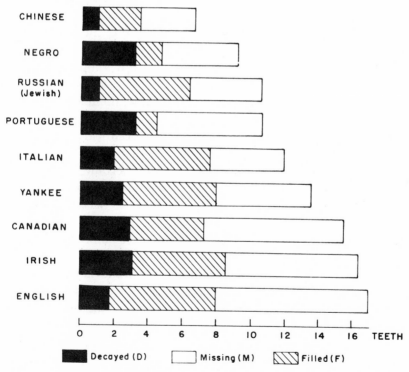

Figure 13. Relation of dental caries incidence to nationality. [Courtesy, *New England Journal of Medicine.*]

size. One would also expect caries incidence to be low in later life, when the more susceptible tooth surfaces in the average mouth have already decayed and when the number of remaining attackable surfaces is significantly reduced. Another factor operating toward lower caries in later life may be the gradual accumulation of fluoride in bones and teeth with advancing age everywhere, as noted in Chapter 16.

If this hypothesis were true, the best place to look for evidence would be among surveys in terms of surfaces, rather than DMF teeth. Large-scale surveys in terms of surfaces and covering a wide enough age span to be of interest are hard to find and are likely to be inaccurate if they do not include x-rays—at least a pair of bitewings. Evidence is accumulating that older teen-age children have more DMF surfaces per DMF tooth than do younger teenagers, a quite natural finding.[18] The work of Hollander and Dunning, among office workers over the age of 17, is expressed in surfaces and shows a gradual decrease in caries incidence with age, the most pronounced decrease occurring in the interval between 25 and 35 years of age. X-ray evidence is included in this study. Fig. 14 shows the data in question. These studies suggest that the greatest intensity of the caries process lies in the period from 15 to 30 years of age. The methods used to compile them are discussed in Chapter 14.

One exception to the trend just described occurs in ages over 60, with the development of *acute root caries,* a process named and described by Bodecker.[19] As root surfaces become denuded by gingival recession in advancing age, vulnerable dentine areas become well situated for the accumulation of bacterial plaque. Occlusal abrasion often contributes by permitting food impaction. If at the same time the patient's oral clearance ability deteriorates and his oral hygiene habits do too, an ideal condition exists for rapid development of caries. Lesions are broad and shallow at first, but if untreated can result in pulp involvement with surprising speed. Considerable tooth loss probably occurs among older people for this reason, but statistical studies to document the amount are lacking. There is evidence, however, that lifelong residence in fluoridated areas is accompanied by reduced root caries. Stamm and Banting have compared such adults with those living in nonfluoridated areas.[20]

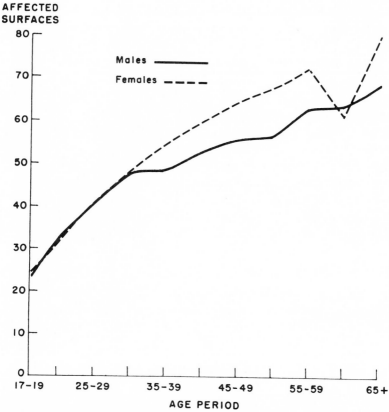

Figure 14. Affected surfaces per person by age and sex. Samples above age 60 are too small for reliable inferences.

Sex

Many statistical studies have been made to differentiate between the dental-caries experience of males and females. In young people, caries has been seen to be higher in the female to an inconsequential extent, but some studies show no significant difference between the sexes, and a few show slightly higher caries for males at certain ages but not at others. Above age 30, where statistical material is far scarcer, the study of the Metropolitan Life Insurance Company employees stands out in that it shows a very marked difference between the sexes (Fig. 14).[15] The difference appears first in the age group 35–39, and widens progressively after that to age 60. This study is impressive because most of the samples composing it are of over 100 cases. The curve for caries experience in females here, if plotted on semilogarithmic paper as in Fig. 15, becomes a straight line, indicating a rate of increase proportional to some overall factor, perhaps the remaining attackable teeth in the mouth. The experience curve for males breaks sharply above the age of 30, as if some real change in caries susceptibility occurred about that time. Further work should be undertaken to substantiate this sex difference among older people, and, if it persists, an intensive study should be made of factors, perhaps physiological, which differentiate the male above 30 from the male below 30 and from the older female.

An impression has long been held that pregnancy accelerates dental caries in the female. No evidence has been found to substantiate this impression, in spite of several careful studies.

Familial Heredity

There is a widespread clinical impression that dental caries varies considerably from family to family, and that inheritance of a char-

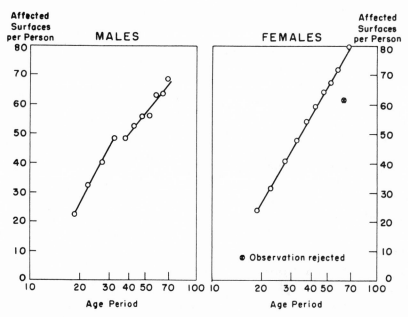

Figure 15. Affected surfaces per person in relation to logarithm of age by sex.

acterisic tooth structure, either good or poor, is common. Good genetic studies of caries incidence are few in number, and in such studies it is difficult to distinguish between true inheritance through the chromosomes and the transmission of dietary and other habits through family indoctrination. Twins offer perhaps the best opportunity for research upon this matter. Mansbridge finds greater resemblance in caries experience between identical twins than between fraternal twins, while unrelated pairs of children show less resemblance than either type of twin.[21] Summarizing the work of several authors on this subject, we may conclude that environmental factors have greater influence than genetic factors but that the latter also contribute to the causation of caries.

Emotional Disturbances

There is a widespread clinical impression that emotional disturbances, particularly transitory anxiety states, influence the incidence of dental caries. Most dentists have patients who have passed through periods of stress and associated high caries incidence, with a later return to a more normal mental health and caries rate. Such cases are extremely difficult to document because of the difficulty of defining stress and of relating it accurately to a chronic disease such as caries, but one such study is available, showing a sharp peak in caries incidence at times of acute stress, with return to previous caries incidence later.[22] Salivary changes have been shown to occur in connection with changes in mental health. Thus schizophrenics have been shown to have an increased rate of salivation, and salivary pH has been seen to rise under temporary emotional stress.[23] One study is available on dental disease itself, attempting to relate dental examinations in terms of DMF teeth to mental diagnosis among psychiatric patients.[24] Four major diagnostic groups were considered: primary behavior disorders and psychopathic personality (considered a continuum), schizophrenia, manic-depressive psychosis, and alcoholism without psychosis. Statistical analysis demonstrated a higher dental-caries experience at all ages among the manic-depressive group than in the baseline hospital population, significant *in toto* though not necessarily so at each age.

Concomitant disease other than emotional has often been considered to affect caries rate. The disease most often thought of in this connection is diabetes, but statistical evidence of increased caries is completely lacking. Reduced dental caries has been demonstrated among controlled diabetics, probably due to the drastic dietary change needed.[25] Beyond this no particular disease seems to have been singled out. The emotional disturbance which so often accompanies systemic disease may turn out to be the common denominator which links these impressions.

Nutrition

Mention was made in the previous chapter of the difficulty of assigning a single logical place to nutrition in the list of host, agent, and environmental factors. Nutrition can be called a host factor to the extent that the individual instinctively selects specific foods from the array available to him, and after ingesting the foods metabolizes or excretes them according to a pattern dependent upon his normal physiology and his current state of health. Some people are natural protein feeders, others are natural carbohydrate feeders. In a civilized community with good transportation facilities, an extraordinary variety of food is actually available. Modern means of preservation and refrigeration in such a country as the United States permit an individual to construct almost any dietary regime he may wish, irrespective of the food-producing potential of the area in which he lives.

Insofar as a population is dependent upon locally grown food, and to the extent that climate and other factors influence the consumption of food in a given locality, nutrition is an environmental factor. Health education, directing a choice among foods, is an environmental factor. Nutrition is so much more often linked with environment than with host that it will be given detailed consideration later among environmental factors.

Variation in Caries within the Mouth

The epidemiologist in the dental field must deal, in effect, with populations of two different types: populations of people and populations of teeth within a mouth. While most of his work is likely to be with groups of people, the dental records which come to him are well suited to analysis of variations of caries within the mouth. Useful observations of this nature have so far grouped themselves under three main headings: (1) observations on types of caries, according to tooth *surface* attacked, (2) observations upon the frequency with which the *different teeth* in the mouth are attacked, and (3) observations upon *bilateral symmetry*.

There are four main types of caries attack by surfaces. *Pit-and-fissure caries* is not only the easiest to detect, but also the first to appear and the easiest to explain in terms of tooth structure. To the extent that pits and fissures often represent actual structural defects in enamel, they constitute the most susceptible surfaces in the mouth. Attack commonly occurs fairly early in life.

Proximal caries is the next to appear. It is seen in the deciduous teeth toward the end of their life span, and in the permanent teeth predominantly between the ages of 15 and 35, after which it becomes less frequent.[26] It is easy to relate this timing of proximal caries to the fact that non-self-cleansing areas exist from the time of tooth eruption beneath the contact points of teeth. In view of the difficulty of restoring carious proximal surfaces, it is of interest that fluoridation is at its most effective in preventing proximal and other smooth-surface lesions.

Cervical caries is the third type of major importance. It occurs more or less uniformly through life, and can be related logically to the progressive changes in the free margin of the gingivae which increase susceptibility to plaque formation, and hence caries, with the advance of years. The fourth type of caries is *acute root caries*, described earlier in connection with the degenerative processes of old age.

Entirely aside from variation in the point of attack of caries, there are marked variations found between the different teeth in the mouth. Thus the lower incisors are far less frequently attacked than any other teeth, and are frequently the only teeth remaining in the mouth after all others are lost. Various articles document this situation. A good modern study is that of Backer-Dirks in Holland, giving details on intraoral variations in children 12 to 15 years.[27] The opening of major salivary ducts near the lower incisors has been advanced as a reason for this resistance to caries, but the opening of the parotid glands near the upper molar teeth has failed to give these teeth similar protection. We shall be much closer to an understanding of the etiology of caries when variations such as these have been explained.

Bilateral symmetry of caries in the human mouth may not help our reasoning processes in tracing the causes of caries, but the knowledge that this symmetry exists is of great help to the public health worker in evaluating topical preventive measures for dental caries. Proof of bilateral symmetry can be found in various articles.[28] Knutson and Armstrong not only contribute materially to the evidence in their studies of the effect of topically applied sodium fluoride, but immediately put the knowledge to practical use by using one side of the mouth as a control against the other.[29]

AGENT FACTORS

Ever since the days of Miller, dental-caries research has been directed toward the identification of a microbial agent for the disease. Two generations ago a number of workers became impressed with the relation which appeared to exist between dental-caries rate and the number of lactobacilli in the mouth.[30] Whether or not these bacilli were causative of caries was not determined. Later, in working with germ-free rats, Orland et al. found that they were unable to produce dental caries in germ-free rats when feeding a diet which was highly cariogenic under normal circumstances.[9] This observation still stands, and has produced renewed attacks upon the microbiology of the oral cavity.

A large amount of information has now been obtained on experimental dental caries initiated by various bacteria in hamsters and rats. Human studies have progressed also, with attention centering on certain strains of streptococci, chiefly *S. mutans*. Gibbons and van Houte sum up current research:

Collectively, the data indicate that *S. mutans* must be considered an important organism in the initiation of carious lesions on enamel surfaces, but unequivocal evidence concerning its direct involvement in human disease has yet to be obtained.

As a consequence of the recent appreciation of the bacterial specificity involved in caries etiology, and particularly because of the apparent importance of *S. mutans*, efforts have been directed towards specifically controlling this organism . . . If enzymes are to be of practical use, difficult obstacles to overcome include: their mode of administration, their short contact time in the mouth, their slow diffusion into the plaque, their specificities, and the avoidance of continuous use.

It is obvious that long term use of antibiotics and other chemotherapeutic agents which are of general medical importance is unadvisable for controlling dental caries. Nevertheless, the possibility exists that short term administration of these agents may be of practical value, particularly in severely infected or handicapped individuals.

It has been possible to immunize experimental animals with vaccines of caries-inducing bacteria, and to obtain a partial reduction in dental caries development under certain experimental conditions . . . Immunization studies offer much promise, but they are still in their infancy, and the immunization of humans is only now getting under way.[10]

Not all agents need to be microbial. In the case of caries it has long been recognized that carbohydrate residues were essential. Workers now realize that these residues are not all equally conducive to plaque formation and multisurface caries. The rate of clearance from the mouth also affects the rate by which bacteria may act upon carbohydrate to produce acid. Foodstuffs with rapid oral clearance seem to be less dangerous than those which remain in the mouth for a long time.

With laboratory science now giving the epidemiologist definite objects for search, the study of agent factors have moved out into the field. Jordan et al. have searched for some of the best-known plaque-forming streptococci in various population groups and found them to be relatively common.[31] Their presence correlates with the extremes of caries activity on a group basis. Many other such studies have added to this picture, and others are to be expected in years to come, as agent factors are gradually linked to host and environmental factors.

ENVIRONMENTAL FACTORS

Major Geographic Variations

So many detailed environmental factors are dependent in one way or another upon geography that it seems of most interest to consider major geographic variations in dental caries first, and proceed from them toward more detailed factors. The writer has made an effort to analyze such major variations and from this analysis most of the material in the succeeding pages is drawn.[32]

In order to study geographic variations in dental disease apart from racial or ethnic variations, it is necessary to select an area for study inhabited either by one racial or ethnic group predominantly or by such a mixture of ethnic groups evenly distributed over the area that variability from this source will be evened out in large samples. The United States is probably the best place to look for such material. A number of reports have been made upon the geographic variations in dental disease found in military populations within the United States. One study of children made by the U.S. Public Health Service was large enough to give regional and often local comparisons, but the fact that this study was based upon questionnaires makes one hesitate to use it for statistical analysis any more than necessary.[33] A few studies are available from other parts of the world showing variations in dental disease within widespread but racially homogeneous groups.

The term "dental disease" is used advisedly because, for lack of more accurate case histories, one cannot exclude teeth lost for reasons other than caries. Above the age of 40 or 50 years the tooth loss from periodontal disease seems to exceed loss from caries. Nevertheless, studies of decayed, missing, and filled teeth among children or young adults, and of military acceptance based upon these conditions, may be presumed to be predominantly studies of caries. The difficulty of obtaining accurate dental data from large geographic areas is tremendous, even when populations are racially and socioeconomically relatively homogeneous. Existing nationwide surveys are far from ideal. The larger the population groups to be studied, the more unknown variables are likely to be present, but also the greater is the chance that these variables will even out. We must do the best we can with the material we have. Any pattern seen consistently in large studies should be taken seriously.

The United States. The large studies of military populations available in the United States have been mentioned. These populations, while not completely homogeneous, represent predominantly the white race and have in common certain cultural and physical denominators that are relatively reliable. Since recruiting and draft standards are national matters, each study group has some uniformity in age composition and physical excellence within itself, state by state. The nationwide transportation of many common food items tends toward a more or less uniform diet. East,

Nizel and Bibby, and others have noted the similarity of the various existing studies as to relative amounts of dental disease found in certain major regions of the country at intervals since the Civil War.[34,35]

The three military studies best adapted to geographic analysis are those of Britten and Perrot, Ferguson, and Nizel and Bibby.[36,37,35] The first of these gives the prevalence of rejectable dental defects among men who were rejected or accepted for limited duty in World War I. The second study gives the average number of decayed, missing, and filled teeth per recruit among 4,602 white naval recruits seen at one induction center in peacetime. The third study gives average numbers of decayed and missing teeth per selectee among 22,117 men at a large Army camp in World War II. Each study has defects from a statistician's point of view. Internal comparisons, however, are justifiable on the basis of a rank list of states from 1, the state with the lowest prevalence of dental disease, to 48, the state with the highest.

Each of these three studies in itself shows a pronounced geographic pattern for the prevalence of dental disease similar to the other in major outline, but with occasional discrepancies. The act of combining the rank lists to give a mean rank seems to preserve the pattern but iron out many of the discrepancies. The mean ranks for states are plotted in Fig. 16. The list contains no number 1 and no number 48, since no state was at the beginning or end of the list in all three studies. Shading has been arranged to group the states of similar rank. It is of interest how clearly these groups cohere in a geographical pattern.

The pattern of prevalence of dental disease which emerges suggests two striking associations: one, latitude, the other, distance from the seacoast. It seems impossible to interpret the map without considering both of these factors. Statistical testing of the correlation between each of the factors and the prevalence of dental disease confirms the significance of the relation. A correlation among the states along the Atlantic coast from Florida to Maine, arranged in order of latitude, shows a coefficient of 0.844, with a probability of less than 0.001 that this coefficient could be the result of chance. A similar comparison among inshore states of different latitude gives a similar result. The states from Texas to

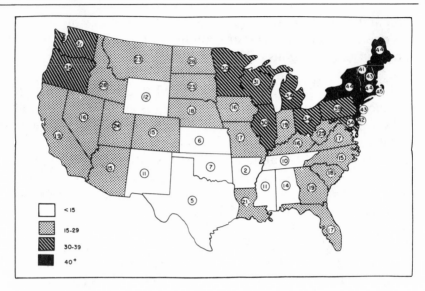

Figure 16. Mean rank of states in dental health from three nationwide military studies.

North Dakota show an almost perfect progression in prevalence of dental disease. The correlation coefficient between mean rank and latitude here is 0.923, with a probability of chance occurrence of just less than 0.01. Corroboration of this increase in dental disease with latitude is found in the U.S. Public Health Service National Dental Caries Prevalence Survey of 1979–1980.[38]

The relation of dental disease to distance from the seacoast in the military groups can be studied on almost any parallel of latitude. The 43rd parallel was chosen, since 11 states from New Hampshire to Oregon abut on or are crossed by this parallel. A correlation coefficient of −0.874 results, with a probability of chance occurrence of approximately 0.001.

South Africa. Ockerse has published a vast amount of data from the Southern Hemisphere which can be analyzed in a manner similar to that used in the United States.[39] His map of percentages of children with dental caries in the magisterial districts of the Union of South Africa gives a pattern which is almost the inverted image of that seen in the United States. Fig. 17 shows a plotting of these figures, with magisterial districts having more than 0.70 part per million of fluoride in the water supply excluded in order to minimize the known influence of fluoride. The shape of the Union of South Africa makes it difficult to separate the influence of latitude from that of distance from the seacoast. For convenience, the latter has been used in a statistical analysis which demonstrates its significance.

The Eastern Hemisphere. Andrews studied 2,000 members of the Royal Australian Air Force, dividing his data by states.[40] He found that counts of DMF (decayed, missing, and filled) teeth vary considerably according to latitude. Analysis of the relation shows a certain amount of significance, particularly between Tasmania and the mainland.

The 1951 Yearbook for the Commonwealth of Australia gives interesting climatological data for the Australian capital cities which help elucidate the Andrews figures for dental caries.[41] Table 17 gives the data and the corresponding rank lists. It is interesting to note that mean annual hours of sunshine, temperature, and relative humidity all vary more or less together, the first two

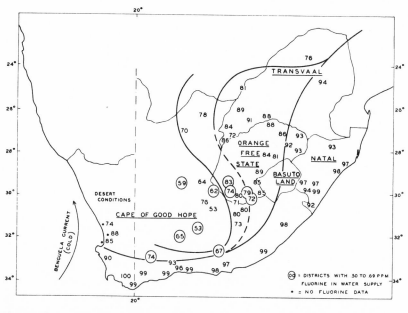

Figure 17. Prevalence of dental caries in districts with less than 0.70 ppm fluoride in the water supply, Union of South Africa. [Adapted from Ockerse.]

Table 17. Ranks of Australian states in dental disease compared with ranks of their capital cities in certain climatologic features.

State and city	Dental disease		Mean daily sunshine		Mean temperature		Mean relative humidity	
	DMF teeth	Rank	Hours	Rank	Degrees F.	Rank	%	Rank
West Australia Perth	17.50	1	7.8	6	64.5	5	62	2
South Australia Adelaide	18.57	2	7.0	4	63.1	3	52	1
New South Wales Sydney	18.66	3	6.8	3	63.7	4	68	4
Queensland Brisbane	19.72	4	7.5	5	69.0	6	67	3
Victoria Melbourne	19.74	5	5.6	1	58.8	2	69	6
Tasmania Hobart	21.98	6	5.8	2	54.4	1	65	5

Rank correlations (Spearman): dental disease-sunshine $r' = -0.771$; dental disease-temperature: $r' = -0.600$; dental disease-humidity: $r' = 0.829$.

rising as the third declines, and that all three are related fairly well to the variations in dental disease. Dental disease correlates best with relative humidity ($r' = 0.829$) and also fairly well with sunshine ($r' = 0.771$). Because of the small number of observations, only the coefficient for relative humidity approaches the 5 percent level of significance.

In other parts of the Eastern Hemisphere, the pattern of low caries near the equator and higher caries away from it seems carried out by studies of the Interdepartmental Committee on Nutrition for National Defense (ICNND), which coordinates nutrition studied in the armed forces and in civilian areas friendly to the United States, and by other related studies reported by Russell.[42] He lists New Zealand and Australia (the latter with greater population centers in the south) as relatively high caries areas; India, China, and Ethiopia are listed as relatively low.

Interpretation of Geographic Variations

The identification of variations in dental disease with latitude and distance from the seacoast will prove most useful if it helps us in a study of individual environmental factors influencing caries or periodontal disease. The largest group of such factors is climatological and includes sunshine, rainfall, humidity, and temperature. These factors are often related to one another, directly or inversely, but they deserve separate study. Chemical composition of water supply and urbanization are other important factors. Any effort to divide all these factors into those associated either with latitude or with distance from the seacoast is arbitrary, for a factor such as sunshine may often be related to both. Such an effort, however, is a necessary part of the analysis of the obvious geographic trends in dental disease and will help us to an understanding of the factors themselves.

Sunshine. One of the factors most commonly thought to vary with latitude is sunshine. The measurement of sunshine is not a simple matter. Total possible hours of sunshine per year actually increase a little as one leaves the equator, since long days in summer compensate for long nights in winter.[43] Actual hours of sunshine in the absence of cloud cover give a better measure and one which generally decreases as one leaves the equator. Even this does not tell as much as it might about sunshine available to human beings, for a given ground area intercepts less sunlight when the sun is low in the sky, temperature falls, and human beings clothe themselves or are driven indoors. The atmosphere, too, intercepts more ultraviolet light when the sun is low.

Mean annual hours of actual sunshine are shown on U.S. Weather Bureau Map No. 13, from which Fig. 18 has been adapted. This map shows a pattern very similar to that for dental disease in the United States (Fig. 16), at least in terms of latitude variation. Corroboration comes from East, who compares dental caries among the rural children reported in Public Health Bulletin No. 226 with the mean annual sunshine where they live and finds an inverse relation which is highly significant statistically.[44] Ockerse gives sunshine figures for certain areas in South Africa.[39] When these figures are compared with those for dental disease in the same areas a high rank correlation of -0.879 results.

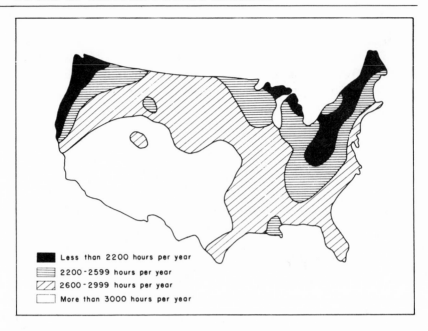

Figure 18. Mean annual sunshine, U.S. Weather Bureau Map No. 13.

This high correlation leads to consideration of the mechanism relating sunshine to caries. Ultraviolet light from the sun is known for its ability to promote synthesis of vitamin D in skin tissues, and thus to reduce caries incidence (Chapter 3). Ultraviolet light is blocked by the thickness of the atmosphere and by the water vapor it may contain. This phenomenon helps to explain several geographical parameters: sunshine (the absence of cloud cover), a high angle of incidence of the sun's rays upon the earth (greatest in low latitudes), nearness to sea coast (relative humidity), and even altitude above sea coast. Barmes in Papua, New Guinea, has observed a correlation of caries with altitude which needs further study.

Temperature. As Fig. 19 shows, temperature varies almost entirely with latitude. The only other factor to vary temperature seems to be high altitude, as is seen in the Rocky Mountain area. Temperature, in turn, acts to vary the caloric requirements and water intake of human beings. Carbohydrate food is not only a quick, but a relatively cheap, source of caloric energy. Our knowledge of the etiology of caries, therefore, indicates a way in which this disease may be related to temperature. Data on variations of civilized diet with latitude or temperature are scarce. One study by the U.S. Department of Agriculture showed the consumption of baked goods (breads, cakes, and pastries not baked at home) to be higher in the North.[45] Consumption of sugar was also found to be higher among northern farm families than among farm families elsewhere in the country, though this contrast was not seen in a later study.[46] Further studies of carbohydrate consumption are needed, as well as further basic studies on carbohydrate nutrition and on methods of refinement.

Relative Humidity. This is the ratio of the amount of moisture in the atmosphere to the maximum amount that can occur without precipitation at a given temperature and barometric pressure. It is a better indication of the dampness of a climate than is actual precipitation. A mapping of the mean annual relative humidities over a period of years in the United States (Fig. 20) shows these humidities to be greatest along the immediate seacoasts, both Atlantic and

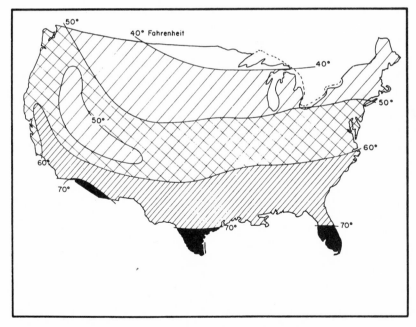

Figure 19. Mean annual temperature; U.S. Weather Bureau Bulletin S.

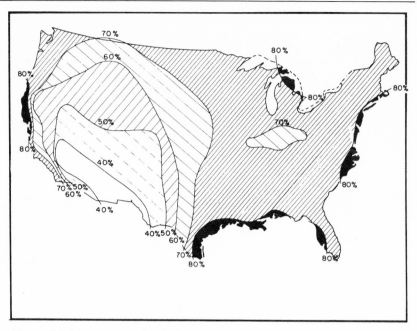

Figure 20. Mean annual relative humidity, U.S. Weather Bureau Bulletin O.

Pacific. From a short distance inshore, east of the Mississippi, most of the area shows little variation from percentages in the middle 70's (the "humid East"). The western states show sharp and regular variations with both distance from the seacoast and latitude, giving an appearance to the map much like that for dental caries. The data for individual weather stations in U.S. Weather Bureau Bulletin O are difficult to compare with state averages for dental caries, since many sharp changes in relative humidity cut across states, especially those on the seacoast. A better study can be done.

The data from Australian states (Table 17) show a higher correlation (0.829) between caries and relative humidity than between caries and any other climatic factor. Relative humidity, for these reasons, needs careful consideration as a factor in the causation of caries.

Rainfall. Another factor is rainfall, which leaches minerals from the soil and blocks sunlight. Fig. 21 shows mean annual precipitation for the United States. Though no latitude relation is evident, there is a regular decrease in rainfall as one proceeds inshore.

Only on the Atlantic coast is this pattern at variance with the one for prevalence of dental disease. Rainfall, though decreasing inland, is greater in the South than in the North. The mechanisms by which relative humidity and rainfall might be linked to dental caries, either together or separately, need further study.

Fluoride. Among nonclimatic factors, fluoride is the one that one would first attempt to relate to geographical variations in dental caries. Van Burkalow's mapping of maximum fluoride concentrations in communal and noncommunal water supplies on a county basis gives the most comprehensive material available for the United States.[47] No latitude variation is evident. Area for area, there are as many counties with fluoride maxima above 1.5 parts per million in the Dakotas as there are in Texas, and a similar situation holds to the east and to the west. Van Burkalow discounts climatic variations and feels that differences in geologic formation are probably more important. There is, however, some relation between fluoride maxima and distance from the seacoast. The coastal states seem to have somewhat fewer high fluoride maxima,

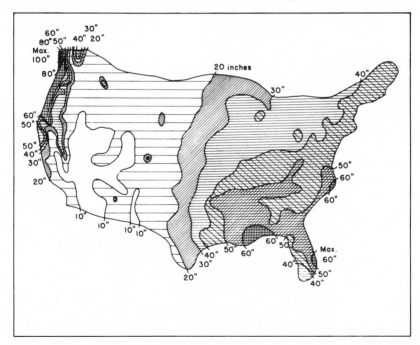

Figure 21. Mean annual precipitation, U.S. Weather Bureau Bulletin D.

though unmapped areas in these states contribute to the impression. Correlation between fluoride and distance from the seacoast is probably much better than is shown on Van Burkalow's map, for one deep-well water supply in a county may provide a high maximum figure, while the bulk of the county uses surface supplies (river, lake, or shallow well) which are almost always fluoride-free. Rivers are larger near the seacoast, the surface water is more commonly used there than it is inshore. Other aspects of the epidemiology of fluoride in relation to caries are taken up in Chapter 16.

Total Water Hardness. Usually measured in terms of calcium carbonate, total water hardness is an etiological factor in caries that has been known for many years. More recently it has faded from sight as attention was focused more sharply on fluorides. Röse[48] and Ockerse[39] are among the authors who have reported an inverse relation. Ockerse's correlation coefficient between calcium carbonate and percentage of caries is −0.811, even higher than his coefficient of −0.662 between caries and fluorides. If his data for calcium carbonate are plotted on a map zoned in hundreds of miles from the seacoast, a significant correlation coefficient of 0.462 is obtained for the increase seen as one proceeds inland. All of this returns our attention sharply to total hardness. Known components of hardness deserve further study. Trace elements must be studied and factors now unknown must be sought.

Trace Elements. A number of trace elements deserve attention, some found in water supplies but most found in greater concentration in common foodstuffs. Epidemiological studies must rely, therefore, not only on studies of local water supplies and perhaps soils, but upon concentration of the trace elements in the urine, hair, or other ultimate repositories. Hadjimarkos has found marked increases in dental caries in areas where selenium was high both in water and foodstuffs and the only environmental factor which could not be ruled out was sunshine. He summarizes this and other work on trace elements:

Selenium is the first micronutrient element shown to be capable of increasing caries, particularly when consumed during the developmental period of the teeth and incorporated into their structure. Epidemiological studies on selenium and caries should be undertaken not only in high seleniferous areas but also in low-seleniferous ones. In the latter areas the element may be present in sufficient amounts to increase caries without producing other symptoms of selenosis which are clearly apparent, as was the case among Oregon children.

The proposed caries-inhibiting influence of molybdenum and vanadium remains unresolved at present. Contrary to common belief, water supplies in general do not contribute significant amounts of micronutrient elements to the daily diet.[49]

Soils. Where populations depend largely on locally grown food products it is logical to look to differences in soil composition to help explain differences in caries experience. A number of studies upon soil have yielded negative or confusing results. The only really suggestive study to date relates to molybdenum content and acidity. Ludwig, Healy, and Malthus noted marked differences in caries between the towns of Napier and Hastings, New Zealand, without any environmental factor other than soil to account for it.[50] Differences in diet, fluoride, climate, and so forth were negligible. The soil of Napier, however, had higher pH, higher molybdenum, and the children there had lower caries. There is enough collateral evidence to justify further study of both these factors. In Hadjimarkos's work on selenium, the most logical source of this trace element was the local soil.[49]

Soil is not likely to prove an important element in programs for the prevention of dental disease, even if further study confirms relationships such as the above. Modern methods of preserving and transporting food products give our markets of today a variety that is bound to neutralize the effect of the local soil under all but extreme conditions.

Urbanization. Ferguson attributed the regional variations he found in caries to the greater frequency of large industrial cities in the North.[37] This claim deserves examination, and Public Health Bulletin No. 226 affords dental data on a number of cities, together with similar data on nearby rural county balances. The defects of Bulletin No. 226 have been mentioned. Nevertheless, errors should be at a minimum when comparing closely adjoining samples within it. Care was taken to select areas of similar distance from seacoast, lake, or major river. Urbanization was found to be accompanied by only an 11 percent increase in caries, which did not prove statistically significant.[32] The National Dental Caries survey of 1979–80 differentiates between regional levels and those of standard metropolitan statistical areas within them, with opposite but probably insignificant results.[38] A careful study by the World Health Organization of metropolitan and nonmetropolitan areas in five cities in different countries shows a consistent but small trend in the opposite direction, with the high caries scores in the nonmetropolitan areas.[51]

A small, but probably accurate, study of urbanization is found in Fulton's report on the New Zealand national dental service.[52] A sample of 4,072 children was selected to include 2,048 rural and 2,024 urban children, all ages from 7 to 14 being equally represented. Small differences are found in DMF teeth, but Fulton states that "neither these differences in average DMF nor any other differences between corresponding figures . . . seem to be significant."

Nutrition

To the extent that broad geographic, cultural, or educational factors influence the food available to a population, nutrition is an environmental factor. Fluoride, available in a water supply, is similarly environmental; this matter is taken up in Chapter 16.

We have already discussed an instance in which temperature may affect food intake within a population able for the most part to make its own selection among a broad array of foods. A more striking example, where the question is not one of choice but of the actual availability of certain nutrients, is that of the Eskimos in their original surroundings. The lack of plant food in the Eskimos' usual habitat makes it necessary to seek animal food and in turn receive a diet consisting largely of protein and fat. The results have been excellent for the Eskimo dentition, as the work of Waugh[5] and others testifies. Only when civilized transport facilities permit the introduction of foods other than native do the Eskimo teeth break down.

By far the most interesting study of caries rates in native population groups throughout the world have come from the ICNND. Russell, working with this committee, reports widely different DMF counts from eight countries, as shown in Fig. 22. In commenting on these very diverse figures, Russell states:

> The lowest prevalence of caries was noted in Ethiopia and the Far East; an intermediate experience in Lebanon, representing the Near East; and the highest experience, paralleling that in the United States, in Central and South America. Sugar consumption as determined by ICNND dietary teams followed the same pattern.

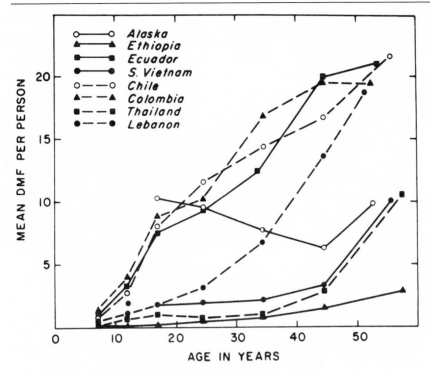

Figure 22. DMF teeth in eight countries, ICNND survey. [Reprinted by permission of Dr. A. L. Russell and *Journal of Dental Research.*]

High carbohydrate diets were not necessarily associated with high caries prevalence, unless sugar was a prominent factor. The principal food in Ethiopia is a cereal called teff, and rice is the staple in South Vietnam, Thailand, and Burma.

There is no suggestion anywhere in the ICNND data that any particular nutritional factor (except fluorine) is caries-inhibitory, or that caries is lessened by adequate nutrition.

It does not follow that starvation or deprivation is necessarily caries-inhibitory; if so, one would expect that within malnourished populations people with caries would be better fed than people without caries; but it is not so.[53]

Social Factors

Good *economic status* and *social pressure* in the direction of good mouth appearance are both strong factors in creating demand for dental treatment. Evidence of these facts can be found in the American Dental Association's findings of differing needs for fillings and other dental operations among different economic groups.[54] The effect of social pressure can be seen on an international basis by comparing dentist-population ratios among civilized countries all well able to afford as many dentists as may be considered important. Neither of these relations is solely a measure of caries incidence, yet evidence does exist here and there that economic or social factors can affect caries incidence too, as may be the case in the major decline in developed countries. A good economic status carries with it a lower caries rate, most pronounced and best documented among preschool and young primary children but extending, in one instance at least, up through high school age.[55] In adults, there is a slight trend in the opposite direction. The National Center for Health Statistics finds low-income whites (but not blacks) to have fewer DMF teeth than their higher income counterparts.[56]

Industrial hazards to the teeth probably belong in the economic category, and will be discussed in Chapter 21. As examples, carbohydrate dust and acid fumes are both known to be deleterious to the teeth, the one promoting caries and the other chemical erosion.

On a broader scale than any peacetime variation in the structure of society is the influence of *war.* The physical surroundings of whole populations are altered by drastic dietary change, and there are many other environmental changes less easy to measure. Impressive evidence has been assembled by Toverud, Mellanby and Mellanby, and others showing reductions in dental caries after the third or fourth year of war in several European countries and continuing for several years into peacetime thereafter.[57,58] Analyzing reports from some ten different European countries, Sognnaes concludes that children's teeth there "show 1) a definite tendency to decrease in caries in the latter part of and following the recent wars. This is 2) most significant in young children, and 3) in those teeth of older ones which have developed or matured during the war years. Finally, and perhaps the most important, the general principle evolved from our analysis is 4) that there seems to be several years' delay in the initial effect of wartime conditions on the teeth, and, following the First World War even a greater delay in the return to prewar dental status."[59]

The predominant environmental modification to which this change in caries might be laid is a reduction in refined carbohydrates. Thus Norway before the war consumed 36.3 kilograms of sugar per person per year, and during the war only 10 kilograms per person. Other countries had comparable caries reductions, as in Fig. 23. In many of the countries where caries reductions occurred, the children were known to have remained in generally good physical condition, and as active as ever. From this and other evidence it is inferred that the children must have ingested more than the usual amounts of available natural foods, including a considerable bulk of less refined carbohydrates—potatoes, kohlrabi, wartime bread of high-extraction flour, and so forth. Sognnaes does not attempt to decide whether the reduction of refined carbohydrates or the introduction of favorable nutrients in the natural foods is the true cause of the caries reduction, but from a

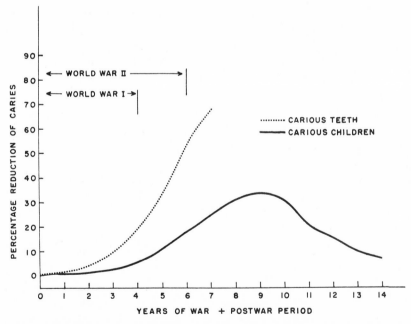

Figure 23. Year-to-year reduction of caries-susceptible teeth and carious children during the two world wars. Data on carious teeth represent averaged findings from Norway, Denmark, Finland, Sweden, and Britain; data on carious children are from Norway, Denmark, Britain, France, and Germany. [Adapted from Sognnaes.]

practical public health point of view the first change made the second change necessary and may therefore to a certain extent be considered causative. He does reason that the favorable influence, whatever it is, acts upon teeth before eruption and produces tooth structure which will withstand the renewal of high carbohydrate intake at the close of the war.

Sognnaes has reinforced this hypothesis by work upon rats and other animals changed at various stages in development from a stock diet to a purified diet high in sucrose and complete in known nutritional essentials. The changes were made at the prenatal period, before weaning, and after weaning.[60] Animals brought up on the sucrose diet from the beginning of the prenatal period had caries scores almost four times as high as those changed from a stock to a sucrose diet after the eruption of the teeth, as seen in Fig. 24. All this does not constitute a denial of the intraoral effect of carbohydrate upon caries. It may show instead a reduction in the reservoir of cariogenic streptococci which we now know are available for transmission from a mother to her offspring, either before or after birth.

Sognnaes's study and those of others in "undernourished" areas make it clear that a diet adequate in known nutrients, and balanced according to ratios currently thought desirable, cannot be claimed to be the only route to a low caries rate. Bacteria need to be present in the oral environment. The importance of the location of bacteria *in the mouth* is borne out by the study of Kite et al. on the tube feeding of rats.[61] Rats fed a cariogenic diet by stomach tube developed no caries at all, whereas their litter mates, fed the same diet by mouth, developed considerable caries.

Current Changes in Caries

During the 1970s a series of reports began to be received from various countries of the developed "Western World" to the effect that children everywhere were getting far less tooth decay than they were a couple of decades earlier. These changes were occurring in both fluoridated and nonfluoridated communities, though previously large decreases in the fluoridated areas left less opportunity for further change. A fairly large number of factors could be involved in these changes, in addition to fluoridation.

Is this a secular change, of the long-term, noncyclical nature seen in the Greek skulls? How can it be reconciled with an opposite

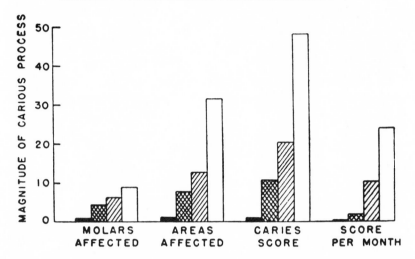

Experimental	Rations	During :
PREGNANCY	LACTATION	POSTERUPTIVELY
stock	stock	stock
stock	stock	sucrose
stock	sucrose	sucrose
sucrose	sucrose	sucrose

Figure 24. Caries incidence in groups of hamsters whose experimental feeding on the purified ration was commenced before, during, or after tooth development. "Sucrose" refers to the purified ration containing 67 percent sucrose; "stock" refers to the Purina laboratory chow. [Reproduced from *Science* by permission.]

trend in developing countries? Whether or not the term *secular* can properly be applied to it, the change needs careful description and further epidemiologic study. An appraisal of the effect of this decrease in childhood caries upon dental practice is attempted in Chapter 13.

The best description of the downward trend is found in the report of the First International Conference on the Declining Prevalence of Dental Caries, held in Boston in 1982.[7] Published as a special issue of the Journal of Dental Research, the report includes papers from Denmark, England, Ireland, the Netherlands, New Zealand, Norway, Scotland, Sweden, and the United States.[62] All tell the same story, whether in terms of DMF teeth, DMF surfaces, percentage of children caries-free (this one, up), restorations placed, or extractions performed. Drops of 30 to 40 percent are common. Typical is that from the United States.[63] A large-scale comparison in DMF surfaces is provided by the National Center for Health Statistics Survey figures for 1971–1973 and the NIDR Dental Caries Prevalence Survey figures for 1979–1980. In this interval of approximately eight years, regional decreases of 28 to 39 percent are reported, with a national average of 32 percent. During this period, approximately one-half of the United States population, chiefly in the urban areas, were receiving fluoridated water.

The extent to which these decreases may be the result of individual fluoride preventive procedures in nonfluoridated areas can be inferred from Horowitz's eight-year study in a nonfluoridated area.[64] A combination of weekly rinses, daily supplement tablets, and a fluoride dentifrice produced reductions in DMF surfaces of 40 percent in 12-year-old children and 62 percent in 14-year-old children.

What factors can be postulated for the causation of this great change? Water fluoridation tops the list, but fluoridated dentifrices may be a close second. The list can also include children migrating from fluoridated to nonfluoridated communities, fluoride rinse programs, topical fluoride applications, better oral hygiene, and better nutrition. A final factor, as yet unmeasured, is the influence of antibiotics. A generation ago Helmut Zander studied a penicillin-containing dentifrice and recorded 48 to 60 percent caries reductions over a two-year period.[65] This dentifrice could never be generally marketed, but according to Gibbons, the increased use of antibiotics in treating childhood infections "has likely contributed to some degree to the decline in caries."[66] The magnitude of this contribution has yet to be determined.

On the other side of the coin is the story from developing countries. The World Health Organization Data Bank records upward changes of from 1.6 to 10.4 in DMF teeth over periods of 9 to 50 years, averaging 20 years.[8] Table 18 gives these figures.

The reasons for these increases can be inferred to some extent from earlier experience in the developed countries. The use of refined carbohydrate foods had increased more rapidly in these countries than the knowledge of oral hygiene and the increase in dental manpower. Native diets with associated low caries had given way to cariogenic diets, and only recently have preventive measures overtaken and reversed the upward trend in caries. Dental manpower increases have usually correlated with an upswing in dental health education as well as in a demand for dental care. Møller reported that seven developed countries showed ratios ranging between 1090 and 2890 people per dentist, whereas six developing countries showed ratios of 5520 to over one million persons per dentist. The rural areas in developing countries must indeed get no dental care at all, owing to the habit of 80 to 90 percent of all dentists to locate in urban areas.

These conflicting trends in caries incidence tend to make one wonder whether the downward trend in developed countries can really be called secular. Barmes observes that among 12-year-old children in developed countries the downward trend was toward 3 DMF teeth, and among children of similar age in developing countries the upward trend was also toward 3 DMF teeth.[67] Is it possible that these figures indicate an approximation to an endemic caries level which will actually be slightly greater than that of previous centuries?

The term *secular* may or may not apply to this situation. According to Webster, the term means "belonging to an age" or involving long periods of time, probably centuries. In practical public health work the term seems to be applied mostly where the factors causing change are unknown. To call the current drop in caries in developed countries secular may be allowable, but it is counterproductive if it discourages further search for specific causative factors.

Table 18. Increase in prevalence of dental caries in children aged 10–14 from selected countries.

Country	Increase in DMFT		Within no. of years
	From	To	
Ethiopia	0.2	1.6	17
Kenya	0.1	1.7	21
Iraq	0.7	3.5	9
Thailand	0.7	4.5	15
Vietnam	2.0	6.3	11
French Polynesia	negligible	7.5	50
Greenland	1.5	10.4	20

The foregoing mass of material, which has been primarily descriptive, is indicative of a variety of causative factors for caries. Fluorides and streptococci have made it possible to advance beyond the descriptive phase of epidemiological strategy (see Chapter 7) into hypothecation, analysis, and finally experiment. It is now important to do similar work in connection with the numerous other factors that will produce certain levels of caries attack in certain people at certain times and at certain places.

CHAPTER 9

Epidemiology: Periodontal and Other Diseases

THE DENTAL diseases other than caries have received far less epidemiological attention than caries. No one of them deserves a chapter of its own in a general public health textbook, though periodontal disease deserves a good half chapter and the material on periodontics is constantly increasing.

PERIODONTAL DISEASE

Diseases which attack the supporting structures of the teeth are of two main types: those which attack the gingivae and are commonly described as gingivitis and those which involve chronic and progressive destruction of the periodontal membrane and alveolus. Though gingival disease may occur as a tissue enlargement or recession of a noninflammatory nature, most such disease is inflammatory and reversible (that is, can be cured). Chronic destructive periodontal disease, on the other hand, is progressive and irreversible, though it can often be arrested.

There are three main types of chronic destructive periodontal disease.[1] Inflammatory disease is the commonest form, usually called *periodontitis,* marginal periodontitis, or Schmutz pyorrhea. Here local causes predominate and not all teeth are equally affected. Destruction of alveolar bone is accompanied by the formation of subgingival pockets which are generally, though not always, sites of chronic inflammation, particularly if they are not cleaned out periodically. The second type of periodontal disease is apparently systemic in origin and is called *periodontosis,* juvenile periodontitis, or diffuse alveolar atrophy. The predominant feature here is bone loss, usually more generalized and serious than with periodontitis, but not always accompanied by pocket formation or inflammation. Local irritants may determine the site of onset for periodontosis, but it soon becomes obvious that forces more generalized and as yet imperfectly understood are at work. The third type is mere *atrophy,* associated with such conditions as old age or disuse. These three types frequently blend in such a way as to be indistinguishable one from another.

The epidemiology of periodontal disease is one of the most important challenges before the dental profession at the moment, but work upon it has been retarded by a number of factors which make it a more difficult subject to study than caries. In the first place, two areas are involved, the gingiva and the alveolar bone, each with its characteristic disease processes. Gingivitis and bone loss often blend in such a way as to make periodontal disease appear as a single clinical phenomenon in the mouth, yet both etiologically and for purposes of treatment it is important to distinguish between them.

In the second place, periodontal disease, unlike caries, has its greatest incidence late in life. This means that valid assumptions are usually impossible as to the reason or reasons for the loss of teeth which are found missing at the time of examination. DMF counts of children's teeth can be interpreted with reasonable accuracy on the assumption that the missing teeth were lost because of caries. Measures of periodontal disease, however, must usually be made without accurate estimation of disease processes in missing teeth.

In the third place, periodontal disease does not lend itself well to objective measurement. Assessment of degrees of gingivitis is almost of necessity subjective and vague. Alveolar-bone loss is very difficult to evaluate clinically without the use of x-ray. Observational errors as to pocket depth accumulate easily, with a bias toward underestimation, and interpretive differences are wide. Impairment of tooth function is also difficult to estimate. The expense and physical difficulty of taking x-rays in field epidemiological surveys, as well as the radiation hazard involved, have resulted in a scarcity of good studies to date in which x-ray data have been included. Detailed discussion of the measurement problem in periodontal disease appears in Chapter 14.

Finally, and in part as a result of the foregoing difficulties, quantitative studies of periodontal disease have been poor and unstandardized. Such indices as do exist (discussed in Chapter 14) are far from perfect. It is seldom possible to compare one investigator's work with another's, though in measurements of the simplest type—percentage prevalence figures—this has been done. Table 19 gives prevalence figures for gingivitis and for bone loss from data from a number of different parts of the world.[2-21] All figures should be treated with caution, as interpretive errors may be large. Some of Russell's findings on severity of periodontal disease appear in Fig. 27.

Periodontal disease repays analysis in terms of the three basic factors of the infectious disease epidemiologist: host, agent, and environment. The practical preventive measures which arise from such analysis are discussed in Chapter 12.

Host Factors

Because of the difficulties in measurement of periodontal disease, epidemiological data have been slow to collect, but enough are available that the major trends connected with such principal host factors as age, sex, and intraoral distribution are becoming quite clear. A number of other factors, both intraoral and systemic, are beginning to come into view but are as yet imperfectly documented.

Chronic destructive periodontal disease has always been associated with the older *age* groups. Andrews and Krogh, in a large study of causes for the loss of human teeth, show periodontal disease accounting for a larger percentage of lost teeth than does caries above the age of 40 years, in both sexes.[22] Bossert and Marks in a study involving not only histories of extraction for periodontal disease but also morbidity data upon teeth still present, find steadily increasing percentages of affected teeth among industrial employees in New York City (Fig. 25).[5] Day and Shourie, in their roentgenographic survey of periodontal disease in India, find an almost equally steady progression in alveolar-bone loss with increasing age. With gingivitis alone, the age progression is not so clear.[15] A gradual increase is probably the most reliable assumption, since bone loss does conduce to gingivitis because of the abnormal contours it produces. Varying interpretation of clinical findings, of terminology, and of many other factors may contribute to the confused picture of age changes in gingivitis, plus the fact that gingivitis is a reversible condition dependent upon varying levels of oral hygiene technique.

One aspect of the age factor is the extent to which heavy loss of teeth from caries at an early age may *mask* periodontal disease later on, or low caries accentuate it. Two or three of the reports

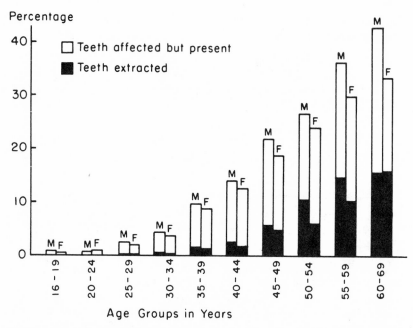

Figure 25. Percentage of teeth affected by periodontal disease among industrial employees, New York City, 1951–1952.

from Australasia mention the masking effect. Further studies of caries, therefore, must accompany our advancing work upon periodontal disease.

In all the above studies, *sex* incidence was studied as well as age incidence. Females were consistently found to have less periodontal disease than males, though the differences, shown typically in Fig. 25, are not very great. Day states that in India females show a significantly lower bone loss of the periodontitis variety than do males, but a relatively high incidence of loss from periodontosis. Since periodontosis is a much less common phenomenon than the local-origin periodontitis, it will be seen that this finding is not of sufficient importance to counteract the general trend. Gingivitis alone seems to be more common in male children than in female.[3] Adult sex differences are similar. In both instances, better oral hygiene technique on the part of females is probably the cause. The American Dental Association 1965 study of dental needs shows white males on the average to require between 0.92 and 1.25 extractions for periodontal reasons in the age period 45–69, while females of similar age required only 0.34 to 1.06 such extractions.[42] The National Center for Health Statistics reports the same relationship for Periodontal Index scores among adults.

Epidemiological data are not sufficient as yet to differentiate *race* from environment in most studies of periodontal disease. Geographic differences in prevalence are becoming fairly obvious, and these are discussed under environmental factors for lack of evidence to the contrary. In the United States, at least four studies indicate a greater prevalence and severity of periodontal disease among blacks than among whites. Russell finds this among urban populations.[23] Rozier et al. find it in North Carolina. The two big national studies conducted by the National Center for Health Statistics, one in the early 1960s and one in the early 1970s, also find it.[24] Even these differences may be due more to educational background than to race, as will be mentioned later under the heading of environmental factors. Russell's ICNND studies from all over the world show certain rough regional groupings of populations with high or low periodontal disease, but little evidence of racial or ethnic trend.[25] On the contrary, Vietnam hill tribesmen show twice the severity of disease found among the regular Vietnamese.

On the subject of *intraoral variations* in periodontal disease,

Table 19. Prevalence of gingivitis and bone resorption in various countries.

Country	Author	Year of study	No. examined	Age (years)	Percent with gingivitis	Percent with bone resorption	Remarks
U.S.	Brucker[2]	1943	1634	4–16	8.7	—	Newark, N.J.
	Massler et al.[3]	1949	804	5–14	64.3	—	Suburban Chicago schoolchildren
	Day et al.[4]	1954	332	13–22	66.2	11.3	A representative cross-section of population, both sexes, Boston, Mass.
			238	23–34	79.4	80.4	
			331	35–48	86.8	98.7	
			286	49–up	91.8	100.0	
	Bossert and Marks[5]	1952	4478	16–24	—	3.8	Industrial employees, New York, N.Y., both sexes
			1973	25–34	—	13.0	
			3323	35–44	—	36.6	
			2164	45–54	—	54.9	
			862	55–69	—	69.6	
	Greene[16]	1958	577	11–17	92.0	0.5	Schoolchildren, Atlanta, Ga.
Canada	McIntosh[6]	1953	398	6–11	—	74.5	Low-income children, Toronto
Virgin Islands	Day and Shourie[7]	1950	823	6–18	57.1	—	Boys and girls, 91% black population
Great Britain	Ainsworth and Young[8]	1925	4063	2–15	60	—	Schoolchildren of England and Wales
Sweden	Westin et al.[9]	1937	1141	—	86.5	—	Schoolchildren
Italy	Schour and Massler[10]	1945	682	6–10	40.0	—	Patients, mostly low-income, examined by nutrition mission
			721	11–20	55.0	—	
			602	21–30	72.0	—	
			702	31–40	87.0	—	
			645	41–50	94.0	—	
			553	51–60	98.0	—	

Region	Author	Year	No.	Age	%	%	Description
Egypt (Cairo)	Dawson[12]	1946	423	15–25	95.9	—	Hospitalized patients
			351	26–35	99.6		
			200	36–up	100.0		
East Africa (Kenya)	Schwartz[11]	1945	89	4–19	18.0	0	Masai natives
			214	20–30	27.1	2.8	
			105	40–up	61.9	3.8	
India	Day and Shourie[13]	1944	613	5–15	73.7	5.7	Schoolchildren
			525	21–30	27.2	62.4	Police constables
			996	5–60	28.5	68.6	Hospital patients
	Day and Shourie[14]	1947	1054	9–17	99.4	—	Middle-class group
			261	6–20	73.6	—	High-class group
	Day and Shourie[15]	1949	95	9–12	—	0	Attending a clinic
			60	13–14	—	8.3	
			30	15–16	—	40.0	
			353	17–60	—	100.0	
China	Greene[16]	1957	1613	11–17	96.9	1.3	Schoolchildren, Bombay
	Anderson[17]	1929	100	15–30+	90.0	—	Male workers, Peiping (3 over age 30)
Australia	Clements and Kirkpatrick[18]	1938	530	—	63.0	—	European preschool and school children
Oceania	Campbell[19]	1939	350	—	50.0	—	Aborigines, all ages
	Williams[20]	1939	243	5–16	53.0	—	Samoan children, European and mixed descent
			712	5–20	54.0	—	Samoan children, Polynesian
	Davies[21]	1953	497	1–40+	45.0	—	Cook Islands, Polynesian (8 over age 40)

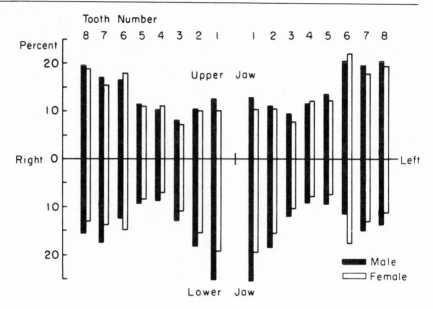

Figure 26. Percentage of individual teeth affected by periodontal disease among industrial employees aged 40–44, New York City, 1952.

Bossert and Marks again give us the best documentation.[5] The pattern they show fits well with clinical impression. Fig. 26 gives in bar-graph form the data pertaining to percentage of individual teeth affected by any form of periodontal disease in the New York sample aged 40–44. This age group is typical of the groups above and below it in that the upper molars and lower central incisors are seen to be the teeth most frequently affected, with the lower molars following closely behind. The teeth least affected are the lower bicuspids and the upper canines. The authors note a strangely consistent series of higher values for the upper left molars than for the upper right molars, which Fig. 26 also reflects. If future studies confirm such a departure from the pattern of bilateral symmetry seen in other phases of dental disease, a search for the cause will become of interest. Right-handed people are often seen to brush the teeth on the left side of the mouth better than those on the right side (though this difference is most marked in the anterior part of the mouth), and gingivitis can often be traced to areas neglected by the toothbrush. This observation would lead one to look for less periodontal disease on the left side instead of more.

In the field of *endocrine changes,* there is good statistical documentation of an increase in gingivitis among children as they approach puberty.[3,23] Similar increases in gingivitis have frequently been reported in individual cases among females at the times of menstruation and of pregnancy. The pregnancy changes are often quite marked and may proceed as far as the formation of small benign gingival tumors which disappear after parturition. Pathological endocrine changes which are reported associated with periodontal disease include hyperthyroidism (Grave's disease) and hyperparathyroidism.[26]

An important local host factor for periodontitis is found in *traumatic occlusion.* The supporting structures of the teeth are best designed to resist forces directed in the line of the long axis of the tooth. Circumstances arise, particularly where long, sharp cusps act as "plungers" or interlock with similar cusps in the opposite arch, in which individual teeth are subject to severe torque upon lateral excursion of the mandible. This situation produces forces destructive of the alveolar bone accompanied by tooth mobility and alveolar resorption. A somewhat similar local factor operates where improper relation between teeth at the contact point, or imperfectly contoured proximal restorations, permit *food impaction.* Here, bulky debris is lodged in the interproximal embrasure, causing chronic gingivitis and eventually destructive periodontal disease. A third factor associated with occlusion is *disuse.* A tooth, the opponent of which has failed to erupt or has been extracted, extrudes in time beyond its neighbors and the crest of the alveolus does not follow it. The result is a loss of alveolar support and susceptibility to periodontal disease. The situation is accentuated by the lack of cleansing action from mastication. The deposits which thus collect so heavily upon disused teeth predispose them to both gingivitis and dental caries.

Certain *occupational habits* and *neuroses* conduce to periodontal disease. The occupational habits include the holding of nails in the mouth, as by carpenters or upholsterers, thread biting among tailors, and the pressure of a reed or other mouthpiece upon the teeth of players of woodwind or other musical instruments. The neuroses include lip biting, cheek biting, bruxism, and the habitual biting of fingernails, pencils, and so forth. The use of tobacco may be classified as a habit. Excess smoking can cause thermal irritation of the gingivae and mucous membranes and over the years may conduce to leukoplakia. Another habit is misuse of the toothbrush, with consequent areas of cervical abrasion and gingival recession where the wear has occurred. A heavy horizontal toothbrush motion is usually the cause of such abrasion.

Concomitant disease is a final host factor for which to look. Diabetes and heavy-metal poisonings are among the commoner diseases predisposing to periodontal disease, chiefly gingivitis and periodontitis. None of these conditions seem likely to initiate periodontal disease but they accentuate it where it has started for other reasons. A rarer condition, but one which should be kept in mind by dental examiners, is leukemia or anemia. Acute monocytic leukemia may produce gingival enlargement, ulceration, and hemorrhage. Pernicious anemia may show an inflamed gingival margin standing out in sharp contrast to adjacent pale gingival mucosa.[27]

A clinical impression has existed that periodontal disease is more common in persons with *emotional disturbance*. Belting and Gupta confirm this impression in an adequately controlled study of over 100 mental patients.[28] Incidence of periodontal disease was significantly higher in all age groups, regardless of frequency of tooth brushing.

Agent Factors

Among local factors causing periodontal disease, the most prominent are bacteria, plaque, and calculus. Löe has demonstrated that *plaque* must be present for bacteria to gain a lasting hold in the periodontal area.[29] *Calculus* gives plaque a firmer hold on the neck of a tooth, defying the action of the toothbrush or dental floss. The process of calculus removal in dental prophylaxis usually takes plaque with it and arrests the disease process.[30,31]

The *bacterial* flora responsible for gingivitis and ultimately for destructive periodontitis are not fully understood. In the field of periodontosis (ideopathic juvenile periodontitis) a unique bacterial flora was found by Newman and Socransky. It was predominantly gram negative and strictly anaerobic at the advancing fronts of the lesions. Bacterial specificity has varied in other forms of periodontitis, but Socransky feels the question is no longer whether organisms cause periodontal disease but whether specific organisms are responsible for specific disease forms.[32]

Acute necrotizing ulcerative gingivitis (Vincent's infection) is a peculiarly destructive form of bacterial invasion, discussed in more detail under environmental factors. A mixed bacterial flora is usually involved, with the Vincent's spirochete predominant. This disease, if allowed to become chronic, can produce considerable periodontal damage through the destruction of gingival papillae, the prevention of proper oral hygiene, and so forth.

Certain *chemical* and *physical hazards* are known for their effects upon the periodontal tissues. Mercury, lead, and thallium, in decreasing order of frequency, have been reported to produce gingivitis accompanied by a dark line parallel to the gingival margin. In long-standing cases alveolar resorption occurs. Good oral hygiene will minimize these phenomena. Radium and other sources of ionizing radiation produce alveolar damage and loosening of the teeth.[33]

Environmental Factors

The study of environmental factors is very greatly dependent upon large-scale statistical studies which will rule out individual variability, particularly that resulting from host factors. For reasons which have been outlined, comparability is poor between those studies which are available. It is only beginning to be possible to say that certain *geographic areas* throughout the world are associated with more periodontal disease than others, and it is not yet possible to analyze what subfactors may contribute to these geographic variations. Table 19 summarizes those studies dealing with prevalence of periodontal disease which can be placed side by side with a minimum of risk. Comparisons of any sort are hard to make from this table, except with the work of Greene in India and in the United States. There is a small, though statistically significant ($p = 0.001$), difference in prevalence of gingivitis and a smaller difference in bone loss (not significant), with the higher figures coming from India.[16]

There is a strong clinical impression in the Harvard University Health Services that students from China, Japan, and the Philippines, as well as those from India, will show severe periodontal disease at an earlier age than will U.S. citizens, and less dental caries. Anderson's observations, showing 90 percent prevalence of hypertrophic gingivitis among Chinese workers aged 15 to 30, are in line with this impression.[17] So also are those of Mehta et al. in India, where a study of dental extractions showed 66.3 percent at all ages and 79.2 percent at ages above 30 to have been necessitated by periodontal disease.[34]

From material of this sort it is difficult to pick trends and also difficult to separate geographic from ethnic factors. Loos, comparing studies of periodontal disease in Europe, has similar difficulties, though he draws a conclusion that such disease is more widespread in southern than in northern countries, and that the southern and Dinaric races are more affected than others.[35] Russell, summarizing experiences from various parts of the world, finds it easiest to describe populations and regions according to whether such disease is relatively high, intermediate, or relatively low.[25] In the relatively high grouping he places Chile, Lebanon, Jordan, Thailand, Burma, some parts of Vietnam, Malaya, Ceylon, India, and Trinidad; in the intermediate group, the United States black population, Ecuador, Colombia, Ethiopia, and other parts of Vietnam; in the relatively low group, the United States white population and the primitive Eskimos of Alaska. Fig. 27 combines these findings with those from some other related studies. A weak generalization is possible to the effect that underdeveloped and dentist-deprived areas show greater scores for periodontal disease than developed countries, but exceptions do exist.

Nutrition is essentially an environmental problem. Aboard the old sailing ships avitaminosis C manifested itself as scurvy and produced acute periodontal disturbance accompanied by loss of teeth. The milder vitamin deficiencies associated with modern civilization are also conducive to periodontal disease over longer periods of time. Vitamin A deficiency may possibly show a positive correlation, though firm evidence is lacking. Niacin deficiency has been found to produce a severe type of necrotic gingivitis with pseudomembrane formation and associated sloughing along the buccal mucosae. Beyond these recorded results in human beings, experimental work in animals has shown other types of nutritional deficiency to affect the periodontium, notably protein starvation and magnesium deficiency.[36] In the ICNND studies, no consistent association was established between periodontal disease and the nutritive items observed. The overwhelming relation which did emerge was between disease and mouth cleanliness.[25]

One encouraging study deals with the possible relation of *fluoride* in the drinking water to periodontal disease. In three fluoride communities with 1.0, 2.5, and 8.0 parts per million of fluoride, respectively, in the drinking water, a weak tendency was found among native schoolchildren for periodontal disease to decrease as fluoride increased.[37] Migrant children served as controls. The differences found were slight, but they served to refute completely any hypothesis that periodontal tissues of children are harmed by use of a fluoride-bearing domestic water. Low figures for tooth mortality found among adults in endemic fluoride areas suggest a similar situation among older age groups.[38]

Degree of urbanization appears to be related to periodontal disease. In two studies of U.S. children, rural children were found to

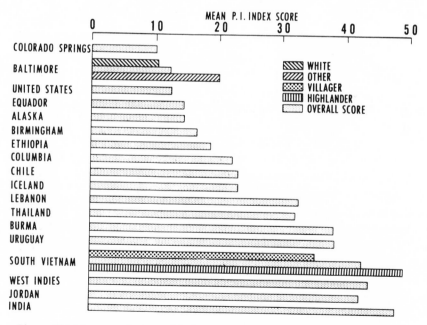

Figure 27. Mean periodontal index scores worldwide for ages 40–49.

have significantly higher group scores (Periodontal Index) than did urban children, particularly at the younger ages.[39] It is doubtful whether the difference can be attributed to rural life as such. Russell[31] feels *educational background* to be more important. He finds degree of education to be inversely related to the severity of periodontal disease once it has started. Mehta et al. suggest a similar situation in Bombay, India, when they report that the severity of disease increases with low socioeconomic groups and decreases with high socioeconomic groups.[16] Perhaps the answer lies in the more systematic home care and dental-maintenance care found among the well-to-do and the educated.

One of Russell's "unexplained and tantalizing enigmas" is his finding that *military* men 20–24 years of age studied in ten countries (not the United States) by the ICNND group showed on the average twice as much periodontal disease as their civilian counterparts.[25]

The epidemiology of acute necrotizing ulcerative gingivitis—*Vincent's infection*—has been of interest ever since World War I, when the disease received the name "trench mouth." Although obviously associated with a mixed infection and controllable in part by antibiotics, the disease no longer appears to be considered contagious. This concept stems largely from the fact that the organisms usually found in connection with this type of gingivitis are normally found in any healthy mouth. The onset of the disease appears to be caused more by environmental factors than agent factors. Whereas most studies of acute necrotizing ulcerative gingivitis have been made on military populations, Stammers has found the same age predilection to occur within a large civilian group.[40] The most important predisposing factor appears to relate to stress. Peacetime military groups appear to show greatest prevalence during or immediately following periods of leave. Giddon et al. found a monthly prevalence of the disease in a college population so timed that it appeared to have some relation to situational factors such as academic examinations or vacation periods.[41] Much more work needs to be done upon the distribution and determinants of this disease.

In programs for dental treatment, it must be realized that although the acute phase of Vincent's infection is easily controlled by antibiotics, a chronic continuance of the disease can usually not be avoided without careful removal of hard deposits harboring bacteria and causing lowered resistance at the necks of the teeth that are involved.

Treatment Needs in the United States

The recent drop in the incidence of childhood dental caries in developed countries has turned the attention of the dental profession quite sharply to the control of periodontal disease. The American Dental Association in its 1965 study of dental needs found only 9 percent of U.S. dental patients in need of periodontal treatment.[42] This probably reflected a lack of alertness to the diagnosis and treatment of periodontal disease.

Since that time, improved research and teaching and a general change of attitude within the profession appear to have increased awareness of periodontal disease. Gingivitis seems to be decreasing in prevalence, as shown in the decreasing oral hygiene scores (OHIS) of adults 18 to 79 years of age.[25] Better oral hygiene and more periodic dental prophylaxes could account for this finding. These same adults, however, show little change in proportions of periodontal disease with pockets. The oral hygiene scores drop more in the debris category than in the calculus category. These findings indicate that a serious treatment problem still remains.[24]

For the future, the drop in caries indicates an increasing retention of natural teeth into middle age and beyond, and the elderly proportion of the population is definitely on the increase. The factors thought responsible for the caries drop (fluorides and antibiotics) may also reduce the incidence of periodontal disease, but hardly enough to compensate for the increase in tooth retention. The best estimates at present indicate an increasng need for periodontal treatment in developed countries in the years to come. Chapter 13 carries more detailed projections on future treatment needs.

This brief presentation may well conclude with a word of hope and a word of warning. Hope lies in the fact that measurements for periodontal disease are improving and the study of the epidemiology of this condition is now attracting widespread attention. The warning deals with the varied nature of the conditions which go to make up periodontal disease and the perplexing way in which these conditions blend. Systemic factors undoubtedly exist about which we are yet unable to reason logically. Glickman's "bone factor" seems to be one of these, and may prove a term covering many factors.[43] The solving of the riddle of periodontal disease will undoubtedly involve cooperative work on the part of all types of research workers in the field of biological science. In addition, dental practitioners and public health workers must devote more effort to control measures for periodontal disease than seems to be made at present.

MALFORMATIONS

The epidemiology of oral malformations is relatively new. Malocclusions, to be sure, have been studied ever since the specialty of orthodontics arose, but the absence of good objective measures for severity of malocclusion and the wide differences in subjective interpretation as to which malocclusions were and which were not considered disabling have hampered comparison between studies and reliable estimates of prevalence. Chapter 14 discusses the indices which are currently coming into use for the measurement of malocclusions. None, however, have achieved enough widespread use to have produced a reliable epidemiological literature. Certain localized studies do permit internal comparisons. Thus Ast in Newburgh and Kingston, New York, and Erickson and Graziano in North Carolina have shown water fluoridation to reduce the incidence of malocclusion.[44] These studies are matched by others in which no differences were found.

Angle's classification is, of course, the best-known means of categorizing types of malocclusion, though offering no information on severity or the amount of disability found. Møller, in an excellent chapter on malocclusion, groups 17 studies of prevalence covering seven countries into one table.[45] The prevalence of malocclusion per study ranges from 42 to 91 percent of population surveys, from which one may assume both that the diagnosis of malocclusion is a somewhat subjective matter and that most malocclusions found are non-disabling. This same author interprets his data to indicate that there is no significant sex difference in prevalence of malocclusion, that blacks and American Indians have less malocclusion than whites, that oral habits such as thumb sucking are probable causes of malocclusion, and that there is a positive association between malocclusion and periodontal disease.

Jago, in a survey of 44 studies covering 18 countries, finds that reports of malocclusion range all the way from 1.0 to 90 percent of the child population.[46] He considers the use of the term *malocclusion*, irrespective of functional disability, to be sufficiently vague to justify abandoning it. He finds no evidence of a relationship between occlusal anomalies and other oral conditions, including caries. Age, sex, and geographical location seem equally unimportant. He finds Angle's classification to be "a qualitative indicator, and not a quantitative index."

Of greater importance in planning aid for severely disabled children and in counseling their parents is the work which has established certain expected frequencies of the occurrence of *clefts of the lip and/or palate*. Greene estimates new clefts to occur at a rate of 6,000 per year, or 1.3 per 1,000 live births in the United States.[47] Cleft lip is somewhat more common in the male, and cleft palate in the female; a combination of both clefts is a little more common in the male. Both genetic and environmental forces appear to be involved and these have not as yet even been well described. Hypothecation as to causation awaits further work. Curtis et al. have made estimates of the probability that further clefts would appear in children born subsequently into families where clefts have already occurred in a sibling or in one of the parents.[48] These figures are of considerable interest in family planning. Greene summarizes other research to indicate that blacks have a much lower rate of clefts than whites, that highest rates are found among Orientals, and that clefts occur more commonly in plural births, children born prematurely or to older parents, and children with other malformations.[49]

ORAL CANCER

The death rate from oral cancer, approximating 3 per 100,000 persons in the United States, in recent years is large enough to demand attention in the public health field. Older persons are naturally more vulnerable than younger, with more than three-quarters of the deaths occurring among persons 55 years of age or older.[50] More males are involved than females. The cure rate for oral cancer does not exceed 30 percent. For this reason, there is a high premium on early recognition and prompt treatment of the condition.[51] Of all sites classified as buccal cavity and pharynx, the chances of survival are best for lip cancer, followed in order by cancer of the salivary glands, mouth, tongue, and pharynx.[52]

The relative frequency of oral cancer compared to all malignancies appears much higher in Southeast Asian countries than in Western countries.[48] In Europe, significantly higher mortality rates are found in France (8.2) and Switzerland (6.4) than elsewhere.[53] Some material on the prevention of cancer is found in Chapter 12, and methods for cancer detection are discussed in Chapter 14.

Among precancerous lesions, leukoplakia is probably the most important. Considerable descriptive epidemiology has been done on this disease, a good digest of which appears in *Dental Abstracts*.[54] On oral cancer itself, a fine comprehensive review appears in Chapter 3 of Pelton's *Epidemiology of Oral Health*.[55]

CHAPTER 10

The Social Sciences

PREVIOUS CHAPTERS have dealt with tools of public health which measure the physical causes and the physical manifestations of disease, and with these there has been some consideration of psychological factors as they might affect an individual patient. The public health worker, however, when he embarks upon organized community effort, is very dependent upon the group behavior of individuals, determined by their culture. *Culture* may be defined as a shared and organized body of customs, skills, ideas, and values which is transmitted socially from one generation to another. Human beings in groups, as well as individually, react to their environment in terms of their culture.

It is often very difficult to realize the strong influence of culture till one sees the difference between one's own reaction to a fairly simple situation and that of an individual from a different cultural background. An illustration of this is in the difficulty experienced by Christian missionaries in making the New Testament understood in Chinese. Jesus, after his resurrection, is pictured as sitting upon the right hand of God—the right side, of course, being the side of honor. To the Chinese, the left is the honored side. Thus the whole implication of this biblical passage becomes reversed if it is translated into Chinese literally.

Public health workers face similar difficulties in program planning. Thus, as previously mentioned, a representative of a district health service, attempting to reduce the incidence of malaria and tuberculosis in rural Peru by inducing the people to boil their drinking water, found her efforts frustrated by a long-standing tradition that only sick people drank boiled water.[1] To do this was to advertise oneself as sick, not well. Long and patient education was needed to overcome this cultural barrier.

It is one of the important developments in public health during the last decade that the social scientists have been called in to aid in adapting new health programs to existing cultural patterns. Culture refers to many items, which in combination form a system, its parts interconnected. A look at other cultures often helps us to understand our own, and an understanding of the whole culture is often necessary in order to change one item. To change one item, therefore, one must often change many. Note, for instance, the difficulty the dental profession has found, and still finds, in restricting refined carbohydrates in patients' diets. The chief offenders are candy or sweets, both so long considered desirable that they have become symbolic of the good things in life. They are given to children as prizes for good behavior, even by physicians following medical visits. In addition, large commercial interests have become involved in their manufacture. Only in the past three decades has the American Dental Association dared to warn frankly of the danger of candy to the teeth. The adjustment of American culture to the limited and wise use of candy by caries-susceptible individuals has constituted a major challenge. Though the adjustment is by no means complete, it seems to be proceeding favorably in certain social groups.

SOCIAL SCIENCES DEFINED

The social sciences, as they are referred to in college curricula, usually include sociology, cultural anthropology, and psychology.

They frequently also include economics and government—and sometimes history as well. The term "behavioral sciences" covers almost the same ground, but is usually considered to omit history, government, and economics and to include more material at the edge of natural science, particularly psychiatry. The disciplines in the behavioral group are of most help in public health planning. Each subject has its subdivisions and its linkages with other subjects. Most helpful at the moment are the workers in the field of social psychology, sociology, and cultural anthropology. Among these, the methods often differ more than the subject matter. As Paul describes it, psychological research tends to lean heavily upon experimental data, with people or animals used as subjects; sociological research leans heavily upon the use of questionnaires and interviews, most commonly single interviews of many people; anthropology leans heavily upon direct observations of behavior and, as a rule, upon repeated and extensive interviews with a relatively few informants who come to be known fairly well.[2]

Lest this listing of scientific disciplines appear more formidable than it really is, an illustration may help to show the commonsense material with which the social scientist has to deal; it is so simple, in fact, that he may overlook it for its very obviousness. A story is told of Dr. John Cassel, an American physician stationed at the time among the Zulus of South Africa.[3] He was called in one day to see an old Zulu man who was severely ill. Dr. Cassel diagnosed the case as one of tuberculosis accompanied by cavity formation in one lung and with a poor prognosis. He advised the man's family to come to the clinic for drugs. This they did not do, but called instead a woman witch doctor, who declared that the man was bewitched by his only son and the son's new bride, who both lived with him in his home. The witch doctor advised sending the young couple away from the home and taking steps to disinherit the son. The old man followed this advice, and soon improved in health, to the surprise of Dr. Cassel, who saw him a month later. Dr. Cassel investigated the situation and found that the son had become a ne'er-do-well, squandering both his father's and his older sister's money, and insisting by Zulu custom that the sister should have no status in the house. This situation had led to tensions, arguments, and eventually blows. The witch doctor had released the old man from all this so that he could recover. In retrospect, Dr. Cassel remarked, "When I was called in to diagnose the case, my total diagnosis consisted of a hole in the lung and I missed all the psychological and cultural factors. The witch doctor, on the other hand, had diagnosed the whole setup, and had missed only the hole in the lung. Of the two, I should imagine that her diagnosis was more complete than mine."

Coming closer to home, Paul calls attention to studies which demonstrate characteristically differing reactions of Jewish, Italian, and Anglo-American patients to *pain experience.* The Jewish and Italian patients are like each other in responding expressively to pain sensations, but they do not have the same reasons for doing so. Italians tend to be more oriented toward the present and to regard pain primarily as an unpleasant state. They respond well to anodynes and have confidence in the doctor. Jews are more oriented toward the future and worry more about the symptomatic meaning of pain; they are sometimes suspicious of pain-relieving drugs and inclined to have less confidence in the competence of doctors. Doctors from an Anglo-American background characteristically assume that the appearance of suffering should be suppressed. Confronted by Jewish or Italian patients whose culture disposes them to express their feelings, these doctors understandably but unjustly think the patients are "exaggerating" and putting on an insincere act.

SOCIAL SCIENCE IN PROGRAM PLANNING

When applied to a practical problem such as dental program planning, social science in effect adds a new dimension to the process of surveying and evaluation. Without the social scientist, it is fairly easy to decide what a given program should attempt to do, and to measure the effort theoretically needed for the execution of the program. It is also possible without his aid to measure fairly well the effect of the program in terms of reduced susceptibility to dental caries or increased amounts of dental care received, or other measures of a similar sort. The social scientist becomes really necessary when effort and effect do not match each other and we want to know why. He helps us in the assessment of the process our program is using or plans to use, in finding out how well this process fits with the sociocultural system of the group with which we are working. This sociocultural system is as important a part of the group's environment as are the physical surroundings which form so much of the basis for the study of epidemiology. This is especially true in the field of chronic diseases, where people's living habits have so much to do with their susceptibility to disease.

An example of social science in connection with dental public health planning is of interest. Jong, conducting the dental phase of Project Head Start for the city of Boston in 1967, sought information about the attitudes and habits of the Head Start families in order to plan suitable referral-to-care facilities for children found in the dental-screening program to have dental needs.[4] An interview schedule was designed with the aid of a psychologist. A team of interviewers—eight dental hygienists and three senior dental students—were then given a 3-day orientation in the use of the schedule. By the end of the summer 646 families had been interviewed, representing 83 percent of the total active enrollment in Head Start that year. The interview schedule comprised data under two main headings: social and demographic measures, and dental care variables. In the former category were questions on residence, number of children in family, welfare recipient status, occupation of the head of the house, educational status, annual family income, and race. The dental care variables included such questions as: Does the respondent have a regular source of dental care? Is it a public or private dental facility? When were dental services last obtained? Were preventive measures used? Was restorative dental care completed? What were the respondent's feelings about going to the dentist as a child and also about going in recent years? What were the dental care costs of the family during the past 12 months?

The findings of this survey made it clear that while over half of the respondents reported a dental visit during the past 12 months, the family approach to dental care had been of the crisis variety, with little attention to preventive services. The population was by no means homogeneous in status or outlook. It appeared that the supply of dentists was not a major factor in the utilization of dental services, and that income, education, and residential stability played important roles. Almost one-half of the families identified dental clinics as their regular source of family dental care. It was found that a considerable number of the respondents left their own community to obtain dental care, and these patterns of travel were recorded. For the families that were interviewed, the interviews contributed largely to a proper orientation, accounting for a good showing of completed dental care cases in subsequent months. General findings were also made, for instance, that because the disadvantaged population of the city depended heavily on clinic facilities, it was of the utmost importance that these clinics offer a full range of preventive services, including prophylaxis, topical fluoride treatment, early diagnosis, and frequent recall.

Social scientists may also play a major role in public health experiments. In Chapter 15 one such experiment in the dental field is presented in which social scientists and health educators have appraised the use of fear in motivating high school children to seek dental care. In the broad field of public health many such cases are available and make excellent reading for the dentist. Paul has assembled a number of case studies of public reactions to health programs in his volume entitled *Health, Culture, and Community,* designed particularly for the teaching of students of preventive medicine and public health.[5] Many of these cases deal with programs that failed, but the analysis of these failures can help us in constructing more successful programs.

ATTITUDES TOWARD TEETH AND DENTAL CARE

Dentists have long been disturbed because their appraisals of dental disease were not taken seriously, and their recommendations for treatment were not followed or were followed only in part. It is obvious that many people do not consider their teeth very important and give dental care a low priority. Why should this situation exist and what can be done about it?

One of the best studies of this problem was made for the American Dental Association by behavioral scientists on the staff of Social Research, Inc.[6] The subjects for study were a group of 126 men, women, and children living in a typical Midwestern community. These people were selected by a quota sampling according to age and sex and according to the social-class distribution then commonly used among sociologists. All were given careful and detailed interviewing on their attitudes toward teeth, dental care, and dentists. Some of the findings of this study are of interest.

One major finding of this study is reassuring: people in this area did consider their teeth to be essential physiologically, whether they were natural or artificial. In addition, people were aware of the relation between teeth and appearance and were quick to associate certain personality characteristics with certain types of teeth. These reactions were elicited by asking interviewees what they thought people might be like if they had a certain characteristic appearance such as even white teeth or a "toothy grin." The interviewees considered that teeth refer to the general state of health of a person and are symbolic of a person's age. As for care, they had apparently learned the tooth-brushing lesson quite well and it seems about the only lesson they have learned. They said in effect that "brushing is the thing," and seemed to feel the more frequent and the more vigorous the brushing the better it was. They were inclined not to attach much importance to preventive dentistry and to associate dentists more closely with the final stages of dental problems than with preventive measures. A very interesting feature of the study is its description of certain *social classes* and the reaction of each to dental care.

The *upper middle class* is defined here as "the professional and business executive group, well educated, living in preferred areas in well-maintained, usually spacious homes." The members of this class "seek out 'expert' advice, and, in areas where they feel it is important, follow the advice with considerable religiosity. They take a long-range view of life and want to feel prepared to know how to prevent or at least to deter as long as possible the unavoidable: aging, disease, decay, death."[6] They value their teeth, are interested in preventive dentistry, and actively pursue various types of dental care. The dentist is visualized as a professional who not only repairs teeth and stops pain, but also prevents decay and loss of teeth and makes a person's teeth more attractive and useful. The members of the upper middle class are much impressed with the desirability of having their own teeth for as long as possible. They "think of themselves as highly rational people, willing to be swayed only by authoritative sources."[6]

The *lower middle class* includes generally the owners of small businesses, minor executives, teachers, salesmen, and white-collar workers. "They are a highly moralistic group, usually with at least a high school education, and live in well-maintained, clean, pleasant neighborhoods."[6] They are inclined to admire and imitate the upper middle class, but their behavior is not necessarily motivated by the same considerations. They wish to be considered *proper* and consider duty a value in and of itself. They are not nearly so individualistic as the upper middle group; they are the most compulsive in their dental care attitudes and practices of any social class. "The dentist is regarded as an authority—not always a friendly authority (as tends to be the case among upper middle class people) but someone who 'fixes' teeth."[6] The dentist is also viewed as one who gives directions as to how teeth should be cared for and who is useful for preventive dentistry. Training in dental health habits begins early in the group and is followed with persistence, though not always with accompanying flexibility. The necessity to be clean, good, conforming, and socially presentable makes for a high standard of dental care among people at this status level.

The *upper lower class* is regarded as "the group which needs to become the objective of major educational efforts regarding dental care, and this is primarily because they are the most accessible to these attempts and offer the best possibilities of behavioral and attitudinal changes."[6] The upper lower class people are generally skilled and semiskilled blue-collar workers. At present they enjoy a high standard of living as measured by income, but they are people of limited education and live in modest neighborhoods; they are law-abiding, respectable, and hard-working citizens. "They set fewer regulations for themselves than the lower middle class and are indulgent of themselves and permissive with their children. In rather sharp contrast to higher-status groups, upper lower class people are resigned to whatever happens and feel there is little they can do to stave off the inevitable,"[6] including the loss of their teeth. On the basis of this attitude, it is probable that they do not receive professional dental care geared to maintaining their own teeth. They acquire artificial dentures at a relatively early age and are reasonably happy with them. "Self-medication, based on popular notions of what illness is and what remedies are apt to relieve or cure it, does interest them. As for physicians or dentists, they typically do not have continuing personal relations with authority figures of this type."[6] They instruct their children how to care for their teeth, but the children are more or less on their own after that.

As a group, these people are often happier receiving their care from a clinic than from an individual practitioner. They acquire confidence in the reputation of the clinic, in part because the clinic was started by a well-known agency or in a certain area to serve them, and in part because they see their friends there. This can lead to what has been called "the clinic habit."[7] These people become so dependent on the clinic that if they graduate from the classification served, as school children do, they find it difficult to adapt to private practice.

The *lower class,* now called *underprivileged* or *disadvantaged,* is estimated to constitute about 20 percent of our urban populations. It consists of the unskilled laborers, people who shift from job to job, have a limited education, live in slum areas, and exhibit (from a middle-class point of view) no stable pattern of life.[6] As a group they are the ones who reveal the most consistent neglect of teeth, and because of their cultural differences from the middle class, they require careful understanding if they are to receive adequate care in public health facilities.

One of the best of the detailed documentations of the attitudes of underprivileged people toward health care is Trithart's summary of two workshops on understanding the underprivileged child, held in 1968 and conducted by Frank B. W. Hawkinshire. So well has Trithart summarized the attitudes of the underprivileged that his listing is given here in full, with my notations in brackets, as an aid to health planners.

Castration complex: There is a reluctance to be at the complete mercy of the health practitioner. This is marked by reluctance to have a general anesthetic or sedation for dental or surgical procedures. [This complex is sometimes offset by a desire on the part of parents to spare their children pain which can not be adequately explained to them. Thus parents sometimes request a general anesthetic for children rather than a local anesthetic, even in fairly simple cases of operative dentistry.]

Contradiction of common sense: Some dental or medical procedures such as the continuation of a drug after acute symptoms have subsided seem to contradict common sense. It is recommended that a common sense approach rather than a scientific approach be used in giving dental advice or dispensing drugs.

Coming in crowds: Disadvantaged people do not like to be outnumbered by the people providing treatment. For this reason, they tend to come in crowds, with family and friends, to private dental offices or public clinics. The privacy of individualized treatment in a dental office may be a terrorizing experience.

The last-ditch effort: The disadvantaged often turn to medical or dental treatment by health professionals as a last resort after all individual efforts have failed. They are in a sense challenging health professionals to salvage something from an almost hopeless situation. [Dummett cites the case of a mother who pointed out that if she went to the clinic at Watts in California it would cost her $2.30 in carfare; she would have to wait six hours in all likelihood, get no treatment, and would be unable to go to her job, thus losing a day's pay of $12. If she went to a private physician she would be charged $10 for the visit and $5 for a shot of penicillin; therefore, it was her custom to "wait until her family was $15 worth of sick before going to the physician."]

If it hurts, you are a quack: This group has the general feeling that medical and dental treatment should be painless and, if it hurts, the health practitioner does not know what he is doing. In those instances in which pain or discomfort will be caused by dental procedures, the patient should be informed so that he can be prepared for it.

Unclean or dirty feeling: The aseptic cleanliness of a dental office or clinic may convey the feeling of personal uncleanliness. This feeling may be reinforced by the dentist washing his hands after he treats the disadvantaged person. Such simple procedures as hand washing should be explained.

The clinic was built there, not here: Since many health facilities, such as hospitals and out-patient clinics, are located at inconvenient places for the underprivileged, many of them tend to think and say, "If you really cared about me you would have built the hospital or clinic here instead of there."

Cold professional attitudes: Many disadvantaged people complain about the cold, impersonal, objective attitude and conduct of health professionals. They value empathy as well as professional competence as an essential characteristic of the practitioner.

Difference in pain threshold: There may be a wider variation in the pain threshold of the disadvantaged than in the population in general. The pain threshold for those in poor health may be low. Patients should be prepared for pain if it is to occur.

Complication of the unknown: Fear of the unknown is a natural human tendency. This feeling is accentuated with underprivileged people since there are so many things that are unknown to them.

The pills don't work: There is a tendency to expect immediate results from the administration of any drug. Any time lag between administration of a drug and relief from symptoms may be considered a failure of the drug and its use may be discontinued.

Appointments not important: Appointments of any kind have never been an integral part of the lives of the underprivileged. There is no reason to expect them to consider dental appointments as a means of conserving their time as well as the practitioner's. Patience and understanding are essential in educating them to the value of keeping appointments.

Teeth lost anyhow: There is a feeling that despite competent and conscientious personal and professional care, the ultimate loss of teeth is one of the natural vicissitudes of life. Patience, understanding, and continuing education are essential to overcome this fatalistic attitude.

Traditions: Contrary to some beliefs widely held by the more affluent segments of our society, impoverished families and neighborhoods have strong and deep-seated traditions. To communicate and deal with disadvantaged people, it is important that these traditions be recognized and understood. It is also important that these traditions not be discredited unless they are actually harmful to health.[8]

Perhaps as an expression of these attitudes, community groups, particularly in underprivileged areas, have very clear feelings about the priorities in the health care field and the way health care is rendered. They realize their lack of expertise in the technical and scientific aspects of health care, but they want a real control in matters of priority, delivery of care, and perhaps even personnel selection.

Whenever consumers or consumer groups express themselves in the United States, a certain pattern of complaint has appeared in recent years. Angevine, speaking for the Ad Hoc Advisory Committee of the President's Committee on Consumer Interests, has summarized the situation by stating that "the average consumer is concerned and frustrated by increasing costs of medical care without a compensating improvement in health care."[9] Over a 20-year period, medical service prices have more than doubled, and an increasing number of Americans are being "priced out" of good medical care. In the United States, where we are spending over 10 percent of our Gross National Product on health care, the lower-income segment of our population is receiving poorer health care than in many European countries that spend only 6 percent of their Gross National Product on health care. Within the federal government, health-care expenditures have more than tripled in recent years, but spiraling costs, fragmentation, and disorganization have prevented the effective use of this money. Consumers feel that the country needs a plan or system for allocating and using the medical care dollar so that better care will be rendered more efficiently than it is now.

ATTITUDES TOWARD HIGH CARIES INCIDENCE

Trithart's remark that the underprivileged consider their "teeth lost anyhow" applies to considerable segments of the United States population which have been faced by high caries incidence and low financial resources. The remark applies also to entire populations regardless of income when faced by disastrously high caries, as in the case of New Zealand.

Early in the twentieth century, Sir Thomas Hunter noted such a severity of caries in New Zealand that it was common for fathers to give their daughters full dentures as a wedding present. Hunter's response was the founding of the New Zealand School Dental Service, whereby over the years dental nurses reduced tooth loss among children almost to zero. Adults who were not reached as children by this service, as well as adults and the dental profession in general, had become so accustomed to removable prosthetic treatment that years after the young children were found to be keeping their teeth, the adults still exhibited an unusually high rate of tooth loss.

In 1976, the Dental Research Unit of the Medical Research Council of New Zealand conducted a thorough epidemiological survey of adult oral conditions, treatment needs, oral behavior, and attitudes toward dental care.[10] They found over one-quarter of persons 35 to 44 years of age to be edentulous, and higher proportions were edentulous above that age. Treatment needs, however, were relatively low. The number of edentulous persons without dentures was extremely small. Efforts to explain the phenomenon of adult tooth loss led only to recognition of an attitude, both professional and lay, favorable to tooth extraction and a "decision to move to the edentulous state." The report concludes that "clearly, the individual considering the future of his or her natural dentition, appears to face, both at the professional and lay level, little positive encouragement to retain natural teeth."

Fortunately, New Zealand is now among the countries reporting lowered childhood caries incidence. Many of its cities are now fluoridated. The dental nurses, still rendering primary care to 98 percent of the elementary school children, can talk prevention rather than spending most of their time on fillings and extractions.[11] The rate of adult edentulism is dropping.

ATTITUDES TOWARD DENTIST

The American Dental Association study casts interesting light upon public attitudes toward the dentist himself. In general, "the dentist occupies a high status in the minds of people and as such he and his profession evoke a feeling of respect from most individuals."[6] This attitude is akin to feelings people have about physicians, yet in general the dentist is seen as someone possessing specialized knowledge and techniques but not as well educated as the physician. The dentist is concerned with a limited and more external portion of the body and is not completely identified with the broad, progressive, developing field of medicine. Though not fully revealed by the present data, there are suggestions that lower middle class people are most favorable in their attitudes toward the dentist. Upper middle class individuals tend to be somewhat critical, though they certainly accept him, whereas lower class individuals give evidence of respecting him as an authority, but at the same time being more intimidated and possibly more resentful of him.

Turning now from the dentist himself to a patient's eye view of dental treatment, such criticisms as were registered during the course of the study seemed to center upon the following points, in decreasing order of importance: (1) pain and the anticipation of pain, (2) high cost (though this factor never seems to be the sole determinant of whether a person cares for or neglects his teeth), (3) the overcrowded nature of many dentists' schedules, and (4) rough handling or lack of personal attention. On the constructive side, patients are more likely to go to their dentist for preventive purposes if the dentist has a recall system, has an assistant, performs dental prophylaxis, x-rays the teeth, has a high-speed dental engine, and, finally, takes a personal interest in his patients.

Certain aspects of the dentist-patient relationship deserve mention because they relate to children in public dental services. Thus

Frankel et al. studying children 3 to 5 years of age found that they reacted more favorably to local anesthetic and restorative dentistry when their mothers came into the operatory and less favorably when separated from their mothers.[12] The mother's own level of anxiety, however, was a factor of importance. Johnson and Baldwin report that children of mothers with high anxiety scores showed significantly more negative behavior during an extraction than did children of mothers with low anxiety scores.[13]

The waiting period for dental extraction was considered in two further studies by Baldwin.[14] Older children about to undergo extraction for orthodontic reasons were compared with a control group not receiving extraction. Children without a waiting period showed a distinctly different pattern in a "draw-a-person" test from that of those with a waiting period. These tests, and interviews, established that extractions did produce stress, but that it was greatly lessened by warning and a waiting period, and that recovery from stress was greatly hastened by these procedures.

ESTIMATION OF INDIGENCE

One very practical problem upon which social scientists can help is the estimation of the proportion of a population in need of public aid in obtaining health care. Where some indigence is thought to exist and to merit aid, the next question to be solved is the economic strength of the community. Here, specific measures exist, most of them applied to "welfare" work rather than health.

In 1967 Wallace et al. examined the availability and "usefulness" of 29 indicators that might be used for characterizing census tracts in an urban area according to their need for medical or social services. To be "useful" an indicator had to be based on reliable data and be "associated with other high indexes in the same tract. It was assumed that the existence of several high indexes pointed to a need for medical or general services." Of 29 indicators examined, the following were judged "useful":

Health Indexes:
  Inadequate prenatal care: Number of live births with no prenatal care or care only in the third trimester, per 1,000 live births.
  Fetal mortality: Infants over 400 grams born dead per 1,000 live births.

Incidence of prematurity: Infants born alive weighing 2,500 grams or less at birth per 1,000 live births.

Tuberculosis incidence: Reported new cases per 10,000 population.

Social Indexes:

Unemployment: Unemployed males in civilian labor force per 1,000 males in civilian labor force.

Low income: Families with annual incomes under $3,000, per 1,000 families. [It would be more than $3,000 today.]

Inadequate education: Adults with 8th grade education or less, per 1,000 adult population.

Overcrowding: Housing units with more than 1.0 persons per room, per 1,000 housing units.

Parental composition: Children under 18 not living with two persons, per 1,000 population under 18 years.

School-age illegitimacy: Illegitimate live births to mothers aged 15–19, per 1,000 live births.

Juvenile delinquency: Boys 8–17 charged with a non-traffic offense by police or juvenile court, per 1,000 male population 8–17.[15]

The work of Wallace et al. is a good example of the localization of need by geographic area and points out clearly the interrelationship of ill health and social pathology. It is interesting to note that several indexes, including neonatal and postnatal mortality, that are reported by others to differentiate socioeconomic areas, were found not to be "useful" in this study.

A good example of the application of such measurement to the problem of health care was made by the Greater Boston area in 1948.[16] A rank list of the various communities was constructed, for use in assigning priorities for public assistance. This rank list was also of great use in appraising the supposed adequacy of the number of public-service dentist hours per 1,000 children per year found to be provided in each community, as shown in Fig. 28.[17]

For estimating the socioeconomic position of a given individual or family, several indexes are used. One good one is Hollingshead's 2-factor index of social position, where the breadwinner's occupation and education are estimated on a 5-point scale, with professional people, executives, and the like in the first position and unskilled and uneducated persons in the fifth, or lowest, position.[18]

From general information of the kind just outlined, and from

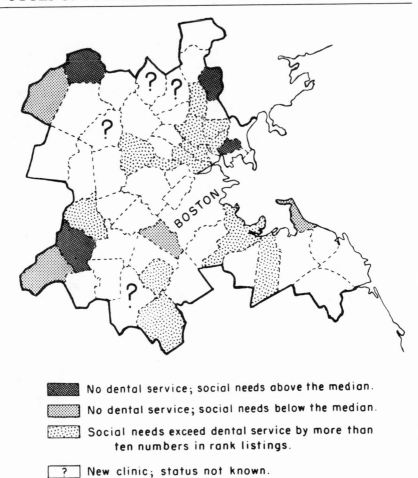

No dental service; social needs above the median.

No dental service; social needs below the median.

Social needs exceed dental service by more than ten numbers in rank listings.

? New clinic; status not known.

Figure 28. Dental services that are apparently substandard as compared with index of social need, Greater Boston area, 1946–1947.

our knowledge of the per capita income of a family, estimates of indigence can be made. The lowest level involves real *indigence*, where welfare assistance is mandatory in order to prevent gross neglect and starvation. Local and state welfare boards have their rules of thumb for such determinations, usually varied in accordance with the recommendations of trained social workers where unusual conditions are found to exist. The next higher level involves inability to pay for large programs of medical care, even though the basic needs of the family can otherwise be met. This situation is termed *medical indigence* and forms the basis for setting up eligibility levels for government medical assistance in such a form as is offered by Title XIX (Medicaid). Chapter 22 discusses this program in further detail.

Where large-scale international studies are being made, much simpler methods must be used. The World Health Organization, in its International Collaborative Study, uses merely the total number of years at school as an indicator of the social position of the adult respondents.[19] However, as educational systems differed between countries, the main purpose of such measurement was to see if there was any intra-area variation connected with the socio-economic and educational distribution of the samples.

FUNCTIONS OF SOCIAL WORKER

The emergence of widespread financial aid to the indigent and medically indigent has brought into being the need for a new professional group to aid the planners of public health programs: the social workers. These people, with special training in the social sciences, are experts at appraising personal and family economic problems and in organizing sensible patterns for health care, education, and home life. They are needed especially where multiple problems exist such as the combination of low income, loss of a parent, and physical disability or mental illness. Careful interviewing is needed to appraise these "hard-core" cases and refer them to agencies where they will receive adequate assistance, professional as well as financial. The social worker can help the public health dentist in appraising the accessibility of low-income patients to health care facilities and the cultural "fit" of the family to the type of care, appointment schedule, and other conditions found in these facilities. We are beginning to realize there is a special "culture of poverty" in which there is not only lack of money, but a helplessness to make use of even those facilities which are within economic reach. A good example of the usefulness of the social worker in a low-income child health clinic in the Boston area is reported by Cowin et al.[20] A small staff of social workers here aided a larger group of public health nurses and pediatricians, and eventually the dental hygienists and dentists of the program.

FLUORIDATION

It is hard to call to mind an issue which has thrown a somewhat retiring professional group into the public arena more suddenly than has the fluoridation issue the members of the dental profession. For decades the dental profession has had little to offer in the way of mass preventive measures requiring community action. Then, within a very short space of years, a powerful preventive procedure has been devised which is effective, inexpensive, and endorsed by the medical profession, public health workers, and groups to which it is of concern. It is the irony of fate that this method cannot be applied to volunteers with more than a fraction of its total cost-effectiveness, but must be applied through a major public utility, the communal water supply. A clearcut governmental decision is needed on every fluoridation program, whether it is made by elected or appointed officials or by referendum to the whole voting population. It is not compulsory to drink from a communal water supply, but it is difficult enough to avoid doing so that a cry of "compulsion" is often raised.

The dentist, suddenly thrown into a community fluoridation controversy, realizes he is dealing not merely with a professional matter where scientific evidence can be weighed objectively, but with a public political problem of very high voltage. He has been expecting to have to educate people on the benefits of fluoridation and also upon its systemic safety. For this scientific task he can be pretty well prepared, thanks to clearcut reports in the dental journals, but for political maneuvering he is not so ready. Even scientifically, he tends to rely upon the opinions of the U.S. Public Health Service, the American Medical Association, and other national associations, rather than upon the factual evidence upon which these opinions are based. He is distinctly not prepared for the proportion of the population which is ignorant of the dosage concept and insistent upon saying "once a poison always a poison." Neither is he prepared for those who would raise the flag of individual and minority rights and insist that their personal freedom is being violated by fluoridation. In addition, he is surprised to note that the antifluoridation cause draws to it not only the fanatics, the paranoid fringe, and the health faddists, among them some very powerful orators, but also a large mass of older, conservative people who simply do not want to adopt a personal health measure on the basis of an incomplete knowledge of the scientific facts.

Opponents of Fluoridation. The vehemence of the anti-fluoridation reaction was such as to attract the attention not only of physicians and other health workers, but of the social scientists too. Social-science studies have been made in several areas. Regardless of their immediate outcome in terms of new communities adopting fluoridation, the dental profession will be much better off because of these studies.

The first efforts of the social scientists on the matter of fluoridation have usually involved studies of communities in which heated contests have occurred, with emphasis upon the opinions of the vocal antifluoridationists. Of greatest interest to them have been such communities as Northampton and Williamstown, Massachusetts, where the controversy reached its heat after the adoption of fluoridation and the measure was later abandoned. In the former community, the Mausners became struck by the pervasive attitude of suspicion among those who oppose fluoridation.[21] There was suspicion not only of scientific organizations, but of the scientists themselves. Some antifluoridationists found it perfectly reasonable to suppose that scientists would lend themselves to a conspiracy with enemies of our country (the Communist "brainwashing plot" theme) and at the same time would permit themselves to be used by a giant monopoly (the Aluminum Corporation of America, which was supposed to be profiting from the sale of fluorides). This attitude of suspicion was so clearcut, so prevalent, and so polarized, that the Mausners named it "the antiscientific attitude" and used that term for the title of their article. Other workers in this field do not feel that real antagonism exists, but merely that the vocal antifluoridationists (who are probably not as large a proportion of the whole group as one might imagine) differ in their definition of science.[22] These vocal enthusiasts may include in the ranks of scientists a number of fringe paramedical groups, and be unable to distinguish between these and the major professional groups responsible for the main mass of evidence in a field such as fluoridation.

In general, the evidence suggests the hypothesis that people who have a sense of deprivation are more likely to oppose fluoridation. The deprivation may be economic or related to prestige, or to a feeling of lower political efficiency. People of these sorts are most receptive to misinformation that will follow the line of their desires, and unfortunately a great deal of such misinformation has been forthcoming. Certain leaders, with more fanatical determination than scientific perspective, have supplied erroneous information to the public, particularly at election time. The distribution of their material has been aided by liberal sums of money contributed by individuals or groups with right-wing or food-faddist leanings, and their tactics are commonly those of flooding the mails, the newspapers, and radio and television stations with fear-arousing statements too late for informed officials to refute them.

The antifluoridationists' arguments are generally understandable and easy to follow. The weaknesses of the arguments are often difficult for a layman to grasp, while the arguments themselves are grounded in some of the most widely held ideas and emotions of our culture: respect for individual rights, fear of poison, and so forth. The Mausners feel that the proponents of fluoridation have too often ignored psychology in presenting their case. They have relied too heavily on the fiat of organized science and have tended to dismiss opponents as "crackpots." As lessons for the future they point to the necessity of avoiding the errors of relying on prestige, of name calling, and of failing to reach people before issues become polarized.

Another type of social-science study on the fluoridation question involves statistical appraisal of the communities that adopt and the communities that reject fluoridation. Paul and his coworkers have done this in 53 Massachusetts communities, 27 of which decided in favor of fluoridation and 26 against.[23] His analyses showed that the communities accepting fluoridation tended to be smaller, wealthier, more educated, growing more, and to have a higher proportion of children under 15 and a lower proportion of people aged 65 or over, than do communities rejecting fluoridation. These factors were found to be interrelated to a considerable degree. The strongest connections were between the percentage of population change from 1945 to 1955 and two other measures, educational level and percentage of population under age 15.

The Massachusetts study also developed some quantitative material on the reasoning of the vocal antifluoridationists. These arguments were found to center upon three main issues: the uncertainty of benefits, the possibility of injurious consequences, and the violation of individual rights. The first argument Paul found to be the least effective and to weaken gradually as additional results of fluoridation field trials became public knowledge. The second argument (poisoning) he found to be more forceful and to be universally used by vocal antifluoridationists. Yet among 22 of these people intensively interviewed, he found only 2 who said they would bother to order bottled water if fluoridation were adopted. The third issue, that of personal freedom, Paul found to be held vehemently by leading antifluoridationists. This argument is important, not because it is demonstrable but because it rests upon an important ethic, or value assumption. This ethic, in the absence of knowledge of the impracticality of reaching our low-income population with any other fluoride technique than water fluoridation, assumes an importance which it is difficult to deny.

Paul's work also included interviews with civic leaders and dentists in order to appraise their roles in fluoridation controversies. In general it was found that the civic leaders, political and otherwise, tended to avoid an open stand even when personally convinced of the merits of fluoridation. They hesitated to split their following over a controversial issue relating to a problem (dental caries) which neither they nor their followers considered to be of grave importance. Not without reason, they preferred to save their influence for issues apparently more vital to the community or to their own continuation in an elective office. The dentists, too, Paul found to be hesitant to go on record on an issue which might antagonize actual or prospective patients. The dentists, moreover, were generally unprepared by training or experience to maneuver adeptly in the political storm in which they often found themselves. Nevertheless, failure upon the part of the dentists of the community to take a firm stand on the fluoridation issue seemed often to be one of the major causes for its defeat.

Weaver, in summarizing the common reasons why fluoridation is so likely to fail in public referenda, lists the following categories:

Psychological
   The antiscientific response (Mausner)
   The deprivation response
Political
   Poor communications

Poor professional support
Poor timing
High turnout of elderly, conservative voters
Lack of long and thorough educational campaign
Demographic
Town meetings are more favorable than public referenda
A low rate of unemployment favors adoption of fluoridation
Migratory populations tend to oppose fluoridation
Upper middle class communities tend to oppose fluoridation
Structural characteristics of the community
Social structure of community including position of officials and lay
opinion leaders
The effect of other concomitant events such as high dental cost for
Medicaid
Cultural factors such as religion, kinship, neighborhood attitudes
and political attitudes
Factionalism left over from earlier conflicts[24]

This list does not mention confusing wording in a referendum text. Though not necessarily a common problem, it needs attention. As Hanlon writes, "It has long since been demonstrated that one can obtain sufficient signatures to get about any referendum before the people, and by adroit choice of words to confuse the voters so that either they do not vote, or vote contrary to their wishes."[25]

One of the large problems in the mind of a voter trying to make up his mind on the question of fluoridation is, "Whom shall I believe? Whom shall I trust?" In spite of the almost universal endorsement of fluoridation by scientific groups, the antifluoridationists can almost always muster a small number of scientists to their cause, and these individuals usually use all their degrees and institutional connections in an endeavor to impress the layman. The layman himself, without scientific background, is at a loss to know which set of scientists to believe. His doubts are enhanced by the fact that every now and then a pioneer, such as Sister Kenney, will fail to be recognized at once by the major scientific organizations and, in fact, may have to battle them. Since the layman himself is not in a position to distinguish between a genius and a fanatic in a field beyond his own competence, he has little choice but to rely upon the decisions of the large professional organizations, studying the way those decisions are worded and doing his best to appreciate the evidence back of them. He must also study carefully the expertise and responsibility of the organizations that have expressed themselves.

As of 1984, an added problem has arisen to retard new fluoridation programs: the sharp drop of dental caries among children in developed countries. Fluoridation is actually to be credited with a major share of this drop, particularly in countries such as the United States where a large proportion of the population receive fluoridated water. The fact that significant drops have also been seen in unfluoridated areas and that dental needs among children are now less urgent than they used to be makes fluoridation harder to promote. On a cost-effectiveness basis, however (see Chapter 19), fluoridation remains by far the best preventive measure for dental caries where communal water supplies exist.

In conclusion it may be stated generally that the social sciences have brought to the field of public health the study of psychology, culture, and other aspects of human behavior, which are as important a part of our environment as the physical environment. As a result, social scientists are prepared to aid public health workers in many phases of their program planning and evaluation problems, and have already begun to do so to a significant extent in the dental fields, particularly as regards the fluoridation issue. Their experiments and their reports should be watched with interest by the dental profession and their assistance sought in program design whenever possible.

CHAPTER 11

Principles of Administration

THE DENTIST with a leadership role in a public health program needs to know many of the principles by which large enterprises are administered, whether they be governmental or private. He will have only small numbers of workers under his control, in all likelihood, and will therefore not need to know the more detailed techniques of personnel management; but the general principles of administrative organization and management are very definitely within his area of responsibility.

There are two main areas into which administrative work may be divided. The first is *organization,* which deals with the structure of an agency and the way people are arranged into working groups within it. The relation of the agency to other agencies and to the public is also a matter of organization. The second area is *management* or executive control. This is concerned with the handling of personnel and operations in such a way that the work of the agency gets done. These main subdivisions of administration will be discussed in the order named.

ADMINISTRATIVE ORGANIZATION

Certain well-established principles of organization are essential to any large endeavor in the field of public health. Dentists who served in the armed forces will recognize them as characteristic of military life; but they are equally applicable to private enterprise. They are essential to the management of any group of people working toward a common goal in a situation involving teamwork.

The first of these principles is that of *centralized authority*. A hierarchy or chain of command must exist, with one person at the top in a position of executive responsibility. This is not a concession to power politics nor does it mean that one person can always be found who is clearly better than his fellows in the administration of an enterprise. The most important single reason for centralized control is efficient communication. Orders dealing with the conduct of the enterprise must come from one source, or else confusion will arise. Subleaders in the enterprise must know to whom they must look above them for orders and guidelines and must also be responsible for communicating clearly with those subordinates who are assigned to them.

Even in a democratic country such as the United States, an executive branch of government must exist. Popular control can be exercised through a legislative branch, the function of which is planning rather than doing. In private enterprise, boards of directors and advisory committees have similar planning functions.

The executive is a clearing house, not only for orders but for information of all sorts. An example of this can be found in any dental school, where one of the main functions of the dean's office is to receive and redirect to the proper source all requests for information wherever the exact person able to supply the information is not known to the inquirer. The handling of such a stream of information going in various directions is in itself an aid in the process of administrative organization. It permits the executive in charge to plan the work of his enterprise with more perspective. It is also a help to the public to know of one individual or one office where responsibility for the conduct of the enterprise rests.

Another principle of organization is that the executive should have a *span of control* no larger than is efficient. The foreman of a group of workers may be able to handle 20 or 30 people who are all performing the same simple operation. An executive, however, can seldom deal with more than 8 to 12 immediate subordinates, each of whom has a different administrative problem to be coordinated with the main effort of the enterprise. Where more than this number of subdepartments or divisions exists, deputies must be appointed, each responsible to the chief for the handling of a group of related subdepartments. Thus, as is seen in Fig. 1, the New York Commissioner has about seven group, office, or division heads directly responsible to him. These second-level heads, in turn, have from three to seven third-level division or group heads responsible to each of them. The smaller operating units are mostly called bureaus or laboratories here, though in other states differing terminology may be used.

In enterprises of any size it is logical to make a distinction between *line* and *staff* services or functions. In a department of public health, such major divisions as disease control, dental health, and sanitary engineering would be considered to be line because they are in charge of units that carry the services of the organization to the public, and are in the direct line of administrative hierarchy. Personnel, finance, and other services applicable to the entire organization but operating entirely within it would be considered staff. These are usually small groups of specialists, responsible quite closely to the chief executive. Some staff services, usually technical, carry their functions outside the organization. A health educator lent by a state to a local area would be an example of this. The health educator while on loan would be responsible temporarily to the line health officer in the locality, not to state headquarters.

The distinction between line and staff is particularly clear in military organizations. Here, the dental officer finds himself working entirely within the organization, alongside the medical officer, the chaplain, the engineer, and the supply officer. His work is only indirectly related to the main task of the organization: fighting. He is therefore a staff officer, not a line officer, in this situation.

Functions of the Executive

The executive of an enterprise has three major functions. The first is to decide the goals of the organization and how it shall be internally organized. The second function is to get the organization to its goal through proper budgeting, proper personnel administration, and other applicable techniques. The third is to act as ceremonial representative and communicating officer for the organization, symbolizing and, where necessary, describing the organization to the world outside. This last function is much more than mere pageantry. People need symbols when they think about organizations, just as they do in many other types of thought. The person who is in charge of the organization becomes by that fact its symbol and the person best qualified to describe it and its activities. He provides the organization with an "image."

It is inescapable in the growth of an enterprise that the larger it becomes the more work will be needed to direct it and operate it, and the smaller the proportion of such work, therefore, that the top executive can handle by himself. *Delegation* therefore becomes necessary, not only of work but of the authority, the responsibility, the pride, and the credit that go with it. Andrew Carnegie is reputed to have made it a policy never to do anything he could hire someone else to do for him. He was careful also to treat his subordinates in such a way that they would take adequate pride in their work and have authority enough to perform it. As Dimock says, "It is generally agreed that in order to obtain best results, the authority must equal the responsibility vested in a person when delegation is made."[1] The supervisory authority, however, must be retained. "There is no substitute for an executive riding herd on his own supervisory functions. He can delegate many other things, but not this one."[2]

The principle of delegation is not without its complications. Subordinates expect a leader to be able and willing to perform, within reason, the tasks he delegates. A military leader, thus, must on occasion expose himself to enemy fire as his men are exposed. In the field of dentistry, the best leader for small teams of dentists is a person who not only is known to be a good operator himself but is willing to take his share of the operating load. Young dental officers do not respect a senior who is using his rank merely as an excuse to sit down behind a desk. The larger the organization, however, the more obvious it becomes that administration is a full-time job and the more natural it becomes for the executive to devote his entire skill and attention to this task.

The attitude an executive takes toward his subordinates can become a matter of administrative policy. In a democratic country it is natural to think of an organization in the same terms as one thinks of the entire country. This involves what Scott and his co-authors call "the citizenship conception of labor." Not only are workers human beings and to be treated as such, but they are also a part of the enterprise to which they have sold their labor: "Just as citizens of the United States automatically have certain inherent rights and a voice in determining and exercising those rights, so are workers, as citizens of the industry in which they are em-ployed, entitled to the same right of having a voice in determining the rules and regulations under which they work."[3]

One of the organization matters of great concern in dental pub-lic health is that of *autonomy*. Dentists operating either as individ-uals or in groups wish to be free of the control of others in matters affecting the professional quality of their work. This attitude has arisen historically from the tendency of some physicians to under-estimate both the physiological importance of dental care and the skill and training needed in order to render it. Military dental services prefer, in general, to be responsible directly to line officers rather than to medical officers. This arrangement has both advan-tages and disadvantages. It gives the dentist the desired operating independence, but it impairs coordination between two important branches of a health service and makes for difficulty in handling cases such as those of maxillofacial surgery where the best both in medical care and in dental care must be brought to bear upon the same patient. In public health, where the emphasis is upon pre-ventive work, the question of autonomy seems to have been less critical. It is important that the dentists have needed control of the professional standards of their work, but when this work is in such fields as epidemiology, health education, or case findings, less misunderstanding seems to arise than when the major atten-tion is upon restorative dentistry. In public health departments, dental autonomy is sufficiently achieved by separate divisional status.

Techniques of Executive Control

There are various techniques for organizational control which de-serve brief mention at this point. The larger the organization the more detailed these techniques will need to be, but certain tech-niques are needed even in the small units commonly seen in dental public health. *Organization charts* are perhaps the first of such devices to deserve mention. They are invaluable aids in depicting the chain of authority in an organization. Such a chart appears in Fig. 1 (Chapter 2) to illustrate the place of the dental service in a large health department. Another chart appears in Fig. 63 (Chapter 17) to illustrate the use of auxiliary personnel in a large dental clinic.

A device of similar general purpose but involving far more detail is that of the *procedure manual.* Here is seen a detailed analysis of the working of the organization and statements are made as to exactly how certain functions are to be executed. The manual will serve a valuable purpose if there are complicated or unusual functions to be performed beyond the easy comprehension of the average subordinate. Procedure manuals, however, are hard work to prepare and can result in a rigidity of operation which sometimes impairs efficiency. An American teacher of medical ethics, back from England, reported recently that at Oxford, "There are no rules, but dozens of 'ways that things are done.' "[4]

On a less formal level, *standing orders* or *guidelines* on certain specific functions are of great value. These may deal with the handling of complex situations involving conflict of two or more operating principles or they may deal with technical matters such as fees or methods of record keeping. Dimock, however, warns of the ease of misunderstanding written communications and also of the time that goes into preparing them. He considers that their use should be confined primarily to issuance of instructions and assignment of duties. They are also clearly indicated in the setting of policies and programs, because the written work can be read and reread when necessary and thus continues to be absorbed over a longer period of time.[5]

Records, of course, constitute a vital organizational technique. In the field of health, records are kept primarily for the benefit of the patient, and next in importance, they serve the purpose of aiding epidemiological study. A third, hardly less useful, purpose is that of evaluation of effort for organizational control. *Summary sheets* by the week, month, or year are most helpful to the executive in appraising the success of his enterprise and the efficiency of his workers. They are of great use in program planning and in budgeting.

Budgeting

The public health dentist, who is ordinarily in charge of a rather small unit, has less concern with the process of budgeting than does the chief of a large enterprise; nevertheless, a few words should be said upon the subject since the budget is probably the single most valuable tool of administration. It has been called "a plan of work with dollar signs attached." The preparation of a budget forces an executive to define first the objectives of his enterprise and then the basic units which will compose it. It makes him think about the share of the total available public money which his enterprise should receive or is likely to receive. The budget, when completed, will describe the enterprise to the public, not in full perspective, to be sure, but at least in terms of the most important medium through which public support is rendered: money.

In accord with the citizenship concept of labor previously alluded to, the budget is a valuable means of describing an enterprise to the workers who compose it. It therefore has value in staff development, education, and coordination. Since the executive lives with his budget during the year for which it has been constructed, it stimulates him to the most efficient use of his resources and yet warns him against overexpenditure. A distinction, to be sure, needs to be made between budgets for supplies and equipment and budgets for salary. The former can easily be displayed to an entire working force. The latter, to avoid envious comparisons, must be treated with discreet restriction, though probably not with real secrecy.

The usual construction of a budget involves attention both to sources of money and to expenditure. On the income side there is often a division into what is called "hard" money and "soft" money. The "hard" is the main supply of funds regularly available, whether from the parent organization, from endowment, or from a conservative estimate of fees or reimbursements for services rendered. Some of this money may be unrestricted as to use; some may be restricted to special purposes. The "soft" money involves gifts or grants for immediate use. In the field of health, research grants are common. They not only are given for special purposes but are usually given for a limited time only, so that indefinite renewals cannot be expected.

Grantsmanship

The process of applying for research grants in terms satisfactory to the agencies which supply them, and of preparing the progress and terminal reports which are usually required, is an art in itself, occupying much executive time. The ever-increasing dependency of health agencies and health educational institutions upon grant money makes it inevitable that the success of an executive in these fields be measured, to some extent, by his success in obtaining such funds. During the past several decades the greatest flow of federal grant money in the health field was for the support of research. Now, with the coming of Medicare legislation, an increasing proportion of the grant money is awarded for service programs and for the solution of problems that are better called development than research, that is, pilot programs and demonstrations. The principles which apply to federal funding also apply to the obtaining of funds from private and from other governmental sources.

In assessing the qualities which go to make up a research or service application which will seem successful in the eyes of a funding agency, the negative approach is sometimes revealing. Allen has analyzed the reasons for rejection of 605 applications for grants of funds to initiate or continue research under the auspices of the National Institutes of Health.[6] He groups reasons for rejection under four headings: problem, approach, man, and environment. Under the first heading, by far the most common reason for rejection was that the study committee believed the problem was of insufficient importance or was unlikely to produce any new or useful information. Other criticisms related to the problem were that it rested upon a hypothesis for which there was insufficient evidence, and that it was more complex than the investigator appeared to realize. Under approach, the most common reason for rejection was that the proposed tests or methods or scientific procedures were unsuited to the stated objective. Other criticisms appeared to center upon failure to think the project through carefully, and failure to design an approach which was clearcut, well focused, and permitted adequate evaluation. Apparently, investigators find it easier to define their goals sharply than to define with equal sharpness the routes they propose to follow toward those goals. The chief objection centered upon the third category, man, appeared to be that the investigator did not have adequate experience or training, or both, for *this* research. Environmental reasons dealt with equipment, personnel, institutional setting, and the other commitments of the principal investigator, but these seemed to be minor matters in comparison with the causes for rejection mentioned earlier.

In preparing an application for grant funds there is always a high premium on imagination and upon careful follow-through. "Knowing the right people" seems of minor importance in the usual political sense but of great importance in demonstrating that the applicant has a clear knowledge of the program for which funds are being made available and the channels through which these funds flow. Applications, of course, must be clearly written with good attention to detail, particularly in regard to the approach to the problem. Any responsible executive may feel that he should be trusted to solve details of approach as he meets them, and should not be required to spell out every move in advance. There is probably much justice to this thought, but a study committee in Washington does not know the investigator, and can judge him only by his ability to spell out such details in a competent manner.

Perhaps the most important matter of all is the ability of the applicant to sense the exact type of research, training, or service the funding agency is most anxious to stimulate. Then the application—and the project—can be concentrated upon this particular area.

Expenses

Expense budgets are usually constructed in terms of salaries for personnel, together with appropriate retirement allowances and sums of money for piecework services, supplies, equipment, and so forth. A variation upon this system, termed *cost accounting*, attempts to allocate appropriate costs to the different functions for which the enterprise is responsible. Thus a dental-health service might wish to estimate how much money goes for health education, how much for case finding, how much for restorative dentistry, and how much for administration. The salaries of personnel performing two or more of these functions would have to be divided pro rata, as would also the cost of supplies, services, and so forth.

Two techniques have arisen to appraise the value of monies expended for health. The first is *cost-benefit analysis,* as described in Chapter 19. Briefly stated, this process involves a series of mathematical calculations to provide an estimate of the potential value of following a given course of action in the health field, either new or revised. The total cost of a disease per case is estimated both directly (in terms of the cost of treating it) and indirectly (in terms of the money lost to the patient and to society as a result of the ensuing disability). The net benefit to society is the gross cost of the disease, less the cost of control or eradication. *Cost-effectiveness analysis,* the second item, is a series of analytical and mathematical procedures which aid in the selection of the most effective method from among various alternative approaches. Here, various models or diagrams of procedures are constructed and compared, and the efficiency of each is estimated. This process involves not only dollars, but subjective judgments as to the quality of the result. The object is not necessarily to select the least costly method of rendering a service, but to select that method which is optimal in terms of attaining its goal without undue cost.

Two general words of warning should be given in connection with administrative work. The first deals with the danger of tailoring an administrative organization to the personality of any one official or member of it, to the exclusion of good long-range planning. Organizations are designed to outlast individuals. They should be planned to function well when staffed by people of the more usually available types of personality and training. It is a mistake to design the structure of the organization to fit an unusual personality such as may not appear again.

The second warning deals with "Parkinson's law" to the effect that "work expands so as to fill the time available for its completion."[7] There is, unfortunately, much truth in this law. An executive who demands complicated records or reports which are really not needed will often give his subordinates comfortable routine jobs with which they will occupy their time to the exclusion of more important endeavors. Administrative procedures for their own sake should be avoided. They produce a top-heavy structure in which the real work of the organization too often suffers.

In program design and implementation a delicate balance is often needed between radical innovations and conservatism (in the best sense of the word). Alexander Pope advises us:

> Be not the first by whom the new is tried,
> Nor yet the last to lay the old aside.

Again, Aristotle has many followers when he states, "It is the middle disposition in each department of conduct that is to be praised, but . . . one should lean sometimes to the side of excess and sometimes to that of deficiency, since that is the easiest way of hitting the mean and right course." This does not mean that research projects and pilot programs should not "try the new." Such efforts are always much needed, and are the cutting edge of progress. The foregoing comments are directed toward organizations that are reponsible for direct service to the public through accepted channels.

This very brief treatment of administrative organization is no more than an introduction to the subject. More material will be found in such chapters as that on public health in practice and in Chapters 1 and 17 to 23. A dentist entering upon administrative responsibility, however, will wish to do a good deal of general reading. Some pertinent textbooks are noted in the references to this chapter. Other sources of information may become obvious as a result of the specific nature of the organization he is joining.

EXECUTIVE MANAGEMENT

A good example of the division between administrative organization and management can be seen aboard naval ships, where the captain is the one who plans the organization of the ship and its relations with the rest of the fleet, but the executive officer is the one who deals directly with personnel and keeps the ship operating. In small organizations both functions are usually vested in one man. This is perhaps fortunate. Administrative organization can often be a lonely job; executive management is a very active and interesting experience in human relations.

One of the most important concepts in personnel management is that of the "worker-in-his-work unit," to which Scott and his coauthors devote a whole chapter of their book on this subject.[8]

The worker is to be thought of in terms of his *capacities* and *interests,* and the *opportunities* he is likely to expect within the organization. The job he has to fill also has its own characteristics. When the worker and the job are put together, an entirely new "chemical compound" results with a character of its own which may or may not have been entirely predictable. Thus if a dentist is taken from private practice and made a member of a public health team he may not react in the same way that he did in his original surroundings.

It is one of the main problems of management to make every worker-in-his-work unit as effective as possible. This involves arranging things so that the capacities, interests, and opportunities of the worker will receive maximum, and preferably equal, emphasis. Good recruitment procedure implies that the training and aptitudes of the worker be carefully studied before employment and be those best suited to the job he must fill. The interests of the worker should be inquired about in advance or predicted by the executive to the best of his ability: not only the worker's manifest desires and ambitions but also his instinctive, impulsive tendencies and those vague yearnings that may or may not stir him to his fullest action in performing his duties. The opportunities of the job should also be carefully considered. Are they sufficient to attract the type of person that is wanted? Does the job lead logically to a higher one, or will the responsibility within the job increase as the worker becomes acquainted with it to the extent that the job will prove ultimately satisfying? An adequate salary is important, but by no means the whole story.

The importance of balance between *capacities, interests, and opportunities* must not be neglected. Most obviously unfortunate, of course, is the situation where a worker with poor capacity attempts to fill a job with considerable interest and opportunity for advancement. The work in this instance will not be performed well, and the worker may feel anxious and uneasy and develop unattractive personality traits as a result. Less obvious are the situations where opportunities for advancement do not exist in an interesting position or where a job which leads clearly to the upper rungs of the ladder is not in itself of real interest. It is the executive's function in such instances to readjust duties to the best of his ability and also to talk with the worker in an effort to motivate him to make the best use of the interests and opportunities which do exist. Before an employee is hired, careful thought should be devoted to the type of advancement he will probably wish and probaby deserve. The matter should be thoroughly discussed at the time of the application interview.

Attempts to measure the interest of the employee in his job inevitably call for an analysis of the *incentives* most educated people find in their work. Dimock, on the basis of interviews, finds four main incentives to predominate: *financial gain, power, prestige,* and *public service,* in order of importance as they have been listed.[9] All incentives may be present at once, but it seems usual for there to be a time progression from one incentive to another. The urge for financial gain seems to occur first; the other incentives develop a little later as the worker matures, coming to feel himself an integral part of the organization in which he works, and later of his community. Good *working conditions* should also be included in this list of incentives. They include attractive quarters, good equipment, congenial associates, good working hours, and fair vacations. An annual *vacation* on full pay should always be planned. A fair handling of weekends and holidays is also important. Undue laxity must be avoided, however, or both the work and the morale of the organization will suffer.

In attempting to list the practical responsibilities of personnel management, five principles stand out: (1) good recruitment and careful selection of workers; (2) sound classification of jobs, not only in order of rank, but also through an accurate written description of duties; (3) equitable pay scales; (4) provisions for tenure, or, at the very least, an understanding as to the length of employment to be reasonably expected; and (5) adequate provisions for separation and retirement.[10] In small organizations these matters can often be handled on an informal basis. In large organizations, particularly governmental ones, it is more usual to find *civil service systems* or *merit systems* in operation. Both are in essence organized objective methods of selecting and advancing employees on the basis of their qualifications and in relation to their aptitudes for particular jobs, and then arranging for them length of tenure and pay which is standardized according to skill or quantity of work. If the plan exists by virtue of a statute, it is commonly referred to as a civil service system; if it exists through administrative ruling it is called a merit system.[11] Civil service is thus a governmental system while a merit system may be either governmental or private.

Civil service or merit systems commonly make use of written examinations and graded experience ratings, with weight given to both in making up a list of competitive applicants for a position. The employer must agree to select from the top, or nearly the top, of this list. In many areas, veterans, particularly disabled veterans, receive preference. Advancement is usually upon a merit basis, with qualifying examinations for certain types of promotion. Permanent tenure during good behavior and retirement upon a pension are usually part of the plan.

There are obviously advantages to the worker in these systems, yet there are disadvantages as well, chiefly to the employer. Life tenure for large personnel groups within an organization imparts a rigidity to the organization which limits its ability to adapt to changing conditions over the years. Tenure can often prove a narcotic to the employee, rather than an incentive. The veterans' preference, introduced for an obviously humanitarian reason, can force inefficient staff selection. Entrance and promotional examinations serve their purpose only when examiners are of good quality and above political influence.

Any good system of employee selection should rest heavily upon the *personal interview*. There is no substitute for a leisurely talk with an applicant during which his character and experience can be drawn out through informal questioning. Such an interview also gives the executive a chance to describe the job to the applicant and answer any questions he may have concerning it. The reaction of the applicant to this information is often very valuable. It is always important to find what sort of a career the applicant pictures for himself. A particularly good leading question is, "What would you like to find yourself doing ten years from now?" It is important to make good notes on the applicant after the interview, particularly if a series of applicants must be interviewed for one position.

Modern efforts to reduce racial and ethnic discrimination have led to "affirmative action" programs designed to attract and employ minority-group persons who have commonly been the victims of prejudice or have not been entering normal recruitment channels. Laws, quota systems, and enlightened employment practices need to be studied in order to give these people a fair chance. It is no kindness to them, however, to place them in positions for which they are inadequately prepared, whether by lack of education, aptitude, or culture.

Reference has been made to equitable *pay scales* for employees. It is common practice that there be a minimum and maximum salary for a given job. A new employee with minimum experience will presumably start at the bottom of the scale and work upward by regular steps, partly according to merit and partly according to length of service. Pay increases should ordinarily be between 5 and 10 percent per year; to give less is meaningless, to give more, often an indication that the original pay was unfair. The top limit should be reached within 6 to 10 years within one grade. If the usefulness of the employee keeps on increasing after such a period it is usually an indication that promotion is deserved to a job of another grade. Maximum pay levels cannot, of course, remain frozen for an indefinite period of time. The system should include arrangement for increases to match an increase in the cost of living, if and to the extent that such may occur.

Program Evaluation

Any health service, or for that matter, any system of operations, requires an initial planning effort followed by periodic appraisal and replanning. The term *evaluation* is the one most commonly used to describe these processes. Chapter 14 deals with the formal approaches to surveying of populations and evaluation of results of service upon these populations. Within an organization, similar though differently structured procedures must occur. Cost-benefit and cost-effectiveness analysis has been mentioned in connection with expense budgets. Good executive management requires frequent hard looks at the internal efficiency of the operations being conducted. The terms *operations research* and *systems engineering* have been devised to cover a large range of techniques which apply in this area. Some items of the input and output of a system are measurable, and for these mathematical models of ideal procedure may be constructed. Graphic models or flow charts will help in other situations. Subjective evaluations as to complex factors bearing on the efficiency of the operation and subjective assessments of quality of output also have their place. This often boils down to "just plain common sense." The executive who relies on common sense to the exclusion of a study of more sophisticated methods of analysis, however, will miss much of the valuable experience of his colleagues. Operations research is essentially an analytical discipline and systems engineering a constructive one, but their techniques and objectives blend.

Flagle, Huggins, and Roy list a wide variety of hospital problems which lend themselves to operations research, and give suggestions on approaches to the solutions of the problems: "Should we adopt a newly developed method for measuring body temperature? How can we reduce delays in caring for pediatric outpatients? With whom should responsibility rest for transporting patients from hospital floors to radiology? How can we reduce labor turnover in the ancillary personnel groups? Can medical records and statistics be adapted for managerial controls? What can be done to raise the upper limit of hospital census? What should be the information content of directors' meetings? What is the optimum interval between deliveries of supplies to their points of use?"[12] The dental equivalents of these problems are obvious.

One specific approach to operations research is called PERT, or Program Evaluation and Review Technique.[13] This involves the preparation of drawings which show the flow of operations in relation to time and to other controlling factors. A network results which can be analyzed for efficiency and then adjusted to minimize the risk of not reaching operational goals on time, within acceptable quality limits, and within acceptable cost. This method has been used with success by the U.S. Public Health Service in organizing dental public health residency programs and in organizing continuing education programs for private practitioners of dentistry.

Programs may also be evaluated by their results in such measurable matters as receipt of dental services (following a referral program) or changes in attitudes or behavior patterns (following a health education program). Questionnaires are often valuable in this latter area. Other chapters touch upon these approaches.

Consultation Work

Persons charged with oversight of other workers are frequently defined as consultants, with advisory functions but no authority to give orders. Such consultation work may often be confined to in-

formal conversations, but a planned structure gives the relationship a lot more meaning. Nowjack-Raymer, outlining the duties of
dental hygienists who were to act as consultants to the classroom
teachers in Project Headstart, lists five stages in the process: 1) an
early contact during the planning stages of the classes, 2) collection
of data relevant to the children's oral health, 3) feedback, and
decision as to recommendations for action, 4) implementation (the
effort to make the teachers self-sufficient in the oral health field),
and finally 5) extension, recycling, or termination of the relationship.[14]

Qualifications and Training of Personnel

It is beyond the scope of this book to discuss in detail the professional education and subsequent field training of personnel for a
dental public health program. Mention must be made, however, of
certain common categories of dental personnel and the qualifications they are normally expected to possess.

The field of dental public health can be approached through
various channels of education and accreditation. For dentists, the
first of these channels is the degree of Master of Public Health
(M.P.H.), involving one or two years of study at a school of public
health. The courses offered there in biostatistics, epidemiology,
behavioral science, and health service administration build well on
the courses offered for a dental degree, and in some instances they
form the health care delivery research track in a 5-year program
leading to the two degrees. With this preparation, the dentist
should qualify for a wide range of health care administrative and
teaching assignments. Equivalent degrees to the M.P.H. provide
valuable, if less general, preparation.

Top-level dental public health directorships usually require certification by the American Board of Dental Public Health.[15] This
Board requires dental graduation, the M.P.H. degree or an equivalent, licensure in at least one state, and a total of at least six years
of graduate education and field experience, including a residency.
The final step is passage of an examination with written and oral
components, accompanied by two project reports. One difficulty
regarding application for certification is the requirement of current activity which is limited to full-time specialization in administration, teaching, and clinical practice or research related to dental

public health or preventive dentistry. This appears to exclude part-time public health activity or certification in any other dental specialty.

Clinical dentists can be recruited for service in public agencies without further qualification than a dental degree. A general practice residency is helpful, but it is not necessary where supervision by a senior operator is available.

Dental hygienists for clinical assignments need only the certificate based upon two years of training. Hygienists for teaching, case finding, and other responsible assignments under general, rather than direct, supervision are best recruited from applicants with four years of training and a Bachelor of Science or Bachelor of Dental Hygiene degree.

Residency for specialists in dental public health is now involving programs with an increasingly careful structure, as with other clinical specialties in medicine and dentistry. The supervisor must be board-certified. The training program must be diversified enough to contain in suitable proportion such matters as program administration, design of preventive, diagnostic, and corrective services, program promotion and consultation, direct teaching experience, and research experience.[16] The American Board of Dental Public Health is working with the Council on Dental Education of the American Dental Association to elaborate and apply accreditation procedures for dental public health residency. Dental divisions in state health departments and university dental schools are agencies well suited to administer such residencies; the best situation of all exists where a health department and a university collaborate on a residency program.

The question of apprenticeship or *in-service training* for subprofessional employees is an important one. It is often desirable to hire an employee with inadequate training or with none at all for a nonprofessional job and then arrange training during the course of employment. This needs planning as well as teaching time during working hours, but the rewards are great in building the interest and the usefulness of the employee. Such a system also permits selection of candidates from a wider field, giving the employer an opportunity to look for character and for interest in work rather than merely for training and experience.

The term *apprenticeship* implies a rather formalized arrangement for indoctrination of a completely new employee over a set period of time, usually 3 to 12 months. In the dental field we hear of it most often in connection with the training of laboratory technicians. It is also used with dental students devoting summer vacations to employment designed to orient them toward a future career: specifically, dental public health. Federal grants have supported these last-named programs. *In-service training* implies a briefer and less formal arrangement. The dentist will find the greatest need for this method in connection with training dental assistants for specific tasks not covered in general training courses. It is important to teach such assistants new techniques at properly spaced intervals and to remember how much the assistant has learned at a given moment. By teaching the commoner, simpler tasks at first the dentist can bring even an untrained worker to a considerable degree of usefulness within a very short time. Another example is found in the training of lay persons, often parents of children, in the supervision of fluoride rinse programs.

For introducing basically trained employees to new tasks there are other types of indoctrination. *Observation* implies a brief experience, lasting 1 day to 1 week. *Orientation* is usually for a period of 1 to 2 months; *field experience* is for 3 to 6 months.

The Executive

No complete listing could ever be made of all the characteristics necessary in a good executive or of the control techniques he might be expected to employ. Both are bound to vary greatly with the personality of the executive and the situation in which he operates. Schell lists a number of qualities of unquestionable value to an executive.[17] Among them are enthusiasm for his work (for enthusiasm is contagious), cheerfulness, calmness in difficult situations, consistency, a receptive attitude toward employees and their problems, frankness, impressiveness (by which he means the ability to impress the mind of another), firmness, tolerance, tact, and finally, a friendliness or kindness based upon a true liking for other people. It is very important to remember people's names and to make them feel at ease so that there will be frankness and complete cooperation between executive and employee.

A principal test of an executive's leadership, according to Dimock, is his or her ability to step in unobtrusively at the right moment and supply an instruction or suggestion when greater knowledge of the overall situation, or a sense of strategy, reveals the necessity: "He must not attempt to do everything himself; indeed he must avoid as much detailed work as possible. His social function, therefore, is to maintain a sense of goals, strategy and timing, and to supply specific instructions and accelerations at the right point. The executive does his most effective work when the subexecutive has contributed everything of which he is capable and needs the extra 5 percent of knowledge and leadership with which to turn out a workmanlike job."[18]

Among techniques for executive control, some have been mentioned under the heading of administration and many more can be learned through observation, general reading, or merely the application of common sense. Two points, both closely linked to the character of the executive, do deserve mention here. The first is the need for clear habits of *communication*. Barnard's four requirements for an authoritative communication are worth remembering in this connection: the communication must be understood; it must seem consistent with the purposes of the organization at the time; it must also seem compatible with the personal interest of the recipient at the time; and finally, if an order, it must be one with which the recipient is mentally and physically able to comply.[19] Sir William Osler gives advice as applicable to the executive as to the physician: "You cannot afford to stand aloof from your professional colleagues in any place. Join their associations, mingle in their meetings, giving of the best of your talents, gathering here, scattering there; but everywhere showing that you are at all times faithful students, as willing to teach as to be taught."[20]

One point deserves the greatest possible emphasis: a subordinate should *never be criticized in the presence of others* when this can be avoided. The person taken to task is thinking so much of the effect this criticism will have upon his standing among his peers that his resentment blocks his understanding of the criticism. There are times, of course, when public correction of a subordinate cannot be avoided, but this correction should take the form of a simple order to do the proper thing, not of a personal criticism. It also helps to apologize afterward when one has been forced to correct a subordinate in public, and to reach an understanding with the employee so that the situation will not recur in the future.

It will be appropriate to close this chapter with a brief word on the nature of executive responsibility. Barnard, in his book *The Functions of the Executive,* attempts to define these by relating responsibility to specific moral codes, and by showing that the executive has a more complicated system of moral codes to deal with than has the ordinary worker:

Every executive possesses, independently of the position he occupies, personal moral codes. When the individual is placed in an executive position there are immediately incumbent upon him, officially at least, several *additional* codes that are codes of his organization . . .

It will be sufficient for present purposes of illustration to take a hypothetical industrial organization, and to suppose the case of an executive head of an important department. The *organization* codes to which he should conform are: 1) the government code applying to his company, that is, the laws, charter, provisions, etc.; 2) obedience to the general purpose and general methods including the established systems of objective authority; 3) the general purpose of his department; 4) the general moral (ethical) standards of his subordinates; 5) the technical situation as a whole; 6) the code of the informal executive organization, that is, that official conduct shall be that of a gentleman as *its members* understand it, and that personal conduct shall be so likewise; 7) the code that is suggested in the phrase "the good of the organization as a whole"; 8) the code of the informal organization of the department; 9) the technical requirements of the department as a whole.[21]

The main function of the executive, Barnard feels, is the reconciling of plans for action with as many of these moral codes as may be involved. The successful executive devises plans which comply with the largest number of codes and are incompatible with the fewest. It is he who must decide fairly between the desire of a secretary to be home with a bedridden child, the need that she accomplish urgent work, and the relative availability of others to take her place either at work or at home. Some of the complexity of an executive's position is shown humorously in a recent New Yorker cartoon (Fig. 29).

This listing of the responsibilities of an executive in terms of moral codes may sound more formidable than it really is. Habit and experience come to the rescue of the executive, as will also the tolerance both of his superiors and of his subordinates. Some complexity does exist, however, and there is a need for endeavor beyond the average level. There is no escaping the old saying "noblesse oblige."

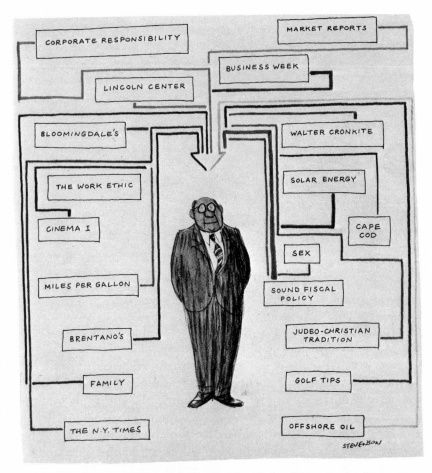

Figure 29. An executive, as seen by *The New Yorker*. [Drawing by Stevenson; © 1976 The New Yorker Magazine, Inc.]

CHAPTER 12

Preventive Dentistry

THIS CHAPTER will attempt to present clinically practical methods of preventing dental and oral disease. It will present as tools for the public health dentist those well-authenticated means of prevention which are also the tools of the private dentist. Experimental methods verging upon the unknown will be referred to only if they give promise of large practical value in the future or indicate a need for revising present methods. Chapters 4 to 9 on biostatistics and epidemiology point the way toward the testing of new preventive measures, but space limitations preclude much speculation about such measures here. Most public health dentists have enough pioneering on their hands when they attempt to apply tried and true methods to new population groups.

The material in this chapter will be presented under major headings which deal with specific oral diseases or abnormalities, beginning with dental caries. The reader is left to combine techniques to the best of his ability in order to anticipate the problems of the area with which he will deal.

LEVELS OF PREVENTION FOR DENTAL CARIES

An interesting concept in thinking about preventive measures for any disease is that of *levels of prevention*.[1] These levels extend through from the prepathogenic period of the disease to the period of rehabilitation after the disease itself has gone by. True or *primary* prevention, according to this scheme, occurs in the prepathogenic period and involves first health promotion and then specific protection. Health promotion includes health education, attention to genetic or environmental factors which might influence the disease, attention to good physical and mental development, and periodic selective examinations. Specific protection includes such immunizations as vaccination, attention to personal hygiene and safety, and the use of specific nutrients such as vitamin D for the avoidance of rickets. A *secondary* type of prevention may occur in the early period of pathogenesis. This involves early diagnosis and prompt treatment. Later in the period of pathogenesis comes disease *control*. This includes disability limitation, which is prevention to the extent that the sequelae and complications of the disease are minimized. Table 20 shows an application of this concept to dental disease. Most of the measures noted are specific for dental caries.

It would be convenient if the primary preventive measures in the field of dental caries could be divided into the epidemiologist's categories of those dealing with host, with agent, and with environment. Such a breakdown, however, will not be meaningful until we have more information upon the exact participation of factors in each of these three areas. It is better to take Sognnaes's division into those measures which affect the oral environment, more simply called oral hygiene; those which involve topical protection of the tooth; and those which involve developmental protection of the tooth.[2] Under the first heading will come oral hygiene, and for its intraoral effects, diet. Under the second heading will come those preventive techniques which fall within the field of operative dentistry and then topical treatment of teeth by fluoride solutions and other chemicals. Under the third heading come water-supply fluoridation (dealt with in Chapter 16) and the nutritional effects of diet operating through the blood stream. These last two measures exert their major thrust during tooth development and maturation.

Table 20. Levels of prevention for dental disease.

Period of prepathogenesis (primary prevention)		Period of pathogenesis (seconary prevention)
Health promotion:	Specific Promotion:	Early diagnosis and
Health education	Good oral hygiene	prompt
in oral hygiene	Fluoridation of	treatment:
Good standard	public water	Periodic detailed
of nutrition	supplies	oral
Diet planning	Topical fluoride	examination
Periodic screening	application	with x-rays
or inspection	Avoidance of sticky	Prompt
	foods, particularly	treatment of
	between meals	incipient lesions
	Tooth brushing or	Extension of
	rinsing after eating	therapy into
	Dental prophylaxis	vicinity of
	Treatment of highly	lesions for
	susceptible but	prevention of
	uninvolved areas in	secondary
	highly susceptible	lesions
	persons	Attention to
	(sealants)	developmental
	Preventive	defects
	orthodontics	Preventive
		orthodontics

In spite of ever-increasing inadequacies, Miller's chemico-parasitic theory of the causation of dental caries still give us the rationale for two of our most used techniques for preventing dental caries after the teeth are formed. The slogan "A clean tooth never decays" may be impractical to the extent that we can never clean our teeth completely of dental plaque, but Miller's theory encourages us, first, to minimize this carbohydrate material by brushing our teeth regularly, and second by avoiding such foodstuffs.

ORAL HYGIENE

Toothbrush Design

Much has been written about toothbrush design. There are brushes with tufted ends, designed particularly for getting to the lingual surfaces of the lower anterior teeth. There are brushes with various slopes and curves, designed to improve access to certain particular brushing areas. Finally, there are straight brushes with all bristles of equal length. Since few persons will use more than one brush at one tooth-brushing session, the straight brush is the one most generally recommended. It gives the best overall efficiency in all parts of the mouth. The American Dental Association used to state in detail that a good toothbrush should have:

A flat brushing surface,
Firm resilient bristles, and
A head sufficiently small to permit access to all surfaces of the teeth.[3]

Modern plaque-control programs often make use of brushes of similar design but with soft nylon bristles.

The Association further recommends that a person keep at least two toothbrushes in use and use them alternately. The brushes should be kept clean, should be kept where they will dry quickly and will not come in contact with other brushes, and should be replaced when the bristles become soft or loose. Small children should in general have brushes one-quarter to one-third smaller than those used for adults but of the same design.[4] Many prefer natural bristles to nylon. They appear to grip the tooth surface better but they do not last as long. Machine testing has shown no essential difference between the abrasiveness of nylon bristle and natural bristle, abrasion depending in general upon the dentifrice used.[5]

Electric toothbrushes offer mechanical aid to the disabled and to many others who are not adept at hand manipulations. The small excursion of the electrically produced motions makes it of relatively minor importance whether these brushes produce motions in line with the handle of the brush or arcuate motions. The hand motions producing major excursions of the brush still remain the most important ones.

At the other end of the spectrum, people in the developing countries of Africa and Asia achieve acceptable oral hygiene by the use of *miswaks,* or chewing sticks. These are twigs of suitable soft wood about the size and shape of a pencil, the ends of which fray and are sometimes known to exude antimicrobial agents. They can be sharpened at one end for interdental cleaning.

Techniques for Cleaning the Teeth

There are many different techniques for the use of the tooth-brush, some adapted for general use, some for special problems such as the abnormal gingival contours which accompany perio-dontal disease.[6] For general use, and particularly among young people for caries control, the one most commonly recommended involves a rolling motion on the outer surfaces of the teeth. The toothbrush rotates from the gingiva toward the occlusal surface, both buccally and lingually. The upper teeth in general are brushed down and the lower ones up, according to the phrase "Brush your teeth the way they grow." Fig. 30 illustrates this motion. Occlusal surfaces may be brushed with a scrubbing motion involving small strokes in almost any direction. Each area should be brushed at least ten times, with particular care to reach the buccal surfaces of the furthest posterior teeth. Current plaque-control programs usually recommend a different motion, a modification of the Bass technique, where a soft multituft nylon brush is vibrated with the bristles pointed in to the gingival sulcus. No significant differences have been found between the effectiveness of this method and that of the roll technique. More important than the technique is the thoroughness of its application.

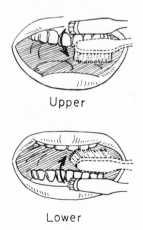

Upper

Lower

Figure 30. Roll technique, a toothbrush motion for general use.

For children, the Fones method of tooth brushing from the outer surfaces of the teeth is a simple one. This involves a circular motion, the brush being carried up, back, down, forward, then up again, without any twisting of the handle. This method is probably easy to learn but has the disadvantage that it often degenerates into a straight horizontal motion backward and forward. Over the years this can notch the cervical dentine on the labial surfaces of the more exposed teeth, chiefly the canines and bicuspids, also abrading the gingivae. Any patients seen with abrasions such as these should be questioned as to the use of a horizontal toothbrush motion.

The recommended *times* for tooth brushing are immediately after eating. Some people like to brush the teeth immediately upon arising in the morning, but this custom is disadvantageous if it discourages brushing teeth after breakfast.

Advertising claims to the contrary notwithstanding, *dentifrices* are aids, not essentials, in oral hygiene. Much good work can be done with a bare toothbrush or one dipped in baking soda powder or a mixture of baking soda and table salt. Beyond this, dentifrices are useful if they provide a mild abrasive and an attractive taste. In the light of current knowledge, the most reliable advice is given by the American Dental Association when it says: "The function of a dentifrice, whether it is a paste, powder, or liquid, is to aid the brush in cleaning the teeth. Don't expect your present dentifrice to do more than this."[7] Their Council on Dental Therapeutics does not consider for acceptance ordinary cleansing dentifrices without therapeutic or prophylactic effect.

Considerable research has been done upon *therapeutic dentifrices* which contain agents designed to inhibit the growth of oral microorganisms or increase the resistance of the dental hard tissues. The major groups of therapeutic dentifrices are those containing ammonium compounds, those containing sarcosinates, and those containing fluorides. Encouraging results have been published following tests with most of these different types and there have also been tests where the results have been inconclusive or negative. The best results so far have been obtained with dentifrices containing stannous fluoride.[8] The Council on Dental Therapeutics of the American Dental Association has concluded that certain such dentifrices can be of significant anticaries value when conscientiously used. Standard generic formulas have not yet been developed, however, and clinical testing of specific preparations is still needed before approval is granted. Fluoride dentifrices probably exert their major influence through the reducing of enamel solubility, a method which would seem to have no disadvantageous sequelae. In contrast, those dentifrices which aim to inhibit bacterial growth or action are always faced with the disadvantage that, after continuous use for a period of years, different strains of bacteria will appear that are resistant to the therapeutic compound.

The efficacy of *tooth brushing alone*, with or without a neutral dentifrice, needs consideration. Good studies are lacking in this area. Fosdick found reductions in caries of 41 percent by explorer and 60 percent with x-ray among 702 young adults, 429 of whom brushed for 10 minutes after ingestion of food or sweets, over a 2-year period.[9] This study has received considerable criticism. Other somewhat similar studies have shown no reduction, or have given inconclusive results. Two cross-sectional studies report higher DMF tooth counts among those who brushed their teeth most frequently.[10] This type of study neglects the stimulus to tooth brushing which known high-caries susceptibility most probably provides. Keyes, considering current microbiological research, states that "there is abundant evidence that the majority of people suffer from poor oral health and loss of teeth because adherent microbial deposits have not been controlled."[11]

The use of some device for entering individual crevices (*dental floss*, rubber tip, balsa toothpick, and the like) is often advisable in connection with tooth brushing, since no toothbrush can reach proximal surfaces of adjoining teeth effectively. Routine use at intervals of between one day and one week is particularly helpful in cases where malocclusion or unusual gingival contour produces crevices not easily cleaned by the toothbrush or where incipient peridontal disease is evident.

Where tooth brushing may be inconvenient after a meal or after between-meal snacks, *oral rinsing* with plain water is very helpful in promoting the clearance of fermentable carbohydrate. Fig. 31 shows the difference in carbohydrate concentration in the saliva in a test group of 50 students and student nurses who were given taffy in connection with the Vipeholm studies of dental caries in Sweden.[12] The subjects were tested twice, with and without a vig-

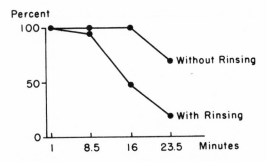

Figure 31. Percentage of subjects showing more than 0.02 percent carbohydrate in saliva.

orous rinsing of 20 ml of water, which was later swallowed. It can
be seen that after a period of 23½ minutes more than three times
as many of the subjects showed high carbohydrate concentration
without rinsing as did these same individuals after rinsing. This
technique can be of great value in situations where tooth brushing
cannot be accomplished after luncheon or after between-meal
snacks, but should not be considered to be a satisfactory substitute
when careful tooth brushing is possible. A mechanical device, the
Water Pic, provides a similar rinsing effect with particular value
for patients with large interdental embrasures, where gingival recession has occurred.

Another aid to oral hygiene may possibly be found in gum chewing, provided that the period of chewing is long enough and ex-
tends well beyond the disappearance of the sugar flavoring so
often incorporated in the gum.[13] In view of the potential danger
of the carbohydrate, however, the most desirable chewing gum
will make use of artificial flavoring instead of sugar. Such gums are
on the market.

Dental Prophylaxis

A thorough dental prophylaxis performed by a dentist or dental
hygienist is probably an aid of some importance in the prevention
of dental caries and an even greater aid in the process of dental examination and the prevention of periodontal disease. It is listed after those techniques which can be carried out by the patient himself,
not because it is less important, but because it is less frequently available and requires professional service. Regular dental prophylaxis

maintains smooth tooth surfaces which can be cleansed at home more efficiently than those which are roughened by stain or calculus. It also facilitates the early recognition of small lesions of caries if performed just before dental examination. More important, it removes those local irritants which are probably the greatest single factor in the causation of periodontal disease. For these reasons, dental prophylaxis is one of the most valuable procedures in a preventive dental-health program whether private or public.

Dental prophylaxis must be viewed today in the light of two facts: first, it is a necessary prelude to effective topical fluoride therapy, and second, prolonged pumice polishing can remove just enough of the outer layer of high-fluoride enamel to leave the remaining surface less protected by fluoride than before. For these reasons, prophylaxis should be performed with an effectively fluoridated pumice and followed routinely by liquid topical fluoride therapy.

DIETARY CONTROL OF DENTAL CARIES

There are two ways in which diet may act upon the teeth and play its role in the prevention of dental caries. The first is through the oral environment, by controlling the lodgment around the teeth of fermentable carbohydrate debris which clears slowly from the mouth. The second is through general nutrition. Essential nutrients carried by the bloodstream from the digestive tract, or, before birth, through the placental circulation from the mother to the fetus, provide the chemical means for the development of strong teeth. These same or other nutrients acting in many ways to produce good general health may improve the physiology of the mouth, reduce deficiency disease which might contribute to caries, and in other subtle ways give beneficial effects. It is often extremely difficult, if not impossible, to separate the local and the general effect of diet upon the teeth.

Oral Clearance of Carbohydrate. The question of improving the oral environment through the prompt elimination of fermentable carbohydrate is considered first, in part because it is involved in the consideration of oral-hygiene measures, in part because it is easier for a dentist to influence than is general nutrition, and in part because it has a more immediate and probably a more important effect upon caries rate after the teeth are fully developed and functioning in the oral cavity.

A classic study upon oral clearance is that of Lundqvist at the Vipeholm Hospital for the retarded in Sweden, where over 600 patients were studied for periods up to 2 years both on the institutional diet (control group) and upon that diet supplemented by various forms of carbohydrate both with and between meals.[14] Dental caries was measured in new carious surfaces per person per year. The mean values for numerous measurements of sugar-clearance time were expressed in percentages of a day when sugar concentration was above a certain baseline minimum.

The principal results are shown in Fig. 32. It will be noted from this bar diagram that caries activity in general was greater with increase in clearance time. It is particularly interesting to note how much more harmful the 24 pieces of sticky taffy were than a similar amount of more directly soluble sucrose.

Another aspect of the Vipeholm studies lies in the distinction made between consumption of sweets with meals or *between meals*. It takes significantly longer for sugar to be cleared from the mouth, and caries increments are correspondingly greater, when sweets (chocolate, toffee, caramel) are consumed between meals. This result has been confirmed by other observers, notably Weiss and Trithart, who found clear increases in affected deciduous teeth with frequency of between-meal eating.[15]

Further data on the sugar clearance of many different foods from the mouth is given at the end of the Vipeholm study report,

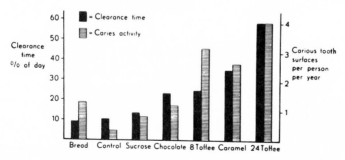

Figure 32. Oral clearance time of certain foodstuffs compared with caries activity induced by supplements of each. [Courtesy, C. Lundqvist, p. 82, Fig. 10.]

and, by adding the times in minutes in which certain concentrations of sugar in the saliva were exceeded, "caries potentiality indices" were worked out for these foods. Table 21 gives an abbreviated summary of the material. Caution must be used in interpreting it, for two reasons. First, the method used in combining facts upon the sugar content of a food and its oral-clearance time is arbitrary. Second, although rate of clearing the oral cavity is possibly the most important factor in the caries potentiality of a food, the likelihood exists that the food may contain protective factors (phosphate ion could be one) which will alter its reaction upon oral microorganisms and hence alter the ensuing carbohydrate fermentation. The application of these facts, however, is

Table 21. "Caries potentiality" of representative foods.

Food	Total sugar content (%)	Sugar concentration in saliva		Caries potentiality
		Maximum (%)	Avg. clearance time (min.) above 0.02 %	
Caramel	64.0	18.8	18.75	27
Honey + bread + butter	19.0	4.6	15.0	24
Honey	72.8	5.6	11.25	18
Sweet cookies (biscuits)	9.0	1.9	11.25	18
Marmalade	65.3	3.5	5.75	10
Marmalade + bread + butter	16.3	1.8	6.25	9
Ice cream	2.4	3.2	5.0	9
Potatoes (boiled)	0.8	1.6	4.5	7
Potatoes (fried)	3.9	0.4	4.5	7
White bread + butter	1.5	0.8	5.0	7
Coarse rye bread + butter	2.3	1.3	4.0	7
Milk	3.8	0.6	4.0	6
Apple	7.5	0.4	3.5	5
Orange	6.5	0.3	2.0	3
Lemonade	9.3	0.5	1.5	2
Carrot (boiled)	2.4	0.1	1.0	1

fairly obvious. If sweets are to be used, those of quickest oral clearance should be selected. Substitutes for sweets should be suggested whenever possible, since absolute prohibitions often defeat their own purpose.

An additional approach to oral clearance lies in the *detergent* properties of certain rough foods. Evidence has already been presented that gum chewing will reduce oral debris; so also will apples, sliced oranges, and some other foods, to a degree reported by one observer (Knighton) to be even superior to that attained by tooth brushing with a dentifrice for 3 minutes followed by water rinsing.[16]

Several large clinical tests have been made of the efficacy of *carbohydrate restriction.* Two of the most important are by Bunting in Michigan and by Becks and Jensen in California.[17,18] The procedures in both instances involved accurate measurements of daily carbohydrate intake, probably not necessary except for research purposes. Bunting's method is of interest in that it involves an initial 2-week period during which carbohydrate intake is limited to 100 grams daily, potatoes, bread, and sugars being excluded, a second period where potatoes and bread are gradually returned, and a final period in which the patient may eat moderate amounts of sugar at any one meal during the day. It is usually true that when sweets are withheld hunger will result in consumption of those foods which provide enough of the essential protein, minerals, and vitamins to improve general nutrition.[19] A brief period of adjustment is often needed. The Bunting method is designed to relax restrictions as adjustment occurs and is also based upon observations that lactobacillus counts do not return promptly to previous levels after a period of carbohydrate restriction. From these studies and others come three major dietary recommendations aimed chiefly at improving the oral environment:

1. Keep the carbohydrate content of the diet as low as possible consistent with satisfactory caloric intake. It is preferable that no more than half the daily calories be carbohydrate.

2. Where carbohydrates are used, select where possible the soluble forms or those that clear the mouth most quickly. Leafy, green, or yellow vegetables are good carbohydrate sources with low retention. Avoid sticky candy and "all-day suckers."

3. Consume carbohydrate at meals so far as possible. Avoid between-meal snacks. Substitute nuts, raw fruits, vegetables, or the like if such snacks are unavoidable.

These recommendations are easy for any layman to put into effect. The main problem lies in recognizing as carbohydrates many common foodstuffs not ordinarily thought of as such. For such information the reader is referred to any of a number of books, pamphlets, or charts commonly available on diet.

Diet for Good General Nutrition. The material on diet so far has been focused upon the control of the oral environment. In approaching diet for good general nutrition, we move on to Sognnaes's third preventive area, developmental protection of the tooth. In Chapter 8 various dietary regimes have been mentioned which seem to produce better teeth through nutrition, aside from any influence they may have on the oral environment. These diets may be classed as (1) containing increased calcium, (2) containing increased vitamin C, (3) containing increased vitamin D, (4) containing reduced carbohydrate, and (5) containing enriched phosphate. Some evidence to support the first four of these categories has been presented in Chapters 8 and 9. The phosphate enrichment has been demonstrated in a number of studies with experimental animals and is only just emerging into the clinical-trial phase among humans. Beyond such specific approaches, it is apparent that a diet which is good for the general health is also good for the teeth. Space does not permit a detailed discussion of dietetics, but the dentist—or, for that matter, the housewife, who is ultimately the responsible person—can do a reasonably good job if two considerations are kept in mind: *balance* and *adequacy in essential nutrients.*

Good balance can best be attained in a diet by including four basic food groups in proper proportion: the milk group, the meat group, the vegetable-fruit group, and the bread-cereal group. Table 22 gives some details on proportioning.[20] If the recommendations there are followed there will be a reasonable distribution of the diet among protein, carbohydrate, and fat. Adequacy in essential nutrients may also be attained, though accurate knowledge on this point usually requires detailed diet analysis. It is important also that the diet be adequately distributed throughout the day, with particular attention to the eating of a good breakfast.

Table 22. Essential daily foods for adequate nutrition.

Group	Daily requirement[a]
Milk	Three to four 8-oz. glasses for children; two or more glasses for adults
Meat	Two or more servings of beef, veal, pork, lamb, poultry, fish, or eggs, with dry beans, peas, and nuts as alternates
Vegetable-fruit	Four or more servings including: a dark-green or deep-yellow vegetable, important for vitamin A, at least every other day; a citrus fruit or other fruit or vegetable, important for vitamin C, daily; other fruits and vegetables, including potatoes
Bread-cereals	Four or more servings, whole grain or enriched

a. The number of servings listed is the minimum foundation for a good diet. Many people will want more than the minimum amounts of these foods, and everyone will eat foods not specified, such as butter, margarine, and fats and oils used in cooking.

Where breakfast is neglected, there is a tendency to get insufficient nutrients at the other two meals and to make up a deficiency in calories through between-meal sweets. It is a general defect of the American diet that it contains unnecessary carbohydrate, and this appears also to have been the case in peacetime Europe.

There are many books and pamphlets of help in practical menu-planning. For the dentist, Nizel's textbook, *The Science of Nutrition and Its Application to Clinical Dentistry*, gives several good chapters on the application of nutritional knowledge to patients of different sorts, particularly those with rampant dental caries and with periodontal disease.[21]

Diet-History Analysis. It is frequently the case that vague reports obtained from patients make it impossible to determine with any accuracy whether an adequate diet is really being obtained. Under these circumstances it is always best to have the patient record his exact food intake for a period of 1 day or preferably 1 week, and then analyze the report for calories, carbohydrate, protein, fat, and certain important minerals and vitamins. Fig. 33 gives a 1-day diet-history form used at the Harvard School of Dental Medicine. This permits the recording not only of the diet itself but also of the analysis, together with notes as to usual food consumption.

In approaching diet analysis, one must guard against three sources of bias, any one of which may produce important inaccuracy in the recommendations to be made to the patient or group of

USUAL FOOD CONSUMPTION

NAME: *Sandra S.*   DATE

		Daily	Weekly
BREAKFAST	Milk, fresh, evaporated		2½ qts.
2 Eggs	Cheese		0
5 slices bacon	Foods made with milk		
1 piece toast	Egg		6
1 tsp. margarine	Fish		1 serving
8 oz. milk	Meat	1-2 servings	
	Poultry		1
	Pork		
	Liver		2-3+
	Legumes		1-2+
	Nuts, peanut butter		
LUNCHEON	Fruits		3-4+
2 bologna	Citrus		1-2+
sandwiches	Canned		
	(Raw) fresh		
1 tsp. mayonnaise	Dried	1+	
8 oz. milk	Vegetables		
	Raw		
	Yellow or green		2
	Tomatoes, cabbage		1
	Others	1+	
	Potato		
DINNER	Cereal		
1 potato	Whole grain or enriched		3-4+
1 carrot	Others		
3 tbsp. string beans	Bread		
steak ½×2½×3½ in.	Whole grain or enriched	3-4 slices	
4 tbsp. gravy	White		
tea - 4 tsp. sugar	Crackers	1-2 tbsp	
1 piece toast	Butter or oleomargarine		3 tbsp.
½ tsp. margarine	Other fats		
	Cream		1 serving
	Sugar in beverages, on cereals, etc.	2-4 tsp.	2-3+
	Ice Cream		1-2+
	Cake		1+
IN-BETWEEN	Candy		2 pieces
1 apple	Pies, etc.		2
	Gum		
	Soft drinks		
	Water		
	Number of glasses daily		
	Amount taken with meals		
	Other foods		
	Cod liver oil		
	Vitamin preparations		

Evaluation of Diet

	Daily	Weekly		Daily	Weekly		Daily	Weekly		Daily	Weekly
CHO			Ca			Vitamin A			Niacin		
PRO			P			Thiamine			Ascorbic Acid		
FAT			Fe			Riboflavin			Vitamin D		
CAL									Sunshine		

SUMMARY:

CHANGE IN DIETARY HABITS:

SIGNATURE ....

HARVARD SCHOOL OF DENTAL MEDICINE   Form No. 2

Figure 33. Sample one-day diet-history form, Harvard School of Dental Medicine.

patients. The first bias is in recording. The patient may remember certain favorite or scientifically favored foods and bias the record by incorrect listing of either items or quantities consumed. The second bias is in the data bank description of the food, where the nutrient data are representative of contributions of the food eaten. There is wide variation in the nutrient content of similar foods, such as the vitamin C content of oranges, and average values are therefore used to "represent" the nutrient. Certain varieties of such common foods as milk, bread, and most "ready-to-eat" foods may be either lacking or couched in language unfamiliar to the patient. The third bias may lie in the interpretation of dietary intake in relation to actual consumption by the particular patient or patient group.[22] The National Research Council Recommended Dietary Allowances, shown in Table 23, disclose the wide differences in such items as energy requirements for persons of different age and sex. These allowances, moreover, are designed for groups of *healthy* people. The most valuable diet recommendations should be based on the characteristics and health needs of the individual case, with particular attention to such common activity levels as are listed by the Food and Agriculture Organization of the World Health Organization.

The analysis of a diet history involves the translation of food servings into weight or units of various nutrients according to food tables such as those compiled by the U.S. Department of Agriculture. Fig. 33 shows a form on which such recording has been made. Computer science has simplified this laborious process and made it easier to tailor dietary recommendations for individual cases. There are now over 60 nutrient data bases or banks in the United States, most of them connected with universities, from which dentists or the patients themselves can get computerized diet analyses via modem. These systems can handle up to 8,000 separate food items and analyze them for as many as 40 different nutrients. The *Nutrient Data Bank Directory* gives exact information on these details and provides contact persons' names and addresses.[23] For persons or agencies with personal computers, software is now beginning to be available for their own diet analyses.

Results are then compared with the recommended dietary allowances of the National Research Council as shown in Table 23 and also with the recommendations in Table 21 for desirable distribution of foods among the four basic food groups.[24] Of the two sets of standards, the latter, simple though it is, may actually be the better for purposes of dental health.

It is helpful for the dentist to know the best sources of minerals and nutrients of particular importance to the teeth. Calcium is much more easily available in milk than in any other food product. Cheese is also an excellent source for calcium. Soybeans, kidney beans, kale, and turnip greens are reasonable sources. For vitamin C, the best common sources are citrus fruit juices and tomato juice. One and one-half oranges will usually supply enough vitamin C for a whole day's requirement if fresh. Broccoli, collards, kale, green peppers, and turnip greens, are good vegetable sources of vitamin D is difficult to obtain in food, though egg and certain types of fresh canned fish will do fairly well. Mackerel and salmon are among the better fish sources. Most milk in public

Table 23. Daily dietary allowances recommended by Food and Nutrition Board, National Academy of Sciences—National Research Council, revised 1980.[a]

| | | Weight | | Height | | Protein | Fat-soluble vitamins | | |
| | | | | | | | Vitamin A | Vitamin D | Vitamin E |
Persons	Age (yrs.)	kg.	lb.	cm.	in.	(g)	(μg R.E.)[b]	(μg)[c]	(mg α T.E.)[d]
Infants	0.0–0.5	6	13	60	24	kg × 2.2	420	10	3
	0.5–1.0	9	20	71	28	kg × 2.0	400	10	4
Children	1–3	13	29	90	35	23	400	10	5
	4–6	20	44	112	44	30	500	10	6
	7–10	28	62	132	52	34	700	10	7
Males	11–14	45	99	157	62	45	1000	10	8
	15–18	66	145	176	69	56	1000	10	10
	19–22	70	154	177	70	56	1000	7.5	10
	23–50	70	154	178	70	56	1000	5	10
	51+	70	154	178	70	56	1000	5	10
Females	11–14	46	101	157	62	46	800	10	8
	15–18	55	120	163	64	46	800	10	8
	19–22	55	120	163	64	44	800	7.5	8
	23–50	55	120	163	64	44	800	5	8
	51+	55	120	163	64	44	800	5	8
Pregnant						+30	+200	+5	+2
Lactating						+20	+400	+5	+3

a. Allowances are intended to provide for individual variations among most normal persons as they live in the U.S. under usual environmental stresses. Diets should be based on a variety of common foods in order to provide other nutrients for which human requirements have been less well-defined.

b. Retinol equivalents. 1 Retinol equivalent = 1 μg retinol or 6 μg β carotene.

c. As cholecalciferol. 10 μg cholecalciferol = 400 I.U. vitamin D.

d. α-tocopherol equivalents. 1 mg d-α-tocopherol = 1 α T.E.

e. 1 N.E. (niacin equivalent) = 1 mg niacin or 60 mg dietary tryptophan.

f. The folacin allowances refer to dietary sources as determined by *Lactobacillus casei* assay after

Table 23. (Continued)

	Water-soluble vitamins						Minerals					
Vita-min C (mg)	Thia-min (mg)	Ribo-flavin (mg)	Nia-cin (mg N.E.)[e]	Vitamin B$_6$ (mg)	Fola-cin[f] (μg)	Vitamin B$_{12}$ (μg)	Calcium (mg)	Phos-phorus (mg)	Magne-sium (mg)	Iron (mg)	Zinc (mg)	Iodine (μg)
35	0.3	0.4	6	0.3	30	0.5[g]	360	240	50	10	3	40
35	0.5	0.6	8	0.6	45	1.5	540	360	70	15	5	50
45	0.7	0.8	9	0.9	100	2.0	800	800	150	15	10	70
45	0.9	1.0	11	1.3	200	2.5	800	800	200	10	10	90
45	1.2	1.4	16	1.6	300	3.0	800	800	250	10	10	120
50	1.4	1.6	18	1.8	400	3.0	1200	1200	350	18	15	150
60	1.4	1.7	18	2.0	400	3.0	1200	1200	400	18	15	150
60	1.5	1.7	19	2.2	400	3.0	800	800	350	10	15	150
60	1.4	1.6	18	2.2	400	3.0	800	800	350	10	15	150
60	1.2	1.4	16	2.2	400	3.0	800	800	350	10	15	150
50	1.1	1.3	15	1.8	400	3.0	1200	1200	300	18	15	150
60	1.1	1.3	14	2.0	400	3.0	1200	1200	300	18	15	150
60	1.1	1.3	14	2.0	400	3.0	800	800	300	18	15	150
60	1.0	1.2	13	2.0	400	3.0	800	800	300	18	15	150
60	1.0	1.2	13	2.0	400	3.0	800	800	300	10	15	150
+20	+0.4	+0.3	+2	+0.6	+400	+1.0	+400	+400	+150	h	+ 5	+25
+40	+0.5	+0.5	+5	+0.5	+100	+1.0	+400	+400	+150	h	+10	+50

treatment with enzymes ("conjugases") to make polyglutamyl forms of the vitamin available to the test organism.

g. The RDA for vitamin B$_{12}$ in infants is based on average concentration of the vitamin in human milk. The allowances after weaning are based on energy intake (as recommended by the American Academy of Pediatrics) and consideration of other factors, such as intestinal absorption.

h. The increased requirement during pregnancy cannot be met by the iron content of habitual American diets nor by the existing iron stores of many women; therefore the use of 30–60 mg of supplemental iron is recommended. Iron needs during lactation are not substantially different from those of nonpregnant women, but continued supplementation of the mother for 2–3 months after parturition is advisable in order to replenish stores depleted by pregnancy.

markets is now reinforced with vitamin D to the extent that the recommended daily dietary allowance can be met from one quart. If one is in doubt as to the ability to obtain vitamin D from natural dietary sources, particularly for young children, it is best to use some of the many vitamin pills or concentrates put out by the drug houses. Consult the U.S. Pharmacopeia or a reliable local druggist.

TOPICAL PROTECTION OF TEETH

Sognnaes's second category for caries prevention, topical protection of the teeth, should rightly include all measures to maintain an intact outer surface for the tooth through treatment of that surface itself. Operative dentistry restores lost tooth structure in time to protect adjoining surface areas. Topical chemotherapy alters intact areas in such a way as to increase resistance to caries. Sealants add a protective layer to occlusal pits and fissures.

Operative Dentistry

In the broad area of preventive medicine, dentists find they enjoy an excellent reputation because of their systematic and successful efforts to bring their patients back for periodic examination and treatment. Any private dental office where long-term maintenance care is an objective depends heavily upon its recall system. Six-month intervals have become traditional for such recalls, and are in fact well suited to the majority of patients, young or old. Although the need for oral prophylaxis is an important factor, the time schedule for such recall visits has been basically governed by the requirements of operative dentistry. Dental caries usually progresses at such a rate that a new carious lesion can be filled with relatively little loss of tooth structure after 6 months, whereas after a 1-year interval the lesion may often have become damagingly large. This operation is correctly termed caries control. It is "secondary" rather than "primary" prevention of dental caries, but prevention just the same.

The term *prophylactic odontotomy* was coined by Hyatt to describe the routine filling of pits and fissures in posterior teeth if they were deep enough to "catch" an explorer.[25] The theory back of this procedure has been documented by one of Hyatt's coworkers, who found that teeth with very deep fissures showed caries at the bottom of the fissure 60 percent of the time while those with shallow fissures showed caries only 20 percent of the time.[26] The deep fissures can easily be filled the first time they are recognized. If they were not filled it might be very difficult to detect caries at the bottom until it had advanced perhaps to a dangerous extent.

Sealants

Modern operative protection of occlusal pits and fissures is making increasing use of sealants. Among the chemical agents that are used, the most common contain as principal ingredients bisphenol A and glycidyl methacrylate (Bis-GMA). Sealants should be applied to noncarious, deep pits and fissures of posterior permanent teeth soon after the eruption of the teeth—seldom more than four years after eruption. Tooth surfaces should be etched with a weak solution of phosphoric acid to ensure retention. As of 1982, the American Dental Association Council on Dental Materials, Instruments, and Equipment had certified six sealant materials as acceptable.[27] The Massachusetts Department of Public Health gives instructions on sealant application in a training manual, which appear in Table 24.[28]

Experience in some programs has shown that sealant application is best done as a four-handed operation, with an assistant monitoring cotton roll isolation to be sure that *no* saliva or other contaminant reaches an etched surface before sealant is applied. Teams of a dental hygienist and an assistant have operated effi-

Table 24. Procedure for sealant application.

1. Tooth selection
2. Clean
   Prophy
   Rinse
   Dry with compressed air
3. Isolate
   Place cotton rolls and absorbent shields or rubber dam
   Dry with compressed air
4. Etch
   Dab etchant for 60 seconds on occlusal surface to be sealed
   Rinse etched surface for 10 seconds/suction
5. Reisolate (only if necessary)
6. Dry
   Dry prepared surface with compressed air for 60 seconds
   Check for dull opaque appearance
7. Resin placement
   Mix universal and catalyst in a 1:1 ratio (chemically cured)
   Apply resin to etched surface
   Apply light source for 20 seconds (light cured)
   Allow to cure (chemically cured), check manufacturer for time
   Check sealant with explorer that it fills all grooves
   Rinse
   Remove cotton roll holder, absorbent shields/rubber dam
8. Check occlusion
   Check occlusion with articulating paper
   Reduce sealant with slow speed burr (if necessary)
9. Educate
   Allow patient to view sealed teeth

ciently in New Mexico under general supervision and with advance training and a written protocol.[29] More teeth suitable for sealant use seem to be available among sixth grade children than in any other grade. Teeth should not be carious, but if an occasional carious tooth is sealed, there seems to be a sufficient reduction in bacterial flora underneath the seal to assume the arrest of caries.

The use of sealants has grown slowly for a number of reasons, including concern that sealants may not last long, that they may not be cost-effective in comparison with small amalgam restorations, that bacteria trapped underneath may cause caries, and that insurance programs may not reimburse for their application. New findings, summarized in a 1984 symposium, set most of these fears at rest.[30] Complete retention has been found to be approximately 85 percent after 5 years. Bacteria, deprived by the sealants of their essential nutrients, do not cause caries. Caries prevention where sealants are retained seems to be over 90 percent. Calderone found in a state program in New Mexico that it cost ten times as much to provide restorative care for the dental needs of children as to provide sealants in advance. In a 5-year study of first permanent molars, children had sealants applied for $10.23 per child per year, whereas a control group had first molars restored for $21.15 per child per year. Trained auxiliaries can apply sealants. Some 33 states allow its application by dental hygienists; some 14 states by assistants. The recall period for evaluation need not be shorter than the customary recall period for caries diagnosis. Dental insurance programs are beginning to reimburse for sealants.

The use of sealants, therefore, offers an important preventive measure for public health use. The indirect or intangible benefits are great: elimination of pain and the fear of pain, intact versus restored teeth, and less dental chair time. The value of sealants is technique-related, to be sure, but this problem can be faced in both public and private dental programs.

In the same technical area as sealants, the use of *fluoride varnishes* may in time prove valuable. There has been considerable use of these varnishes in Europe, using both natural resin and polyurethane bases. Preliminary work in Canada suggests particular value in buccal surface caries. Official approval of these varnishes is beginning to occur in the United States.[31]

Any program for operative protection of the teeth requires early periodic screening, as well as diagnosis and treatment. Private dental practices have long been organized to provide periodic recall; a federal program implemented by grants to states under the acronym EPSDT has aided government efforts to the same end.

Topical Fluoride Therapy

During the past half century several methods have been in vogue for the topical treatment of exposed surfaces in order to increase their resistance to dental caries. The older of the methods were based upon protein precipitation. It was postulated that if the protein in the organic matrix of the enamel were coagulated it would become unavailable for the growth of microorganisms, would be more likely to remain physically intact, and would also protect the sides of the enamel rods from decalcification. Ammoniacal silver nitrate precipitated by formalin or eugenol has been used for many years for this purpose. Studies upon the efficacy of the method have produced conflicting answers.

With the advent of the knowledge of fluorides, topical therapy turned quickly in that direction. A mixture of equal parts of sodium fluoride powder, white clay, and glycerine was introduced in the 1940s for the desensitization of sensitive cervical dentine areas. The mixture is still occasionally used under the name of Lukomsky paste. Then came Knutson's epochal work with aqueous *sodium fluoride* solutions.[32] Following dental prophylaxis, a 3-minute application of 2 percent sodium fluoride was spread liberally over the teeth of first one side of the mouth and then the other, under cotton roll isolation. The application was repeated 5 times, at intervals of approximately one week. This series of applications was repeated every third year, at the recommended ages of 3, 7, 10, and 13. A 40 percent reduction in dental caries was the usual result.

So successful was this technique at first that federal funds were made available to local dental organizations for pilot programs. A decade later, however, Muhler developed a *stannous fluoride* method by which similar results could be obtained with one or two applications per year, timed to coincide with the periodic recall of children for dental examination and treatment.[33] It was necessary to make a fresh solution each time of 0.8 gram of solid stannous fluoride dissolved in 10 ml of distilled water. Each quadrant of the mouth received a 4-minute immersion. The easier scheduling and equal effectiveness of this technique caused it to replace the Knutson technique, though there was some trouble with the pigmentation of precarious lesions and defective anterior fillings.

A final development was that of Brudevold, who introduced an *acidulated phosphate fluoride* solution.[34] This was an aqueous solution containing 1.23 percent sodium fluoride and 0.1 m orthophosphoric acid at a pH of about 3.0. The method had two advantages: the solution was stable and did not stain teeth. The teeth were kept moist by reapplication every 15 to 30 seconds for a 4-minute period. One annual treatment appeared to be sufficient to achieve on average the 40 percent caries reduction that seemed common to all three of the topical fluoride techniques.

The Brudevold solution has also been incorporated in a *gel* which is suitable for home application in acrylic resin impression trays made to fit the mouth of the individual patient. Striking results have been obtained with this gel when a small group of children on a research basis made use of it several times per week.[35] When the gel is used only semiannually or annually in the dental office, however, the results are less than with the aqueous solution similarly applied.[36] A possible reason for this decrease in efficiency lies in the fact that once the gel has been placed against the tooth surfaces it does not circulate, and the supply of fluoride cannot be replenished, as is done during the application of a fluid. The use of fluoride gels has largely replaced the use of solution in recent years. The gels can be applied in trays adapted to the upper and lower arches of the patient, thus eliminating cotton-roll isolation and the reapplication of solutions.

Considerably more research needs to be done on the use of topical agents, with emphasis perhaps on certain small details of operative procedure which may spell the difference between success and failure. For example, if cotton rolls fall out of position in the child's mouth during the period of application, fluid may be blotted away from the teeth before the fluoride can be properly absorbed from it. Again, dental prophylaxis, as noted earlier in this chapter, may have been so prolonged as to remove enough of the high-fluoride outer enamel layer of the teeth to negate the increase in caries resistance, which the new fluoride application would otherwise have produced.

Fluoride Mouth Rinses

A newer method of topical fluoride application is supervised mouth rinsing. This permits frequent use without professional personnel in such locations as elementary schools, though well-trained lay supervisors must control the programs under the direction of a dentist or dental hygienist. Though daily rinses have been used in some studies, the commoner and more practical interval is once a week. Studies of sodium fluoride solutions have usually involved a 0.2 percent concentration for weekly use. Benefits have ranged from 16 to 49 percent caries reduction over test periods of 2 or more years. Acidulated phosphate fluorides have also been used, with somewhat similar results.

The American Dental Association Council on Dental Therapeutics, concerned about accidental overingestion of these solutions, has limited acceptance of single containers of mouth rinses to 264 mg of sodium fluoride. This is within a reasonable safety limit for ingestion at one time. The usual amount dispensed for rinsing is 100 ml.

Horowitz explains the technique for fluoride rinses, using 0.2 percent sodium fluoride in paper cups.[37] The dental caries reduction associated with these rinses has approximated 30 percent in a number of studies, such as those at Stony Brook, New York, in 1980 and at Biddeford, Maine, in 1981.[38,39]

Many aspects of rinse programming beyond mere DMF reductions are important, particularly their educational and psychological aspects. The rinses give children something to do while the reasons for so doing are being described. This is far better education than mere talk. Psychologically, rinses operate best when they are novelties and in areas where professional personnel are scarce. Messer, serving a large area of Labrador for the Grenfell Regional Health Services, established 54 rinse programs in remote villages only occasionally visited by dentists.[40] Public health nurses managed the program, and children participated on a voluntary basis. No costs were involved beyond $2.00 per child per year for supplies. From 88 percent participation in 1978 when the programs started, participation dropped to 54 percent of the eligible elementary school children in 1984. Evaluation has not yet been made in terms of teeth saved, but community attitudes toward dental health, and to dental care when available, have changed for the better. Bentley, Cormier, and Oler similarly found that rinse programs in an area served by both private and public dentists made no difference in the utilization of private dental care.[41] Where private dentists were providing chairside education, elaborate outside educational and rinse programs seemed not to be worthwhile. Where public dental care was brought to the schools in mobile facilities, however, enriched health education and fluoride rinses increased utilization considerably. The mere presence of the facility was not enough to do so alone.

Another aspect of fluoride rinsing and other group preventive measures is the value of novelty. In Portland, Oregon, where rinse programs had become an old story, the city preventive program switched over to fluoride tablet supplements.[42] In New Mexico, rinse programs also were not popular, but participation in them rose sharply when a sealant program was offered as a tangible accompaniment.[29]

DEVELOPMENTAL AIDS TO TOOTH RESISTANCE

This third category of Sognnaes for methods of preventing dental caries includes only two items at present: water fluoridation (a form of nutrition) and general nutrition. General nutrition has already been dealt with in connection with the influence of diet upon the oral environment. Water fluoridation, in its community aspect, is dealt with in Chapter 16. It remains, therefore, at this point merely to mention current efforts to bring fluoride dietary supplementation to individuals.

Where water-supply fluoridation is not as yet available to the public, the Council on Dental Therapeutics of the American Dental Association endorses the carefully supervised use of fluoride tablets designed to give equivalent dosage.[42] Since this group feels that these solutions are far less desirable than community water fluoridation, it is suggested that prescriptions be given only to responsible individuals or health agencies in areas where community fluoridation is not easily possible.[43] Table 25 gives the facts and rationale for a generic prescription but proprietary products are often more easily obtained. It should be realized that the best approximation available in the home provides a less evenly distributed dosage than does community fluoridation and is far less practical; also, that few statistical studies are available to prove that the two methods do in fact produce similar results. Further discussion of dietary supplementation programs and other alternatives to fluoridation is found in Chapter 16.

An additional disadvantage to the methods just outlined is cost. In 1956 Baumgartner estimated the cost for fluoride tablets at one cent per child per day, on a group-purchase basis.[44] Individuals making retail purchases from their pharmacist would undoubtedly have to pay much more. Even so, further study may vindicate the methods, where communal water supplies do not exist.

In closing this consideration of the various methods of using fluorides for prevention of dental caries, a rough effort at comparison will be of some value. Table 26 gives very rough figures for expected caries reductions, practicality, and approximate cost per person per year of the four major types of fluoride prevention now available. In urban areas, the higher cost-levels are to be expected and cost efficiency may be reduced because of existing lower caries levels. Preventive measures should be targeted to the caries levels found locally. They will be more cost-efficient in areas where dental care providers are not easily accessible.

Table 25. Supplemental fluoride dosages.

1. Prescription form for use by individuals over age 13

        Rx Sodium fluoride tablets 2.2 mg.
          Dispense 120 tabs.
        Sig. One tablet each day to be chewed and
          swished before swallowing.
        Caution: Store out of reach of children.

2. Supplemental fluoride dosages based on fluoride concentration of drinking water, to be used in prescriptions for children age 13 and under (mg. F/day)[a]

	Concentration of fluoride in water (ppm.)		
Age (yrs)	<0.3	0.3–0.7	>0.7
Birth to 2	0.25	0	0
2 to 3	0.50	0.25	0
3 to 13	1.00	0.50	0

a. 2.2 mg. sodium contains 1 mg. fluoride.

CARIES-SUSCEPTIBILITY TESTS

No consideration of the prevention of dental caries would be complete without mention of those tests which are supposed to indicate the activity of dental caries at a given moment. Several such tests have been used or proposed, but only two, the lactobacillus count and the Snyder test for acid production, have achieved important recognition. Even these two tests are not beyond controversy. Some authors have reported fairly high correlation between test results and subsequent recognition of new carious lesions, but other observers have failed to find even a reasonable degree of correlation. Both tests are made upon free saliva and involve the assumption that such saliva reflects fairly accurately the bacterial situation or degree of acid formation under the mucin plaque or in other protected areas of the mouth where the surfaces of teeth are being attacked.

The *lactobacillus test* involves the spreading of measured quantities of saliva, undiluted or diluted, upon a plate containing an appropriate medium.[45] Incubation then occurs for a period which

Table 26. Relative benefit, practicality, and cost of different fluoride-preventive measures.

Preventive measure	Expected caries reduction (%)	Practicality	Approximate cost per person per year ($)
Water fluoridation, community[a]	35–50	Excellent	.20–.50
Fluoride supplementation	35–50		
Individual[a]		Poor	10.00–20.00
Group		Excellent	8.00–12.00
Topical fluoride therapy (liquid)[b]	20–40	Fair[c]	20.00
Fluoride dentifrice, approved type[b]	10–20	Good	c. 15.00
Fluoride rinses[b,d]	20–60	Good	2.00–5.00

a. Operates preeruptively and posteruptively.
b. Operates posteruptively only.
c. Requires approximately one hour professional chair time per year.
d. Once a week at school with paid supervisors.

is usually 96 hours. At the end of this period, the number of lactobacillus colonies appearing upon a given area of the culture medium is counted, with multiplication where dilution has occurred. From this an estimate is made of the number of lactobacilli per milliliter of saliva. Interpretation of the lactobacillus count is usually made according to Table 27.

The *Snyder test* measures the ability of salivary microorganisms to form acids from a fluid carbohydrate medium.[46] An indicator dye, bromcresol, is contained in the carbohydrate medium in such a way that when a given concentration of saliva is incubated in the medium the acid-producing potential of the saliva will be measured by the length of time it takes to turn the green indicator to a yellow color. If the color change occurs within 24 hours, caries activity is said to be marked; if within 48 hours it is said to be definite; and if there is no color change at the end of 72 hours, caries is believed to be inactive.

The reliability of current susceptibility such as those just described does not justify their inclusion in the ordinary public health dental program. They may, however, be of considerable value in the treatment of individual cases where carbohydrate restriction is part of the plan.

Disclosing agents, though not actually tests of caries activity, do give an indication of potential danger, through coloring plaque on the teeth and directing attention to neglected deposits. Erythrosine is the dye most commonly used as a basis of tablets that can be used either at the dental office or at home.

OTHER ORAL DISEASES AND MALFORMATIONS

Periodontal Disease

There are three main methods by which periodontal disease may be minimized. These involve (1) dental prophylaxis, (2) dental home care (chiefly tooth brushing), and (3) the systemic strengthening of gingivae through proper nutrition and the elimination of systemic disease. It is to be assumed, in addition, that certain dental conditions predisposing to periodontal disease will have been dealt with as part of a general program of dental care. These conditions include prevention of loss of teeth through caries, the

Table 27. Lactobacilli in saliva as related to probable caries activity.

No. per milliliter of saliva	Symbolic designation	Suggested caries activity
0–1,000	±	Little or none
1,000–5,000	+	Slight
5,000–10,000	+ +	Moderate
>10,000	+ + + or + + + +	Marked

replacement of missing teeth if loss does occur, and the correction of traumatic occlusion.

Dental prophylaxis has even more importance in the control of periodontal disease than it does in the control of caries. This is because deposits of salivary and serumal calculus are highly conducive to periodontal disease and cannot be removed by the patient in the course of home care. Patients with a tendency to gingivitis must be observed until it is known in how many months the accumulation of hard deposits upon the teeth will pass beyond the control of home care. Many periodontal patients must receive dental prophylaxis every 3 months or every 4 months in addition to whatever more extensive treatment may be necessary at the hands of the dentist. Posterior bite-wing x-rays should be taken at yearly intervals and studied for incipient bone loss.

Home care for the periodontal patient is somewhat more exacting than home care for the control of caries. *Tooth brushing* must be carried out with a particular effort to reach those interproximal embrasures which so often accompany periodontal damage.[47] The standard technique used earlier is usually satisfactory for this, but certain specialized methods are also available, of which the Charters vibratory method is one of the best.[48,49] In this method, the toothbrush bristles are placed in contact with the tooth enamel and gingivae with the ends pointed at about a 45° angle to the plane of occlusion and toward, not away from, that plane. Lateral and rootward pressure is then placed on the brush and the brush is vibrated gently back and forth. The tips of the toothbrush bristles then slide into the embrasures with a positive cleaning action. The sides of the bristles massage the gingival papillae.

In cases of periodontal disease where abnormally large embrasures exist, the flat balsa-wood toothpick or the small rubber tip often found at the base of the handle of present-day toothbrushes is particularly useful. The toothpick or tip slips easily into such an embrasure and a slight push-and-pull or circular motion of the handle of the brush will produce a massaging action in the embrasure which is beneficial to the gingival tissue. Patients should be instructed as to which embrasures in their mouths justify this technique on a daily basis.

The *systemic control* of periodontal disease lies chiefly in adequate nutrition with vitamin C and in the control of blood dyscrasias, heavy-metal poisonings, and other conditions which impair the health of the gingivae. Vitamin C requirements have already been discussed in connection with diet and dental caries. It will be remembered that avitaminosis C, when marked, produces scurvy, the curse of the old sailing ships, characterized by bleeding gums and loosening of the teeth. The heavy-metal poisonings to be looked for are chiefly those of lead, mercury, bismuth, arsenic, and thallium, some of them occurring as a result of industrial exposure, some as a result of drug therapy. The question of blood dyscrasias does not justify treatment in the present text. If gingivitis does not yield to the control measures just described, a text on oral pathology should be consulted, or, better yet, a specialist in the field of periodontology.

Malocclusion

Textbooks on pedodontics devote considerable space to preventive orthodontics.[50] Few of the techniques described in these chapters are within the usual range of the general practitioner of dentistry and fewer yet are seen in the average public health program. Those procedures which seem to justify inclusion in the present text deal with space maintenance where teeth are lost, the control of thumb sucking and mouth breathing, and the "jumping" of incisors by home therapy in the case of crossbite.

Space maintainers may be either removable or fixed. The simplest and most reliable devices for the general practitioner to construct are fixed space maintainers based upon orthodontic bands. Fig. 34 illustrates typical designs. Space maintainers are seldom necessary where the permanent successor to the tooth which is lost is expected to erupt within 1 year.

Thumb sucking and *mouth breathing* can produce malocclusion of the anterior teeth, although the evidence in connection with mouth breathing is somewhat questionable. Most thumb sucking disappears before the eruption of the permanent teeth and the effects are generally self-correcting. Mouth breathing may be the result of a nasal obstruction which should be treated by the otolaryngologist. It may also be habitual. The breaking of persistent habitual thumb sucking or mouth breathing is a matter for careful cooperative work with the parents of the child involved and perhaps for consultation with a clinical psychologist. Persuasive efforts must be undertaken, but not to the extent of driving the child to worse habits of a different nature. In extreme cases a plexiglass oral screen may be constructed which will extend over the buccal and labial surfaces of all the teeth from about the first molar forward and up into the mucobuccal folds both above and below to about half of the length of the roots of the permanent teeth. Such a screen is worn at night. It can be so constructed as to bring pressure upon labially malposed incisor teeth and may thus accomplish a small amount of corrective orthodontic treatment.

Several types of minor malocclusion are within the ability of the general practitioner to correct, and hence are within the scope of some public health dental programs. Cross-bite, arch-length management, and incisor crowding are in this category. A good reference on this subject is in Barber's chapter in Caldwell and Stallard's *Textbook of Preventive Dentistry.*[51]

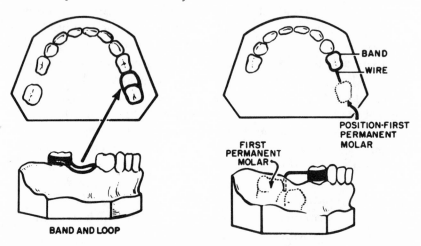

Figure 34. Two types of fixed space maintainers. [From S. B. Finn, ed., *Clinical Pedodontics* (Saunders, Philadelphia, ed. 3, 1967).]

Some of the best "preventive orthodontics" lies in the field of the preservation of the natural dentition. Timely operative dentistry to prevent the loss of teeth, particularly the permanent teeth, and water fluoridation, again with the same end in view, can probably do more than all of the interceptive techniques just listed. Documentation is poor on this matter, but studies have been cited in Chapter 9 to indicate the probable effect of water fluoridation.

Oral Cancer

One of the great contributions the public health dentist can make to the public health team and one which draws him more closely than any other to his medical colleagues is the early recognition of systemic disease or neoplasm. All dental inspections or examinations should be made with a watchful eye for abnormalities in soft tissue or bone. This is particularly true when examining the mouths of the older patients, now constituting an ever-increasing proportion of the population. Another stress group includes excessive users of alcohol and tobacco.[52] The function of the dental-health worker when he finds an abnormality is not necessarily that of diagnosis but that of suspicion and referral. For this reason no attempt will be made in this text to describe and differentiate different forms of disease or neoplasm. A good textbook on oral pathology should be available wherever dental inspections or examinations are routinely conducted.

In the field of oral cancer a simple tool for the public health worker is exfoliative cytology. Oral smears of suspected areas have given effective indication of certain types of cancer and precancerous lesions of the mouth, and the technique is a fairly easy one to apply in large screening surveys. Oral cytology, however, is intended as an adjunct to biopsy and not a replacement.[53] For clinical examination it is important to have a good checklist of those early signs and symptoms which are cause for suspicion. No better such checklist has come to the writer's attention than that published by the American Cancer Society in its pamphlet *Your Family Dentist Can Detect It*. This leaflet lists seven critical areas, noting the signs and symptoms to look for in connection with each. Table 28 gives the list. A more detailed booklet for the dentist is entitled *The Challenge of Oral Cancer*.

It is equally important for the public health worker to be alert to the predisposing factors to oral cancer. Among these may be noted ill-fitting dentures, broken or rough teeth, excessive use of tobacco (including smokeless tobacco), poor diet, and syphilis.

Any lesion suspected of being neoplastic in origin should be observed over a short period of time, the patient being recalled for this purpose. It is important to be sure that any lump, sore or swelling suspected of being cancerous is not the result of some transitory infection or injury that will soon heal. Since numbness or loss of sensation is also a sign of neoplasm, it is important to be sure that this too is not a transitory condition. Do not wait for long, however. Ten days to two weeks is enough. If in doubt, get a biopsy or refer the case to a specialist.

ACCIDENT PREVENTION

Traumatic injury to the teeth has always been an important problem among children and young people, but accidents occur in such a variety of circumstances that many cannot be anticipated or prevented. In recent years, however, there has been growing awareness of the high frequency of injuries to anterior teeth among those engaged in body-contact sports. Football and hockey are the greatest sources of danger, since they are participated in by a large number of young people, but boxing, wrestling, and other sports also deserve attention. School and college health services are beginning now to realize their responsibility to provide mouth protectors for those young people whose risks to the teeth are greatest.

Mouth protectors are of three types: (1) custom-made protectors, fabricated on a model of the player's upper arch, using resilient acrylic resin or vinyl plastic; (2) mouth-formed protectors, in which a rubber tray is filled with a (heated) plastic material which sets after the player bites into it; and (3) stock unfitted rubber protectors, against which the player clenches his teeth in order to retain the guard in place. This last-named type is usually attached by a rubber strap to the chin strap of a football helmet. Fig. 35 illustrates the three designs.

Of these types, the first is the most reliable since it distributes a blow evenly over a large number of teeth. It is constructed of a semirigid material which possesses slight flexibility at mouth temperature and even greater flexibility when held under the hot-water tap, but is rigid at ordinary room temperatures. It is con-

Table 28. Signs of oral cancer.

Site	Appearance and symptoms
Lips	Lump with bluish-white edges and rugged bases, painless
Tongue	Irregular, deep sore on edge or underside of tongue, far back, usually accompanied by radiating pains and speech difficulty
Cheek	Flat ulcer with hard edges, usually inside cheek near corner of mouth, causing difficulty of movement of jaw, slight bleeding
Tonsil	Flat, hard enlargement causing swelling of tonsil, difficulty in swallowing, speech impediment, bleeding
Floor of mouth	Raised and ulcerated and with grayish skin tissue, usually extending into jaw, usually painless
Hard palate	Hard lump, later with raised edges, usually in center or near roof of mouth, usually painless
Gums	Flat or raised lump between teeth, usually in lower jaw, painless

structed over a model of the athlete's upper jaw but also possesses flexibility enough to receive small indentations on the underside, which stabilizes the lower teeth. A fiberglass stiffener is commonly inserted, since prolonged clenching of the teeth or a sharp blow under the chin can cause the player to bite through a protector. Construction of such a protector requires only an alginate impression of the upper arch, from which a model is poured. The protector is easily retained in the mouth, even in such active sports as football, and interferes very little with speech.

Where group programs are providing custom-made protectors—and in individual cases too—the name of the person should be inserted in typed letters within the plastic.

Before the advent of face bars or mouth protectors, dental and mouth injuries constituted one-half of all football injuries. There was a 10 percent chance per year that a player would sustain such an injury. Face bars, when introduced, reduced the number of injuries by almost one-half. Mouth protectors have virtually eliminated the remainder among those players who have used them. In 1962 the National Alliance Football Rules Committee made the wearing of mouth protectors mandatory. This committee had authority over a large majority of high school football teams, but only

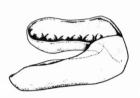
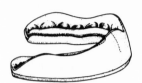
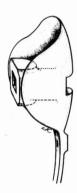

CUSTOM MADE   MOUTH FORMED   STOCK

Figure 35. Three types of mouthguard for body-contact sports. [Courtesy, *Journal of the American College Health Association.*]

a portion of the college teams. Nevertheless, Heintz estimates that from 25,000 to 50,000 players were protected during the 1967 football season alone, and injuries to 83,000 individual teeth were prevented.[54] In addition, there is evidence that mouth protectors were effective in reducing the incidence of concussion following a blow on the chin. Accident insurance underwriters in at least one state have lowered their rates because of this favorable experience and the reduced damage in those accidents which do occur. Penalties are occasionally assessed for failure to wear mouth protectors. These penalties may range from a yardage penalty to the team where an infraction is found, to refusal to pay a damage claim if an accident occurs.

Because of the lower cost, mouth-formed mouth protectors have come into use at a more rapid rate than the custom-made type. As a result, many protectors are uncomfortable, and players and coaches resist using them. The cost of mouth protection, however, is still inconsequential when compared with that of other protective equipment for the football field. The use of mouth protectors is increasing rapidly. The National Collegiate Athletic Association now makes them mandatory (1977).

A full consideration of accident prevention should also include a listing of those hazards to the teeth and oral structures which are found from time to time in industry. These receive further consideration in Chapter 21.

CONTROL OF TRANSMISSIBLE DISEASES

A problem of increasing importance in which dentists share responsibility with physicians is the control of transmissible diseases. Health care providers and consumers alike are endangered by a long list of viral and bacterial disease, whose recognition is essential and whose control is possible. Heading a list of such diseases prepared by the American Association of Public Health Dentistry are hepatitis (types B, A, and non-A/non-B) and acquired immune deficiency syndrome (AIDS). Included also are syphilis, gonorrhea, influenzas and pneumonias, tuberculosis, herpes, and several common childhood infectious diseases.[55] Private practice and public health programs alike share responsibility for education and preventive action in this area, while providing minimum interference in the rendering of needed health care.

A growing literature is available upon these diseases. One article on hepatitis lists groups at high risk of contracting hepatitis B and discusses immunization against this disease.[56] Another article examines the implications of AIDS for dental public health.[57] It includes color illustrations of Kaposi's sarcoma and other oral conditions secondary to infection by the AIDS virus.

Concern about and knowledge of these diseases and their control is growing rapidly, so that dentists must keep up with the current literature. Of particular interest epidemiologically will be the pronouncements of the United States Center for Disease Control in Atlanta, Georgia. In arranging for safe patient care, dentists should also watch for the pronouncements of the American Dental Association Council on Dental Therapeutics.

IMPLEMENTATION OF PREVENTION

A number of educational approaches, as detailed in Chapter 15, are applicable to preventive dentistry, but practical matters in the dental office are also of importance. There is a great need to improve the standard of dental fees which relate to preventive procedures. Restorative services are visible to the patient without explanation and fulfill recognized needs, so they are paid for willingly. If the patient could be made equally aware of the even greater importance of the preventive services, fees could be charged which would not only induce the dentist to spend more time on these procedures but also induce a greater respect for them on the part of the patient. What is well paid for is more likely to be appreciated.

The Committee on Preventive Service of the American College of Dentists noted in 1959 not only the indifference of many dentists to preventive dentistry but also a tendency to delegate both education about prevention and preventive-service procedures to auxiliary personnel.[58] They concluded that, "unless dentists dignify the status of preventive measures by participating personally in such education of patients, the patients are not likely to appreciate sufficiently the importance of this part of their dental service. Dentists should be encouraged to undertake at least the introduction of preventive measures which may then be followed by supplementary training by auxiliary personnel." This statement must be taken in the context of the sharp increase in concern about and knowledge of health matters by the American public which has occurred in recent years. The implementation of preventive dentistry has thus become a two-way matter, in which the profession and the public can cooperate, each listening to the other.

PART III

Dental Health Programs

CHAPTER 13

Dental Needs and Resources

THE DEFINITION of dental public health as that phase of dental health to be achieved through organized community effort leaves the specific objectives of public health dentistry in any given area unstated. Careful studies of dental disease and the facilities for dental care are needed in order to answer a number of leading questions about the function of a public dental health program. The more important of these questions are:

1. What are the dental *needs* of the community or population?
2. To what extent will *prevention* of disease obviate the need for treatment?
3. How large is the *demand* for dental treatment in the population at current or at different prices?
4. What dental *manpower* is available to serve the population and how efficiently is it used?
5. What is the prevailing philosophy of the people regarding

the extent of health care they expect to receive from *government?*

   6. What *scope* of service shall be offered in the public program?

   7. Who *shall receive* the service?

   8. How can the service, if new, be adjusted to the customs and *culture* of the population?

The answering of these questions in a given instance requires extensive thinking and a great deal of hard work in terms of surveying and steering-committee activity. It involves listening to the voice of the community and motivating its cooperation. Careful preparation, however, will pay for itself many times over in the ultimate efficiency of the program.

DENTAL NEEDS

There are various ways for expressing the damage done by dental disease, the most common of which is a listing of decayed, missing, and filled (DMF) teeth. Data of this sort, however, will not of themselves measure dental needs in terms of dollars or man-hours, the ultimate figures needed in order to implement a dental public health program. In order to complete the chain of reasoning, *comprehensive* dental service must be defined and perhaps differentiated from *primary dental care.*

Primary Dental Care

In many developing countries it might be considered adequate primary dental service merely to alleviate acute dental pain—an objective which would require very little help from the dental profession. Elementary exodontia requires very little of a dentist's time and is an operation which can be performed under stress by a physician, a nurse, or even a layman. These people often do exodontia with considerable skill. The people they serve, to be sure, are often unhappy that missing teeth cannot be replaced, but the usual cosmetic urge toward replacement of teeth is reduced by the fact that all members of the community are "in the same boat." A situation such as this does not preclude a certain amount of dental education, which may lead to the prevention of dental disease. Instruction on oral hygiene and nutrition can be given, and even water fluoridation may occasionally be possible.

Dental care of this sort frequently accompanies what in medical circles is called primary health care. Physicians are located in health centers, but the actual care is rendered in outlying areas by auxiliaries under general (not direct) supervision. The "barefoot doctors" in China are reported to be trained and equipped for the relief of dental pain. The World Health Organization outlines training for such auxiliaries under the heading of *health aides*.[1] In Alaskan communities many miles from any dental office, lay persons, preferably with nursing or dental assisting experience, have received brief training to enable them to give dental first aid, place temporary fillings, repair dentures, and make intelligent referrals to urban dentists.[2]

In this sort of primitive situation detailed measurement of dental needs in teeth per person serves little purpose. Yet even here some rough estimate of needs is important, related in a realistic way to human demands. The basic demand of any population that it be kept alive and free from acute pain can be met by the most elementary public health or medical service, almost without the aid of dentistry as a specialty. Since man has been able to cook food, he has usually been able to nourish himself without the restoration of missing teeth. At some point, however, the demand for restorative dentistry begins to be felt. Even before this time, the potential culture and economic resources of a primitive area may justify efforts at health education in order that a demand for modern dental service be created. Demand often arises sooner than one would expect. The writer remembers his first summer with the Grenfell Mission, when he was entrusted with the responsibility of spending for dental equipment some $300 which had been collected among the villagers of the Canadian Labrador through church fairs and voluntary contributions. This was a large sum of money; it represented the living expenses of one family for an entire year on that coast. The demand in this instance was for prosthetic dental service, and the cosmetic motive had a lot to do with it.

The term *primary dental care* could well be applied to the foregoing situation, but most public health dentists would add simple operative and periodontal treatment and even endodontic treatment. Comprehensive dental service need hardly be much more than this. Time will be needed for a real differentiation between primary and comprehensive care. One attribute of primary care is quite definite, however—no gold work.

"Blood and Vulcanite"

The next stage in the evolution of a dental service is what used to be known as "blood and vulcanite dentistry." It is still seen among many low-income or ill-educated groups in the United States. Whether because of lack of education, lack of dental manpower, or lack of economic resources, these groups neither prevent dental disease nor conserve affected teeth. Extraction of broken-down or painful teeth is performed at the local hospital dental clinic or in private dental offices, after varying periods of disfigurement and dental sepsis for the individual patient. Toward the end of the process, a number of good teeth are usually sacrificed. By the time all teeth are gone the patient has saved up enough money to afford full dentures—of vulcanized rubber in the old days, of acrylic resin now. The need was quite foreseeable, and the dentures are visible pieces of property for which the patient with a minimum of resources is willing to pay. In rapid caries areas such as New Zealand a generation ago, a culture may evolve where young people expect—and wish—to lose all their natural teeth in early middle life.[3]

The estimation of dental needs in an area where "blood and vulcanite dentistry" is the rule needs more care than in a primitive and underdeveloped area. Dental manpower, to be sure, must be present to some degree, but the problems of the individual patient are merely those of exodontia and prosthodontia. As always, an effort must be made to assess the readiness of the area for better dental service and to provide dental health education as soon as it may be reasonably expected to achieve results. Prevention and early control of dental disease can be emphasized, for a new generation to be taught to save its teeth.

Systemic Infection of Dental Origin

Since the great advances in bacteriology of the nineteenth century, enlightened people, both lay and professional, have realized that dental health could not be defined only in terms of restored teeth. Concepts such as the focal-infection theory and, later, an appreciation of the mouth as a portal of entry of agents of disease have made it clear that dental infection could not be dissociated from systemic disease. Today, in spite of a decline in recognition of the focal-infection theory, the association of decayed teeth with systemic disease is taken very seriously. *Streptococcus viridans,* for instance, has been identified as one of the most common inhabitants on infected teeth. Burket, in a study of 206 teeth with positive periapical cultures, recovered streptococci from 89 percent of the teeth, 61 percent of the streptococci being of the viridans type.[4] These same streptococci are the predominant cause of acute and subacute endocarditis, a disease grouping which claims the lives of several hundred persons a year in the United States, even since the advent of antibiotics. Since both bacterial endocarditis and caries are chronic diseases, it is very difficult to prove that the germs which cause the former disease have come from lesions of the latter. Nevertheless, physicians who have studied the matter are much impressed with the frequent histories they find of a dental operation, as for the removal of infected teeth, and an attack of bacterial endocarditis shortly thereafter.[5] There is also considerable evidence that transient bacteremia is common following tooth extraction. The American Heart Association is sufficiently impressed with the situation to recommend routine antibiotic premedication where dental operations are performed upon patients with damaged heart valves.[6]

Another disease often thought to be associated with dental caries and its sequelae is rheumatic fever, also a streptococcal disease.[7] A number of other chronic diseases and disabilities have been associated with infected teeth at one time or another, but, perhaps because of the difficulty of obtaining proof in a matter of chronic disease, statistical evidence is usually lacking. Most dentists have seen iritis, acute maxillary sinusitis, and neuralgic and muscular pains of various sorts close to the oral cavity cleared up after the removal of infected teeth. This subject has been discussed at some length because dentists so often think they can establish the importance of dental treatment by merely citing the frequency of dental disease. It is the writer's impression that even an intelligent public will often become impressed with the need for dental health only when a role of a healthy mouth in the control of systemic disease is properly demonstrated.

Dental Needs in Terms of Comprehensive Dental Care

With this new dimension added to the importance of dental disease, we are now ready to consider the estimation of dental needs in an economically capable, civilized society. We shall be thinking not only in terms of the elimination of pain and infection but in terms of the restoration of serviceable teeth to good functional form, the replacement of missing teeth, maintenance care for the control of early lesions of dental disease, and, most important of all, preventive measures, educational and otherwise, so that the population may experience a lower prevalence of disease. Good quality work, using the best of modern restorative techniques, is postulated. This is *comprehensive dental care* in a true sense.

Surveys in terms of needed fillings, fixed bridges, full and partial dentures, periodontal treatment, and so forth, have been made both at the local and at the national level throughout the United States for many years. Best known in this field has been the work of the American Dental Association. The Bureau of Economic Research and Statistics in a survey published in 1966 includes records on almost 12,000 dental patients throughout the country, with a breakdown into subgroups according to region and patient's income.[8] An illustrative graph from this survey is reproduced in Fig. 36, in part to show the type of material collected, and in part because the great peak in the need for fillings shown by this

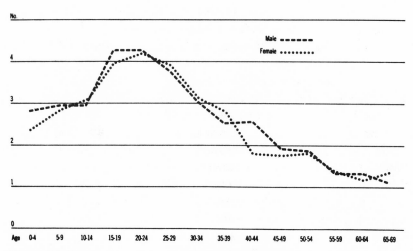

Figure 36. Average number of fillings needed per dental patient by age and sex, United States, 1965. [Copyright by American Dental Association. Reprinted by permission.]

graph—from ages 15 to 24—is one of the important phenomena in the recent American scene.

The extent to which this peak of over 4 fillings per person per year still exists is an open question. Certainly the left-hand slope of the curve must now be much lower, but the present 20- to 24-year age group may well have developed a lot of caries before the current drop in incidence occurred. Dental patients, on account of their perceived need for care, may well have needs above the average for the whole country.

Douglass and his associates, for example, using the National Center for Health Statistics surveys of 1960–62 and 1971–74, which give nationwide values for DMF teeth among adults, have projected the trends shown in these surveys to produce estimates of the true needs for *operative dentistry* in the years 1980 and 2000, in millions of operator hours per year.[9, 10, 11, 12] These figures indicate the *market* for care. They assume 100 percent access to care and 100 percent demand—both of them practical impossibilities. Using life tables and estimates of population growth, the authors have postulated a large increase in the number of middle-aged and older adults who will be present in American society and will *have teeth* over the next 20 years. As to caries incidence, the researchers had two possible paths open before them: to assume a continuing decrease in childhood caries below current levels or to assume stabilization at current levels. They chose both paths, and their graphs do not differ as much as one might imagine. For the year 2000, the graphs peak at over 40 million operator hours per year for each of the groups centered on ages 30 and 40. Table 29 gives the formula for arriving at these estimates.

It is anyone's guess which course will be followed in the developed countries where the big caries drop has already occurred. The graph in Fig. 37, devised by David Barmes of the World Health Association, postulates a stabilized rate.[13] Barmes wonders if the developed countries are not headed downward to a stable endemic caries level, which has now been largely attained, and if the developing countries are not headed up to the same level. He cites a number of countries where real increases in caries incidence have occurred, which probably show the effects upon their populations of an influx of civilized food without the professional manpower to treat the resulting disease. If each of the one-year

Table 29. Conversion formula used to determine hours of coronal amalgam treatment need for permanent teeth.

$$T = \Sigma(a_i \cdot b_i \cdot c_i \cdot (0.5)) + \Sigma(a_i \cdot b_i \cdot d_i (0.1) \cdot (0.5))$$

where T = total treatment hours needed

a_i = age-specific population in a given year

b_i = age-specific proportion of dentulous persons in the same given year

c_i = age-specific mean number of decayed teeth per person in the same given year

0.5 = one-half hour of service time needed per amalgam

d_i = age-specific mean number of filled teeth per person in the same given year

0.1 = proportion of amalgams (filled teeth) needing replacement in a given year

---

averages is multiplied by 10 to give an age-group total, the first two groups show a decrease in need of 29 million hours and the last six groups show an increase of 53 million hours, for a net increase of 24 million hours.

As the picture of dental caries changes and the growing ranks of the elderly keep more and more of their natural teeth, the problem of periodontal disease will assume a larger part of the sum total of comprehensive dental care. This matter has attracted increasing attention among dental researchers and teachers for several years. Douglass and his associates have attempted to estimate future needs in this area, too.[14]

As a basis for their estimates of unmet needs for *periodontal treatment,* they used the National Health and Nutrition Survey (NHANES I), made in 1971–74, in which almost 21,000 non-institutionalized United States citizens received detailed dental examinations, including both Russell's Periodontal Index determinations and a clinical judgment as to advisable treatment.[15] Next, from a study of the work of 873 participating dentists made in 1976–77, describing the operating times needed to perform periodontal operations all the way from routine dental prophylaxis to periodontal surgery, they extrapolated the estimated hours of periodontal treatment actually provided by American periodon-

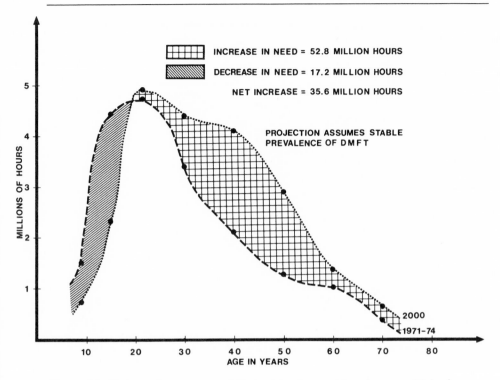

Figure 37. Hours of unmet need for operative services by age, United States, by 1971–1974 and 2000. (Reprinted by permission, Chester W. Douglass).

tists, general dentists, and dental hygienists to the public in a year.[16] The final step was to apply the Nash hourly figures to the NHANES I operation numbers in order to get the total hours necessary to clear up all the unmet needs of the country. As a result, they figured that the dental professionals of the country were furnishing about one-third of the needed periodontal care for the country: the general dentists in 2 percent of their time, the hygienists in 78 percent of their time, and the periodontists in 90 percent of their time. Some 53 million hours of care were being rendered out of a total of 180 million needed.

All this adds up to an enormous market for both operative and periodontal care, which will increase as the proportion of elderly in the population grows larger. One interesting feature of the periodontal analysis is the future importance of the general dentist. With the periodontists 90 percent busy and the hygienists not available for surgical periodontal treatment and extractions, the general dentists are the chief remaining resource. They can, and should, devote more than 2 percent of their time to periodontal disease, and they should learn the techniques involved in the more serious periodontal operations. These operations, which are beyond the scope of the hygienists, comprise 46 percent of the unmet needs, according to the Douglass estimates.

Dental Needs by Sex and Race

The need for fillings shows small and, on the whole, inconsistent variation between the sexes. Women need only slightly less periodontal care than men, but this figure is contradicted by the National Center of Health Statistics finding that men have a score for periodontal disease half again as high as the score for women.[17] Women, however, are more attentive to the health of their teeth and are more anxious to prevent cosmetic disfigurement than are men, and hence may demand more care proportionally than men. The need for extraction is consistently lower among women than among men, especially in the upper age groups. The proportion of women needing both upper and lower dentures also is lower than the proportion of men needing them.

A differentiation between whites and blacks shows greater accumulated needs among the black patients in spite of evidence to the effect that dental-caries incidence actually is lower among blacks than among whites. More blacks required fillings than did whites, and those blacks who did require fillings needed more than did the white patients with similar needs. The important differences, however, occurred in the need for periodontal treatment, for extraction, and for prosthesis. This gives the picture of a group which neglects its teeth either through choice or through necessity and seeks dental service by the "blood and vulcanite" method previously described.

Studies of dental disease and of draft-rejection rates for dental causes give a number of interesting contrasts between other racial and ethnic groups, which have been discussed in Chapter 8. The studies shed some light, by inference, on the probable need for dental treatment. In racial groups other than white, notably in

India and China, it is beginning to appear probable that periodontal needs far exceed those in the United States and that need for treatment of caries is smaller.

Frequency of Treatment

The American Dental Association study shows the patients who had not seen their dentists for more than 3 years to be in far greater need of care than those who had seen the dentist more frequently.[8] The typical patient in the former category required 5.09 fillings and 3.28 extractions. A total of 29.1 percent of this group needed at least one complete denture, and only 2.1 percent needed no treatment other than prophylaxis.

The average patient in the 6 to 11 months' group, by contrast, needed only 1.75 fillings and 0.26 extraction. He had fewer missing teeth to begin with. Only 1.5 percent of this group needed complete denture prosthesis, and 29.7 percent had no dental needs other than prophylaxis.

Patients who had never seen a dentist often exhibited lower needs than the "3 years or more" patients. The "never" group probably includes accident cases among patients with high resistance to dental disease, and in the age group 14 and under it includes the very young children making normal first visits.

Dental Needs by Income

Dental needs are generally lower among patients with high income. This may be due to better preventive measures, toward which the high-income group is better educated. It is also correlated with more frequent visits to the dentist by this group. Fig. 38 shows clearly the sharp and regular decrease in decayed and missing teeth per person 12–17 years of age in the United States, as family income increases from less than $3,000 to more than $15,000. These figures, collected before 1970, are not relevant today, but the contrasts shown probably are.

Even though the total DMF tooth counts for each person in a sample of young people of varying income studied by the National Center for Health Statistics did not differ from each other significantly, the components of their DMF counts told a different story.[18] The low-income individuals showed a far lower count of filled teeth than those with high income; the low-income people

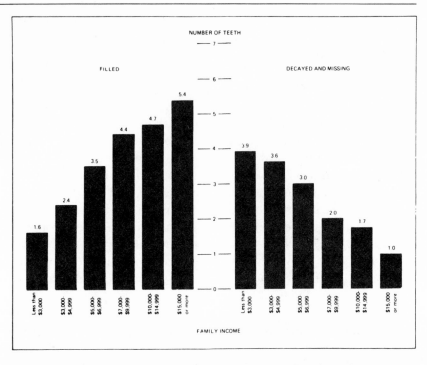

Figure 38. Average number of filled and of decayed and missing permanent teeth per person age 12–17 by family income, United States, 1966–1970. [From National Center for Health Statistics, "Decayed, Missing, and Filled Teeth among Youths 12–17 Years, United States." *Vital and Health Statistics,* Series 11, No. 144. DHEW Pub. No. (HRA) 75–1626.]

had a correspondingly higher count of decayed teeth, showing greater dental need.

Dental Needs by Region

Regional variations in the need for dental care within the United States are not as sharp as they used to be, thanks to fluoridation and other factors in the caries decrease. It is important to remember that dental needs are the resultant of two forces: disease susceptibility and previous care. A great many factors may operate to alter the balance between these forces. One of the largest factors is the state of sociological development of the country. The marked downward trend in childhood caries seen in *developed* countries is noted in Chapter 8. An equally marked upward trend in *developing* countries is discussed in Chapter 25. Whether or not these trends will meet at a stable endemic level remains for the future to disclose.

DEMAND FOR TREATMENT

The foregoing material on needs for dental care has involved a good deal of discussion of the level of civilization for which needs are being computed, and a brief consideration of factors influencing demand for care is now in order.

The cause of health is not a very popular one, even with civilized man. One cannot escape the fact that the public will usually choose present enjoyment in preference to future health unless strenuous efforts are made to persuade them to the contrary.

In terms of visits, only 45 percent of the population was estimated in 1969 to have seen the dentist in the previous year. This figure rose to 50 percent in 1981. Among families with incomes of over $15,000 in 1969 the percentage was 67; among families with incomes of less than $3000 it was 27. Thirteen percent of the population had *never* seen a dentist.[19] In 1981, 14 percent (almost 32 million) of the United States population were below the poverty level. Even when financial barriers are removed, as they have been in some subsidized group-care programs, utilization of dental service is far from complete.

Demand for dental care can be influenced by a number of factors and can vary widely as a result of manipulation—witness the activities of advertising agencies and fashion designers. The American Association of Public Health Dentistry has studied this matter and much of the following material is taken from their report.[20]

Only careful estimation can supply the criteria for determination of the demand for dental services in the future. Not only the portion of the population that will demand these services will have to be estimated, but also the kind of services that will be demanded. In underdeveloped countries demand may exist only for the relief of pain, and this demand can be satisfied by an exceedingly small number of persons trained in a few simple procedures. The next increase in demand will be for dentistry that has been called "blood and vulcanite" service, to supply a prosthesis only. In an area where people consider their teeth expendable, one dentist might be able to meet the demands of as many as 5,000 people. Only when demand develops for the refinements of modern dental treatment will a dentist-population ratio of one to less than 2,000 be approached. The situation in the United States today has been produced by a combination of these various levels of demand.

Two principal questions demand our attention. The first concerns those factors which will increase the quantity of demand for dental care automatically, regardless of the thinking of dentists. The second question concerns the extent of dentists' efforts to stimulate demand for dental services and the probable effect of such efforts.

Pelton has listed the *automatic factors*.[21] First, of course, comes the gross increase in population. Next comes *urbanization*. City dwellers have more social need for dental services than their country cousins, and they are closer to the dentists who can supply this need. In 1930, 56 percent of the population of the United States consisted of urbanites; in 1958 the proportion had risen to 65 percent; and by 1982 it was 74 percent. *Education* is a factor repeatedly found linked with demand for dental care, and the proportion of the population completing high school has risen rapidly throughout the United States. *Occupational changes* have accompanied increased education. White-collar workers can demand more care than blue-collar employees, and the white-collar proportions have been increasing. The final, and probably the most important, automatic factor is *income per capita*. It has correlated positively with the purchase of dental services and has risen in the United States from $576 per capita in 1940 to $11,107 in 1982—an increase of 1928 percent.[22]

High *prices* for dental care, especially where the patient's perceived need is less than the dentist thinks it should be, tend to depress the demand for dental care. Thus economists tend to call dental care "price elastic."[23] There are other factors in price besides the dentist's fee, among them cost of travel, cost of time lost from work (including waiting-room delays), and cost of child care in families with more than one child. Control these factors, and demand should rise significantly.

The reasons why individuals may elect not to ask for needed

dental treatment are often a subject for psychological rather than economic analysis. A discussion of attitudes of people toward dental care appeared in Chapter 10.

Effective education for dental health may be on the threshold of a new era. A conference held in May 1966 in Woodstock, Vermont, brought together teachers, school superintendents, health educators, dental health directors, dentists, and knowledgeable lay people from the six New England States.[24] All of these diverse groups expressed a strong interest in oral health, yet each group was surprisingly ignorant of the problems faced by the other groups in their efforts to attain oral health. This conference demonstrated that interdisciplinary efforts were required in order to translate the language of the dentist into the language of the nondentist and to start educational activity in state departments where it may do the most good. Few states now make health a required subject in the curriculum of elementary and secondary schools. Until they do, the teaching of health, including dental health, will be, as one school committeeman from Massachusetts actually called it, a "frill."

How well is the dental profession adjusted to meet current demands? The American Dental Association in its 1975 survey of dental practice found 32 percent of the dentists it studied to have overloaded practices, another 46 percent to have practices just above or below good volume, and 22 percent to have not enough patients.[25] Five years later, the story was entirely different. Inflation was soaring and the economy was becoming depressed. Federal fiscal policies were separating the rich from the poor more sharply. The costs of dental education and the equipping of a dental office were rising sharply, and dental fees were rising, too. Health care charges of all types were rising more rapidly than any of the items in the Consumer Price Index. Since 1950 the dental fee index has in general risen at very nearly the same rate as the Consumer Price Index, but since 1982 it has risen more quickly. By November 1984 the cost of dental services was showing one of the sharpest annual rises even in the health field: 7.6 percent.[26] Physician services had risen 6.2 percent in the preceding year, hospital room rates 7.7 percent, medical care 6.2 percent, food 4.0 percent, commodities 2.8 percent, services 5.4 percent, and all items 4.0 percent. Faced with these changes, the middle- and low-income segments of the population decreased their demand for dental care.

The cry now arose that there were too many dentists in the country. Dental school applicants dropped sharply. The established dentists, however, were not doing too badly. In 1982, for example, the mean annual net income of all general dentists in the United States was $57,000. The specialists were netting $87,000.[27]

MANPOWER

The supply of dental care available in a given area, and to a certain extent also the demand for dental care, are linked inescapably with the number of people in the dental profession and the way they make use of their time. The dentists themselves, of course, are the most important people to consider, but in order to gauge their total output we must also consider the auxiliaries that make up the rest of their team and the work habits of the team as a whole. Most of the material which follows is based upon the United States, since very little detailed information is available from elsewhere.

Dentists

In 1982 it was estimated that there were 127,000 professionally active dentists in the United States, or one dentist to every 1827 persons in the population. Of this total, the American Dental Association estimates 116,200 to be in active private practice. The rest are in government service, teaching, or research. These estimates neglect the extent to which many dentists combine a private practice with other activities on a part-time basis. Among practitioners, there are estimated to be 3.8 general operators to one specialist.[27]

Twenty-one percent of the dentists in the United States are specialists in the sense that they are diplomates of specialty boards, members of recognized national specialty societies, or licensed as specialists in the states in which they practice. The largest group comprises the orthodontists, the next comprises the oral surgeons. The pedodontists, periodontists, endodontists, prosthodontists, public health dentists, and oral pathologists follow in decreasing frequency. It is interesting that since 1966, the endodontists have moved ahead of the prosthodontists in number.

The American Dental Association in 1984 found wide regional differences in population per dentist, the greatest concentration of dentists being reported in the Eastern and the Pacific states, as shown in Fig. 39. In 1984 improvements appeared in the ratios for most states in the Deep South. Dentists tend also to be concentrated in urban areas. The Bureau of Economic Research and Statistics of the American Dental Association has made a continuing task of surveying dental practice and practitioners in the United States once every three years. The 1983 survey formed the basis of the *Dental Statistics Handbook.*[27]

The overwhelming majority of American dentists are in independent practice, either as individuals or in groups. Less than 10 percent are in salaried positions. The median net income for independent dentists was reported as $61,170 in 1982; that for specialists was $87,490. In an earlier survey of 1975, the income of dentists was found to vary slightly with the region of the country (highest incomes in the West South Central), the size of the city in which the practice was conducted (highest incomes in cities of 100,000 to 1,000,000 population), and the type of practice (specialists made more than general practitioners).[25] Of greater public health significance is the fact that income also varied sharply with the number of employees retained by the dentist. There was a steady progression in income from the dentist with no employees to the one employing 4½ persons or more, the latter having a net income two and a half times that of the former. Teamwork pays.

The number of specialists in dentistry has been increasing more rapidly than the number of general practitioners. The definition of a specialist is a difficult matter and criteria are subject to change. The American Dental Association *Dental Directory* carries in each issue the definition currently in use.

The number of patients seen per nonsalaried dentist per year varies widely and is perhaps among the less reliable of the figures presented by the survey. The median figure of 1,004 patients (1970), however, is thought to be a reasonable description of the facts. This represents an increase of 36 percent over a median number of 724 reported in 1952. Somehow or other the American dentist has been increasing his capacity to treat patients, whether through better personal efficiency, better teamwork, or more complete utilization of his time it is hard to say. Hollinshead, combin-

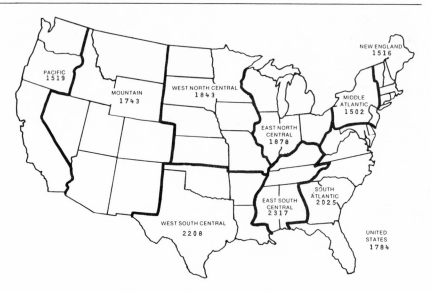

Figure 39. Population per professionally active dentist, United States, 1982. [Adapted from American Dental Association.]

ing such figures for earlier years with others in the U.S. National Survey of Dentistry (1960), projected into the future a 3 percent increase in efficiency per year for the dentist.[28] This has been a reassuring thought, though the result is nearer 2 than 3 percent. With increased attention to the mounting problem of periodontal disease, however, more dentist time will be needed for good periodic care per patient per year. For this reason, estimates of the total number of patients a general dentist can care for in a year need not be changed.

The *Handbook* shows other recent changes in American dental practice.[27] Thirty percent of the independent general practitioners now advertise, and their average annual expenditure for this purpose is $2,037. The group as a whole reports that 59.1 percent of their patients carry at least some private dental insurance and 5.9 percent of their patients are on public assistance programs. Aside from actual dental patients, it is important to realize that, in 1983, an estimated 35,266,000 persons, or 15.2 percent of the entire United States population, were living at poverty level.[29]

Table 30 presents an interesting contrast between the various types of dental practice in patients per week. The median figure of 1,004 patients per year cannot be applied to the dental specialties. Oral surgeons and pedodontists see many more than this number of patients per year; other specialists apparently see fewer.

Another variable in the number of patients a dentist can see per year is the result of caries susceptibility in the region in which he practices. The studies of the U.S. Public Health Service in providing complete dental care for children in certain trial cities have shed valuable light upon this problem.[30] The dentists working in Woonsocket, Rhode Island, where caries was high, were able to provide initial care to only 384 children per year per dentist, while in Cambridge, Maryland, a natural fluoride area much farther south, a dentist under similar working conditions was able to provide initial care for 750 children. Here is an almost 100 percent increase in the population one dentist can serve. Seventy-five percent of that increase may be due to water fluoridation alone. In the field of maintenance dental care, one dentist was able to handle only 848 patients per year in Woonsocket, Rhode Island, whereas in Cambridge, Maryland, he would probably be able to handle 2,000 children annually: an even more striking increase.

Increases in numbers of patients handled per dentist per year must indeed occur if more than the 50 percent of the population reported earlier is to receive care each year. Even the 50 percent, moreover, is larger than the proportion of the population receiving comprehensive dental care. No survey of adult care programs, to the writer's knowledge, has reported "completion" on a nationwide basis. Many of the patients included in the 49 percent un-

Table 30. Median number of patients of nonsalaried dentists by type of practice, 1975.

Type of practice[a]	Median no. of patients per week
General practitioners	60.1
Oral surgeons	73.5
Orthodontics	119.6
Other specialists	70.3

a. Figures on prosthodontics were too few for reliable analysis.

doubtedly made only one visit during the year, and that for an emergency condition.

Supply of Dentists

The dental profession generally had felt itself underutilized in the late 1970s, for a variety of reasons. Some of these reasons may have been: too heavy a concentration upon sophisticated private practice rather than more economical public service; maldistribution of dentists in relation to areas of greatest need; and the fact that the economic pressures of inflation had reinforced the generally low priority placed by the general public upon dental care. Nevertheless, the very large amount of untreated dental disease in the United States has indicated to public health workers and to government agencies that the supply of dentists must be maintained and more dental auxiliaries need to be trained if American dental health is to be raised to acceptable levels. The recruitment of professional personnel therefore needs continuing attention.

In years past the health professions have experienced difficulty in attracting qualified applicants. Both medical and dental schools have found it necessary to engage in new procedures for recruitment. Most of the unfilled places now have been eliminated, but the techniques of recruitment must be continued not only to maintain high quality of applicants but to fill the expanded facilities for dental education in the future. Recruitment may demand both personal contacts and the use of some forms of mass media.

The private practitioners of dentistry can, through their example and through personal advice to young patients, accomplish more than anyone else to insure a good quantity of qualified applicants. The American Dental Association, through its component and constituent dental societies, and professional groups such as the American College of Dentists and the International College of Dentists can serve as agencies to stimulate recruitment.

Faculties of schools of dentistry must continue to recruit through the channels where they have gained attention. The departments of science in colleges, and particularly the premedical and predental groups, should be visited by deans, assistant deans, or members of admission committees. The college premedical advisers must be made aware of new developments in the career of dentistry and provided with literature that will emphasize such development for interested students. The use of mass media apparently can be expanded. Some leaflets are now available on careers in dentistry, and new ones must constantly be prepared. Motion pictures, such as *The Challenge of Dentistry,* developed by the American Dental Association, should be distributed more widely, perhaps by dental societies.

Once college students have made up their minds to enter dentistry, applications present problems which perhaps could be solved at the national level. As of 1976, 2.3 applicants were applying for dentistry per student enrolled. In 1982 it was only 1.4. It has been suggested that a national clearinghouse for applications would prove valuable in ascertaining the acceptable applicants who had failed to be admitted to certain schools because of the popularity of these schools. No applicant can afford to apply to one school only, but he cannot tell in advance where the best openings lie. For this reason, some computerized service which will match applicants to unfilled educational places in schools might prove as important in the future as the service which now matches medical school graduates to hospital internships.

The cost of dental education so far exceeds the monies available to dental schools from tuition and the fees of patients that new schools almost require a federal subsidy. The federal government, itself a large user of dental manpower, has in the past accepted responsibility for this situation and made considerable sums of money available through such channels as P.L. 88-129.[20] Other monies have come from state treasuries. Even so, students must take out large loans and graduate deeply in debt. This load is discouraging. Dunlevy and Niessen have figured that the average 4-year direct cost for tuition, fees, and living expenses in public and private schools combined is $43,483.[31] Against this sum only $2,576 in scholarship aid can be applied, and the student's average total indebtedness after four years is $26,340.

A final, possible source of new dental manpower should be mentioned, although there is no indication yet at either the state or the federal level that it will be accepted. The examination and licensing of dentists trained outside the United States could become a source of manpower. State boards of dentistry construct careful examinations and demand an opportunity to examine personally the desirability of individual dental graduates as practitioners after they complete their study at accredited dental schools. In view of this existing mechanism, the members of state boards might be persuaded to assume the determination of the competence of foreign dental graduates. Such a mechanism already exists for physicians. The physician supply of the United States in 1972 included over 63,000 foreign medical graduates.[32] They constituted one-fifth of the active physicians, about one-third of the hospital interns and residents, and a similar proportion of newly licensed physicians. In the past 10 years the number of foreign medical graduates has increased at a faster rate than domestic production. State dental licensing boards, however, have been unwilling until recently to examine foreign-trained dentists for full licensing. Several states now do so, and more may follow.

Auxiliary Dental Personnel

Taking all types of auxiliaries from the professionally trained down to those requiring no formal training, the American Dental Association estimated in 1956 that "for the first time in history dentists in private practice are outnumbered by the auxiliary personnel."

Although the 1956 figures represent at least a 20 percent increase in auxiliary personnel since the survey in 1952, a comparison between the medical profession and the dental profession shows that the dentists still had a long way to go to match their medical confrères in this matter. Ten percent of the dental profession in the United States still appeared in 1971 to operate with absolutely no assistance at all. A comparison between the dental profession and the medical profession in the use of professionally trained auxiliaries is of interest. The figure of 98,000 practicing civilian dentists in 1976 can be set against rough figures of 41,000 dental hygienists (over half of them part-time) and 45,000 laboratory technicians; this gives a ratio of about 1 to 1. A 1965 figure can be taken for 282,279 nonfederal physicians, and this set against a contemporary figure of 663,000 for nurses, physiotherapists, occupational therapists, x-ray technicians, dietitians, medical social workers, and so forth.[33] This gives a ratio in the medical profession of approximately 1 to 2.3. Figuring of this sort is vague at best, for many workers of marginal training are excluded. Thus the over 160,000 dental assistants, secretaries, and receptionists of 1976 have been omitted from the dental ratio. On the medical side, nurses' aides, medical secretaries, and many others have also been omitted. Pharmacists, who help both physicians and dentists, are excluded. The general figuring, however, is probably pretty close to the truth: physicians use almost three times as many professionally trained assistants per person as dentists do. There are reasons for this situation, to be sure. Physicians have a large proportion of bed patients to deal with, and much of the daily care and the treatment they prescribe can be delegated quite satisfactorily to assistants. These differences aside, dentists have much to learn from the medical profession in their use of auxiliary personnel.

The ways in which the various types of auxiliary personnel contribute or may in future contribute to teamwork in the practice of dentistry will be discussed in Chapter 17.

Dental Manpower in Other Countries

Table 31 shows the number of dentists and the ratio of population to dentists in some typical countries of the world. These ratios vary all the way from 1,100 people per dentist in Norway to the figure for Chad, where two dentists are set among a population of 4 million people. The levels of dental service in these countries can often be inferred from mere inspection of the population-dentist ratio. "Civilized" dentistry is obviously available in the Scandinavian and many other countries. No dental service is apparently available to the vast majority of the inhabitants of such areas as Chad or Indonesia. In between are such countries as Spain or Turkey. Here one would need to know whether the small amount of available dental service is evenly distributed or whether an upper class receives adequate restorative care, and the rest of the population no dental service at all.

One study of seventeen Asian countries may well prove typical of many underdeveloped parts of the world. It concludes: "For many years dentistry in the vast areas of Asia has been practiced in an elementary way. In recent years there has been a desire to raise the standards of dentistry, but considerable difficulties are experienced in attracting sufficient men and women of satisfactory

Table 31. Number of dentists in countries of the world, 1978.

Continent and country	No. of dentists	Population per dentist
Africa		
Republic of South Africa	1,767	14,400
Chad	2	2,015,000
Egypt	2,083[a]	17,900
Nigeria	103	610,900
Asia		
India	8,750[b]	68,400
Indonesia	1,900	71,600
Israel	1,789[c]	1,900
Japan	39,486	2,800
Turkey	4,750	8,200
China	30,000[d]	33,300
Europe		
England and Wales	14,200[a]	3,500
Federal Republic of West Germany	31,613	1,900
France	25,069	2,100
Italy	8,700	6,400
Norway	3,667	1,100
Spain	3,613[c]	9,800
Sweden	7,000	1,200
Switzerland	2,582	2,500
North America		
Canada	8,487	2,700
Cuba (1968)	1,451	6,300
Mexico	5,101	11,800
United States	126,985[e]	1,827
Oceania		
Australia	3,477	3,900
French Polynesia	23	5,600
New Zealand	1,006	3,100
South America		
Argentina	4,620[f]	5,500
Brazil (jungle areas excluded)	27,553	3,900
Peru	2,542	6,100
Venezuela	3,093	3,900
Union of Soviet Socialist Republics	101,600	2,500

a. Government service only.
b. Includes non-university dentists.
c. Registered personnel, not all in the country.
d. Some 10,000 are graduate dentists, the rest less thoroughly trained.
e. 1982 figures.
f. Hospital personnel only.

education to undergo dental courses of university standard. The fact that the traditional dentist has a low status also makes the profession less attractive. In most Asian countries the economic condition of the people is poor and they are therefore unable to support the increased costs associated with modern dentistry."[34] The types of personnel available to give dental first aid in those countries are discussed in Chapter 17.

New Types of Dental Manpower

The existence of large developed areas throughout the world where little or no dental health care is available is beginning to attract attention. Various nations are making strenuous efforts to establish dental schools and much attention also is being devoted to the training of auxiliary dental personnel designed for semiindependent duty under no more than general supervision by dentists. New Zealand has had *dental nurses* for over 50 years, each assigned to 500 to 1,000 children, and doing simple operative dentistry and extractions for these children. This program will be described in detail in Chapters 17 and 20. A number of other nations are now training similar dental nurses or therapists.

The World Health Organization, through an expert committee on auxiliary dental personnel, recommended in 1958 the establishment of two new types of auxiliary for areas where properly trained dentists are not available.[1] The first is a so-called *dental licentiate*, whose training is postulated to be not less than two calendar years. This individual would have a degree of dental knowledge and skill approximately the equivalent of the New Zealand dental nurse but would work under a wider variety of conditions and probably for all age groups. The second is a so-called *dental aide*. This person would be given training approximately 4 to 6 months in duration and would be sent out among native populations to render elementary first aid, including dental extractions under local anesthetics. Both types of auxiliary would be superseded as fully trained dentists became available, and their training programs would be of a flexible nature, permitting improvement when it becomes possible. Both types would work, when this is possible, in dental health teams. The philosophy behind these recommendations is discussed in more detail in Chapter 17.

SCOPE OF SERVICE
Comprehensive Dental Care

Barring the complete prevention of dental disease, an objective toward which the present state of dental science permits us to advance only part way, the next highest objective in the field of public health dentistry is *comprehensive dental care*. By this is understood the meeting of accumulated dental needs at the time a population group is taken into the program (*initial care*) and the detection and correction of new increments of dental disease on a semiannual or other periodic basis (*maintenance care*). Preventive measures aimed to minimize disease are a part of comprehensive dental care. How close can we come to this objective, and what rewards await us when we get there?

Dental needs such as those reported by the American Dental Association give us operations which can be translated into man-hours, and man-hours in turn can be translated into men.[8] Klein, performing these calculations 35 years ago, estimated that it would require some 300,000 dentists to meet the accumulated dental needs of the population of the United States in 1 year, and another 130,000 to provide annual maintenance care for the correction of new defects.[35] These figures were to be set against an estimated 65,000 dentists in active practice at the time. Since that time, only minor changes in dentist-population ratios have occurred. It is obvious that our dental manpower, working with the methods of today, is hopelessly inadequate for comprehensive care for the entire population of the United States.

What might the actual situation be today as to scope of service rendered in the United States? The estimates of the Commission on the Survey of Dentistry in 1960 give us a clue.[36] This group concluded that a little over 40 percent of the American public received periodic, perhaps comprehensive dental care; 30 percent more received "some care," perhaps of the "blood and vulcanite" variety; and the rest received "virtually no care." Reasoning from this, one can imagine how the 127,000 dentists estimated to be active today might be employed. Table 32 provides such a projection.

The hopelessness of this situation on a nationwide basis, however, need not discourage us from planning comprehensive dental

Table 32. Probable actual relationship of dentists to population in United States, 1976.

Population	Status	Percent	No. of dentists	Population per dentist
90,800,000	Receive "periodic care"	40	91,000	1,000
68,100,000	Receive "some care"	30	36,000	1,892
68,100,000	Receive "virtually no care"	30	0	
227,000,000			127,000	

care for an ever-increasing range of population groups. We will in fact lighten our ultimate load by doing so.

Initial Versus Maintenance Care

The relation between initial care and maintenance care becomes of interest at this point. One of the objectives of the previously mentioned study (1943) at Dental Health Service in New York was the differentiation of these two types of care.[37] Fig. 40 presents the findings both in terms of chair hours and in terms of cost. The correction of accumulated dental needs cost the average patient at this clinic $52.66, while annual maintenance cost was only $10.05 during a study period which covered at least 5 years. The figures would be different today in view of the decreased value of the dollar, but there is no reason to believe that the 5-to-1 ratio demonstrated by the study would be essentially altered. The contrast between initial and maintenance care in terms of chair time at the clinic is less striking, but even here the ratio is 3.5 to 1. These were adult patients. Another study made by the U.S. Public Health Service at Richmond, Indiana, showed initial care to have required an average of 2.88 man-hours per child as against 0.75 man-hour per child for maintenance care at the final treatment series.[38] This gives a ratio of 3.8 to 1, which is strikingly similar to that found for adults at the Dental Health Service. It is true that in both instances the average interval after the last previous visit to the dentist is not reported. The total chair time needed to get rid of the backlog of accumulated needs for a group of patients at the end of a period of neglect may not be any greater than that which would have been needed over the years if annual maintenance had occurred (that is, comprehensive dental care), but two facts are obvious: (1) the high cost of initial care is a

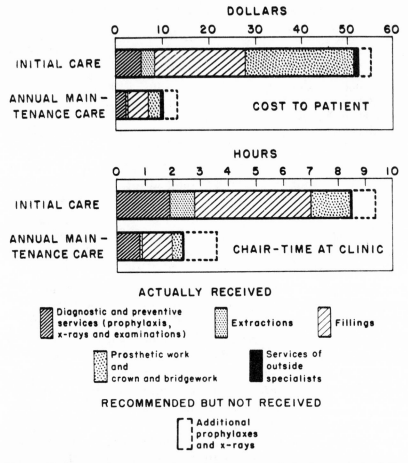

Figure 40. Average cost to patient and average chair time required for initial and annual maintenance care. Dental Health Service, New York. [Courtesy, American College of Dentists.]

tremendous hurdle to be overcome in the initiation of a dental care program for a new group of patients, and (2) comprehensive dental care results in a substantial saving of teeth in good health and function for the average patient, an advantage well worth striving for and not to be measured in terms of actual dollars.

Figures on the saving of teeth as a result of comprehensive dental care and on other benefits of good annual maintenance are hard to come by. The Metropolitan Life Insurance Company, where periodic recall for prophylaxis and examination has almost doubled the amount of restorative dentistry received by home-office employees, can demonstrate a saving of almost 6 teeth per person in contrast with national levels for tooth mortality, and a saving of 2 teeth per person in the group itself during the maturation of their program between 1928 and 1942.[39]

A wide variation is bound to occur between the manpower needed to accomplish maintenance care for different age groups under different operating conditions of dental need. The U.S. Public Health Service found itself able, with standardized operating techniques, to handle about twice as many children per operator per year in a natural fluoride area as in one lacking fluoride, as has been mentioned earlier. Pelton estimated a few years ago that for a cross section of the population at all ages treated in the private offices of U.S. dentists, it would require one dentist working full time for a year (2,000 hours) to handle 250 persons.[40] This suggests a need for *8 hours per patient*—6 hours for accumulated defects, and 2 hours for those occurring during the year. Thereafter, at 2 hours per patient per year, the dentists could be expected to take care of 1,000 persons for annual maintenance. As periodontal diseases take the time formerly devoted to caries, these figures may continue to be valid.

Prevention Versus Treatment

The foregoing discussion of dental needs and resources makes it obvious that attainment of comprehensive dental care for the entire population of the United States is an impossibility at current levels of dental disease, even with the adoption of improvements in the supply and utilization of manpower and improvements in the financing of dental care which currently seem possible. How can the gap between dental care and dental disease be bridged? One answer is obviously in prevention.

Chapter 12 discussed in detail the means we now have at our disposal for the prevention of dental disease. No complete preventive has been discovered, either for dental caries or for periodontal disease. The best hope lies in a combined attack using water fluoridation, dietary improvements, oral hygiene, early correction of dental defects, control of concomitant disease—everything we can think of—and then proceeding the rest of the way toward dental health through the rendering of comprehensive dental care.

The city of Philadelphia is one of many with just such a plan in operation at the present time.[41] Prior to 1954 only 48 percent of the children seen in the city clinics received completed care. Ages 6 to 9 received highest priority, but a preschool group was also included. Fluoridation of the water supply then occurred. By 1966 dental care had been extended to all ages through 12, and in two health districts extended all the way through high school. The preschool children had been dropped from the priority list because needs for care had become minimal in that group. By that time care was being completed for almost 100 percent of the children seen. The decayed and missing proportions of their DMF counts had dropped to almost zero and the filled-tooth proportions had risen to almost 100 percent.

This brings us to our two questions on the scope and beneficiaries of a public health dental program. With the reduction of government payment for work in private dental offices and with the continued existence of high caries among people in underserved areas, community dental health programs still have functions they are best suited to perform. What are these functions?

Public Program and Private Office

Since public health has its major concern with prevention and with those phases of prevention and care to which teamwork can best be applied, it would be of interest at this point to set down the more common dental services as seen from a patient's point of view. The picture will be all the clearer if services are listed in the order in which a patient might experience them. Such a list is shown in Table 33.

This list needs some explanation. The placing of oral prophylaxis under the heading of case finding may seem strange, and, to be sure, it might almost as well be listed under preventive measures or periodontic treatment. In practice, however, dental prophylaxis is a necessary prelude to good dental inspection or examination. If a dental hygienist is doing the inspection work, as is so often the case in a public health dental program, prophylaxis and inspection become one process. Another arrangement which

Table 33. Dental services in sequence as a patient might experience them.

Preliminary services
1. Dental-health education, including nutrition
2. Palliative emergency treatment at the first-aid level
3. Preventive measures
   a. For the individual
   b. For the community (water fluoridation, rinses, etc.)
4. Case finding
   a. Dental inspection or dental examination, perhaps including x-rays
   b. Oral prophylaxis
5. Referral to source of treatment

Treatment services
6. Diagnosis and treatment planning
7. Corrective services
   a. Oral surgery
   b. Orthodontics
   c. Periodontics
8. Restorative services
   a. Operative dentistry
   b. Prosthetic dentistry

may seem curious is the separation of dental examination from diagnosis and treatment planning. This is done on a realistic basis. Dental examination can often become part of a teamwork program, and findings may be prepared for transmission to a private dentist *without any attempt to reach a final diagnosis.* It is quite possible to tell a patient that a cavity is found upon such and such a tooth, and that the operator who performs the final treatment will decide what type of restoration is best suited. It is also possible to show the patient an x-ray with a radiolucent area at the apex of the tooth, and explain that this picture shows bone loss, but that the operator responsible for definitive treatment will make both the final diagnosis and the plan for treatment. This allows dental examination in a public health program, but permits the dentist in charge of treatment (who may be either a public employee or a private practitioner) to do his own diagnosis and treatment planning. Such division of labor makes not only for more efficient treatment, but for better public relations.

A study of this outline for dental services as a patient might experience them shows immediately that the *preliminary services* are those which are most concerned with prevention, and which lend themselves best to teamwork. The *treatment services* are those which take large blocks of time. There is far less inducement for team-work here, though group practice does have its advantages both in the rendering and in the financing of dental care, as will be dis-cussed later. The order in which the services are listed also has its significance. Dental health education must precede dental treat-ment to the extent at least that the patient knows that dental treat-ment exists and can help him. For the uneducated patient, palliative emergency treatment may of necessity be his first experience, and this may lead in time to dental health education and to compre-hensive care. In an ideal program, preventive measures should be first on the list and emergency treatment might not have to exist at all, but the present listing is a more probable one in society as we see it today.

To date, the *ethics* of the dental profession has prohibited the individual dentist from soliciting patients. A recent Supreme Court decision now forbids restraint upon advertising by professional personnel, but it is doubtful if this legal change will soon alter our ethical habits to any great extent. There are many good reasons for our traditional code of conduct, chief among them the fact that the dentist should be in an impartial position when it comes to the rendering or not rendering of treatment, and should never be put in the position of having to "sell" a "product" for his own financial gain. He is treating a highly variable human being—not manufac-turing a product—hence he cannot "guarantee" his results. He should be very obviously in the position of placing the patient's interests ahead of his own. For these reasons the influencing on the public rests best in public hands. Dental societies can urge the public to seek dental care, but always without influencing choice of the individual dentist or program. Between the dentist and the public lies a large area for the action of government, and for the action of communitywide voluntary agencies. The preliminary ser-vices listed in Table 33 are in effect health promotion, and can stimulate treatment services beyond the ability of either the private or public service dentists.

The old concept in the United States that dental care was the responsibility first of the individual, then of the community, then of the state, then of the nation, in that order, was sharply altered in 1966 by the Medicare and Medicaid amendments to the Social Security Act (Titles XVIII and XIX). The first of these amendments established the principle that for one age group, at least, health care, to the extent available, was a "right," and the second enlarged very greatly that segment of the population entitled to receive immediate financial aid in the receipt of health care. Further details of both these amendments are discussed in Chapters 22 and 23.

The dental care that goes with Title XIX is altering profoundly our approach to dental public health and is giving traditional health agencies, in addition to their usual tasks of prevention and epidemiological research, the task of administering large programs for direct dental service. These programs either may represent reimbursement for services rendered in the private dental office, or may be group programs utilizing clinics. There is no single "best answer" as to which of these methods should predominate. The dental profession in general prefers to see care rendered in its own private offices with reimbursement afterward. For patients of an educational and economic level high enough to adapt to private-office routine, this is indeed probably the best solution.

With low-income populations, and particularly with the residents of poverty areas, both rural and in the city ghettos, a number of considerations often point to a different answer. There is, indeed, a "culture of poverty," which has already been discussed. Poor people often lack not only the funds to pay for dental treatment, but the funds to transport themselves to the dental office and to care for other children in the family while the mother is away from home. In addition, poverty means more than mere lack of money. It is actually a helplessness to make use of opportunities, even if they are available without cost. For these reasons, and also because poor people are accustomed to and actually often prefer clinic services to those of the private dental office, clinics must frequently be called into being. These clinics should be located as close as possible to the actual residences of the people to be served. Both the city ghettos and the rural areas are likely to be places where private dentists have not cared to locate their offices. If freedom of choice of dentist is somewhat restricted for the population groups served by clinics there, it is doubtful if the restriction is greater than would otherwise have occurred because of the economics of transportation. Moreover, a clinic is an obvious team enterprise, with the prestige of a university, some charitable agency, or a governmental agency back of it. This situation inspires confidence to an even greater extent, perhaps, than can the private office of a dentist who is not well known to the people he serves.

It is interesting to see how these current developments in the United States resemble the changes seen in other parts of the world. Many European countries in the wake of the Industrial Revolution resorted to compulsory health insurance in a form more far-reaching and rigid than that seen by the current amendments to our Social Security Act. First was Germany in 1883 under Bismarck.[42] The plan here was no dictatorial decree, but the result of years of debate and compromise in the Reichstag. Austria and Hungary followed suit within a few years. Norway started compulsory health insurance in 1909, and Great Britain in 1911, later expanding its program in 1948 to the National Health Service program embracing all phases of medical and dental care, with which we are now familiar. The USSR, Japan, Greece, Italy, France, New Zealand, Mexico, and Brazil are among the more important countries which have adopted health insurance since World War I. All of these countries, so far as is known, still have room for the private practice of medicine and dentistry, but the dominant philosophy is that the major costs of health care should be spread over the entire population rather than concentrated on the individual or small group. The result is called compulsory health insurance, but more of the money comes from general taxation than from insurance premiums. In England it was recently estimated that nine-tenths of the nation's $1 billion health bill came from general taxation, and one-tenth from insurance contributions.[43]

There have been many criticisms of the medical care which results from compulsory health insurance. The intervention of government authorities in such a way as to interfere with the doctor-patient relation, and the overloading of practitioners and hospitals with trivial complaints owing to the absence of any economic barrier, are among the criticisms most often heard. The people of the United States have probably heard these complaints most often in connection with programs in England and Germany, yet both countries continue their plans in the apparent conviction that service rendered through them is better than that which could be rendered in any other way. In the United States, on the other hand, compulsory health insurance has been widely opposed, and recent cutbacks in Medicare and Medicaid services have accentuated health care needs among low-income people. It is difficult to predict the equilibrium which will result from rising public demand for dental care at government expense. The reluctance of the public to pay the new taxes which will be necessary to finance such care and the forces supporting individual initiative which have always been so strong in this country will act as deterrents to change.

A final question relating to government responsibility for comprehensive dental care concerns the *cost effectiveness* of the government dollar. Obviously, a given number of dollars devoted to water fluoridation will produce far greater dividends in dental health than an equal number of dollars devoted to dental treatment. Shall the government deny subsidy for dental care to those areas where fluoridation and other preventive measures are possible but not utilized? Cultural and economic situations must be carefully considered, but the taxpayers of the country do have the right to insist upon efficient utilization of their dollars. The federal government has as yet been unwilling to deny financial assistance to communities which could, but do not, fluoridate.

Dental Care for Children

State and local governments in the United States, usually with federal aid, administer a great variety of programs designed to care for special groups. Children are perhaps the most important such group. They are gathered together at school, and the correction of physical defects there and the control of communicable disease are matters of group importance if education is to accomplish its aim. Children with chronic defects, either physical or mental, deserve special attention. The value of health education, too, is peculiarly great in the child population. Medical and dental care for the indigent comes at an early stage in public health programming, and the extent of care rendered varies with need and recognition of need in each community. Never, however, does dental care in the United States reach an entire child population, as it does in such countries as Norway, Sweden, and New Zealand.

Whether or not a government decides to take care of all children in the community or only the indigent, two important decisions still remain to be made: (1) shall available funds be used to provide as much care as possible for all children, even if it is only filling per child, and (2) if the answer to the first question is negative, and funds will not permit adequate attention to all applicants, which age groups or socioeconomic groups shall receive dental care?

The first of these questions is usually answered in the negative throughout the United States. Comprehensive dental care for a limited group is usually thought to be a better objective than scattered, incomplete care for a larger group. To treat only part of a mouth on other than an emergency basis is to invite the undermining of one's work through the ravages of caries elsewhere in the mouth, and it also fails to demonstrate the advantages of comprehensive care to the child. Almost always, an effort is made to select a group of children, usually a school grade or grades, for whom comprehensive care will be rendered. The children thus selected will be sent off to a good start, both therapeutically and educationally. In these days, with the striking drop in childhood caries so apparent, the selection of stress groups is not as difficult as it used to be. City slum areas, on the one hand, and isolated rural areas, on the other, are occupied by children who have very little access to care but also have had more disease than the average.

Incremental Care

Incremental care may be defined as periodic care so spaced that increments of dental disease are treated at the earliest time consistent with proper diagnosis and operating efficiency, in such a way that there is no accumulation of dental needs beyond the minimum. In private practice, 6 months is the commonest, though not the only, interval between visits. In public health programs, 1-year intervals are usually implied.

There is no doubt that this represents the ideal pattern for care where appreciable incidence of new dental disease is to be expected each year. Lesions of caries are treated before there has been a chance for pulp involvement. Periodontal disease is intercepted at or near the beginning. Topical and other preventive measures can be maintained on a periodic basis. Bills for dental service are equalized and regularly spaced. Incremental care, however, to be effective, must represent a real system of human behavior, faithfully maintained.

There are also several disadvantages to the principle of incremental care. One trouble with the system is that operative dentistry is more time-consuming on a piecemeal basis than upon a wholesale basis. A large operative program can be handled on the *quadrant* basis under local anesthesia. This makes for rapid cavity preparation and easy isolation of teeth for filling procedures. Five or six tooth surfaces can thus be filled in the time required for only two or three surfaces if these are scattered in various parts of the mouth.

Another trouble with incremental care relates to the effort usually made to implement it at the earliest available age, which coincides with the entry of a child into some public health or public school program. The result of this timing is that financial resources are usually exhausted even before the elementary school population has been cared for, and the high school child receives no maintenance care at all. Thus the tremendous peak in the need for fillings shown by the American Dental Association between the ages of 15 and 24 occurs entirely outside the age range for incremental care. Adolescents receive no aid in stemming the massive onslaughts of dental caries upon the permanent teeth.

Most public dental-care programs have been based squarely upon the recommendations made in 1960 by the Commission on the Survey of Dentistry in the United States, a group sponsored by various private and governmental agencies including the American Dental Association. The assumption of the Commission, as stated in its summary report, is that increments of dental disease occur so regularly in the child population that the maintenance costs per year for young children can be considered applicable up until the end of the high school period.[36] Chapter 20 presents strong reasons to doubt the psychological validity of a plan which is based on the expectation that all the children of the United States will become systematic recipients of dental care to the exclusion of heavy masses of initial care following periods of neglect.

Under these circumstances is it justifiable to devote the bulk of the resources of a given program to the restoration of deciduous teeth? The answer almost always given is that premature loss of deciduous teeth is conducive to malocclusion, and that malocclusion in turn conduces to greater susceptibility to dental caries and to periodontoclasia in later life. This may be true, but it seems to the writer that adequate evidence accompanied by untreated control groups is lacking. Existing studies are inadequately controlled, and, though correlations between malocclusion and increased caries have occasionally been found, there are also strange reversals reported. Thus Adler, reporting on malocclusion and caries in five Hungarian cities, found that patients with "covered bite" show less caries than do patients with normal occlusion, and patients with Class II division II malocclusion show no variation from the normal occlusion group.[44] There are some studies, to be sure, showing that premature loss of permanent teeth is associated with malocclusion, but the proponents of incremental dental care usually cite the malocclusion resulting from loss of deciduous teeth and not the malocclusion resulting from loss of permanent teeth. Much additional work remains to be done upon this problem before an easy answer can be given.

Chronically Ill and Elderly

A large category commonly receiving medical care at the expense of state or local governments in the United States is that of the chronically ill. This group deserves attention in part because it is often confined in public institutions, and in part because the chronic nature of the illness involved creates acute financial problems even for people normally in the middle-income brackets—a condition frequently called medical indigence. Sufferers from tuberculosis, cancer, mental disease, arthritis, and the like are commonly cared for at government expense. Hospital inpatient dental service is usually a part of the medical care program for these people, and restorative dentistry should be performed to a far greater extent than is seen in other hospitals, since the patients have no opportunity for elective dental care outside. Details of dental health programs for the chronically ill are presented in Chapter 21.

Special problems of disease, access to care, and psychological attitude toward care occur among the elderly. *Geriatric dentistry* is becoming a field in its own right, perhaps even a specialty. Problems of access and home care are such that dental hygienists have a marked advantage over dentists as scouts for the dentists themselves. This matter is discussed in Chapter 21.

Industrial and Consumer Groups

Not all large-scale group dental care need be rendered by government. There are many voluntary agencies that advantageously maintain public health dental programs. These include consumer groups, industrial employers, labor unions, fraternal organizations, and so forth, maintaining services for their own members, the majority of whom are not readily classed with the medically indigent. Also included are "service clubs" and other philanthropic organizations maintaining dental services for the indigent in their own areas. These services may have originated either as public health programs of the preventive type or as straight efforts to purchase dental care on a group basis. Financing varies all the way from division of all costs among the recipients of service to complete financing by dental health insurance. A primary inducement to group dental care is frequently the economic and other benefits to be realized from group practice. Chapter 17 will describe this benefit in further detail, and Chapter 21 will take up the specific reasons for industrial management and labor groups to become interested in dental care.

In some of the larger cities especially, a new problem has arisen: health care for the *homeless,* among whom males outnumber females by a wide margin. In a study of over 100 persons, aged 18 to 65, at a shelter in Boston, 97 percent were found to need some form of dental treatment.[45] Eighteen percent required emergency treatment for pain or infection. Periodontal and prosthetic problems were common. Thirty-four percent did not own a toothbrush.

MATCHING PROGRAMS TO NEED AND DEMAND

The foregoing discussions make it clear that the fitting of dental health programs to need and demand, at least in the United States, is far from a simple matter. Different levels of dental care can be designed for varying degrees of civilization, but if the United States—a relatively civilized area and a world leader in dentistry—

were to demand the highest level of care, the need for such care would far exceed the ability of present manpower to meet it. Demand now seems insufficient to lead the public to avail itself either of the full amount of needed dental treatment or of the preventive measures necessary to cut the disease rate down to a level where it can be controlled. Demand will prove easier to alter than manpower, as our experience with government-assisted health care (Medicaid) is demonstrating. The effort to increase manpower requires long-term action on a number of fronts, such as recruitment, training places in dental schools, licensing, geographical distribution, auxiliary utilization, and others, if present population-dentist ratios are to be maintained, much less improved. In the field of prevention of dental disease, the need for increased understanding and action is clear and strong.

Granted that public programs have a vital function to perform in the preventive phases of dental health work, and also have an obvious place in the rendering of dental care to certain segments of the population, where shall they be established in a free society? The answer is dependent not only on the ability of the dental profession to achieve proper working conditions, but on local political thought as well. No exact rules can be laid down for type, scope, and availability of service, but a few general principles do seem of value:

1. *Search for real stress groups* in the population, where the need for education or for care clearly exceeds ability to obtain it. Beyond such conventionally accepted groups as young children and the indigent, the stress groups now most in evidence in the United States are single-parent families, teen-agers, the chronically ill, and the aged.

2. *Do not be afraid to educate* for fear demand will exceed manpower supply. The demand is of economic value in encouraging utilization of the profession, and any immediate excess can be diverted to preventive measures if treatment is unavailable.

3. *Be attentive to public demand*, particularly in the field of group care. It is easy to underestimate the health-care knowledge of consumer groups. In matters of personnel selection and priority planning for care, their skill may equal or surpass that of the dentist.

4. *Learn team leadership* for the more efficient use of auxiliary personnel. (See Chapter 17.)

5. *Concentrate the public program* on those services where *prevention* of disease can best be obtained and where *teamwork* is of greatest value.

6. *Blend financial aid* from private and from government sources, making most efficient use of the principles of insurance, prepayment and postpayment. (See Chapter 18.)

CHAPTER 14

Surveying

IT IS NOW time to pass from the background material and the general principles of public health to the practical planning of dental health programs. The writer well remembers the remark of his predecessor when he was taking over the chairmanship of a community health council a few years ago: "You will generally find yourself doing what people want done." How does one find out what people want, or what people need, and how does one go about doing it? The best first steps usually involve a survey and its analysis.

Surveying is generally taken to imply a collecting of facts, and analysis or *evaluation* the interpretation of facts once they have been collected, comparisons being made between the current survey data and comparable data from other times or places. In effect, the processes of surveying the evaluation are hard to separate. Evaluation has, however, become associated with quality-control procedures to such an extent that a number of new techniques have arisen of a nature rather different from methods used in typical survey work. Evaluation procedures, therefore, deserve a chapter of their own, Chapter 19.

Dental health program planning, like any other form of action, is best stimulated by a simple statement of needs and objectives. No matter how complex the array of facts confronting a planner as he enters a new community may be, the facts must eventually he boiled down into simple form. One of the most important procedures in survey analysis is the separating of relevant from irrelevant facts. This process should start right from the beginning of the survey.

This chapter will take the form of an outline which is in effect a checklist of things to look for and yardsticks to be applied. There is no though that all items in the outline will demand equal attention in a survey of a given community, particularly a small community. Many items may be of minor importance, or perhaps require no attention at all. It will be noted that the outline omits many details which would go to describe the preexisting dental health program in the community. This omission is intentional. Later chapters will deal with actual program planning, and it is best during the survey phase to concentrate attention upon general community attitudes, manpower resources, disease conditions (dental and otherwise), and health programs *other* than dental. These constitute the framework within which the dental health officer must operate. The planning of his own specific service comes later.

SURVEYING OF ATTITUDES AND MANPOWER

The previous chapter has outlined in general the way in which the dental needs of a community, the demands for dental treatment within that community, and the manpower and other dental resources available within the community bear upon construction of a dental health program. It is the function of a survey to select those yardsticks which will best measure these rather intangible items in a specific community and then to use them. Information should probably be sought in most or all of the areas dealt with here.

Community Attitudes and Economic Resources

The attitude and economic status of a community should be studied with a view to estimating its willingness to assume responsibility for the solution of the dental health problems it may contain. First a general estimate should be made of the degree of *interest in dental health* in the community. This interest should probably be tabulated as superior, moderate, or little. Think of the interest in terms of the type of dental care you feel the community should really be receiving. Do the people wish to save their teeth? Do they make the best of the resources available to them for comprehensive dental care? Ideally, a careful survey of consumer expenditures for medical and dental care might be made, with estimates of cost effectiveness. The techniques for such surveying are difficult, however, and in most instances an "educated guess" must suffice.[1]

It is important at this stage to appraise the needs and interest of subgroups within the population. Particular attention should be given to urban versus rural subgroups and those with distinctive ethnic or religious customs or dietary habits. Differences in educational level are also important.

Community Agencies and Professional Resources

Next assess the community for the *voluntary or lay organizations* to be found within it capable of furthering education and health. Parent-teacher associations should be sought first. Service clubs (Rotary, Lions, Kiwanis, and so forth) may often be making a valuable contribution to a better standard of living for the community. Chambers of commerce, civic associations, and health councils should also be studied.

Another item of importance under attitude is the quality and quantity of *pediatric supervision* available to the children in the area. An alert group of physicians impressed with the importance of prenatal and pediatric supervision can accomplish a tremendous amount of preventive medicine, and preventive dentistry as well. Their greatest contribution to dental health will probably come through the establishment of sensible standards of nutrition and the prescription of fluoride supplements where fluoridation is not available. It is the writer's impression that children brought up under systematic pediatric supervision will show the first onset of dental caries years later than children who have not had similar advantages.

Another measure of attitude may be found in the *objectives and budget of the local health department*. How much money does the community spend per capita per year for health? Current national and local statistics should be consulted upon this matter. In 1967 the people of the United States were estimated to have spent approximately $1.44 per capita for local health services.[2] This sum was subject to regional variation, and so also was the proportion of it devoted to dental service. In many areas it used to be estimated that dental health got about 10 percent. The proportion of local funds is probably less today, where Medicaid provides restorative dentistry for eligible children. The proportion of the health dollar which goes to dentistry will also vary according to dental needs, and the amount of actual dental care included in the current program.

Financial figures on dental health programs should be given no more importance than they deserve. They tell nothing of the wisdom of the programs concerned or how far these go toward the attainment of their objectives. Good programs, too, may operate on hidden budgets. We are told of one program in Massachusetts "which is a joy to behold, at a cost which cannot be identified with any item called 'dental' in the budget, the cost being hidden in the water department budget (fluoridation) and the school health services budget."

Social Needs

The general *social* and *economic level* of the community will determine to a large extent the proportion of its population likely to need dental health education or dental care at government expense. Chapter 10 has described some of the factors which enter into social need. An index for the status of a community (Wallace's) was described which makes use of a number of suggestive factors such as fetal mortality, juvenile delinquency, unemployment, crowded housing, and tuberculosis incidence.[3] In spite of the wide divergence of specific causes of these factors, the fact remains that they correlate well one with another in most instances, and are very helpful in providing a picture of the economic status of the community. For individuals or families, the Hollingshead 2-factor

5-level index is of value.[4] No formal index need be used in most instances, but estimates help us to gauge the proportion of the population likely to need government assistance.

If a new survey is needed to define public appraisal of health or social needs, care must be taken to prepare a valid interview questionnaire and to follow well-established sampling techniques. The National Health Survey prefers the use of lay rather than medically trained interviewer such as nurses or hygienists. The Survey summarizes its position as follows: "In obtaining answers to certain questions by the questionnaire, the interviewer performs a function that is simply one of reporting what she hears. This function does not include any element of interpretation. For this reason, lay interviewers are generally preferred to medically trained interviewers, despite the nature of some of the information that is being handled. A person with a medical education is trained to interpret what the patient says, and this interpretation is difficult to standardize for statistical purposes."[5]

Objective determination of social needs is not the only factor in predicting the load on a government-financed dental care facility. Pride and custom play their part, often leveling out the local variations which might be expected. Thus the Division of Dental Health in Massachusetts has considered it almost a rule of thumb that 10 percent of a local population will avail itself of free service in that state. New cultural patterns may be expected to emerge as Medicare and Medicaid become stabilized, and if national health insurance emerges.

"The Voice of the Community"

The recent rise in the cost of health care and the efforts of the Republican administration to shift federal health programs to state or private agencies has resulted in an increasing divergence between independent and dependent population groups. The dependent groups need particular attention, and questions of access to care, local community customs, and community pride need study. Urban underserved areas (ghettos) and rural areas where professional personnel are lacking present the most urgent problems. In both, the community groups must be listened to and encouraged to think their problems through.

In New York City, certain areas showed severe levels of racial imbalance, social and economic disadvantage, poor relationships between providers and consumers, drug abuse, alcoholism, corruption, and other barriers to good health care. A series of seminars was organized in three of these areas under the title "The Voice of the Community."[6] Leading lay and agency people were encouraged, under a skillful and empathetic coordinator, to discuss the history and current aspects of the community. The lifestyles of minority ethnic groups and the interpersonal and interprofessional communications between providers and consumers were then discussed. Finally, specific information was presented on nutrition, social service, dental and medical care, and expressed consumer demands. Further details on these seminars appear in Chapter 15, since they are as important in the field of health education as in the field of surveying.

Environmental Preventive Services

There are not many community services or programs which contribute directly to the prevention of dental disease, but *water fluoridation* and a good *school lunch program* should be looked for these days. Both involve community action rather than individual action.

The very large dental benefits and low cost of fluoridated water make it likely that some consideration will have been given to fluoridation in almost any community except a very small one. It is useful to study not only the facts but the attitudes toward this matter. Further material is given in Chapters 10 and 16.

A constructive attitude on the part of the school department toward the provision of a school lunch program adequate in quantity and quality will make a great difference in the ease with which common concepts of preventive dentistry can be put into effect. Particularly important here is the control of excess refined carbohydrates. Is candy sold on school premises? Are acceptable substitutes for candy sold on the school premises? An adequate and attractive school lunch program, with candy substitutes available, can provide an example of good nutrition and discourage the purchase of sweets out of school hours.

School Health Education Programs

The mere fact that no specific program for dental health education exists on paper at the time a dental survey of the community is made does not mean that many principles of dental health are not being taught throughout the school system. The careful study of existing health-educational practices will be well worthwhile, first, because it will probably uncover some degree of good work which need not be duplicated, and second, because those engaged in health education directly or indirectly will prove better allies in future dental program planning if they are given credit for what work they are actually doing.

Specific headings under which dental health education may be studied are as follows:

1. The role of *classroom teachers* in the elementary schools (How much do they know about dental health? How much effort do they make to transmit this knowledge?).

2. The *grades* at which most dental health education is concentrated.

3. The role of *health educators, nurses,* physicians, physical education and science teachers, and others for whom one would expect health education to be a primary responsibility.

4. The role of the *dental personnel* already existing (Do they get away from the chair side for educational purposes? Are they recognized as an integral part of the school faculty or not?).

5. The quality and quantity of dental health *educational materials* available for distribution to classroom teachers and others concerned.

Chapter 15 presents evidence that school health education programs are far more important in professionally underserved areas than in areas where there is a good supply of physicians and dentists.

School or Neighborhood Health Care Programs

At this point an initial appraisal of public health care facilities must be made. Such general questions as the following need answering:

1. What groups or school classes are eligible for care?
2. What is the scope of care?

3. What are the quality and outcome of care? (See Chapter 18.)

4. How accessible and available is care?

5. How effective is continuing care, including the recall system if any?

6. What proportion of the needy population is actually served?

Dental Manpower

A listing of the private sector workers in the field of dentistry and health education should be made as part of any survey.

Dentists. List the number of private practitioners in the community and the time (if it is possible to estimate this) which they commonly give to the treatment of children. A population-to-dentist ratio should be computed and compared with national and regional standards. The various dental specialists in the community should be listed, with particular attention to the orthodontists, pedodontists, periodontists, and oral surgeons available. The dentists in public programs in the community should be listed, with some estimate of the time they give to public service (if they are not on full time) and beyond that an estimate of how they divide their time between case-finding activities, dental treatment, and dental health education.

One very important fact to be recorded in connection with dentists in public employment is their pay. Good salaries in a health department usually attract good personnel and vice versa. If the median net income of the average dentist in the United States during a given year is divided by the approximately 2,000 hours he works per year, an hourly figure can be arrived at which might be a fair basis for a salary. If a dentist is on part-time employment with many items of his private-office overhead such as rent continuing even when he is working elsewhere, it is only natural that he should expect to be paid at a rate above that for median net income. Part-time dentists do in fact seem to command slightly higher pay per hour in most localities. A final factor of interest in listing dentists in public employment is the amount of time and the quality of opportunity available to them for in-service training.

In considering recruitment of dentists for the program it is important to remember the nonfinancial rewards of public service. Young dentists or others newly moved to a community may welcome an opportunity to become known and to fill time currently unoccupied. Valuable practice in pedodontics and preventive dentistry may also prove an inducement. For dentists of any age, part-time salaried public service gives a good change of pace and valuable contact with colleagues.

Dental Hygienists. The number of dental hygienists available in private offices throughout the community is of some interest, but the number of hygienists in public employment is far more important. An estimate should be made of the time any publicly employed dental hygienists devote to case-finding activities, dental prophylaxis, and dental health education. Health-education work deserves particular attention because of the opportunity for group instruction in the classroom, and because of the increased job satisfaction of this work for the hygienists themselves. Average salary levels for dental hygienists will be of interest in the community, as will also the opportunities available to dental hygienists in public employment for in-service training. The efficiency of public service hygienists is vastly improved if they are permitted to work under general rather than direct supervision.

Health Educators. These specially trained people are of great value to a dental health program not only for the direct teaching they may do, but for the services they may render in the distribution of literature on dental health and in the relaying of information on the need for such literature. Their function is discussed in the following chapter.

Geographic Factors. The size of the community and the usual modes of transportation employed within it have much to do with the location and administration of dental clinics. Will a central dental clinic suffice for that portion of the community to receive public dental care, or should there be a series of separated school-based clinics so as to minimize the transportation of children from one part of town to another? The accessibility of the community to other communities is also of interest. An American Dental Association survey shows that about 23 percent of dental patients live in towns different from their dentists' and travel an average of 22 miles to see them.[7] These are composite national figures, behind which are important regional and local variations. The conclusion is obvious, however, that the dental manpower resources of a community cannot be estimated wholly within its own confines.

INDICES FOR DENTAL DISEASE

The real focus of any dental health survey, and the part from which the dental needs of the community will be computed, involves the measurement of dental disease, or morbidity. The teeth and their surrounding structures are so definite, so easy to observe, and carry with them so much of their previous disease history that the measurement of dental disease is easier than the measurement of many other forms of disease. There are still many unsolved problems in this area, however. The dental conditions common enough to justify inclusion in a survey of community dental needs can usually be grouped under the headings of caries, periodontoclasia, and malocclusion. Other disease conditions such as cancer, to be sure, justify the best efforts at detection as part of a service program. The early detection of malignant neoplasm may save a life. Surveys for rare diseases are important aspects of a service program, but they need not form a part of an initial survey.

The development of an index of any disease condition depends upon accurate definition of terms. Some of the basic terms used in biostatistics have already been defined in Chapter 4. Definitions referring specifically to dental conditions are found in texts on oral pathology or may be phrased by the researcher, provided he is careful to state his exact terms. A most useful publication, since it invites standardization of terminology on a worldwide basis, is the booklet of the World Health Organization on basic methods for oral health surveys.[8] This booklet makes a valuable distinction between prevalence of various disease conditions and their intensity, severity, or extent. In general, the indices used there are very simple. The booklet may be expected to reappear in revised editions from time to time, but in view of its widespread use in underdeveloped areas, simplicity will continue to be an important aspect. Fig. 41 gives on two sheets the combined oral health and treatment assignment form recommended in the booklet. The boxes following the questions are each to receive a number from 0 to 9, for later transfer to punch cards or other coding devices.

WHO COMBINED ORAL HEALTH AND TREATMENT ASSESSMENT FORM   Sheet 1

Note: 1. No codes to be changed.   2. Unused sections to be cancelled by diagonal lines

(1) [J] [2] [ ] [ ]   (5)   (6) [ ][ ]   (7) Registration (8) [ ][ ][ ][ ]   (11) Examination Number (for (12) duplicates) [ ]
Study Number   Date 19   Number

PERSONAL AND DEMOGRAPHIC INFORMATION

Sex M = 1   F = 2 . . . . (13) [ ]   Name . . . .
                                                              family   other

Age in years . . . . (14) [ ] (15)   Geographic location . . . . (18) [ ][ ] (19)

Ethnic group . . . . (16) [ ]   Examiner . . . . (20) [ ]

Occupation . . . . (17) [ ]

SERVICE UTILIZATION

Q. 1 Did you obtain dental care in the last 12 months?

                              NO = 0   (21) [ ]   CODE CATEGORIES FROM RESPONSE (1 to 6, 9)
                              YES = 1   See list in criteria (p. 1)

If YES Q. 1(a) For what reason?   (22) [ ]   CODE CATEGORIES FROM RESPONSE (1 to 5)
                                                        See list in criteria (p. 1)
        Q. 1(b) Who treated you? (23) [ ]

If NO Q. 1(c) Why not?   (24) [ ]   CODE CATEGORIES FROM RESPONSE (1 to 9)
                                                        See list in criteria (p. 2)

Q. 2 Is anything wrong with your teeth, gums or mouth now?

                                  (25) [ ]   CODE CATEGORIES FROM RESPONSE (0 to 4, 9)
                                                        See list in criteria (p. 2)

Q. 2(a) Do you want any dental advice or treatment?

                              NO = 0   (26) [ ]
                              YES = 1

If you do Q. 2(b) What sort of advice or treatment do you want?

                                  (27) [ ]   CODE CATEGORIES FROM RESPONSE (0 to 9)
                                                        See list in criteria (p. 2)

DISORDERS OF MUCOSA TEETH AND BONE AND OTHER CONDITIONS

            ABSENT = 0, PRESENT, NO TREATMENT
        RECOMMENDED = 1, PRESENT, TREATMENT
                  RECOMMENDED = 2   OTHER CONDITIONS
ORAL MUCOSAL DISEASE   (28) [ ]   Titles to be entered as needed, from results of pilot study
Specify
Disease . . . . (31) [ ]
Treatment . . . .
DEFECT OF TEETH   (29) [ ]
Specify
Defect . . . . (32) [ ]
Treatment . . . .
DISORDERS INVOLVING BONE
Specify   (30) [ ]   (33) [ ]
Disease . . . .
Treatment . . . .

PROSTHETIC STATUS   **DENTURE REQUIREMENTS**
     NO   DENTURE = 0, DENTURE WEARING = 1   NIL = 0, NEW DENTURE REQUIRED = 1
          DENTURE NOT WEARING 2   REPAIR, RELINE OR REMODEL 2
     UPPER JAW   LOWER JAW   LOWER JAW   UPPER JAW
(34) [ ]   (35) [ ]   (36) [ ]   (37) [ ]   (38) [ ]   (39) [ ]   (40) [ ]   (41) [ ]
     full   partial   full   partial   full   partial   full   partial

WHO 5297 ORH (6/76) - 40000

Figure 41. World Health Organization form for detailed study of an individual case, Sheet 1. [Courtesy, WHO.]

WHO COMBINED ORAL HEALTH AND TREATMENT ASSESSMENT FORM   Sheet 2

Note: 1. No codes to be changed.   2. Unused sections to be cancelled by diagonal lines

(1) J 2   (5) Date 19   (6)   (7) Registration (8)   (11) Examination Number (12)
Study Number   Number   (for duplicates)

PERIODONTAL STATUS	Absent = 0 Present = 1			PERIODONTAL TREATMENT REQUIREMENTS (66)
SOFT DEPOSITS	max. (42)	(44)	NONE	0
	mand. (45)	(47)	Oral Hygiene Instruction	1
			Prophylaxis and OHI	2
CALCULUS	max. (48)	(50)	Periodontal therapy (no extraction)	3
	mand. (51)	(53)	Treatment with 1 or more extraction	4
INTENSE GINGIVITIS	max. (54)	(56)	Full extraction	5
	mand. (57)	(59)		
ADVANCED PERIODONTAL INVOLVEMENT	max. (60)	(62)		
	mand. (63)	(65)		

NB. Central segments include cuspids and incisors left and right segments include molars and premolars

DENTOFACIAL ANOMALIES

WHO Criteria condition (specify)	(67)	
treatment	(68)	
Other criteria (to be specified) condition (specify)	(69)	
treatment	(70)	

CONDITIONS NEEDING IMMEDIATE ATTENTION   ABSENT = 0   PRESENT = 1

RELIEF OF EXISTING PAIN OR INFECTION   (71)   TREATMENT OF PULPALLY INVOLVED TEETH (73)

TREATMENT FOR LESIONS LIKELY TO CAUSE PAIN OR INFECTION IN THE IMMEDIATE (72) FUTURE   OTHER (SPECIFY) . . . . (74)

. . . .   CARD NO.   (80)   3

DENTAL CARIES STATUS AND TREATMENT OF TEETH

		55 54 53 52 51 61 62 63 64 65																
		18 17 16 15 14 13 12 11 21 22 23 24 25 26 27 28																
CARIES	(13)																	(28) CARIES
TREATMENT R	(29)																	(44) TREATMENT L
		85 84 83 82 81 71 72 73 74 75																
		48 47 46 45 44 43 42 41 31 32 33 34 35 36 37 38																
CARIES	(45)																	(60) CARIES
TREATMENT	(61)																	(76) TREATMENT

DENTAL CARIES	PRIMARY	PERM.	TREATMENT	
SOUND	A	0	NONE	0
DECAYED	B	1	RESTORATIONS	
FILLED & CARIES FREE	C	2	1 surface	1
FILLED WITH PRIMARY DECAY	D	3	2 surface	2
FILLED WITH SECONDARY DECAY	E	4	3 surface	3
PRIMARY TEETH MISSING DUE CARIES < 9 yrs	M	–	> 3 surface or crown	4
PERMANENT TEETH MISSING DUE CARIES (UNDER 30 YEARS ONLY)	–	5	EXTRACTION FOR	
PERMANENT TEETH MISSING ANY REASON OTHER THAN CARIES (UNDER 30 YEARS ONLY)	–	6	caries	5
			periodontal disease	6
			dentures	7
PERMANENT TEETH MISSING ANY REASON (30 YEARS & OLDER)	–	7	other reason	8
UNERUPTED TOOTH	–	8	OTHER (specify)	9
EXCLUDED TOOTH	X	9	CARD No. (80)	4

Figure 41 (cont.) World Health Organization form for detailed study of an individual case, Sheet 2. [Courtesy, WHO.]

Tooth Numbering

Dental records have long depended on letters or numbers for quick identification of specific teeth. Several methods have been in common use. Perhaps the oldest is the so-called Set-Square or German system, adapted to hand-written records:

R $\quad \dfrac{\underline{8|}\ \underline{7|}\ \underline{6|}\ \underline{5|}\ \underline{4|}\ \underline{3|}\ \underline{2|}\ \underline{1|}\ \|\ \underline{|1}\ \underline{|2}\ \underline{|3}\ \underline{|4}\ \underline{|5}\ \underline{|6}\ \underline{|7}\ \underline{|8}}{\overline{8|}\ \overline{7|}\ \overline{6|}\ \overline{5|}\ \overline{4|}\ \overline{3|}\ \overline{2|}\ \overline{1|}\ \|\ \overline{|1}\ \overline{|2}\ \overline{|3}\ \overline{|4}\ \overline{|5}\ \overline{|6}\ \overline{|7}\ \overline{|8}}$ $\quad$ L

The permanent teeth receive numbers from the mid-line outward; the deciduous teeth are usually lettered A to E, also from the mid-line outward.

When numbers alone become essential, as with typewriters, a system was devised from 1 to 32, which is still in use in the United States in many government and other programs:

R $\quad \dfrac{\begin{array}{cccccccc} 1 & 2 & 3 & 4 & 5 & 6 & 7 & 8 \end{array}\ \left|\ \begin{array}{cccccccc} 9 & 10 & 11 & 12 & 13 & 14 & 15 & 16 \end{array}\right.}{\begin{array}{cccccccc} 32 & 31 & 30 & 29 & 28 & 27 & 26 & 25 \end{array}\ \left|\ \begin{array}{cccccccc} 24 & 23 & 22 & 21 & 20 & 19 & 18 & 17 \end{array}\right.}$ $\quad$ L

Computer programming and other analytical processes have found a combination of single-digit and double-digit numbers to be awkward. The Federation Dentaire Internationale and the World Health Organization have therefore combined to devise a double-digit system which preserves the old concept of 1 for a central incisor to 8 for a third molar:

Permanent teeth

R $\quad \dfrac{\begin{array}{cccccccc} 18 & 17 & 16 & 15 & 14 & 13 & 12 & 11 \end{array}\ \left|\ \begin{array}{cccccccc} 21 & 22 & 23 & 24 & 25 & 26 & 27 & 28 \end{array}\right.}{\begin{array}{cccccccc} 48 & 47 & 46 & 45 & 44 & 43 & 42 & 41 \end{array}\ \left|\ \begin{array}{cccccccc} 31 & 32 & 33 & 34 & 35 & 36 & 37 & 38 \end{array}\right.}$ $\quad$ L

Deciduous teeth

R $\quad \dfrac{\begin{array}{ccccc} 55 & 54 & 53 & 52 & 51 \end{array}\ \left|\ \begin{array}{ccccc} 61 & 62 & 63 & 64 & 65 \end{array}\right.}{\begin{array}{ccccc} 85 & 84 & 83 & 82 & 81 \end{array}\ \left|\ \begin{array}{ccccc} 71 & 72 & 73 & 74 & 75 \end{array}\right.}$ $\quad$ L

Take your pick.

Dental Caries

Although unfilled carious lesions constitute the largest item of dental need to be faced by any dental service, at least in the United States, a count of open lesions actually measures two processes: dental caries (a plus factor), and prior dental treatment (a minus factor). An accurate view of community needs requires separation of these factors, hence dental-caries experience is usually measured on a cumulative basis in such a way as to include all evidence of caries both past and present. Accurate measurement of caries is easy as long as one deals with decayed and filled teeth, but measures involving *missing teeth* must be interpreted in the light of all causes, either known or surmised, for the loss of teeth. In early life there is little inaccuracy in assuming that a count of missing teeth is almost entirely a result of caries, even though in youth a few teeth may have been lost owing to trauma or to extraction as part of orthodontic treatment. Later in life periodontal disease becomes an important factor. A count of missing teeth then becomes a composite picture. The cause of missing teeth can sometimes be assigned accurately, if the patient remembers his own dental history well enough, or if the presence of one form of dental disease in the mouth to the exclusion of other forms makes inference very obvious. Most survey procedures, however, make no attempt to evaluate the history of missing teeth. They are included in surveys of young patients as the probable result of dental caries. In surveys of older people, missing teeth are often omitted entirely, survey procedures for disease being confined to those teeth still in the mouth. When large groups of teeth or all natural teeth are missing, *edentulousness* becomes a subject of interest in connection with prosthetic restorations.

Caries must be *defined accurately* for the purpose of any study. The commonest definition postulates that a sharp explorer (design and sharpness to be described) catch in a cavity with a detectably soft floor and/or some undermined enamel or a breakdown in the walls of a pit or fissure. The World Health Organization recommends in addition that where doubt exists, caries should *not* be recorded as present.[8] The stages of caries that precede cavitation, as well as other similar conditions, are to be deliberately excluded because they cannot be diagnosed reliably.

A confusing situation occurs when areas shown on one survey to be carious are noted on a subsequent survey to be sound. Such *reversals* may be the result of differing interpretations of a minimal explorer catch, but if seen frequently, they are more likely to be the result of careless examination. Remineralization is sometimes considered to have caused reversals, but of a number of studies of remineralization, all but one appear to have been made where particular chemicals were used *in vitro*. The one clinical study of remineralization showed it to have occurred only where enamel surface softening had occurred, never where actual cavitation had occurred.[9]

There are five major measures for dental caries.

1. Percentage of population showing any evidence of caries (prevalence). This measure is useful where caries is low or where, as in the study of ancient skulls, so many teeth have been lost for reasons other than caries that the existence of one or more carious teeth is the best criterion to use in differentiating affected individuals from those with no evidence of dental disease.

2. DMF (decayed plus missing plus filled) teeth. This is perhaps the commonest measure in use today, and was developed by Klein of the U.S. Public Health Service.[10] It reaches its greatest usefulness in areas where, as in much of the United States, the proportion of individuals with some evidence of caries is so high that changes in this proportion are meaningless and it becomes necessary to have a quantitative measure of caries severity within the average person's mouth. Large surveys measured in DMF teeth can be made by explorer examination without x-ray support, and constitute a standardized, though incomplete, picture of caries status. A defect in the method—and one reason for not taking x-rays in connection with it—is that, once a tooth has found its way into the DMF count, further caries on the tooth is not measured. For young children, where deciduous teeth form most of the dentition, a "df" tooth count, to be described later, is used.

3. DMF surfaces. This is a more sensitive measure of dental conditions per person, reaching its greatest usefulness where accurate work is to be done involving the use of dental x-rays. Surface counts have an advantage over tooth counts in that changes in caries experience can still be seen easily in mouths having such high caries already that almost no completely unattacked teeth remain.

4. Carious lesions. This is a sensitive measure involving new points of entry of caries, more sensitive than surface counts since there are often two or more possible points of entry for caries on a given surface. It is of value where short-term studies are to be made involving such methods of prevention as topical application of fluoride, but on the whole it is a measure inferior to DMF

surfaces since differentiation between a new lesion and extension of an adjacent old lesion is often very difficult.

5. Number times size of lesions. This is a very sensitive method where estimates can be made of the volume of the lesion. Much of the experimental work done upon rats and other small animals has been scored in this manner, after sectioning of teeth, giving a total figure which is far more descriptive of the invasion of caries in a given mouth than would be the mere number of lesions or surfaces involved. Human studies can be made this way too, with subjective estimates of size of lesion usually on a scale of from 1 to 3 or 4.

Two statistical concepts come into play at this point: *experience* and *incidence*. The sum total of all decayed, missing, and filled teeth (or surfaces) seen in an individual today represents his *dental-caries experience*, though of course there is the possibility that some of his missing teeth may represent conditions other than caries. It is impossible to tell from this single figure how fast the caries has occurred or is occurring. *Caries incidence,* on the other hand, is a *rate* and must always be expressed in terms of time. It involves repeated examinations at regular intervals such as 1 year and is usually expressed in terms of new findings per unit of time. Dental-caries experience is all one can find from a cross-sectional survey of a group on a single occasion. Incidence is the finding par excellence in a longitudinal survey of the same individuals at different times. Estimates of incidence can be made, however, from cross-sectional surveys by noting how much more of the observed condition is found in one age group than in another. Thus, if 10-year-old children in a fairly large DMF survey proved to have 5.1 DMF teeth per person and 11-year-old children proved to have 6.2 DMF teeth per person, one would say that caries incidence in the 10-year-olds was 1.1 teeth per year.

There are various interrelations among the five main measures for dental caries, and these in turn lead to shortcuts in survey procedure. These interrelations will be discussed later in the chapter.

Periodontal Disease

The measurement of disease conditions, in the supporting structures of the teeth is a far more difficult problem than the measurement of dental caries. There are three main reasons. First, two areas are involved in most instances: the gingiva, where gingivitis is usually a reversible process and easy to observe; and the alveolus, where bone loss is the best measure of damage and is almost always chronic, cumulative, and hard to observe. Second, periodontal disease, unlike caries, has its greater incidence late in life. A patient seen at this age will probably have lost teeth for reasons other than periodontal disease. This means that valid assumptions are usually impossible as to the reason or reasons for the loss of teeth which are found missing at the time of examination. Except in longitudinal studies, measures of periodontal disease must usually be made without including missing teeth. And third, subjective measurement of the severity of the disease is usually necessary. The only real quantitative measure—an estimation of the severity of chronic periodontal disease in terms of linear bone loss—can often be misleading and is extremely difficult to obtain without taking x-rays.

Many studies, such as those reported in Table 19, have been made upon the proportion of a population showing some evidence either of gingivitis or of chronic destructive periodontal disease. These *prevalence* studies cease to be revealing in high-prevalence areas. Studies of severity then becomes necessary, with reliance on some "index" thought to be most descriptive under the circumstances.

Gingivitis is difficult to measure in an objective way. Subjective measures range from a simple yes or no to a numbered scale, usually from 0 to 3. The most commonly used index today is the *Gingival Index of Löe.*[11] Its criteria are:

0 = normal gingiva.
1 = mild inflammation, with slight change in color, slight edema, and no bleeding on probing.
2 = moderate inflammation, with redness, edema, glazing, and bleeding on probing.
3 = severe inflammation, with marked redness and edema, ulceration, and tendency to spontaneous bleeding.

Each of the four gingival areas of the tooth is given a score of 0 to 3; this is the GI for the area. The scores for the areas may be averaged to give the GI for the tooth. The scores for individual teeth may be averaged within a group of teeth (incisors, premolars, and molars) to give a GI for a group. Finally, by adding the indices for the teeth and dividing by the total number of teeth examined, one obtains the GI for the individual. Scoring requires good light, drying of the teeth and gingivae, a mirror, and a pocket probe. Pocket depths, if any, are not recorded.

Alveolar-bone loss is easier to quantitate, especially when radiographs can be taken. Day and Shourie have elaborated one of the first indices for bone loss.[12] The number 10 is assigned to the full root length of a given tooth, and the degree of bone resorption is then measured in tenths from zero (no bone loss) to 10 (complete loss of all bony support). Figures for bone loss are summed to give area totals, and the various area totals then averaged to give a "resorption" figure for the individual patient.

A measure, the *Periodontal Index,* which combines bone loss with gingival disease has been devised by Russell.[13] Here each tooth studied in the mouth is assigned a score between zero and 8. Zero describes a tooth negative for all criteria and 8 describes a tooth with advanced alveolar-bone loss, gingivitis, and loss of masticatory function. Intermediate numbers describe various combinations and degrees of gingivitis. The values for all teeth in the mouth are then averaged to give the patient's whole-mouth score. Table 34 gives details.

In careful epidemiological study more detail would be desirable than that provided by the Periodontal Index. If experience with DMF counts for dental caries can be taken as a guide, future large-scale surveying will be done in such a way as to provide figures for both gingivitis and chronic destructive periodontal disease, as shown by bone loss, as separate entities.

Table 35 describes an index to permit the differential recording of gingival and bone conditions.[14] Subjective measurement of gingivitis is made on a 0-to-3 scale for each tooth and proportional measurement of bone loss is made on a 0-to-5 scale. Whole-mouth mean scores are then added together to obtain what is called a gingivabone or *GB count.* This count weights gingivitis and bone loss on a 3-to-5 basis: an arbitrary relation, but a realistic one in terms of the threat each makes to the usefulness of the tooth. Since the whole-mouth means for gingivae and bone are separately recorded, the conditions making up the GB count can always be

Table 34. Criteria for field scoring of Russell's Periodontal Index.

Score[a]	Description	Criteria for field studies
0	Negative	There is neither obvious inflammation in the gingival epithelium nor loss of function due to destruction of supporting tissues.
1	Mild gingivitis	There is an obvious area of inflammation in the free gingiva, but this area does not circumscribe the tooth.
2	Gingivitis	Inflammation completely circumscribes the tooth, but there is no apparent break in the epithelial attachment.
6	Gingivitis with pocket formation	Epithelial attachment has been broken, and there is a pocket (not merely a deepened gingival crevice due to swelling in the free gingiva). There is no interference with normal masticatory function, the tooth is firm in its socket and has not drifted.
8	Advanced destruction with loss of masticatory function	Tooth may be loose or may have drifted; may sound dull on percussion with a metallic instrument or may be depressible in its socket.

a. When in doubt, assign the lesser score.

known. No attempt is made to evaluate the missing teeth in the mouth. If a prevalence figure for periodontal disease is desired, the cases with a GB count of zero can be compared with those having counts above zero. The GB count and the Periodontal Index resemble each other in a number of ways, including the fact that each carries a maximum possible score of 8 per tooth. Fig. 42 clarifies this relationship.

For whole-mouth appraisal, the World Health Organization[8] recommends scoring the presence or absence of four conditions: *soft deposits, calculus,* intense *gingivitis,* and advanced *periodontal disease.* The mouth is divided into six segments for recording: anterior from canine to canine and right and left position, upper and lower. Each condition assessment for each area should be made separately. Sheet 2 in Figure 41 gives spaces for such recording.

Table 35. Gingiva-bone count: a periodontal scoring system.

Observation	Score
Gingivitis[a]	
Negative	0
Mild gingivitis involving the free gingiva (margin, papilla, or both)	1
Moderate gingivitis (involving both free and attached gingiva)	2
Severe gingivitis with hypertrophy and easy hemorrhage	3
Maximum	3
Bone loss[b]	
Negative	0
Incipient (not > 2 mm) bone loss or notching of alveolar crest	1
Bone loss approximately ¼ root length or pocket formation on one side not > ½ root length	2
Bone loss approximating ½ root length or pocket formation on one side not > ¾ root length; mobility slight[c]	3
Bone loss approximating ¾ root length or pocket formation on one side to apex; mobility moderate[c]	4
Bone loss complete; mobility marked[c]	5
Maximum	5
Maximum GB count per tooth or person	8

a. One score is assigned for each tooth studied, and a mean is computed for the whole mouth.

b. One score is assigned for each tooth studied visually or by x-ray, and a mean is computed for the whole mouth.

c. If mobility varies considerably from that to be expected with the bone loss seen, the score may be altered up or down one point.

For detailed appraisal of needed periodontal treatment, measures of *pocket depth* and *mobility* can be made for individual teeth.[15] A tooth diagram can bear figures in millimeters around each tooth for sulcus or pocket depth in as many as six localities: mesial, mid-root, and distal on the buccal side and on the lingual side. Mobility can be marked on the crown of the tooth using figures from 0 to 3.

For specific research purposes and perhaps for limited general surveys, more detail may be desired than is involved in the previously mentioned indices. *Ramfjord* has devised an index which records seven different characteristics for each of six typical teeth, if present in the mouth.[16] These teeth are the maxillary right first molar, left central incisor, and left first bicuspid, and the mandib-

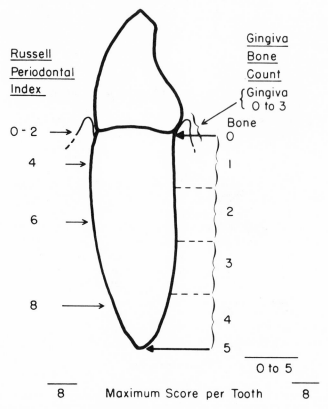

Figure 42. Scoring of periodontal disease by two indices. The approximate bone loss corresponding with each score must also be interpreted by the criteria found in Tables 34 and 35.

ular right first bicuspid, right central incisor, and left first molar. A dry field is required. The characteristics recorded are:

1. Gingival findings. A subjective scale is used from G-0 (absence of inflammation) to G-3 (severe gingivitis characterized by marked redness, and so forth).

2. Calculus. This is recorded on a subjective scale from C-0 (absence of calculus) to C-3 (an abundance of supra- and subgingival calculus).

3. Periodontal pockets. Measurements in millimeters are secured from the free gingival margin to the cemento-enamel junction and from the free gingival margin to the bottom of the gingival

crevice or pocket on the mesial, buccal, distal, and lingual aspects of each tooth. Specific directions for obtaining and recording these measurements must be observed.

4. Occlusal and incisal attrition. A subjective scale is used from A-0 (no attrition) to A-3 (extreme attrition: the occlusal surfaces are worn flat and "inverted" cusp pattern is present).

5. Mobility. A subjective scale is used from M-0 (physiologic mobility; firm tooth) to M-3 (extreme mobility; a "loose" tooth that cannot be used for normal function).

6. Lack of contact. A subjective scale is used from D-0 (normal contact; not open) to D-3 (opening more than three millimeters).

7. Plaque, after application of disclosing solution. A subjective scale is used from P-0 (no plaque present) to P-3 (plaque extending over all interproximal and gingival surfaces, covering more than one-half of the entire clinical crown).

In general, formal scores are obtained by adding the values for each characteristic and dividing by the number of teeth present. Detailed instructions are given for certain phases of this process.

The World Health Organization now carries analysis a step further, estimating community needs for periodontal treatment. The Russell index is simplified and disease status is converted into four treatment categories as follows.

The Community Periodontal Index of Treatment Needs (CPITN) is based on the examination of six segments of the dentition, from second molars to first premolars and from canines to canines. One recording only is made for each of these sextants. In epidemiological surveys the recording can be based on examination of the two molars in each posterior sextant and one central incisor in each of the two anterior sextants. The alternative procedure, also suitable for the screening of individual patients, is to base the recording on the worst condition found around any one of the four or six teeth comprising the sextant.

The use of a special WHO designed periodontal probe is recommended. This probe has a colour coded band 3.5–5.5 mm from the tip. If this disappears into the pocket during probing, the pocket depth is 6 mm or more and gives the sextant a code of 4. If the coloured area remains partly visible, the pocket depth is 4 or 5 mm and Code 3 is given. If the entire coloured band remains visible, Code 2 is given if supra- or subgingival calculus is present. Correspondingly, Code 1 is recorded if the pocket depth is 3 mm or less and there is no calculus but bleeding occurs after gentle probing of the pocket or sulcus. Absence of any sign of disease in a sextant qualifying for recording (two or more functioning teeth) is indicated with Code 0. Disease status codes are easily converted into four treatment categories: complex treatment (III) for sextants with 6 mm or deeper pockets (Code 4); scaling (II) for Codes 3 and 2; improvement of personal oral hygiene (I) for Code 1; and no treatment for absence of disease. Treatment category III also requires treatments II and I, and treatment category II also requires treatment I.

The CPITN facilitates rapid assessment of the mean disease status of a population group as well as the prevalences of the various grades of periodontal involvement. After determination of the time needed for treatments III and II per sextant and treatment I per subject, the total treatment time can be calculated.[17]

The only example so far available of the use of this index is Ivan Curson's report of a dental health survey in the Grenfell region of northern Newfoundland and Labrador, Canada, in 1984. A sample of 781 adults was divided at age 40, and percentages of the population falling into each of the four treatment categories, were recorded for each of six regional groups. Below age 40, zero scores (healthy gums or *no teeth to score*) ranged from 25 to 62 percent. The largest treatment categories were categories II and III. Over age 40, the zeros ranged from 42 to 91 percent, with most areas above 80 percent. Treatment categories II and III again prevailed for such teeth as remained. No control studies were available for comparison.

Oral Hygiene Appraisal

Occasions arise frequently where careful measurement of oral hygiene status helps in epidemiological study of periodontal and other problems. The Greene and Vermillion *Oral Hygiene Index* (OHI) has become standard for the purpose.[18] Each dental arch (upper and lower) is divided into three segments: (1) the segment distal to the right cuspid, (2) the segment distal to the left cuspid, and (3) the segment anterior to the bicuspids. Scores are recorded for calculus and for debris on both buccal and lingual surfaces of the areas mentioned, the score representing in each case the worst area found in the segment. Subjective scales from zero to 3 are used. For debris, zero means no debris or stain present, and 3 means soft debris covering more than two-thirds of the exposed tooth surface. For calculus, zero means no calculus present and 3 means supra-gingival calculus covering more than two-thirds of the exposed surface and/or a solid, heavy band of subgingival calculus around the neck of the tooth. Separate indices for debris and for calculus are determined by averaging scores for the various regions. The same authors in 1964 proposed a *Simplified Oral Hygiene Index* (OHIS) in which only 6 surfaces from four posterior and two anterior "index" teeth are examined for debris and calculus, whereas 12 surfaces are examined for a regular Oral Hygiene Index.[19] Both methods are now widely used. Neither needs to be used where the new World Health Organization regional scoring for periodontal disease has been carried out (see Figure 41, sheet 2).

Malocclusion

The measurement of malocclusion as a public health problem is extremely difficult, since much orthodontic treatment is undertaken for aesthetic reasons only and it is very difficult to estimate the extent to which malposed teeth or other dentofacial anomalies constitute a psychological hazard. The World Health Organization suggests that one or more of the following subjective conditions be present for anomalies to be deemed to require treatment in a public health program:[8]

1. A significant and unacceptable effect upon facial appearance.
2. A significant impairment of speech and mastication.
3. A gross defect such as cleft lip or palate or an injury requiring plastic surgery.
4. An occlusion predisposing to tissue destruction through caries or periodontal disease.

The space for treatment recommendation (see Figure 41, sheet 2) is to be coded: 0 for no treatment necessary, 1 for extraction of teeth only, 2 for removable-appliance treatment (active tooth movement with or without extraction), 3 for fixed-appliance treatment, and 4 for surgical or other treatment for gross defects.

Some surveying of malocclusion has been done according to Angle's classification. Work of this sort may be valuable from an anthropological standpoint, but is almost meaningless in terms of those treatment needs serious enough to warrant attention in a public dental health program, since Angle's classification measures type of malocclusion but is not weighted to indicate disability.

In recent years a number of attempts have been made to devise indices for malocclusion which would be of aid in making priority decisions in public assistance programs. Draker devised an index to measure "handicapping labiolingual deviations" and introduced the concept of small weighted scores for specific occlusal defects.[20] More recently, two new indices have appeared. Salzmann devised a *Handicapping Malocclusion Assessment Record,* which assigns weights of 1 or 2 to instances of intra-arch deviation (missing teeth, crowded teeth, and so forth) inter-arch deviation (overjet, crossbite, and so forth) and posterior-segment deviation.[21] Fig. 43 illustrates the

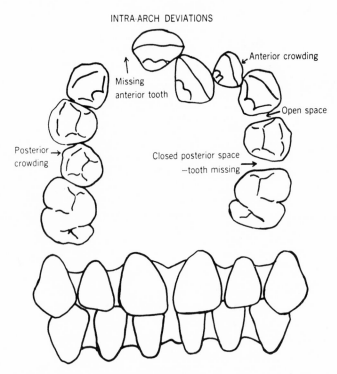

INTRA-ARCH DEVIATIONS

Figure 43. Intra-arch occlusal deviations from Salzmann's Handicapping Malocclusion Assessment Record. [Reprinted by permission, *American Journal of Orthodontics.*]

intra-arch deviations recorded. Additional unusual dento-facial deviations such as clefts or facial asymmetry are given an arbitrary weighting of 8 points each. This index has received praise from the Board of Trustees of the American Association of Orthodontists, and commendation from the Council on Dental Health of the American Dental Association.

A more sophisticated approach to the analysis of malocclusion has been taken by the Burlington Orthodontic Research Group of the University of Toronto.[22] Through the use of multiple-regression equations, the findings from the field examination of 375 12-year-old children have been combined to produce an *Orthodontic Treatment Priority Index* (TPI) consisting of ten objective components which are weighted and summed to a single number on a 10-point scale of case severity. The components include upper and lower anterior overjet (in millimeters), overbite (in crown thirds), open bite, congenitally missing incisors, distocclusion, mesiocclusion, number of teeth in posterior crossbite to buccal or lingual, and tooth displacement score. Provision is made in the Index for arbitrary weighting of other additional defects not included in this list. Careful statistics are presented to relate the measurements for all the various specific occlusal defects to the subjective evaluations made by orthodontic consultants as to degree of handicap. A computer program for data processing is included. Experience is still needed to test both the general validity and practicality of these two indices and others which may succeed them. Carlos reports a study of 100 dental casts by 5 examiners in which the TPI proved to show highly reproducible results, in terms of both ranks and scores.[23]

An additional factor which has yet to be measured and incorporated into any index is the level of *anxiety* created by a malocclusion. Certain preliminary studies are available on the relation of malocclusion to manifest-anxiety tests, but the reliable application of such material to specific cases is still lacking.

Cancer and Oral Manifestations of Systemic Disease

Any good dental health service must recognize its responsibility in the detection of oral neoplasms and the oral manifestations of systemic disease. The personnel of the service must be adequately trained and examination procedures must allow for the recognition of unusual oral abnormalities. Since these conditions are rare, however, they are not best looked for in the randomly selected populations seen at initial surveys. One excellent method is to offer cancer screening on a volunteer basis, perhaps first to persons over 40 years of age, using oral exfoliative cytology reinforced by expert clinical examination. The self-selection involved in this method gives a high early yield which contributes to the success of the program, but constitutes a bias in any statistics which may be derived. The examiners for the program need special indoctrination. Oral exfoliative cytology is of little use in detecting certain types of malignancy, and is an effective aid to the dentist in his clinical examination rather than a definitive test upon which he can rest his diagnosis.

INTERRELATION OF DISEASE INDICES

All the indices just described are interrelated to some extent with other indices for the corresponding disease, and fall into a scale of progressive refinement. First comes prevalence, then, the various measures that describe extent or severity of disease. The best gradation of refinement is seen in the indices for dental caries. It was this concept which led Knutson to develop his curve relating caries prevalence to DMF tooth counts: a curve which is occasionally useful but also carries with it serious possibility for error.[24]

In practice, each measure for caries has its own area of high sensitivity and these areas differ in relative placement. Fig. 44 shows a plotting of three different measures for a given population. All are upon one graph, where the vertical axis reaches a peak of 100 percent, or the total possible caries involvement. The horizontal axis is the logarithm of age, the log scale giving increased sensitivity during the early years of caries development. Two continuous series of observations have been plotted, each representing an age span from 6 to 60 years. The first is from the relatively low-caries area of Aurora, Illinois.[25,26] The second is from the relatively high-caries area of Nicollet County, Minnesota, and New York City—the two placed in juxtaposition not for any theoretical reason whatever, but merely because they do form a continuum.[25,27]

Fig. 44 shows clearly that measurements of prevalence—percentage of population showing any evidence whatever of dental

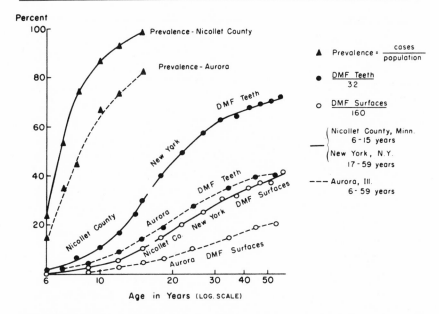

Figure 44. Measures of prevalence and severity of dental caries, expressed as a percentage of the possible total involvement. [Courtesy, The New York Academy of Sciences.]

caries—are very sensitive in the early years after emergence of the permanent teeth and much less sensitive a little later on when values over 80 percent have been attained and far smaller changes occur each year. With the Nicollet County material it is obvious that values approximating 100 percent have been reached by age 15 and that full 100 percent involvement will be the expectation in older age groups. This situation is true in many parts of the country, so much so that prevalence figures are almost never recorded for adults. Aurora, with its relatively lower caries rate, shows a sensitivity for prevalence which is somewhat greater in the older childhood period. If the really low caries levels of primitive populations were being measured, it might be that prevalence would be a sensitive measure throughout the entire adult period.

Measures of DMF teeth can be seen to rise sharply and give great discrimination after measures of prevalence have ceased to do so. A plateau is eventually reached, however, between 60 and 70 percent of the possible DMF total in New York City after age

35, and a similar plateau is reached at a lower level in the adults of Aurora. Both plateaus appear to recognize the fact that certain teeth, such as the lower anteriors, appear to resist the onslaught of caries almost completely, even after other teeth in the mouth have shown initial involvement so universally that further measurement of DMF teeth as units is useless.

Measurements of DMF surfaces seem to show less evidence of plateau formation. Graphed as they are in this instance on a percentage scale, which minimizes numerical totals, it looks as if totals of DMF surfaces did not change very much in adult life. When expressed in pure numbers (that is, numbers of surfaces per person), the values rise much more sharply and there is much better discrimination even in the two samples reported here. Greater discrimination yet is theoretically possible in samples showing higher caries intensity, since it is obvious that after one decayed surface has brought a given tooth onto the DMF count, four more surfaces remain for caries attack and for measurement in terms of DMF surfaces.

Bilateral symmetry within the human mouth is another relation which has its usefulness, both in surveying and in clinical research. Bilateral symmetry cannot be relied upon to any great extent as between individual teeth on the right and left sides of the mouths of individual patients. When entire mouth quadrants are considered, however, reliability becomes much greater. Hadjimarkos has conducted surveys using only one-half of the mouth, and his results are accurate to within about one-tenth of one tooth when checked against surveys of the whole mouth, even in samples as small as 33 persons.[28] Knutson and Armstrong, in their studies of the efficacy of topical fluoride therapy in Minnesota, not only demonstrated bilateral symmetry convincingly in their control group of children but used this fact effectively in comparing controls and experimentals.[29]

PERFORMING THE SURVEY

Since any survey of dental disease should be available for external as well as internal comparison, it is obvious that an accurate statement should be made of the methods, instruments, and aids used in a dental examination or inspection. Failure to do this is an invitation to error and to misrepresentation. The reader may remember the occasion, perhaps 5 years after the Newburgh-Kingston study on water fluoridation was started, when antifluoridationists claimed surveys to be showing less dental caries in Kingston, the control city, than in Newburgh. Investigation disclosed that an explorer survey of Newburgh, expressed in terms of DMF teeth per person, was being compared with the results of a routine tongue-depressor screening of Kingston. No wonder the latter city showed less caries!

Classification of Types of Inspection and Examination

The American Dental Association has standardized four main types of examination and inspection.[30] Not only is this classification a logical one, but it is likely to be widely used because of its sponsorship. The classification is as follows:

Type 1. Complete examination, using mouth mirror and explorer, adequate illumination, thorough roentgenographic survey, and when indicated, percussion, pulp-vitality tests, transillumination, study models, and laboratory tests. This method can seldom be used in public health work.

Type 2. Limited examination, using mouth mirror and explorer, adequate illumination, posterior bite-wing roentgenograms, and when indicated, periapical roentgenograms. This method is of great value where public health programs combine service to individual patients with population survey work, and gives superior results for pure survey work where time and money permit.

Type 3. Inspection, using mouth mirror and explorer and adequate illumination. This is the most-used method in public health surveying.

Type 4. Screening, using tongue depressor and available illumination. This method identifies individuals in urgent need of treatment, but is too unreliable for most public health surveying.

Planning the Survey

The professional and auxiliary manpower available will determine in most instances the type of examination or inspection to be used. Samples must be large enough to overcome unavoidable variability, as is discussed in Chapter 5. Beyond this size, which is usually from 100 to 200 cases per age group in most caries work, it is seldom necessary to survey an entire school or other population. *Stratified sampling* methods may be used in order to select typical age, economic, or other groups which are meaningful. Thus, if the community contains well-defined upper and lower income groups or well-defined ethnic or neighborhood groups, it is important to see that sampling methods give proper weight to each. It is much better to do accurate work among a series of stratified samples than to do inaccurate work in an entire population.

Easy methods of sampling include examining every other or every third child on an alphabetical class list, examining certain important grades only instead of all grades in a school, and examining only certain schools in properly distributed neighborhoods rather than all schools in a large community. "Random numbers" from a statistical table of such numbers may be used in selecting children from a regularly numbered list. Randomization is most necessary when the list of suitable cases, with as many unwanted variables eliminated as possible, exceeds the minimum sample sizes postulated in Table 11. The list must also be too large to survey in its entirety.

Age groups need careful selection. The World Health Organization recommends single-year age-specific samples up to age 19, 5-year age groups from 20 to 34, and 10-year groups from 35 to 64.[8] Where not all these groups can be included, WHO has used three typical groups: 8 to 9, 13 to 14, and 35 to 44. The use of these particular groups is especially recommended where international comparisons are to be made. For schoolchildren WHO sometimes uses age 6 and age 12 instead of the 2-year groups.

When the samples have been determined it will be time to obtain *consent,* first from local or other officers of government, including school officials, and then perhaps from parents of children and from the adults as individuals. *Informed consent* is particularly necessary where radiographs are to be taken or where restorative care will follow the survey through public facilities. It is a good idea to alert local dental societies or local dental practitioners. Good public relations requires this, and the cooperation of these groups is often invaluable.

Where the survey is part of a clinical trial or some preventive or therapeutic measure, local and national policies on use of human subjects must be conformed to. The balance between the need for trial of agents which have not been tested in human subjects and the need to protect those subjects from harm is a delicate one, requiring careful thought. The American Dental Association has adopted (1972) an ethical policy to govern such situations; so also have various state health departments and universities.[31]

The *selection of examiners* is the next problem. For an initial survey in a community, local dentists who will volunteer their services can often be found. The question of probable examiner errors must then be considered. Table 5 shows what widely divergent figures may be obtained by different examiners even in the same cities and working with the same age groups. This table perhaps represents an extreme situation, but unexpected differences in interpretation can arise even between examiners who think they are familiar with each other's standards. The following precautions are usually wise:

1. Keep the number of examiners to a minimum.

2. Discuss interpretation of borderline problems carefully in advance, particularly the distinction between noncarious and carious pits or fissures.

3. Use only one make and design of explorer, making rules for discard as explorers become dull.

4. Have all members of the team examine a few cases in sequence and then exchange cases until each examiner has examined each patient. Divergences of opinion or of observation can then be discussed and minimized.

5. Type and circulate among the examiners any rules or systems which may seem pertinent.

6. The supervisor should recheck an occasional case throughout the entire survey.

7. Subtle changes in interpretation should be guarded against. Grainger and Sellers remark wisely that "unconscious subjective influences such as gradual refinement of examination techniques, an acquired tolerance for certain defects, or even bias resulting from desire to be unbiased are almost always present in data such as these."[32]

Where the same examiners are used over repeated yearly examinations, the *reversal rate* of each demands attention. A reversal occurs when a tooth or surface originally recorded as decayed is later reported as sound. A certain number of reversals are understandable with lesions of questionably small size. A large number of reversals, especially when colleagues report lower numbers, is usually an indication of carelessness upon the part of a bored examiner.

Careful thought must be given to the delegation of as many procedures as possible to *properly trained auxiliaries*. Dental hygienists, with adequate instruction, can perform Type 3 explorer inspections which correlate well with those of dentists.

For maximum efficiency recorders should be provided. Dental assistants or hygienists are preferable, but parents or other volunteers can often help if properly instructed. Monitors and other lay assistants may be needed to assure an even flow of subjects to and from the place of examination, according to a plan worked out with local authorities.

The *number of examinations per hour* should be carefully planned. One state health department expects a dentist to perform from 25 to 40 Type 3 inspections per hour.[33] This figure is probably too high in areas of rampant caries or where inexperienced personnel are doing the work.

Construction of a Prevalence Survey

After the dental examinations or inspections have been performed, the tabular presentation of the findings of the survey is the next problem.

The prevalence method of tabulation is by far the simplest. It also gives the best presentation of a situation where an appreciable proportion of the population is free of any disease or of the defect or treatment under study. In caries work where the percentage of population with any history of dental caries is above 70 or 80 percent, however, there can be great variations in the severity of the disease (that is, the number of DMF teeth per person) without any very marked change in percentage of population. For most areas in the United States, therefore, prevalence tabulation of survey data is inadequate.

The data most commonly recorded in a prevalence survey include:

1. Percentage of population with any history of dental caries.
2. Percentage of population with any permanent fillings.

3. Percentage of population with any deciduous fillings.

4. Percentage of population with any presently decayed teeth.

5. Percentage of population with any extractions or indicated extractions.

Fig. 45 shows a typical record form for material of this sort. Note the use of pluses or zeros to indicate presence or absence of a condition which may be widespread, and the use of more exact symbols for less common occurrences, such as extractions. Note also that no column is included for noting decayed teeth, though a plus in the DMF column and zeros elsewhere do indicate the presence of caries. A negative record on this point, following inspection or screening only, might be misleading.

In the realm of pure shortcut, one of the most useful devices involves the construction of a percentage prevalence survey through the use of Type 4 screening (tongue depressor) to eliminate those cases where one or more DMF teeth are obviously present, and then Type 3 inspection (mouth mirror and explorer) for those cases whose status is not readily apparent. This combination of methods produces the accuracy of Type 3 while retaining much of the speed of Type 4, particularly in areas of high caries prevalence. It is of no use in procuring a count of DMF

COUNTY _____ SCHOOL _____ EXAMINER _____

CITY _____ ADDRESS _____ DATE _____

NAME OF PUPIL	AGE	SEX	PERMANENT TEETH (EXCEPT FOR FILLINGS)						
			DMF	FILLINGS		MISSING			REMARKS
				P	D	EXTRACTION INDICATED	EXTRACTED	TOTAL	
White, Linda	9	F	+	+	0	0	꜀6	1	
Green, Jonathan	9	M	+	+	+	6/	16	2	
Epstein, Henry	9	M	0	0	0	0	0	0	
Johnson, Lorna	9	F	+	0	0	0	0	0	13 congenitally absent
Kelly, Mary	9	F	+	+	+	꜀6	0	1	
P—Permanent, D—Deciduous									

Figure 45. Form for dental caries prevalence survey.

teeth, unless low prevalence permits the use of the Knutson curve for prediction.

Recording DMF Tooth and Surface Findings

The common procedure followed by dentists in examining patients is to record carious areas by the surface on which they occur and the missing teeth by location. It is an easy step beyond this to record the location of existing satisfactory restorations. From such information, it is possible to construct the DMF tooth index (DMFT) or DMF surface index (DMFS) for caries in permanent teeth or the "def" or "df" index for deciduous teeth.[34,35] It is also possible to perform a number of simpler measurements, such as those recommended by the World Health Organization, and others to be described later, which lend themselves to computer data processing in various phases of caries research. The original record form is relatively unimportant, and hundreds have been designed that are satisfactory. Standard Form 603 is illustrated in Fig. 46 because it is used by the U.S. armed forces and in many other federal programs such as those of the Office of Economic Opportunity. The form is conservative in its design and fits very well with the experience of most practicing dentists. The numbering of teeth upon it, however, is in some ways inferior to that used by the World Health Organization (see Fig. 41, sheet 2).

Modern methods of optical scanning have encouraged the design of forms from which the data can be fed directly into data processing machinery without the expenditure of time and possibility of error which occurs when manual transfer must be made from a sheet such as Form 603 to an IBM punched card or computer tape. Fig. 47 shows a single 8½" x 11" sheet of paper which contains on the front (upper arch) and the back (lower arch) spaces for marking all of the surface data for all 32 teeth in one mouth, for preparation of the DMF surface index or other measurements of tooth or surface status. This sheet, prepared for Forsyth Dental Center, Boston, enters a scanning machine, but does not actually become the punched card or tape which enters the computer. It should be noted that each tooth box contains a spot for marking whether the tooth is permanent or deciduous, whether it is sound, unerupted, or extracted, and whether any one or a combination of

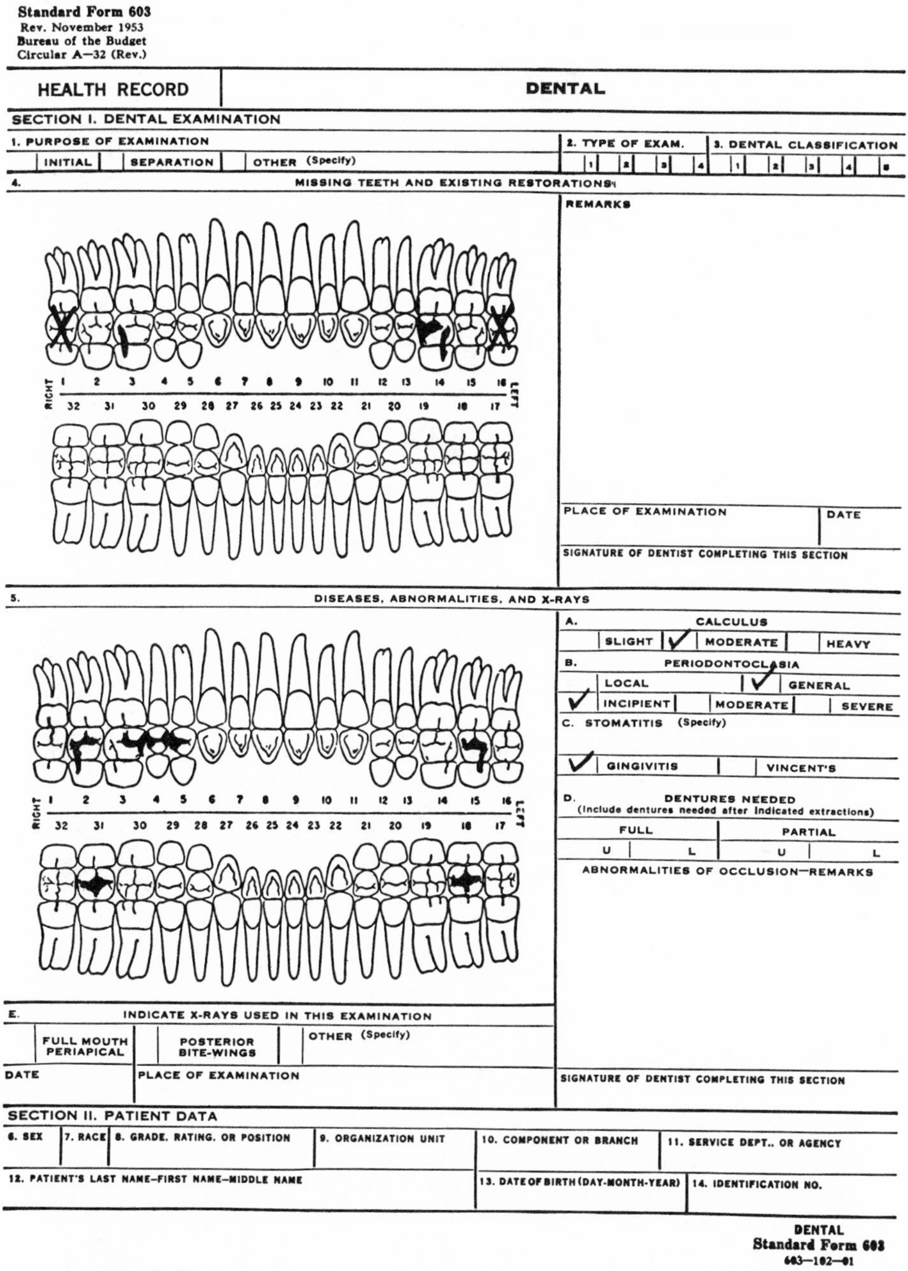

Standard Form 603
Rev. November 1953
Bureau of the Budget
Circular A—32 (Rev.)

HEALTH RECORD | DENTAL

SECTION I. DENTAL EXAMINATION

1. PURPOSE OF EXAMINATION — INITIAL | SEPARATION | OTHER (Specify)
2. TYPE OF EXAM. — 1 | 2 | 3 | 4
3. DENTAL CLASSIFICATION — 1 | 2 | 3 | 4 | 5

4. MISSING TEETH AND EXISTING RESTORATIONS

RIGHT 1 2 3 4 5 6 7 8 9 10 11 12 13 14 15 16 LEFT
32 31 30 29 28 27 26 25 24 23 22 21 20 19 18 17

REMARKS

PLACE OF EXAMINATION | DATE

SIGNATURE OF DENTIST COMPLETING THIS SECTION

5. DISEASES, ABNORMALITIES, AND X-RAYS

RIGHT 1 2 3 4 5 6 7 8 9 10 11 12 13 14 15 16 LEFT
32 31 30 29 28 27 26 25 24 23 22 21 20 19 18 17

A. CALCULUS — SLIGHT | ✓ MODERATE | HEAVY

B. PERIODONTOCLASIA — LOCAL | ✓ GENERAL

✓ INCIPIENT | MODERATE | SEVERE

C. STOMATITIS (Specify)

✓ GINGIVITIS | VINCENT'S

D. DENTURES NEEDED (Include dentures needed after indicated extractions)

FULL — U | L
PARTIAL — U | L

ABNORMALITIES OF OCCLUSION—REMARKS

E. INDICATE X-RAYS USED IN THIS EXAMINATION — FULL MOUTH PERIAPICAL | POSTERIOR BITE-WINGS | OTHER (Specify)

DATE | PLACE OF EXAMINATION | SIGNATURE OF DENTIST COMPLETING THIS SECTION

SECTION II. PATIENT DATA

6. SEX | 7. RACE | 8. GRADE, RATING, OR POSITION | 9. ORGANIZATION UNIT | 10. COMPONENT OR BRANCH | 11. SERVICE DEPT., OR AGENCY

12. PATIENT'S LAST NAME—FIRST NAME—MIDDLE NAME | 13. DATE OF BIRTH (DAY-MONTH-YEAR) | 14. IDENTIFICATION NO.

DENTAL
Standard Form 603
603—102—01

Figure 46. United States standard dental record form no. 603. [Bureau of the Budget.]

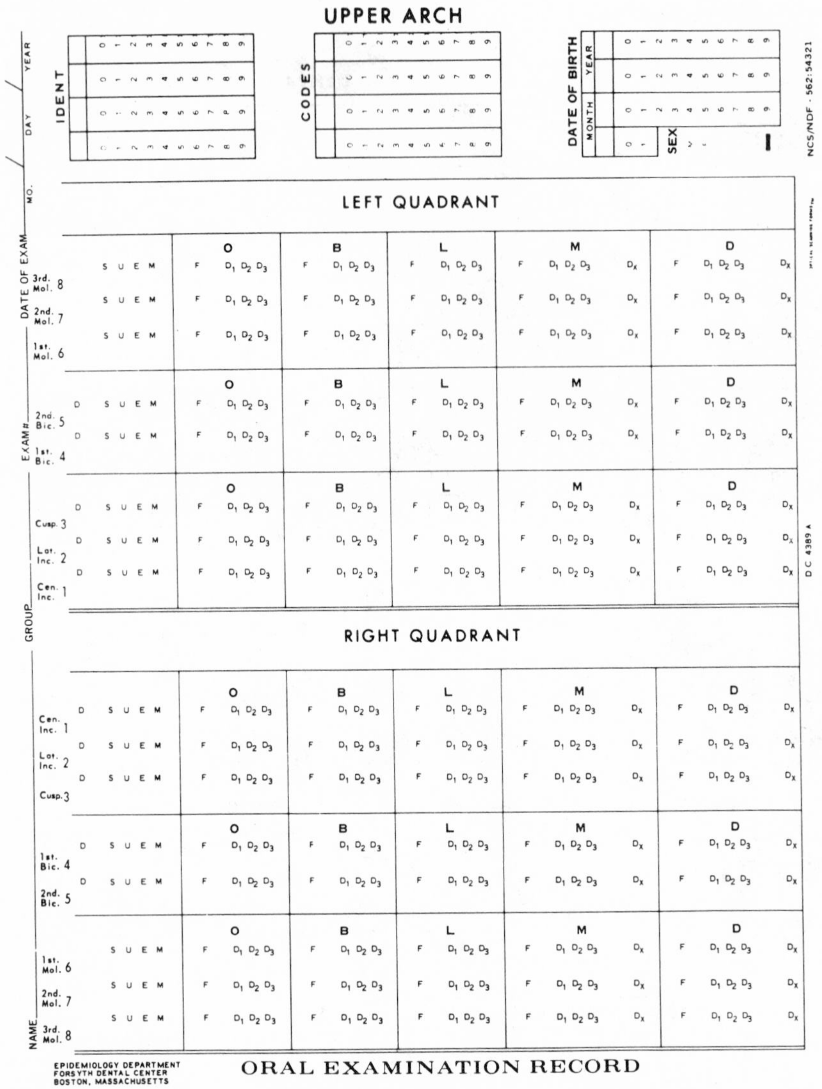

Figure 47. Optical scanning form for surface data, upper arch of one case, one line per tooth. Lower arch is recorded on reverse of sheet. O-occlusal; *B*-buccal; *L*-lingual; *M*-mesial; *D* (in column heading)-distal; *D* (in left margin)-deciduous; *S*-sound; *U*-unerupted; *E*-extracted (presumably for caries); *M*-missing (for other reason); *F*-filled; $D_{1,2,3}$-decayed to degree noted; D_x-decayed (x-ray finding only). Boxes are filled by ordinary pencil. [Reproduced by permission, Forsyth Dental Center, Boston, Massachusetts.]

the various five surfaces of the tooth is either filled, decayed, or both.

Rules for DMF Tooth or Surface Indices

Counts of DMF teeth or surfaces in the permanent dentition or of "df" teeth or surfaces in the primary dentition all have certain characteristics in common.[34,35] They are designed to represent a cumulative total of the effects of dental caries to the time of examination. There are certain simple rules to be used in constructing a DMF or "df" count. Most important are the following:

1. No tooth or surface should be listed more than once in the count. A tooth with present caries as well as a filling should be listed under D (decayed) since in this way it will be included among those needing treatment. Some authors count a tooth which is both decayed and filled as belonging to both these categories but count it only once in the final DMF count. If this procedure is used, it should be so specified. Teeth to be extracted immediately are listed under M (missing).

2. In surveys primarily for caries, care must be taken to avoid as far as possible listing as missing those teeth which are unerupted or are known to be missing or altered for reasons other than caries. Histories should be taken where it is suspected that teeth have been lost for reasons other than caries, and notes made upon the chart of any pertinent findings.

3. Decayed, missing, and filled teeth should be listed separately at first, since the components of the DMF count are of great interest.

4. Deciduous teeth are not to be included on a DMF count, nor permanent teeth in a "df" count. They should be graphed separately, as shown in Fig. 48.

5. Where counts are made of DMF surfaces, crowns, remaining roots, or teeth missing because of caries are counted at four or five surfaces each (be sure to state which). Five is theoretically the full number of surfaces, but three or four represents a better average, in the writer's experience, for the number of carious surfaces actually seen on extracted teeth. Doyle and Horowitz emphasize that the DMF surfaces on extracted teeth should not be ignored, even though doing so made no difference to their own illustrative stud-

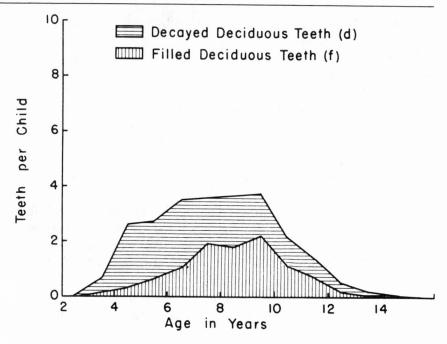

Figure 48. Decayed and filled deciduous teeth per child by age, Greater Boston area.

ies.[36] The best system is to make local studies of extracted teeth and use a figure for DMF surfaces per tooth that actually represent the population under study.

6. Third molars are best excluded from counts of permanent teeth or surfaces, since the status of these teeth is so often unknown unless x-rays have been taken.

7. A total count is taken for the affected teeth or surfaces in each mouth. Counts for a group of individuals are averaged.

Other Measures of Caries Status or Increments

It is by no means necessary to base caries-research findings on changes in the full DMF status of a group of cases. Findings may be focused upon those teeth or surfaces which have been present and "at risk" during the entire period of the study, or have both erupted and become carious during the study. The history of individual teeth can thus be followed in a cohort study. Teeth or tooth surfaces are listed simply according to whether they were unerupted, sound, carious, filled, or extracted at the beginning, and in one of these states or missing at the end of the study.

The "observed increment" of caries is usually considered to be the total of those teeth which were either sound or unerupted at the beginning of a period of time and were either decayed, filled, or missing because of caries at the end of that period. A transition from unerupted to missing in the same tooth is usually discarded because of the difficulty of distinguishing reliably between these two states. The "net increment" of caries is usually taken to include the observed increment less those teeth or surfaces which through error, varying interpretation, or perhaps abrasion have changed from carious to sound. This last category represents the "reversals" which are commonly seen in all studies involving incipient caries, but which should not exceed certain recognized limits if the study is to be considered accurate. Either the observed increments or the net increments may be corrected by covariance analysis so as to eliminate the variability which might have arisen from different numbers of erupted, sound teeth or surfaces in the two samples at the beginning of the study. Computer programs are available to prepare and correct increments very quickly from records of two sets of dental examinations, both introduced into the computer as part of the same process of analysis.

Influence of Bite-wing X-rays on Survey Findings

Public health surveys seldom make use of x-rays because of the cost and other difficulties involved, though statements are frequently made that accurate surveying should include the use of x-rays. It is of interest, therefore, to examine the extent to which x-rays may alter dental-examination findings made by mirror and explorer. Most of the literature available on this subject deals with bite-wing x-rays since films of this sort represent by far the greatest case-finding efficiency for a small expenditure of effort. Under certain conditions, bite-wing pictures are to be preferred to apical pictures, as for the diagnosis of proximal lesions of caries and early alveolar-bone loss.

Fig. 49 shows the effect of one pair of posterior bite-wings upon dental-explorer findings in a large group of school, college, and military samples from ages 13 to 23.[37] It will be seen here that the bite-wings have a relatively small and also fairly predictable effect

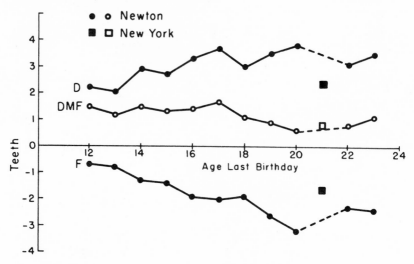

Figure 49. Changes in count of D, F, and DMF teeth per person found by bite-wing x-ray, Newton, Massachusetts, and New York City. [Courtesy, *Journal of the American Dental Association.*]

upon the DMF tooth count for each sample. Increases approximating one tooth per person occur throughout the entire age range. There is a much greater effect, however, upon findings of decayed teeth (D), with increases of from two to more than three teeth per person. There are decreases in the number of filled teeth (F), since many of these teeth were found upon x-ray examination to have additional cavities on previously unattacked surfaces. Such teeth were retabulated as D instead of F. One can reason from these findings that where the purpose of a survey is to determine susceptibility to dental caries, and the DMF tooth count itself will be the most important result, x-rays are of little necessity. Where immediate treatment needs, however, are under study, and particularly where survey findings are designed for the treatment of the individual person surveyed, bite-wing x-rays achieve far greater importance.

New carious surfaces provide a far more accurate measure of the need for dental treatment than do new carious teeth, and a much more realistic one as far as the dental practitioner is concerned. In the tabulation made by Dunning and De Wilde of new carious surfaces per person found by bite-wing x-ray alone, no age group showed an average of fewer than 3 new carious surfaces per person, and the maximum shown was 7.01 for age 17.[37] This tabulation also shows a well-defined variation in the efficiency of the bite-wing x-ray in regard to the *age of the patient*. A fairly sharp peak in efficiency was found at age 17. This peak can be explained in terms of the posteruptive life of the permanent teeth. For the first few years after eruption the proximal surfaces of these teeth, because of their regular enamel structure, seem not to succumb to caries as readily as do surfaces with pits and fissures. Then comes a time, in the late teen-age period, when proximal caries is beginning to occur but is not detectable by explorer. After that time, carious lesions become larger, and hence are easier to pick up by explorer alone. The placement of fillings also decreases the efficiency of the x-rays by overshadowing recurrent lesions. As a result, these lesions can more frequently be detected by explorer than by x-ray.

In public health dental surveying circumstances may arise in which x-rays can be made easily and explorer examinations cannot. It is therefore of interest to know how many of the total carious surfaces of the entire mouth can be found *by bite-wing x-ray alone*. Fig. 50 shows the percentages of carious surfaces so found at

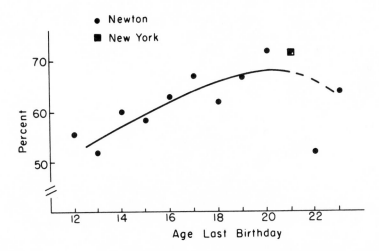

Figure 50. Percentage of carious surfaces for the entire mouth found by posterior bite-wing x-ray, Newton, Massachusetts, and New York City. [Courtesy, *Journal of the American Dental Association.*]

different ages in the studies reported by Dunning and De Wilde. A steady increase in the efficiency of the bite-wing method is seen up to age 21, when almost three-quarters of the total caries observations (72 percent) can be picked up by one pair of posterior bite-wing x-rays alone. Only 40 percent of the total observations of this age group resulted solely from explorer examination. Twelve percent of the total were found by both explorer and x-ray. Above age 21 the efficiency of the bite-wing seems to fall off, but the samples upon which these studies are based are so small that further study would be needed before any valid conclusions could be drawn. Fluoridation, also, has affected proximal caries.

There are various advantages to public health bite-wing x-ray surveying among the population groups where the efficiency of these films is likely to prove high. Among such advantages may be mentioned the fact that in the absence of third-party reimbursement x-ray examinations are still enough less common than explorer examinations in the private office that public health survey x-rays are likely to produce a larger proportion of really new findings than will explorer examinations. Again, x-rays leave a permanent record for future study. Finally, x-rays are easily transmitted to a private dentist without diagnosis and yet with enough explanation to the patient that they act as a far more powerful stimulus to the seeking of treatment than will a mere verbal statement that treatment is needed. In this last way x-rays often bridge the gap between the public health dentist and the private practitioner in such a way as to avoid impairment of public relations. The high number of findings per film in bite-wing x-rays and the safety precautions now available in dental x-ray work combine with the low radiation hazard to make dental x-raying, at least of the bite-wing variety, a thoroughly acceptable modern survey technique where films are later to be used for patient treatment.

A word needs to be said about the influence of x-ray findings upon indices for the severity of periodontal disease (Periodontal Index, GB count, or Ramfjord Index). Evidence is accumulating that posterior bite-wing x-rays will increase total findings of periodontal bone loss, much as they do the findings of proximal caries, and also that bite-wing x-rays are more efficient in this matter than are apical films.[38] The trouble is that a pair of posterior bite-wing films provides information on only those teeth which appear without distortion, usually the second bicuspids and first molars. The number of teeth to show clearly on each film is not standard. A source of variability is thus added to those whole-mouth indices where only a variable portion of the mouth has received study by x-ray. Whole-mouth x-ray surveys, even with bite-wing films, are impractical in the public health setting and usually unnecessary for the anterior part of the mouth. For these reasons x-ray supplementation is proving difficult in the whole-mouth periodontal indices—the Periodontal Index and the GB count. In the Ramfjord Index, however, and in certain modifications of the Periodontal Index, a smaller number of teeth is involved, and full study of these teeth by x-ray is easier. In these indices, the bite-wing or apical x-ray film may thus find its place.

The question of standardization of angulation of x-rays also deserves a word. Backer-Dirks is one of several researchers who have designed devices for positioning an x-ray film in the mouth so that it will relate in a reproducible manner to the teeth it depicts and to the angulation of the x-ray beam.[39] These devices are probably of considerable usefulness in longitudinal studies where the same patients are reexamined after a period of time. Their use in cross-sectional studies or in x-ray work performed primarily for service to the patient seems doubtful.

Safety Factors in Dental X-ray Work

In view of the attention currently being given to the hazards of radiation, it is of interest to examine the radiation dosage received from dental x-rays—particularly from the two films per person taken as part of a typical public health bite-wing survey. We must be on the alert for two types of damage: damage to the tissues closest to the x-ray machine, where a large measure of recovery can be expected, and damage to the reproductive organs, which is cumulative and may show up in future generations.

The tissues closest to the dental x-ray machine, particularly the skin, might show damage in the form of burns if x-rays were taken in great numbers indiscriminately. Partial recovery of these tissues, however, occurs between doses. Many dentists for years have used a 14-film dental x-ray survey as part of their routine maintenance program to be repeated once a year for each patient. No local damage has ever been reported as a result of this routine. It is estimated that the entire series of 14 films could be repeated after a 2-week rest without danger of skin damage. However, no exposure to ionizing radiation should be permitted without the expectation of a commensurate benefit.

The mechanism of inheritance is more sensitive than any other biological system to the effects of radiation. There is no recovery from damage to the reproductive organs, and thus the cumulative lifetime dosage of the patient becomes of interest. A yardstick in common use today is that given in the report of the National Academy of Sciences in 1956 on the biological effects of atomic radiation.[40] Measurement is in roentgens (R), often expressed in the same number of roentgen equivalents in man (rem).

The 1972 report did conclude that the guides adopted in 1956 provided an unnecessarily large cushion. If the medical and dental exposure could be reduced further without impairing essential medical or dental services, then the present standard is unnecessarily high. A maximum of 10 R is suggested as that dosage which can be received safely before the age of 30. Within this figure, about 4.3 R must be allowed for background radiation (cosmic rays and so forth) and an additional small amount, perhaps of the magnitude of 0.2 R, should be allowed if weapons testing were continued for 30 years at the rate of the two most active years (1953 and 1955). Current studies indicate that a series of 14 dental x-ray films produces an approximate dosage of 0.00042 R (0.42 mR) of scattered radiation to the reproductive organs of the male and less to those of the female. This figure is to be compared with the dosage of approximately 0.3 mR received by the male gonads from natural background radiation every day. The practitioner must take into consideration somatic risks when ordering x-rays. Cancer induction is considered to be the only source of somatic risk that needs to be taken into account.

An indication of the small size of the radiation dosage expected from diagostic dental x-rays may be seen from the recommendations of the National Council on Radiation Protection and Measurements for maximum accumulated occupational dose for those in daily contact with sources of radiation (that is, dentists). Their formula permits 5(N-18) roentgen equivalents in man, where "N" is the age in years and is greater than 18. This means in effect that an adult during his working years may receive 100 mR per week to the whole body, gonads, blood-forming organs, or lens of eye without danger. Exposures of only a very small fraction of this amount are the rule in most dental offices, as those who wear film badges will know. Nevertheless, the chance of leakage from, or accidental short-circuiting of, an x-ray machine is sufficient to make film badges important for dental personnel. The National Council on Radiation Protection and Measurements indicates what the practitioner should be concerned with regarding the design and operational aspects of dental x-ray equipment and matters relating to structural shielding design.[41]

As a result of careful study, the American Dental Association Council on Dental Materials has published a series of eleven recommendations on the dental-radiation problem.[42] It is summarized as follows:

1. Radiographic examination is a diagnostic procedure. The dentist's professional judgment should determine the frequency and extent of each radiographic examination, using a minimum number of films.

2. Use the fastest speed film available. Request film of an ANSI (ASA) speed group rating of "D" or faster.

3. When a cylindrical collimated x-ray machine is being used, the circular beam striking the face should not be more than 2.75 inches in diameter. Further restriction of the beam to reduce radiation is preferred and can be obtained by rectangular collimation.

4. Make sure the x-ray machine contains filtration of 2 mm of aluminum equivalent if operating at less than 70 kilovolt peak (kvp), and 2.5 mm of aluminum equivalent if operating at 70 kvp or above.

5. Use only shielded open-end cones to reduce scatter radiation.

6. Use leaded aprons on all patients as an additional precaution to prevent radiation of the gonads and thyroid glands.

7. Use film holders, bitetabs, or other methods to position film during exposure. The dentist or assistant should never hold a film in place for a patient and should stand at least 6 ft. from the patient or behind protective shielding.

8. Have periodic radiation protection surveys made of your office.

9. Properly expose the x-ray film. Overexposure with under-

development subjects the patient and office personnel to unnecessary radiation.

10. Follow manufacturer's instructions for processing x-ray film.

11. Continue your education in the area of radiology as well as in other areas of dental practice.

Every physician and dentist asks himself these days whether the pictures he is taking are actually necessary. In this connection, a survey of entering students at Harvard University is of interest. Sixty-seven percent of the 2,218 entering students x-rayed in 1956–57 showed dental defects of one sort or another. One hundred unselected dental patients from this group showed the following results from two films apiece: 299 cavities of ordinary size; 47 cavities approaching the pulp; 36 teeth with definite periodontal bone loss; 50 impacted teeth; 16 cases of very heavy calculus.

On the basis of such findings as these, it is felt that bite-wing x-ray surveying is both justified and thoroughly safe as part of a dental public health program where the findings are also of service to the patient. Nevertheless, any subject in doubt as to his cumulative dosage or recently x-rayed by his own dentists can easily be excused from the survey pictures on request.

PUTTING THE FACTS TOGETHER

Once the examination procedures of a survey have been completed, the work of assembling the material and interpreting it begins. In large surveys where detailed findings are to form the basis of clinical research, transfer to punched cards may prove advisable. Studies of the conditions of individual teeth give the greatest reason for the making of punched cards. In small public health surveys where findings per patient are more important than findings per tooth, punched cards are seldom necessary. Tally sheets can be set up in such a way as to produce frequency distributions, that is, numbers of cases showing the different categories of findings. From these frequency distributions, means and standard deviations can be computed. With modern calculating machines so commonly available, however, data can be handled so quickly under single-score heads that there is a little inducement to group the data. Problems of statistical analysis have been dealt with in Chapters 4 to 6. Where punched cards are to be used, some statistical service or a computer center will have to render assistance. Such organizations should be consulted about the arrangement of the original record form or of a suitable transfer sheet so that coding can be adapted to the needs of the data processors. The World Health Organization can assist in analysis, where their forms are used and they have been consulted in advance as to modus operandi.[8]

In tabulating DMF material for any one sample, the figures of interest are the mean values of decayed, missing, filled, and DMF teeth per person, and finally, the percentage composition of the DMF mean when taken as 100 percent. These can be combined in tabular form as shown in Table 36.

The mean values of the various components of the DMF count give actual figures for treatment need, tooth loss, and so forth, which are of self-evident value. The DMF total is descriptive of *caries susceptibility* in the sample, entirely independently of any dental treatment which may have been rendered. It is from a study of the components of the DMF count that one learns the amount of treatment that has been rendered to the patient in the sample and the efficacy of that treatment.

The D column gives *treatment needs* in terms of teeth to be restored. In the columns for percentage composition, the first column (D teeth divided by DMF teeth) is a better measure of the failure of dental treatment in the community than is the actual

Table 36. Dental caries experience in permanent teeth among children aged 12–14 at last birthday, 1951.

Area	No. of cases	No. of teeth per child				Percentage composition of DMF			
		Decayed	Missing	Filled	DMF	D	M	F	DMF
Newton, Mass.									
Weeks School[a]	791	3.82	0.31	3.93	8.08	47	4	49	100
Day School[b]	412	6.81	0.52	2.82	10.14	67	5	28	100
Massachusetts									
28 communities[c]	3740	6.33	0.62	3.39	10.34	61	6	33	100

a. Harvard School of Dental Medicine survey, 1950.
b. Harvard School of Dental Medicine survey, 1951.
c. Commonwealth of Massachusetts Department of Health, 1951.

number of D teeth per person, since there is little credit to be gained from a low D count where the DMF total itself is low.

The M column, in young persons at least, represents predominantly the end result of caries. The ratio of missing teeth to DMF teeth has been termed *tooth fatality* since the ratio represents that proportion of affected teeth which are lost.[43] Similarly, a medical fatality rate measures deaths not among an entire population but among patients with actual cases of a disease. *Low tooth fatality is also the best ultimate measure of the success of a dental treatment program,* for the same reason as that given for proportion of decayed teeth.

The number of filled teeth per person indicates the amount of restorative dentistry done among members of the group surveyed, but an allowance must also be made for fillings present in teeth called "decayed" because they have both filled and unfilled cavities and cannot be listed twice. A surface count gives less difficulty on this score than a tooth count. In the percentage column, the ratio of filled teeth to DMF teeth has been termed the *filled-tooth ratio.* This ratio measures in direct proportion the success of a treatment program for dental caries.

The standard deviations for observations of DMF teeth are often included in the table. These enable readers to perform their own significance tests upon differences without imposing upon the publisher of survey data the task of printing detailed frequency distributions for all samples surveyed.

Classification of Treatment Needs

A useful classification of individuals according to their treatment needs may be employed at this point. The American Dental Association's "Dental Classification of Individuals," published in its *Official Policies on Dental Health Programs,* is as follows:

Class 1. Individuals apparently requiring no dental treatment related to the type of examination or inspection performed.

Class 2. Individuals requiring treatment but not of an urgent nature, such as:
  a. Moderate calculus.
  b. Prosthetic cases not included in Class 3.
  c. Caries—not extended or advanced.
  d. Periodontal diseases—not extensive or advanced.
  e. Other oral conditions requiring corrective or preventive measures.

Class 3. Individuals requiring early treatment of such conditions as:
    a. Extensive or advanced caries.
    b. Extensive or advanced periodontal disease.
    c. Chronic pulpal or apical infection.
    d. Chronic oral infection.
    e. Heavy calculus.
    f. Surgical procedures required for removal of one or more teeth and other surgical procedures not included in Class 4.
    g. Insufficient number of teeth for mastication.

Class 4. Individuals requiring emergency dental treatment for such conditions as:
    a. Injuries.
    b. Acute oral infections (periodontal and periapical abscesses, Vincent's infection, acute gingivitis, acute stomatitis, etc.)
    c. Painful conditions.[30]

Evaluation of Dental Care Delivery

The term evaluation can be applied to any reasoning process based upon fact, but in public health practice the term has acquired a more specific meaning. It usually refers to a comparison between the survey findings in a given locality and similar findings of earlier date in the same locality or in other localities at the same time. The evaluation of a dental health program should concentrate attention upon the main survey findings and also upon certain revealing facts to be found from the annual reports of previous dental health staff, reports of school nurses, studies of the quality of dental service rendered, and various other relevant items. Table 36 shows the first stage in the evaluation of DMF data. Here one area in the city of Newton, Massachusetts, is compared with another area in Newton and also with the state as a whole. One area is of fairly high socioeconomic status with relatively low caries susceptibility, low decayed-tooth ratio, and high filled-tooth ratio. The other area, of somewhat lower socioeconomic status, approximates in most characteristics the baseline data obtained by the Massachusetts Department of Public Health. No sharp differences in tooth fatality are seen here, but they frequently appear in comparisons of this sort.

Percentage-prevalence data should be compared with those of other areas if they were part of the survey, and so also should data on *classification of dental needs*. Rules of thumb may often be obtained from the state department of public health as guides to what one may expect in a local area. Thus in Massachusetts it is common to find 30 percent of a school population falling in Class 1 (no apparent treatment needs), 45 percent in Class 2 (treatment needed at convenience), 25 percent in Class 3 (early treatment needed), and no significant percentage at all in Class 4 (emergency treatment needed for pain or injury). In practice the distinctions between Classes 1 and 2, and between Classes 3 and 4 are harder to make than between Classes 2 and 3. In one study at least, therefore, Classes 1 plus 2 have been contrasted with Classes 3 plus 4. Thus a 4-year screening program in a Boston low-income area showed 60 percent of fourth-grade children to fall into Classes 1 plus 2 in 1968 and 82 percent to fall into these two classes in 1971, with a corresponding drop in the urgent or emergency classes (3 plus 4).[44] As the screening program was accompanied by a health education program, referral of children to sources of care, and actual care for some in a neighborhood health center, this change in classification of need was taken as an indication of success of the whole program. A corresponding rise in the *filled-tooth ratio* (F/DMF) from 32 to 48 percent occurred in these same children during the same interval.

From dental-service annual reports perhaps the most interesting commonly available material is the *filling-extraction ratio*. This, to be sure, is not a pure measure either of caries susceptibility or of dental treatment, but a composite of the two, affected very greatly by the resolve on the part of the school dentist(s) to render comprehensive care. The computing of this ratio involves merely a comparison between the number of fillings placed during a given year with the number of extractions performed. In Labrador, where Grenfell Mission dentists are only infrequently available to a primitive population with a high caries rate, it is a good dentist who can do one filling for each extraction he must perform. In Boston, Massachusetts, a 1948 community survey showed public dental programs to be placing 2.7 fillings for each extraction performed.[45] The private practitioners in Boston at the same time were placing 5.9 fillings for their child patients for each extraction performed. The closer approach to comprehensive dental care in private offices is obvious and understandable. Some public dental services rendering comprehensive care have recorded far better results than this. In Philadelphia, for instance, where careful operative dentistry is available for a population already receiving the benefits of water fluoridation, only one extraction is reported for every 100 treatment visits.[46]

Another item of interest usually available from annual reports is the number of *patients seen per day* by the dental service. This figure, again, can be interpreted only in the light of a number of general facts as to the type of care being rendered and the caries susceptibility of the population. A small number of patients seen per day, if coupled with good totals for the various restorative operations, shows a closer approach to comprehensive care than does a high number of patients seen. The proportion of "permanent" fillings to temporary fillings also helps in an appraisal of the extent of comprehensive care, as does a subjective appraisal of the quality of care being rendered.

An overall appraisal of the proportion of cases with treatment needs which are carried to *completion* is a very important part of any evaluation. Percentage of completions may be obtained sometimes from the records of school nurses, sometimes from classroom teachers, and sometimes from the dental health services themselves. It is important that cases referred outside to private practitioners be tabulated as well as those treated in the school clinic. This involves a "certificate" system with proper follow-up as described in Chapter 20. Certificate forms, on their way to the family and the family dentist, may perform a valuable function as mere memoranda that dental supervision is needed, but, unless energetic means are taken to assure that the certificates are returned properly signed, it is misleading to draw conclusions from those which do find their way back to the source. Completed certificates must also be interpreted in the light of the ability of the child to obtain needed dental treatment. For this reason *report forms* are coming into increasing use, where the progress of treatment may be recorded and also the family's inability to obtain care from a private practitioner. The facts found from such reports may prove valuable in the design of the dental health program.

The foregoing material deals chiefly with the evaluation of the quantity of dental care. This is an aspect of the quality of service, to be sure, but a fuller discussion of quality of care is found in Chapter 19.

Final Report

The final step in survey procedure should probably be the construction of a report, with or without a set of recommendations. Clearness and simplicity should be sought here. For purposes of broad community action the recommendations should probably deal only with major objectives. Minor points, though noted for the benefit of the actual or future director of the program, should probably not be included in any public document, since they tend to obscure the major issues.

If a formal written report is to be prepared, the World Health Organization gives an excellent outline.[8] It is abbreviated as follows:

> Statement of the purposes of the survey
> Materials and methods:
>
> 1. Description of area and population surveyed
> 2. Types of information collected
> 3. Methods of collecting data
> 4. Sampling method
> 5. Examiner personnel and equipment
> 6. Statistical analysis and computational procedure
> 7. Cost analysis
> 8. Reliability and reproducibility of results
>
> Results
> Discussion and conclusions
> Summary

Surveying, in the thorough fashion outlined in this chapter, is far more than a collecting and arraying of facts. It is a task through participation in which many key people in a community become aware of the dental needs of the community and what can be done about them. These people are the ones who will subsequently rally popular support for the program, and some of them, the dentists particularly, may participate in it personally. The survey procedures themselves, though not designed for year-after-year dental case finding, may also lay the foundation for the case-finding phase of the ensuing program.

Dental Health Education

IN A FIELD such as health, it is natural that "helping people to help themselves" should be as important as direct service. Indeed, if one concentrates upon prevention of disease and the attainment of positive health habits rather than upon the cure of disease, self-help is much more than half the battle. Health education is therefore a major endeavor for the public health worker. It is interesting also to realize that health looms large to the educator among the major categories of subject material of importance in a public school program. A commission of the National Education Association, reporting as long ago as 1918 upon "Cardinal Principles of Secondary Education," placed health at the top of a list of seven major objectives of education, the others being command of fundamental processes, worthy home membership, vocation, citizenship, worthy use of leisure, and ethical character.[1] Health education thus has become a field for mutual endeavor in which educators, too, have a large stake.

Dentists face the subject of health education at somewhat of a disadvantage. They deal with a very common condition which many people feel is not a disease at all but just a fact of life: namely, teeth decay. Treatment is time-consuming and exacting. As a result, an attitude has risen within the dental profession to the effect that if a dentist is talking, he is not working. This has inhibited proper dental health education of the patient. The situation has been further complicated by the fact that, until recently, we have had few good preventive measures to talk about, and the changes in the behavior of the public which we have been endeavoring to promote are difficult changes in a number of ways. As Young describes it, "there is no clear-cut immediate cause and effect relationship between the incidence of dental caries and recommended health practices. Instead, personal actions must be taken regularly over a long period of time before results can be clearly demonstrated."[2]

Health education is far more than a process of transmitting information from a teacher to a learner. It is a complex process of interactions set in motion by the educator by means of which he hopes to influence first the attitudes and then the behavior of the learner. The learner may thus achieve for himself a desired goal in the field of health. Young's diagram illustrates some of these interactions, as seen in Fig. 51. Note that the learner may easily have set dental health goals for himself which include having his teeth

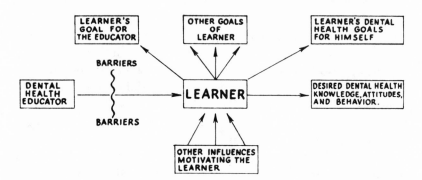

Figure 51. Conceptual model of the educational process as related to dental health. [Copyright, American Dental Association. Reprinted by permission.]

removed as soon as possible so that he can acquire dentures and have no further pain and inconvenience. The learner may also have a goal for the health educator, namely, for him to conclude his complex and boring message at the earliest possible moment. The educator must realize that the learner has many other influences brought to bear upon him with which dental health must compete. Somehow the learner must be made to see that the dental health goals can be fitted in among the others in such a way as to seem practical and desirable, thus placing him in a position to achieve them. He must become convinced that teeth are worth saving.

Part of the educator's problem is the penetration of a screen of barriers between him and the learner. The list of these barriers can be long and varied. Some typical ones are:

Differences in meanings assigned to scientific terms by the layman and the professional.

Difficulty of making and keeping dental appointments.

Poverty (in which lack of money may be secondary to helplessness in the wise use of money and facilities, even when available).

Ethnic and cultural conflicts.

Habits contrary to those desired.

Lack of faith in treatment.

Differing opinions as to treatment plan.

Language and illiteracy barriers.

Attitudes toward "charity" (public clinics).

Convenience (availability of baby sitters, and so forth).

Fear of pain or injury.

Poor administration of services, including lack of personal attention to patient.

Personalities of those connected with dental offices or agencies.

Only in recent years has a body of knowledge upon such matters as oral hygiene, nutrition (including fluoridation), and early control of dental caries been built up to the extent that it constitutes a respectable item in a school curriculum. In times of high demand there are many both within and outside the dental profession who fear education about dental health because they feel this will stimulate an additional demand for dental treatment which cannot be met. These persons, the writer feels, neglect the full value of preventive techniques currently available. If treatment facilities do not exist for all the dental disease which might occur in an uneducated population, education for prevention really becomes more important, not less.

Books on health education customarily devote considerable space to a discussion of the subject material to be transmitted and the health habits to be developed: the "big problems" of greatest current importance. In this book, such subjects are found mostly in Chapter 12. The present chapter, therefore, deals with such problems as methods, media, personnel, and the types of people for whom health education must be designed. The goal of dental health education is the promotion of oral health. Current activities, as Horowitz observes, are often directed toward affluent segments of society, whereas health promotion should be aimed at everyone, not just those who are favorably disposed.[3] Society-wide norms and standards for action must be created. Mere descriptions of the actions themselves are no more than a beginning.

METHODS

The section on methods will deal primarily with school dental health programs since these follow a fairly predictable pattern and are likely to represent the major effort in any one community.

The primary distinction in method, in the field of dental health education, is between individual instruction and group instruction. In an ideal program both should exist. *Individual instruction* is best built around experience in healthful living. In dentistry these opportunities come through school dental inspection, dental prophylaxis or fluoride treatments, visits to the dental office, and individual dietary instructions. All of these fields, because of the specialized knowledge involved, are best handled by professionally trained personnel: the dentist, dental hygienist, dental therapist, or some other auxiliary with specific training. Each should give attention to child psychology and to some of the elements of the learning process, but the problem is essentially the same as that encountered in the private dental office where the ordinary principles of patient handling apply. Individual instruction gives the highest possible interaction between pupil and teacher, and the highest degree of personalization. Dentists and dental hygienists should recognize their unique opportunities—and responsibilities—in this type of instruction.

In the handling of *groups,* special educational experience becomes necessary. Dentists, unless they have taken educational training and had teaching experience, will do best to remain in the role of consultant or perhaps, on occasion, lecturer before familiar groups, such as parent-teacher associations. The dental hygienists employed in a school system should attempt no more than is justified by the amount of training or experience in education which they have received. They can always, and must always, act as a resource person, supplying dental health facts and material to the teachers in their school system, but the extent to which they can do actual classroom teaching varies greatly with their training and with the rapport they are able to establish with school administrators and classroom teachers. No one staff member is likely to possess all the resources which will be needed in a broad and effective educational program. Specialization in the various fields of health (of which dentistry is but one) is inevitable, but specialized teachers not sufficiently coordinated tend to confuse children, divide their attention and loyalties, and invite irresponsible behavior. Dental personnel, therefore, should be careful to coordinate their work with that of others in the health field.

Types of School Curriculum

A brief consideration of the major types of school curriculum in use at present in the United States is of interest in order to visualize the frame into which health education must fit. The National Education Association recognizes three major types: the curriculum of isolated subjects; the broad-fields curriculum; and the core curriculum.[1] More recently, the *open classroom* has introduced new approaches within the core-curriculum pattern.

The curriculum of *isolated subjects* has the longest tradition in this country and is represented more extensively in schools today than any other plan. Health instruction finds its way into this type of curriculum only by being given a specific time allotment. In fact, there is little likelihood of its being effective unless it is accorded time comparable to that given other major areas of the curriculum. In this type of plan, health is taught primarily as a *subject,* like reading, arithmetic, or history. This has a distinct advantage, particularly in connection with the more detailed work necessary for senior high school students, but in general, treatment as an isolated subject discourages both teacher and student from feeling that the study of health is truly vital. The best that seems possible under the circumstances is to give health concentrated consideration for one or two years.

The *broad-fields curriculum* helps pupil motivation by grouping subject material into real-life patterns. Thus history, economics, sociology, and political science are combined into "social studies." An organized approach to health instruction can easily be worked out within the broad-fields curriculum. Such isolated subjects as personal hygiene, disease prevention, community hygiene, and health care of children can be combined into a single course. This program encourages both teachers and children to make correlations more frequently than does instruction in isolated subjects.

The *core-curriculum* concept has arisen recently as a reaction against sterile instruction organized around subjects. It implies in essence that a group of children spend an important portion of the school day with one teacher who is responsible for the core of their experience. For younger children the time may amount to as much as three-fourths of the school day. For the older children, one-third to one-half of the total hours in school may be spent with the "core" teacher and program. Special teachers in health may exist within such a framework and work as specialists, particularly with high school students, but the basic features of the total program are planned by consultation between the core teachers and the special, or resource, teachers. The content of instruction in the core is not given any subject label. The immediate needs and interests of children are given careful attention in planning for health. Nutrition is taught in connection with choosing a meal in the cafeteria. The emotional problems of the older children are studied by the direct observation of younger children, and so forth. There are risks connected with the core-curriculum system. It depends very heavily on the individual teacher, who may be dull. It concentrates often upon complex current phenomena in such a way as to hamper the logical presentation of any one subject.

The *open classroom* represents a child-centered approach to learning rather than a teacher-centered authoritarian approach. There is no predetermined curriculum design, but there are clear general educational goals, among which is the achieving of competence in basic skills in language and in mathematics. There is considerable freedom in the open classroom for children to pursue activities of their own interest within the area of study, including the design and carrying out of projects. Each child advances at his or her own rate, with the teacher as guide and leader. Albertini et al. describe an interesting application of dental health education in the open classroom, including role playing, inspection of each other's teeth, and simple biochemical projects.[4]

From the foregoing consideration of curricula it will be obvious that dental health can seldom be treated as an isolated matter. It makes little difference who does the ultimate teaching, provided the dental subject material is not considered a "stepchild," but is transmitted with understanding and devotion.

Educational Principles

At this point the objectives of education should be considered, including the difference between *education* and *training*. In dental public health the immediate goal is the stimulation of *behavior* designed to minimize dental and oral disease. This could be a mere training problem, and modern plaque-control programs make it so, with a strong emphasis upon the learning and correct repetition of technical procedures. Correct repetition ad infinitum will occur, however, only in the presence of strong motivation. This requires education, even before the technical writing.

Education, almost by definition, involves arousal of curiosity, which can then be satisfied by the learner with or without the guidance of a teacher. Education for health is a general process which at best begins very early. Fourth- and fifth-grade children have a great latent curiosity about their bodies—as do people of all ages to a lesser extent. This curiosity must be stimulated and, so far as possible, satisfied. A large part of a teacher's role is listening to students trying to teach themselves. In the long run education has much larger goals than mere stimulation of technical actions. As an example, adults who may have been only moderately expert with the toothbrush and dental floss may have developed an interest in the delivery of health care which will make them invaluable consumer members of a Health Systems Agency board.

A few isolated hints are in order as to the transmission of dental health information. *Fear arousal* may be considered first. A classical study on the effect of fear, done by Janis and Feshbach, was conducted in the field of dental care.[5] Three 15-minute illustrated lectures on the causes of tooth decay were recorded, each with 20 lantern slides to accompany it. The first lecture played heavily upon fear, emphasizing the painful consequences of tooth decay; the second lecture used moderate fear appeal; while in the third, most of the fear-arousing material was replaced by neutral information upon growth and function of the teeth. The first lecture even mentioned paralysis and total blindness as possible consequences. The freshman class of a large high school was divided into four sections, three receiving the recorded lectures just described and the fourth section serving as a control. It was later ascertained how many children visited their dentist in the week following the lecture. Of those who heard the first lecture, 10 percent visited their dentist within a week. Of those who heard the second lecture, 13 percent visited their dentist, while of those who heard the third lecture (the one with least fear arousal), 18 percent did so. Of the control group, only 4 percent made visits. From this it is apparent that some kinds of fear arousal retard health education. Strong fear and anxiety can block attentiveness and comprehension. It can even cause rejection of the communicator's statements and, as a result, avoidance of the recommended health habits.

A valuable method when working with groups is that of *group decision*. Facts are appreciated less and remembered less if they are merely taken on the authority of the individual who is speaking to the group. If people can be induced to decide for themselves that a change in health habits is needed and that there are specific courses of action open to them, an important step has been achieved toward changing existing health attitudes. This method should be borne in mind in all discussion-group and activity-project work. One way of using it is to present the facts and the problem, then ask questions as to what should be done about them. Learner activity, in almost any form, is a help to the individual as well as to the group. While group decision is of value in the school setting, it is of even greater value in the community setting, upon such matters as fluoridation or the delivery of public health care.

When dentists or dental hygienists are working with individual patients they should *talk more about what they are doing*. Many professional people tend to underestimate their patient's ability to understand the details of, or the reasoning behind, an operation which is being performed. They may also feel it below their dignity to transpose into lay language the terms in which they customarily speak of their work. The resulting lack of communication tends to arouse fear and a feeling of inferiority in patients, and at the same time causes the loss of a golden opportunity for health education. Patients—even very young patients—should be made part of the reasoning process connected with their own treatment wherever possible. Dentists should not become monologists when their patients' mouths are full of cotton rolls; they should take every opportunity possible to engage their patients in intelligent conversation. People learn best when they *participate actively*, either through conversation or some practical project.

Health education, like any other aspect of learning, applies certain general psychological principles. One set of concepts of particular interest is that known as Lewinian field theory.[6] It conceives of the child as situated within his life space or *immediate environment*. We see him, as in Fig. 52, in a space of free movement where he can take part in certain activities, where he receives instruction either personally, in groups, or through mass media, where he receives home care and also services as from the family physician or dentist, and where he is in contact with an environment to which he attempts to adapt himself. This environment, for the purposes of health education, includes such items as the health habits of his contemporaries, the school lunch programs, and the fluoridation program of the community.

In his space of free movement, social facts are as real to a child as physical ones. Vast realms of values, ideologies, style of living and thinking, and other cultural facts come to earth on specific problems. As Lewin puts it, "The behavior of a person depends above all upon his momentary position. Often the world looks very different before and after an event which changes the region in which a person is located. This is why, for instance, a *fait accompli* is so feared in politics."

An intermediate concern of education is with the *attitudes* the person may have toward health as a result of all of these interacting forces. Health facts may change rapidly, but many health hab-

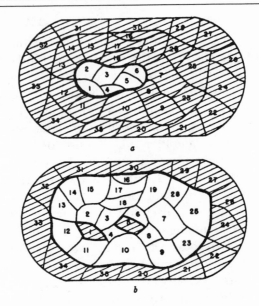

Figure 52. Comparison of the space of free movement of child and adult, showing actual activity regions. Accessible regions are blank; inaccessible regions are shaded. (*a*) The space of free movement of the child includes regions 1–6, representing activities such as getting into the movies at lower rates and belonging to a boys' club. Regions 7–35 are not accessible, representing activities such as driving a car, writing checks for purchases, political work, and performance of adult occupations. (*b*) The space of free movement of adults is considerably wider, though it too is bounded by inaccessible activities, such as shooting enemies or entering activities beyond their social or intellectual capacity (regions 29–35). Some of the activities accessible to the child are not accessible to the adult, such as getting into the movies at children's rates or doing things socially taboo for an adult (regions 1 and 5). [From K. Lewin, *Field Theory in Social Science* (Harper & Brothers, New York, 1951).]

its are deeply culture-rooted, and the total environment of the person—psychological, social-emotional, and physical—must be considered when attempting to make any change. The final objective of health education is suitable *behavior.*

These health education methods must all be used in the light of the attitudes toward the teeth and dentists discussed in Chapter 10. Few people are interested in health except as it affects them directly. Dental caries is often not considered a disease. Treatment of dental disease and payment of the dentist are both resented a little, always, because dental disease was not only unwanted but inevitable. Unless such attitudes can be overcome, favorable dental health habits are hard to produce.

One method of increasing interest in dental health is to *link dental problems* with matters known to have greater urgency in the eyes of the public, or better yet, the individual patient. Maternal and child health is a matter of high urgency; so also are nutrition and heart disease. Appearance has high urgency. Dental health can be linked to all of these in one way or another, and to other personal problems the individual patient may be found to have. Efforts must also be made to overcome the more obvious barriers to the seeking of dental care. These include the negative aspect of dental care just mentioned, the difference in status level often found between dentist and patient, the fear of inadequate attention to the pain problem, the complicated vocabulary of science, and many other attitudes or circumstances which may block or distort the process of communication in health education.

Lastly a word about *semantics,* or just plain honesty. Words must be chosen that will convey the exact thought desired. We must take caution from the plight of the small girl sitting in the school playground, mourning two broken incisor teeth and saying, "But this *couldn't* happen to me. I've been using a toothpaste which makes a shield on my teeth!"

MEDIA

The term *media* should theoretically include all vehicles for communication, whether by example or by word. Any such list should begin with the environment, where examples of healthful living around us and the provision of good sanitary facilities influence our health habits without conscious education. Next, of course, would come the spoken word with all of its implications both in person-to-person counseling and in speaking before groups. Media, however, are more usually understood to be the specific tools used for formal teaching, other than the human voice. These tools are best grouped in two categories: the written and audio-visual aids used in teaching individuals or small groups, and the mass media used in reaching the public.

Audiovisual Aids

In this category are usually included video tapes, motion pictures, film strips, slides, models, charts, exhibits, and the like. In part, they bring information of a specialized nature to a selected audience, without assimilation and representation on the part of the teacher. In part, as so often in television, they present characters with whom the audience would like to identify themselves and show these characters applying the health habits we wish to instill. In part they bring to our aid the picture which is "worth a thousand words" or the three-dimensional model which has the same advantage in transmitting facts. In part audiovisual aids involve techniques which are attractive for audience participation. Thus children can make their own posters, models, or even film strips, and in an attempt to teach others, teach themselves.

One associates *models* primarily with the teaching of dental anatomy and with primary-grade children. Extracted teeth can be used with care, as well as the open apex teeth of rodents, and other natural materials. Primary-grade children also like to make their own models with clay. Models with sufficient scientific detail to attract older children are seldom available outside of science museums, but high school students are sometimes very ingenious in making models even of such a complex subject as a water-filtration plant equipped for fluoridation.

Videocassettes, motion pictures, and *film strips* are adapted to the teaching of almost any age. For elementary teaching, motion pictures are probably more valuable. Simple stories of a child's first visit to the dentist are available in many forms acted out either by children or by cartoon characters. The facts of dental anatomy and physiology are also transmitted in this way. For older children and for adults the story of dental care, the acting out of the health habits that go to make up preventive dentistry, and the stories of community approaches to health problems such as water fluoridation all lend themselves to motion picture presentation. In selecting motion pictures for distribution to schools it is important to be very careful in accepting recommendations as to their quality, and always to *preview* them. The reception accorded a motion picture will vary from audience to audience and the dental health specialist who wishes to persuade classroom teachers to use a given picture must have his convictions well established in order to "make the sale."

Slides are the media of choice for the teacher who has his own story to tell. Slides lend themselves to presentation of detailed fact: exposition rather than narrative. Science teachers, particularly, will use slides, building collections they can use in various ways before various audiences. The dentist, speaking to older children or to parent-teacher groups, will do well to build his talk around a very few well-chosen slides or a film strip.

Posters should convey a simple message, preferably illustrated with figures with which the viewer would like to identify himself. It is a mistake to expect posters to transmit a long and complicated story. It is also a mistake for illustrations on posters to be so grotesque or unattractive that the viewer will have a hard time imagining himself in a similar situation. There are a number of production techniques known to advertising specialists which also go into the makeup of a successful poster. They include warm and attractive coloration and figures with whom members of the audience can identify, as well as the proper relations of space, figure, and color. Posters in essence are attractive temporary reminders rather than original informers.

Posters present perhaps the best opportunity for do-it-yourself projects in the school environment. Children in the intermediate grades will most likely have the greatest interest in making posters. Art teachers should be provided with factual dental material and should be encouraged to have children express ideas on health habits for the benefit of their contemporaries. Poster exchanges or competitions can sometimes be arranged among a group of schools.

Charts are primarily conveyors of information, more detailed than slides and designed for long-term exhibit. Initially, they require teacher explanation. Charts may show tooth anatomy, methods of tooth brushing, foods of various sorts arranged in categories, or, for older children and adults, the graphs and diagrams connected with such complex subjects as disease processes.

Mass Media

The mass media in common use today are pamphlets, newspapers, radio, and television. Each is launched widespread to an audience which, though selected to a certain degree, is unseen and must be both attracted and informed in the same operation. Pamphlets can occasionally be used for high school children, and radio and television programs of course reach all ages. Mass media can convey simple facts fairly well, but because of their impersonal nature, such media may form, but seldom change, basic attitudes and motives. Most commonly they remind people of needs already felt and understood.

The quality and variety of *pamphlets* on dental health have both been greatly improved in recent years. Pamphlets can occasionally be distributed by mail or by placement where people who are interested are likely to congregate, such as the public health clinic or dental waiting room. Their best use, however, is in response to specific inquiry, or in contrived situations where the way has been paved for them, such as following a talk at a parent-teacher meeting. Pamphlets vary a great deal in their approach. Certain ones, like *Why We Recommend Fluoridation, Diet, and Dental Health,* and *Cleaning Your Teeth and Gums* are extremely simple and designed for widespread distribution.[7] Booklets like *Fluoridation Facts* and *American Dental Association Guide to Dental Health* are much more comprehensive and appeal only to the careful reader. The latter type of book, because of both cost and the need for careful assimilation of facts, should be distributed to well-selected and well-motivated audiences.

In *newspapers,* news articles, feature articles, and advertisements all fill sporadic needs. News stories break only occasionally, but when a good one comes along, such as the initiation of a school dental health survey, health authorities and the dental society should get together in advance on an adequate *news release.* This release should be simple and accurate and be placed in the hands of all newspapers and radio and television stations impartially a proper time in advance of the event. Unexpected news events call for careful handling so that accurate and diplomatic information may be given to the press. If in doubt call your local dental society for advice.

Newspaper or magazine *feature articles* need good preparation. The best ones are deceptively simple, written by individuals who have devoted at least as much attention to writing techniques as to the subject material they are presenting. If a dental society or other group wishes to sponsor a feature article, it is usually best to team up a trained writer with one or more sources of authentic professional information. *Advertisements,* too, are jobs for the expert. Production techniques leading to proper relation between headline, body copy, and illustration count for a great deal. Advertisements cost money. They can seldom be afforded by groups other than those which stand to gain financially from good health habits on the part of the public. Dentifrice and drug manufacturers gain thus; so also do insurance companies, dentists, and dental societies.

Radio and *television* programs carry special messages at special times, such as National Children's Dental Health Week, but are also very valuable on a periodic basis throughout the year. The use of specialists in preparing scripts and visual effects is recommended. Spot announcements for radio are often available in advance through the American Dental Association or other sources. Care should be taken in placing the spots so that as wide an audience will be reached as possible. Armstrong quotes an example by suggesting that if there is sufficient promotional appropriation to buy, say, four spots a week, a much larger audience will be reached by spacing those four spots throughout one day of that week than by running them on the same time on four different days.[8]

The public service aspects of some regular television shows must be recognized and encouraged. Small children report that *Sesame Street* not only tells them to brush their teeth but also warns them not to let the water run while they are doing it.

In an introductory text it is impossible to give detailed consideration to the techniques for use of the various media which have been described. More detailed material can be found in textbooks especially devoted to the field. Better yet, experts in the field of health education should be sought out and asked to help when specific problems arise.

SOURCES OF MATERIAL

As a source of dental health educational material for public programs, the American Dental Association has become by a wide margin the best in the United States. State departments of public health probably come second, for these departments frequently design educational material with a local slant particularly adapted for use within their own confines. Inquiries for state material should be directed to the division of dental health of the state department of public health. The U.S. Public Health Service does an impressive amount of research upon public health methods and issues many scientific articles and monographs for professional consumption. Because of their remoteness from the problems of the citizens of any one area, however, federal agencies are inclined to leave the production of lay health educational material to states.

Certain voluntary associations and commercial concerns have worthwhile educational material. Citizens' committees, particularly those devoted ad hoc to a cause such as fluoridation, often print valuable material. Such concerns as dairy councils and food and nutrition bureaus often have well-designed material, supplied in reasonable quantity without charge. Some of these pamphlets bear the approval of the American Dental Association, a valuable endorsement to look for when you are making use of commercially sponsored material. Dentifrice manufacturers and insurance companies may also be looked to for pamphlets and other aids, but care must be used in avoiding those firms which advertise their own wares in an unethical manner. If no satisfactory material can be located, design and write your own; it is good fun and aids in formulation of program objectives. As you do so, however, remember both your reader and your aim. Who is your reader? What does he think? Do you talk his language? Are your facts straight and your suggestions workable? Finally, can your reader react as you wish him to, and can you find out if he does?

Any dentist or dental hygienist approaching the teaching of dental health for the first time would do well to obtain the latest editions of the American Dental Association set of four teaching guides entitled *Learning about Your Oral Health*.[9] These discuss the proper approach to dental health education at certain ages and give elementary material such as classroom teachers might wish to use. They also have bibliographies and duplicating masters to keep children active. District dental societies and community health councils can do a valuable service by purchasing and distributing to classroom teachers booklets of this sort.

Here are some addresses that will be helpful in securing material:

American Dental Association, 211 East Chicago Ave., Chicago, Illinois 60611 (ask for catalogue).

National Institute of Dental Research, N.I.H., Room 2C33, Bethesda, Maryland 20205 (ask for catalogue; in other countries contact the national health service).

Division of Dental Health, Department of Public Health, your state capital city.

Oral Hygiene Service, Hesketh House, Portman Square, London W.1, England (as an example of many private national groups).

Swedish Association for Prevention of Dental Disease, Kungsgatan 53, Stockholm C, Sweden.

Fédération Dentaire Internationale, 64 Wimpole St., London W1M 8AL, England (address the secretary), and British Dental Association, same address.

Dental Health Foundation, Australia, University of Sydney, Sydney NSW 2006, Australia.

National Dairy Council, 6300 North River Road, Rosemont, Illinois 60018-4233, and their state or local affiliates (considerable free dental literature is usually available).

PERSONNEL

In any discussion of an educational program, the personnel doing the work must be carefully considered. A brief listing of the various members of a dental health education team, together with a few words on the qualifications of each, is in order.

Dentist

In the field of dental health education the dentist has two functions: first, that of ultimate arbiter as to the quality and type of factual material presented in the program, and second, that of chair-side teacher in the course of any examination or treatment which may be rendered. Large cities are able to employ full-time dental directors as chiefs of service in a health department. Such dentists should have devoted considerable study to health education, along with their other studies in the field of public health. In smaller communities, however, practicing dentists usually have to carry the load as a part-time activity. These dentists may be called dental health consultants, dental directors, or merely school dentists. They may or may not have had training in education. They will usually be appointees of the local health department but could also be employed by the department of education in a community where health education activities are separated administratively from health services. They may also be appointees of their state or district dental society acting as volunteers. The individual general dentist, however, if he is sympathetic with children, need have no hesitation to respond to an invitation to enter the classroom as a friendly expert, without having to represent formally any society or agency.

In the dentist's role as consultant and professional resource person, he should be reasonably familiar with dental health education methods, definitely familiar with the authentic material available in this field. He must work both with school administrators and with school or community health councils to organize an educational program which will reach all age groups. He must support the dental hygienists and dental hygiene teachers in his area, and should have studied carefully the dental health materials available locally so that he can stimulate the distribution of these to classroom teachers and to all others who can use them. He should work with his state or district dental society to secure most efficient use of such school and community opportunities for dental health education as occur throughout the year.

The dentist will seldom find himself in a direct teaching relation with groups of children, but if he does he should study the vocabulary of the age group he is addressing and check his techniques against some such guide for speakers as that published by the American Dental Association.[10]

Dental Hygiene Teacher

Dental hygienists with additional training or experience in the field of education can function extremely well as a school dental health coordinator and can take part in actual educational activities to an extent to be determined by the degree of their training and of their acceptance by the local teaching fraternity. The usual level of training for such a position involves a Bachelor's degree

(A.B. or B.S.) with a concentration in education, or at least some courses in the principles of education, food and nutrition, mental hygiene, casework techniques, and health education. Dental hygiene teachers function best under general rather than direct supervision. They have a powerful opportunity for the referral of children to sources of dental care, both public and private, particularly where they can perform the screening of individuals.

Dental Hygienist, Dental Therapist, or Dental Nurse

The professionally trained dental auxiliary without specialized training in education can do a great deal as a resource person and even as a coordinator of school dental health programs. Her main job will be as consultant on professional matters, and in the absence of a regular dental hygiene teacher, she may be very valuable on school health councils. She should know and talk to as many classroom teachers in her area as she can, and keep them supplied with relevant literature. She may also talk directly to the children in their classes, where permitted to do so, and may be much more successful in "leveling" with the children than a graduate dentist would be. If she performs dental prophylaxis or topical fluoride therapy or takes part in dental inspection or treatment of schoolchildren, she will have opportunities for individual dental health teaching. She can have brief discussions on problems of dental hygiene and dental care with many children, and perhaps devote intensive effort to difficult cases.

Classroom Teacher and School Nurse

Authorities both in the field of education and in the field of health agree that the classroom teacher must carry a major share of the task of dental health education. In the words of the National Education Association, "regardless of the extent and quality of school dental services, the teaching of oral hygiene is and must be a primary responsibility of the classroom teacher ... The teacher's interest in securing dental corrections is a major factor in developing pupil interest and action. Teachers properly instructed in the principles of oral hygiene and gifted with enthusiasm and persistence can stimulate children to seek dental service as effectively as dentists or dental hygienists. Whether or not these specialists are available, the teacher is the keystone of the arch of dental health education."[1]

This statement carries weight because of the numerical preponderance of classroom teachers over health specialists in the school system and also because of the number of hours per year the classroom teacher is in contact with the pupils. An additional important reason, of course, lies in the educational training of the classroom teacher and her constant practice in the understanding of the minds and motives of her pupils. Nyswander goes further in saying that "the child cannot be helped to assume responsibility for his health through campaigns carried out by specialists. Sound attitudes can only be developed through unified teaching and through one source of instruction—the teacher."[11]

Stoll, approaching the problem from a dental background, gives a much less optimistic point of view. "It has been the experience of the author," she says, "that classroom teachers left to their own devices and without strong motivation from dentists and dental hygienists accept a defeatist attitude toward the health problems of their pupils."[12] They are inclined, she says, to think of dental health teaching only in terms of the remedial care which is so often difficult to attain. They do not have the facts or the initiative to teach prevention of dental disease. Stoll goes on to cite, however, a class in health education attended by a group of classroom teachers. In discussing dental problems they came to recognize the necessity of teaching about prevention and the application of preventive measures as well as about the correction of dental defects.

These two points of view, one elevating the classroom teacher to a position of key importance in the education of the child and the other viewing her as a pessimistic nonexpert, are not really as incompatible as they appear. Combined, they lead to the conclusion that the classroom teacher must be stimulated and aided by the dental health specialist in order to become an effective tool. The dentists and dental-hygiene teachers must therefore realize that their chief function is more to teach teachers than to teach pupils.

The dental health specialists also rely on the *school nurse* for knowledge of a child's home condition, when there are financial or other barriers to the obtaining of dental care. This aids them in referral to sources of care other than private practice, if necessary. In many instances the classroom teacher or the nurse can administer the referral system, including collection of returned "certificates" where dental treatment has been completed.

Health Educator

Health educators have a specialist's responsibility in all fields of health and are usually found serving school districts rather than individual schools. State Education Departments usually have requirements for certification in health education, including a baccalaureate degree. Courses in the principles of education, psychology for teachers, and teaching methods and materials are essential, as well as student practice teaching experience. Health subjects should include human anatomy and physiology, growth and development, health and hygiene, food and nutrition, safety and first aid, health aspects of home and family life, health counseling, and the organization, administration, and supervision of a school health program. For professional health educators at the supervisory level, the American Public Health Association recommends minimum requirements that specify academic training at the Master's level from an accredited institution with a major in health education.

There can be no set rule as to how the load of dental health teaching and resource work can be divided between the dentist, the dental auxiliary, and the health educator. In many instances the dental hygiene teacher will work as an assistant to the health educator. In any case, the health educator will be a good ally whose intelligent interest and help should be solicited.

Other Personnel and Opportunities

A number of other school people may be of assistance in a dental health education program. The *science teacher* should be supplied with facts on dental development and dental disease for use in biology classes. Fluoridation gives an excellent topic for science study, both biological and social. The *physical education teacher* must know how to prevent accidents to the teeth. The home economics teacher or *nutritionist* is in a position to help put dietary recommendations into action. The *dietitian* can arrange meals which will set a good example. The *guidance counselor* in a secondary school can assist in personal health counseling. Even more important, he or she should know the opportunities for careers in dentistry and dental hygiene so as to give information and encouragement to promising young people who are looking for such careers.

The variety of school personnel who may be involved suggests the variety of possible approaches to dental health education in the school setting. Whenever the dental professional has a good rapport with a classroom teacher, enjoys the approval of the school's administration, and likes to talk with children, the lack of more formal educational qualifications may well be unimportant, and should not prevent anyone who is enthusiastic from pursuing an opportunity.

Dental Society

District and state dental societies are playing an increasing role in the dental health education of the public. An alert *council on dental health* in either society will be able to answer inquiries from citizens and be able to promote an understanding of dental health in a great variety of situations. There are many opportunities for contact not only with schools but also with the public through the use of the mass media, including television. Poster exchanges or contests can be stimulated in the schools, and school dental hygiene teachers or others can be informed of new teaching aids which will enliven their programs. Information on careers in dentistry can be sent to school guidance counselors. Information on water fluoridation can be broadcast, and citizens' committees working for the adoption of this measure can be aided through the furnishing of speakers, literature, and the answers to vexing questions.

Interdisciplinary Problems

The various types of personnel just listed as possible teachers and the administrators controlling their programs have a number of different specialized vocabularies. Thus they do not always understand one another's problems, at least as far as the inner essence is concerned. This was brought out recently when the health councils of the various state dental societies in the New England area organized an interdisciplinary dental health education conference. Each state sent representatives in four major categories: (1) teachers and health educators, (2) parents and school committee members, (3) dentists and dental directors, and (4) administrators (state level) and superintendents (local).

A format was organized for the conference by which, after a few introductory talks, each of the four groups in turn centered its members around a large table in the middle of the room. This "spotlight group" developed and discussed the health education problems of special interest to them, while the rest of the audience sat around them, joining the discussion occasionally.

The teachers and health educators deplored the fact that planned curricula in school health are few in number. Even where school health services are reasonably well organized, health education seems to fall into an abyss between departments of health and departments of education, with neither group taking the responsibility for the program. School committeemen emphasized that there was "just so much time in a school day," and that it was necessary to teach certain subjects for college entrance and certain other subjects because of popular social demand. Health was often crowded out and considered a "frill." Administrators cited the lack of teacher preparation in the field of health education, with a resulting lack of awareness of the problem. They also cited the low priority of dental health among health needs, and of health among social needs. They thought there was too much emphasis on treatment and too little on prevention. Treatment is often expensive or not available. All the nondental groups expressed surprise at the scope and seriousness of the dental disease problem, since most of them had never before attended a professional dental meeting. The dentists and dental directors discussed their role in health education and acknowledged that they need to participate in community affairs more than they usually did, and particularly to serve on school committees and other administrative groups.

This conference made no specific recommendations except to suggest that a continuing regional committee on dental health education be formed. Several suggestions for further action arose, however, and were reported in the proceedings of the conference:

State departments of education, along with local school committees or boards, should be urged to make health education a required part of elementary and secondary school curricula.

These departments and boards should be urged to clarify and improve the qualifications for health educators.

These departments and boards should be urged to endorse the teaching of the facts on fluoridation in elementary and secondary schools, and should prepare teaching materials for this purpose, in cooperation with organized dentistry.

The basic facts concerning maintenance of dental health should be taught in all teachers' colleges, schools of nursing, schools of dental hygiene, schools of dental assisting, and to all dentists themselves, both in dental school and through continuing education courses afterwards.

The American Dental Association should be urged to:

a) take a more active role in stimulating dental health education in institutions such as those listed above;

b) extend their own production of dental educational materials, particularly for Grades 4 and 5;

c) develop outlines of specific action suggestions for local school board consideration.

Dentists should be urged to:

a) become more active in community programs for dental health education, including serving on school boards where possible;

b) give more dental health education to patients in the chair;

c) become more active in promoting community water fluoridation.

Obstetricians, pediatricians, and other medical personnel should be urged to give better dental health advice, particularly to mothers, both prenatally and postnatally.

Creative thought should be given to new aproaches to oral hygiene in such a way as to increase its popularity and enlist commercial support.[13]

GROUPS TO BE REACHED

One of the first items in an educational program is the adaptation of materials and methods to the group to be served. Learning occurs best in response to a recognized need. The psychological characteristics of the various age and social groupings in the community, therefore, must be studied in order that suitable material may be brought to each group in a suitable manner. The dental needs of each group should be carefully studied, as should also the social problems which are likely to arise in meeting these needs.

Schoolchildren

By far the largest and most important organized group for health education to reach is to be found in the school systems of the country—public, parochial, and private. Not only are children the best learners, but they are at the beginning of their dental health problems and, with malocclusion and caries, experience the peak of these problems during childhood. Material on children's dental needs is found in Chapter 13. Much has been written on educational approaches to the schoolchild, yet Kasey states that little attention has been given to the findings of research into the health interests of children.[14] Most of the materials from kindergarten through intermediate grades are devoted to tooth structure, development, or decay, she reminds us; yet some researchers indicate that children in grades 4, 5, and 6 have relatively high interest in learning the correct way to brush teeth but much lower interest in tooth development, anatomy, and function.

Dental health education, like education on any other subject, depends on the child's ability to learn and his stage of development. Kasey suggests some examples of age-specific dental subject material. These are not to be viewed as too age-specific, since classes and individual children vary greatly.

Kindergarten–First Grade—Teach keeping the mouth clean, brushing the teeth and washing out or rinsing the mouth. If possible, reach the parent to encourage tooth brushing at home and to stress importance of "baby teeth." Discuss the role of the dentist.

Grades 2–4—Teach the importance of preservation of the teeth through *proper* care, and the importance of visits to dentist and keeping teeth clean. Teach simple facts about diet, especially candy and the need for rinsing mouth after eating.

Grades 5–6—Teach the importance of good dental health to overall physical health. Introduce tooth structure, and the importance of proper tooth brushing technique. Give more detailed information on the seriousness of dental diseases; on the importance of dental care and good oral hygiene and diet.

Junior High—This is the "scientific age," and the beginning of interest in appearance, chemical aspects of tooth formation, importance of preventive measures, study of community dental resources, the pros and cons re fluoridation. Report studies in dental research. Nutrition, especially diet, is important, and how to distinguish facts from fads. Emphasis can be made on dental health care and the prevention of periodontal disease. Include dental health in other courses.

Senior High—Stress the importance of making decisions based on reliable data. Teach the scientific causes of dental disease, including periodontal disease and oral cancer, as well as preventive measures. Stress the importance of adult attitudes toward dental care, and the importance of nutrition especially during pregnancy. Teach how teeth develop in the embryo, and their importance in later life. Teach how to evaluate mass media information and to interpret research findings.[16]

As already mentioned, the American Dental Association has a set of four teaching guides entitled *Learning About Your Oral Health*, which cover this same age range in considerable detail, with hints for student-participation projects.[9]

Age is not the only variable of importance in planning educational programs for children. Sources of dental care are also crucial. In a careful study of rural school-based programs, Bentley, Cormier, and Oler found that those children who received their care from family dentists were so little affected even by enriched dental health education at school as to make it a waste of time.[15] The dentists were the authority figures and did the job on a one-to-one chairside basis.

The children who received dental care that was delivered right to the school by mobile facilities served either by dental teams or by solo dentists, however, profited greatly from an enriched educational program. Utilization of dental care by these children increased by multiples of from 30 to 100. This study indicates the advisability of concentrating dental health education programs in schools where private care is least available and where care, public or private, is brought *to* the schools. These utilization figures parallel those found in the New Zealand, Australian, and Saskatchewan dental therapist programs.

Adult Groups

There are many adult groups within most communities which, under certain circumstances, may be important objects for dental health education. *Expectant mothers* and *mothers of infants* are almost always in need of dental health information and are motivated to make use of it. This group can usually be reached through board of health prenatal or well-baby clinics. A dental health consultant who has access to such a clinic can learn how to make herself useful to the young women who attend, through watching her colleagues in their approach to other health problems there.

Dental health should be part of any health education program among *industrial workers*. The managements of industrial concerns vary greatly in their receptivity to health education, but good opportunities often exist in the larger plants if members of the management have a strong enough sense of community responsibility. A recent study of health education in the industrial setting shows dental care to be one of ten top problems in which industrial employees are interested.[16] The opportunities for "audience participation" in industry are very different from those available in the school system. Group activities are usually not possible, but individual interest can be aroused in connection with visits to any dental service either the plant management or a labor union may provide. This matter is discussed further in Chapter 21.

A large and particularly important community group to reach is the local *parent-teacher* association or associations. These organizations naturally attract the more progressive parents in the community. The question of the dental health of their children is always of interest. Dentists or dental auxiliaries are at less of a disadvantage in speaking before parent-teacher association meetings than they are in teaching children, since in the absence of formal training in the field of education less adjustment is needed to the point of view of the audience. Parent-teacher associations usually meet at regular intervals and are glad to listen to qualified speakers on health subjects.

One of the most important dental health education problems of the present day is that of preparing the *voting population* of a community for intelligent decision when a health matter such as the health department budget or water fluoridation is up for action. Referenda are not to be encouraged on a complex scientific question like fluoridation. It is far easier to educate a small number of community officials to whom adequate authority has been delegated than to educate the entire mass of the voters. In a democratic society, however, the right to referendum cannot be denied. If one must occur, dental health education should be begun as long as possible in advance of the referendum vote and should cover as many different community groups as can be reached by the citizens' sponsoring committee. With water fluoridation, parent-teacher associations are particularly important to reach since the benefits of fluoridation will first be seen among young children. Education should deal with dental health and dental disease in its broadest aspects as well as with the dental benefits of the safety of fluoridation. It is unrealistic to expect public interest in a measure such as fluoridation if the need for it has not been adequately established in advance.

Community Agencies

Health education is not a one-way street. Properly designed and motivated health programs require full input from community agencies and key individuals. The planners must listen. Chapter 14 describes a series of seminars conducted in three New York City ghetto areas under the heading "The Voice of the Community."[17] Each of these areas needed improvements in disease prevention and delivery of health care. Seminars were held there weekly over a three-month period on such matters as local historical background, current social conditions, specific disease problems (dentistry among them), life-styles of ethnic minority groups, and interpersonal and interprofessional relations. The objectives of the seminars included better communication between provider and consumer groups, the development of local leaders and a sense of community pride, on-the-spot problem solving, and better access to outside sources of aid. It proved important to invite key local agency personnel and individuals to the *first* planning meeting of each seminar series and to have a skillful and empathetic seminar coordinator and staff.

EVALUATION OF PROGRAMS

It is extremely difficult to measure in any exact way the effect of education, for ideas sink into the human mind at speeds varying with motivation and are received from many different sources. In a field like dental health, where the goal of the educational program is an alteration in human behavior, factors other than education may affect the behavior changes. A few isolated formal attempts at measurement have been made, however, and these are worth reporting as a guide to possible future attempts. By "formal" it is implied that attempts were made to study characteristics which could be measured and that biostatistical methods were applied to the results.

Changes in Behavior

The work of Janis and Feshbach has already been mentioned as a careful attempt to differentiate between varying health education methods in terms of their short-term results such as making appointments with the dentist.[5] The longer-term results of dental health education have also been studied in several ways. One method involves measurement of the frequency of seeking of dental treatment and receiving dental care. The writer has reported an instance where industrial employees who had had the benefit of a dental health service involving dental prophylaxis, chair-side dental health education, examination, and referral to a private practitioner received 1.7 times as much dental care as did the highest-income group studied a few years earlier by President Hoover's Committee on the Costs of Medical Care.[18] One result was that these people had saved many more of their teeth than people of similar ages in the population as a whole. A somewhat similar attempt at measurement was made by Grainger and Sellers in Canada, both before and after a dental health education program that involved dental examination, health education, and "a few simple preventive measures," including referral to the private dentist.[19] After the educational program, increases in the percentage of children having no cavities were found at certain ages. Decreases were found in the number of untreated carious surfaces per child and the percentage of children needing fillings or extractions but having no evidence of such in their mouths. A number of other measures also indicated improved dental status as a result of the program over a 4-year period.

Questionnaires may be used to test changes in behavior. At the community level, Jordan, Neal, and Valento made a questionnaire survey of several hundred public and parochial schools in Minnesota before and after an educational campaign designed to show that the practice of selling candies and soft drinks to children interferes with proper nutrition.[20] Of 244 schools reporting such sales before the campaign, 152 reported discontinuance by the time of the second questionnaire.

Changes in Attitude

Psychological tests are available to study changes in attitude. For example, Moosbruker and Giddon studied changes in attitude among Tufts senior dental students who cared for chronically ill and disabled patients during a 3-day period.[21] They used the Attitude toward Disabled Persons Scale (ATDP) for this determination. ATDP scores after this experience were compared with scores before it and with scores from another dental school where the experience was not afforded. An improvement in attitude approaching statistical significance was found. Standardized tests may be supplemented by questions directed to the specific problem, as was done in the study just cited, or the tests may be completely replaced by a specially designed questionnaire.

Whatever difficulties may exist in the way of formal evaluation of educational programs, there is no doubt that efforts, either formal or informal, pay for themselves in terms of the improvement of good programs and the elimination of poor ones. Further criteria for evaluation, not necessarily connected with education alone, are found in Chapter 14.

CHAPTER 16

Water Fluoridation

WITH OVER 123 million people in the United States drinking fluoridated water as of 1983, the physiology of fluoride has become not only a subject of intense scientific interest to the public health dentist, but a nationwide political issue as well. Fluoridation may profitably be examined from a number of points of view: the epidemiology of fluoride intake both in respect to dental fluorosis (mottled enamel) and in respect to caries reduction, the safety of fluoridation, the dental benefits of fluoridation in both the endemic and the test areas, fluoridation as an engineering project, and finally the legal, political, and economic impact of fluoridation. Voluminous literature is available on all of these facets of the problem, but space limitations permit only brief considerations of most of it here.

EPIDEMIOLOGY OF FLUOROSIS

The effect of fluoride on man constitutes a story which has unfolded over more than half a century in the United States and has attracted widespread attention from the epidemiologists. There are in fact two stories, which form a continuum: the story of the harmful effects of fluoride in large doses, which came first, and the story of dental benefits from small doses.

The first important mention of the brown stain known now as dental fluorosis occurred in 1902 in El Paso County, Colorado, although in 1888 a family emigrating from Mexico to Germany had been recognized as having the same condition. In Colorado, Frederic S. McKay gave systematic attention to the mottling and brown staining he found on the teeth of many of his patients and even hypothesized that the defect was due to the water supply. By 1908 he had studied enough cases and interested enough of his colleagues in the problem to invite Dr. G. V. Black, then Dean of Northwestern University Dental School, to join him in a local study. Black's visit to Colorado gained national attention for the brown staining of enamel, and cases were reported soon thereafter from many parts of the country. The name "Colorado brown stain" eventually gave way to that of mottled enamel. The process soon became associated with communal water supplies, usually (though not always) from deep wells, but at that time analysis of water supplies for small quantities of fluoride had not been perfected and the etiologic agent was not identified till more than two decades later. Various degrees of mottling were identified, from the mild mottling which involves only a few chalky white spots on the surface of the enamel, to moderate mottling where large areas of white are mixed with brown, and finally to the severe mottling where brown predominates and hypoplasia of the teeth becomes evident.

As mottled enamel became documented in an ever-widening geographical area, confirmation of the deep-well hypothesis was found in several localities. In Britton, South Dakota, in 1916 a study revealed uniform mottling of enamel among the children brought up in the town since a new deep well had been added to the communal water supply in 1898. In 1925, citizens of Oakley, Idaho, where mottling was prevalent, undertook to test the deep-well hypothesis by changing from a warm spring-water supply (artesian water) to another shallower water supply. In succeeding years, the children on the new water supply developed no mottling, but the children brought up on the old supply were not cured.

It is interesting to note that in 1925 also, McCollum, Bunting, and others, who were studying the elements known to occur in teeth by feeding them in excess to rats, developed staining in incisors of these animals following ingestion of large quantities of fluoride. This fact remained for several years unrelated to the occurrence of mottled enamel in human beings.

Studies initiated in 1928 in Bauxite, Arkansas, led to the final discovery that mottled enamel was associated with fluoride in water. An exceptionally high incidence of mottling occurred in this town, and action upon the problem was more far-reaching than usual because of the presence there of a plant of Republic Mining and Manufacturing Company, a subsidiary of the Aluminum Corporation of America. Samples of Bauxite water eventually came to the laboratory of H. V. Churchill, chief chemist for Alcoa, who initiated spectographic study. Thirteen and seven-tenths parts per million of fluoride were found in the Bauxite water, a finding which impressed Churchill and was eventually transmitted to McKay in 1931. McKay then arranged for reanalysis of the water supplies in Britton, South Dakota, Oakley, Idaho, and elsewhere. Reports of high fluoride were soon assembled. Subsequent rechecking in many parts of the United States soon developed a striking correlation between mottled enamel and a fluoride content of public water ranging from 2 to 13 parts per million. It is interesting to note that two other sets of observers (the Smiths in Arizona and Velu in France) also connected fluoride with mottled enamel about the same time as did Churchill, though their ideas did not happen to spark such extensive further study.

The coexistence of low dental caries and mottled enamel had excited comment from McKay, even in the early years of his investigation. After the discovery that fluoride correlated with mottled enamel in 1931, several other investigators also noted this inverse relation. It remained for Dr. H. Trendley Dean, on duty with the U.S. Public Health Service, to make a thorough documentation of the degree of mottled enamel and degree of caries at different concentrations of fluoride in order to permit reliable statistical analysis. Dean's studies took him all over the United States. The magnitude of this task can be imagined from inspection of Fig. 53, which shows the situation in map form. Populations on natural fluoride water were in 1977 estimated at about 10 million. As it became obvious that large reductions in caries incidence were associated with the occasional appearance of enamel opacities that were in no way disfiguring, the term *mottled enamel* gave way to the more exact term *dental fluorosis*.

Dean developed a classification for dental fluorosis which has become a standard in epidemiological work.[1] From it, an index of dental fluorosis can be computed for a group. The classification which is illustrated in Fig. 54, can be abbreviated as follows:

Normal enamel. Weight 0.0.

Questionable mottling. Normal translucency is varied by a few white flecks or white spots. Weight 0.5.

Very mild mottling. Small, opaque, paper-white areas are scattered over the teeth, involving less than 25 percent of the surface. Sum-

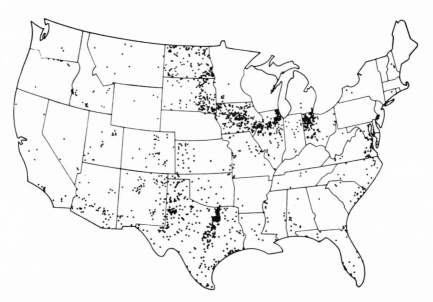

Figure 53. Communities using naturally fluoridated water with 0.7 ppm fluoride or more, 1957. [Public Health Service, National Institute of Dental Research.]

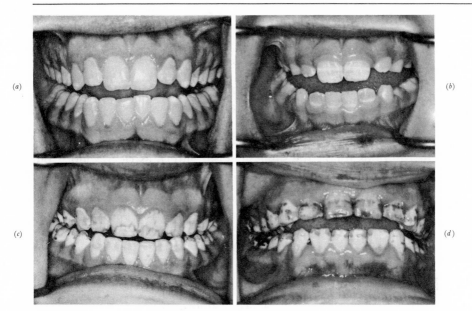

Figure 54. Types of dental fluorosis: (*a*) very mild; (*b*) mild; (*c*) moderate; (*d*) severe.

mits of cusps of bicuspids and second molars are commonly affected. Weight 1.0.

Mild mottling. The white opaque areas are more extensive but do not involve more than 50 percent of the surface. Weight 2.0.

Moderate mottling. All enamel surfaces are affected and those subject to attrition show marked wear. Brown stain is a frequent disfiguring feature. Weight 3.0.

Severe mottling. All enamel surfaces are affected and hypoplasia is so marked that tooth form may be altered. A major diagnostic sign is discrete or confluent pitting. Brown stains are widespread and the teeth often present a corroded appearance. Weight 4.0.

The *Index of Dental Fluorosis* of a group is computed by averaging the weights assigned to the individuals in the group: one weight figure per person. Since scores are easiest to tally in groups, the formula becomes:

$$\text{Index} = \frac{\text{sum of } f \times w}{n}$$

where f is frequency, w is weight, and n is number of cases examined.

A more sensitive index has recently been devised and applied by Horowitz et al., which is called the *Tooth Surface Index of Fluorosis* (TSIF).[2] They use a score scale of 0 to 7 and record it for 2 surfaces on each anterior tooth and 3 surfaces on each posterior tooth. The percentage distribution of scores is then computed for either an individual or a group of individuals. These percentage distributions follow the same general pattern as Dean's index but allow greater discrimination as to the public health effect of fluorosis in a given locality. The index has proved sufficiently sensitive to distinguish between communities with four different fluoride levels as to both prevalence and severity of fluorosis.

The scores are as follows:

Numerical score	*Descriptive criteria*
0	Enamel shows no evidence of fluorosis.
1	Enamel shows definite evidence of fluorosis, namely areas with parchment-white color that total less than one-third of the visible enamel surface. This category includes fluorosis confined only to incisal edges of anterior teeth and cusp tips of posterior teeth ("snowcapping").
2	Parchment-white fluorosis totals at least one-third of the visible surface, but less than two-thirds.
3	Parchment-white fluorosis totals at least two-thirds of the visible surface.
4	Enamel shows staining in conjunction with any of the preceding levels of fluorosis. Staining is defined as an area of definite discoloration that may range from light to very dark brown.
5	Discrete pitting of the enamel exists, unaccompanied by evidence of staining of intact enamel. A pit is defined as a definite physical defect in the enamel surface with a rough floor that is surrounded by a wall of intact enamel. The pitted area is usually stained or differs in color from the surrounding enamel.
6	Both discrete pitting and staining of the intact enamel exist.
7	Confluent pitting of the enamel surface exists. Large areas of enamel may be missing and the anatomy of the tooth may be altered. Dark-brown stain is usually present.

The next step forward involved more accurate studies in areas where fluoride in water supplies was low enough not to cause mottling as a public health problem. Comparisons were therefore made between white children aged 12 to 14 years in Galesburg, Illinois, with 1.9 parts per million fluoride, and in Quincy, Illinois, a nearby city on the Mississippi River, with no appreciable fluoride.[3] Later, a series of studies was made among similar children in Chicago suburbs, some of them using Lake Michigan water with no appreciable fluoride and others using deep-well water with fluoride contents ranging from 0.5 to 1.8 parts per million.[4] These studies showed surprisingly regular decreases in dental caries in the temperate zone as fluoride concentrations increased from zero up to about 2 parts per million. These data, coupled with Dean's earlier data on endemic fluorosis, are shown in graphic form in Fig. 55. A low spot shows where the two curves on this figure cross

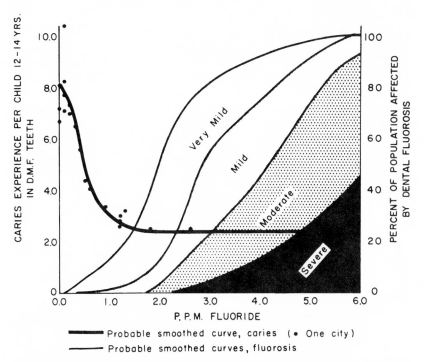

Figure 55. Dental caries and dental fluorosis related to fluoride in public water supply. [Adapted from H. T. Dean, New York Symposium (1945); *Int. Dent. J. 4,* 311–337 (1954).]

near 1.0 part per million. At this concentration most of the benefits in caries reductions at all ages have already been realized through the addition of fluoride, while mottling as a public health problem has not yet appeared. On the basis of such evidence the U.S. Public Health Service later recommended the fluoridation of water supplies with from 1.0 to 1.5 parts per million.

The descriptive and analytical epidemiology of fluoride was now fairly complete. Certain points, of course, still remained to be proved. Dean stated quite frankly in his report on Galesburg and Quincy that he had demonstrated no more than a correlation between fluoride and low caries, and that trace elements or other factors correlated with fluoride content in the water might easily be the causative factor in the caries reduction. The next step lay in an attempt to benefit mankind through the prevention of dental caries. In order to do this, it was necessary to demonstrate (1) that fluoride at a concentration approximating 1 part per million in the water supply was safe and (2) that added fluoride did in fact produce the dental benefits associated with natural fluoride in the endemic fluoride areas. Only when this last attempt had been made could it be said with assurance that fluoride caused, and was not merely associated with, low caries. Trials of water *fluoridation* thus became necessary. Fluoridation was *defined* as the adjustment of a water supply to a fluoride content such that reductions of 50 to 70 percent in dental caries would occur without damage to teeth or other structures. A more current definition omits any reference to specific percentages of reduction. The sharp drop in caries incidence among children in developed countries has reduced the further benefits now possible in newly fluoridated areas. Fluorides in various forms and community water fluoridation in particular, however, have received the probable credit for these reductions; they are not to be construed as indicating lesser efficacy in areas still showing high caries. The definition should now include reference to *significant* reductions.

SAFETY OF FLUORIDATION

Any plan for alteration of the fluoride content of a communal water supply requires a thorough understanding of any possible harmful effects upon human beings of the doses likely to be used or of the accidental overdoses which are possible. The importance of the matter is underlined by the fact that concentrated sodium fluoride powder is known to the public as a rat poison. Fluoride actually produces a wide spectrum of physiologic activity, both normal and abnormal, in the human being. It can be considered a nutrient, a drug, or a poison, entirely on the basis of the dosage used. This same statement, of course, can be made concerning many familiar elements. Small quantities of iodine act to prevent a deficiency disease, goiter, and to this extent are an essential nutrient. Tincture of iodine applied to a wound serves the purpose of a drug. Iodine if swallowed in large quantities constitutes a poison, and iodine bottled for the medicine cabinet is therefore so labeled. Even table salt (NaCl) and water can be fatal in gross overdose to the exclusion of other substances. In short, *the best definition for a poison is "too much."*

The mechanism by which fluoride acts on teeth is considered to be chiefly a replacement of hydroxyapatite by less soluble fluorapatite in the crystalline structure of the enamel. Possible additional mechanisms are indicated by the fact that fluoride favors the precipitation of calcium phosphate from saturated solutions and that it inhibits some and apparently stimulates other types of enzyme action.[5] Catalytic action upon enamel crystallization may also be involved. The probably higher concentration of fluoride in bacterial plaque close to the tooth surface permits reactions not typical of the concentrations of fluoride found in saliva or other body fluids.

Fluoride is present in small quantities in practically all common foods. Exclusive of drinking water, the average diet in the United States has been calculated to provide 0.2 to 0.3 milligram of fluoride daily.[6] Diets involving large quantities of seafood or tea will rise above this level. One cup of tea alone supplies approximately 0.12 milligram of fluoride. Geographical variations in the fluoride content of a normal diet, however, appear to be unimportant in most areas, since they are small in comparison with fluoride available from drinking water. One liter of water with a fluoride content of 1 part per million contains 1 milligram of fluoride ion. Average daily water intake in the temperate zone may be estimated at from 1 to 1.5 liters per day, hence a dosage of from 1 to 1.5 milligram of fluoride. This is five times the quantity normally available from food.

Table 37 gives a broad and approximated picture of the physiological and pathological effects of fluoride at a wide variety of doses, both chronic and acute.

A mass of literature exists on the safety of water fluoridation. There are several competent recent reviews of this literature, among which are those of Hodge, Smith, and McClure.[7,8,9]

The metabolism of fluoride involves rapid absorption of 90 percent or more of soluble fluoride, the reappearance of perhaps half this fluoride in the urine, and the storage of the rest in bone and teeth. There is no evidence for storage of fluoride in soft tissues. Urinary excretion is prompt and responds in sensitive fashion even to low doses of fluoride. Gradual accumulation of fluoride does occur in bone and tooth structure as age advances. Bone

Table 37. Human responses to fluoride.

Concentration of fluoride dose[a]	Medium	Time	Effect
In man			
1 ppm[b]	Water	Lifetime	Dental caries reduction
2 ppm or more	Water	During tooth formation	Dental fluorosis
5 ppm	Water or air	Years	No osteosclerosis
8 ppm	Water	Years	10% osteosclerosis
20–80 mg/day or more	Water or air	Years	Crippling fluorosis
In animals			
50 ppm	Food or water	Years	Thyroid changes
100 ppm	Food or water	Months	Growth retardation
>125 ppm	Food or water	Months	Kidney changes
2.5–5.0 gm	Acute dose	2–4 hours	Death

a. Attainment of these doses of fluoride ion requires approximately twice the weight of sodium fluoride.

b. In temperate zone, less in tropics.

fluoride content is also greater at a given age in communities where there is fluoride in the water, though a slowing or cessation of accumulation appears to occur some 10 years after the initiation of a water-fluoridation program.[10] Recognizable bone changes do not appear in significant proportions of a population until the fluoride is from 4 to 8 ppm, and then take the form of increased or decreased bone density, with or without coarsened trabeculation, excluding osteoporotic change.[9] Larger fluoride exposures, estimated at 20 to 80 milligrams or more per day inhaled as an industrial dust for periods of 10 to 20 years, produced crippling fluorosis in cryolite workers.[11]

One function of fluoride in the system appears to be to improve calcium balance and delay deleterious excretion of calcium.[12] As a result, there appears to be less osteoporosis, or decreased bone density, in fluoride areas than in fluoride-deficient areas.[13] Visible calcification of the aorta is also reduced. This leads to the hypothesis that optimal fluoride ingestion may in time prove to be helpful in the partial and highly beneficial prevention of osteoporosis, as well as other associated problems among older citizens.

Practical use has been made of this hypothesis in the treatment of osteoporosis. Parkins lists several instances where doses up to 60 milligrams of sodium fluoride per day, coupled with calcium and sometimes vitamin D, have led to the deposition of new normal bone in persons with osteoporotic lesions, without toxic effects.[14] The positive value of this therapy is still open to controversy, however, and further study is needed.

A number of large-scale studies have been made over the years of the morbidity and mortality of populations exposed both to natural fluoride near the optimum level of 1 part per million and to fluoridated water at the same level. The most comprehensive of these seem to have been made in the period from 1950 to 1960. The Bartlett-Cameron study contrasted a natural low-fluoride community with one having 8 parts fluoride per million in the water supply.[9] The medical study accompanying the Newburgh-Kingston fluoridation trial followed the populations of these two cities—one on fluoridated water and the other a fluoride-free control.[9] A large study was made of autopsy material from communities with 1.0 to 4.0 parts per million in the drinking water, both natural and adjusted. A comparison of mortality rates was made for 32 cities whose water supplies contained more than 0.7 part per million from natural sources.[15] Each of these cities was randomly paired with a neighboring city containing less than 0.25 part per million. The total population for all cities exceeded 2,000,000. All these studies agree in showing no abnormalities, pathologic effects, or mortality changes that can be related to fluoride in the drinking water, aside from possible dental fluorosis, as discussed below.

More detailed studies of specific pathologic conditions show a similar result. Diabetes and nephritis have been studied without any evidence of fluoride correlation. In the state of Wisconsin the Department of Public Health found no evidence of any correlation between the diabetes death rates in cities with varying amounts of natural fluoride in the water supply. Studies with laboratory animals in which kidneys have been damaged have indicated no disability in the excretion of waterborne fluorides at levels as high as 15.0 parts per million. Hagen et al. also found no difference in the frequency of death from nephritis in fluoride communities and in non-fluoride areas.[15] An increase in the death rate among cancer-susceptible laboratory animals exposed to high-fluoride waters has been noted and has given rise to a fear that cancer might be accelerated in man. There is no evidence among human beings to support this theory, and the cancer mortality in the 32 fluoride cities already referred to is slightly though not significantly less than that in the control cities of the same study.[15] Fig. 56 illustrates the more important findings of this study. A similar study of 22 fluoridated and 22 nonfluoridated cities in the 1970s shows similar results.[16]

Abnormalities of growth, as in height, weight, bone formation as a result of fracture experience, or in other areas as a result of Down Syndrome, have been carefully investigated, and no evidence of a causative relation with fluoride has been found.[17] Needleman et al. report no relationship with Down Syndrome in Massachusetts.[18] Another study shows similar results in England, where recording of the frequency of Down Syndrome and other birth defects is more complete than in the United States.[19]

It is generally agreed that the earliest sign of abnormality due to fluoride in the drinking water is enamel opacity or more serious *dental fluorosis*. Evidence from many areas has been combined in

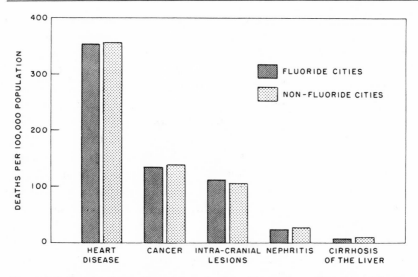

Figure 56. Deaths from five causes in fluoride and nonfluoride cities by age, race, and sex, 1940–1950. [Public Health Service, National Institute of Dental Research.]

Fig. 55 to show the gradual increase of these conditions with increasing fluoride concentration *after* the major reductions in dental caries have been attained. The figures are based upon water consumption characteristic of the North Temperate Zone. A concentration of 1 part per million marks an obvious low point in the two sets of curves; a higher mean temperature, with greater daily water consumption, would move all curves to the left and produce a low point (hence an optimum intake) at a lower concentration, perhaps 0.7 part per million, a concentration actually used in some Southern states. Extensive studies at optimum levels indicate that perhaps 10 percent of those whose teeth were formed on fluoridated water show some degree of mild enamel opacity above the questionable level. Typical of such studies is Russell's report on dental fluorosis in Grand Rapids during the seventeenth year of fluoridation.[20] Eight percent of the white children in this community showed either very mild or mild fluorosis, and 14 percent of the black children showed similar conditions. It is to be remembered that these mild opacities are not unattractive from an esthetic point of view and are matched by nonfluoride opacities and by the early signs of formation of dental caries in the nonfluoride areas. The nonfluoride opacities are usually found in even greater frequency. Thus, 32 cases of very mild or mild fluoride opacities in addition to 36 nonfluoride opacities were observed among 438 Newburgh schoolchildren after 10 years of fluoridation (a 15 percent rate), whereas 612 Kingston children showed 115 nonfluoride opacities (a 19 percent rate). Water fluoridation at optimum levels has never produced positive discoloration of the yellow or brown variety commonly associated with the term mottling. The teeth of children in fluoridated communities in general appear more attractive than the teeth of children in nearby control areas. Even in areas of excess natural fluoride, the stains of moderate fluorosis can be "erased" by the new bonding techniques of operative dentistry.[21]

Where fluorosis is reported in fluoridated areas, it is important to take careful case histories. Some years ago the dosage of fluoride recommended for supplementation, often with vitamins, for children in the first two years of life was .5 milligram per day. Moderate fluorosis was occasionally caused by this dosage, and the dosage was later dropped to .25 milligram, as shown in Chapter 12. Opponents of fluoridation are likely to blame fluoridation for the fluorosis thus caused. Another phenomenon occasionally blamed on fluoridation is the diffuse yellowish discoloration of a number of teeth resulting from heavy dosages of tetracycline for severe illness in early childhood.

The literature on nonfluoride opacities is scanty, but Zimmermann reports some distinguishing characteristics as a result of a study in Illinois and Maryland:

Appearance. Ideopathic (nonfluoride) opacities are more opaque and more oval, often involving the summits of the cusps of posterior teeth. Fluorosed teeth more commonly exhibit horizontal striations, or striae extending down the cuspal ridges of posterior teeth.

Distribution. Ideopathic lesions are not ordinarily found in a definite symmetrical pattern: fluoride lesions are usually bilaterally distributed.

Frequency. Ideopathic lesions seldom affect more than 1 or 2 teeth; fluoride lesions usually involve several teeth.[22]

Reports in years past described a few cases in which symptoms of systemic disability were attributed to the ingestion of fluoridated water of a concentration in the region of 1 part per million.

Typical complaints include "gnawing sensations in the stomach after eating," "stiffness and pain in the spine," "severe muscular pain in the arms and legs," "fingernails brittle," and so forth. It is claimed that some of the symptoms were promptly relieved by a change to water containing no fluoride. Evidence of direct causation is lacking in these studies, and they are not matched by controls. If cases of this sort are to be taken seriously, causation by, not mere association with, fluoridated water must be shown, as well as systemic damage comparable to that arising from dental disease. In July 1971, the Executive Committee of the American Academy of Allergy stated unanimously: "There is no evidence of allergy or intolerance to fluoride as used in the fluoridation of community water supplies."[23]

The attitude of the Commission on Chronic Illness (1954) toward the whole question of the possible toxicity of water with 1 part per million of fluoride is worthy of quotation: "The collection of negative evidence such as this [on excretion patterns for damaged kidneys] for an absolute determination of no possible effects of fluorides in persons suffering from chronic illnesses is an endless and extremely complicated undertaking. Generally speaking, consideration of the primary factors in the causation of such illnesses far overshadows any minor or secondary effects which, in the light of present knowledge, could be assumed from ingestion of trace amounts of fluoride in drinking water." The Commission concluded that "extensive research into the toxicology of fluorine compounds has revealed no definite evidence that the continued consumption of drinking water containing fluorides at a level of about 1 part per million is in any way harmful to the health of adults or those suffering from chronic illness of any kind."[24] It therefore urged American communities to adopt this public health measure "as a positive step in the prevention of the chronic disease dental caries." This recommendation has been consistently confirmed in the subsequent three decades.

Acute Toxicity

It is well known that fluorides in solid form are used as roach and rodent poisons. Acute toxicity in man probably begins about the level of 250 milligrams of sodium fluoride in one retained dose, although this amount has been taken at one time without harm.[25]

Nausea and vomiting are among the first signs of acute morbidity to be expected. A lethal dose for an adult would probably represent from 5 to 10 grams (5,000 to 10,000 milligrams). With such concentration, acute gastrointestinal irritation would develop almost immediately. Nausea, vomiting, diarrhea, and a state of shock would soon follow. Death would be expected within 2 to 4 hours, but if the victim survived beyond 4 hours recovery would be probable. Prompt kidney excretion of fluoride occurs if cellular mechanisms are not overwhelmed. Since 5 grams of sodium fluoride would produce only half that weight of fluoride ion, it can be seen that drinking water fluoridated at 1 part per million, and consumed at the rate of approximately 1 liter per day, carries with it a safety factor of about 2,500 in respect to death.

The question of the danger inherent in the breakdown or sabotage of fluoride-addition machinery is raised from time to time. Recognizable intoxication might be anticipated if a concentration of fluoride in the drinking water were reached sufficient to provide 250 milligrams of sodium fluoride in an 8-ounce glass of water. To obtain this concentration would require more than 4 tons of sodium fluoride per million gallons of water processed.[26] Since the average hoppers in water-treatment plants providing several million gallons per day usually contain only 200 to 500 pounds of powder, the virtual impossibility of such an accident is obvious. A saboteur intent on harming a population could find far easier ways to accomplish his objective.

Fluoride as a Nutrient

Exactly opposed to its status as a toxic agent is the status of fluoride as a nutrient. No human bones or teeth have ever failed to show fluoride when analyzed for it. More than this fact is needed, however, before fluoride can be termed an essential nutrient. Evidence is beginning to accumulate. Complete resistance to dental caries is attained so rarely in areas of fluoride-deficient water, perhaps because dietary fluoride accumulates so slowly in children and young adults, that caries appear to be, in part at least, a fluoride-deficiency disease. Bone structure, too, appears to suffer in fluoride-deficient areas, as has been mentioned.

Taking these facts and others into consideration, the National Research Council, as early as 1958, termed fluoride a "nutrient important for formation of caries-resistant enamel." In 1980 the Council defined the ranges of "estimated safe and adequate" intake for fluoride.[27]

Topical Fluoride Therapy

Since topical therapy involves no planned systemic ingestion of fluoride and operates only on erupted teeth, considerations of chronic toxicity, including possible alteration of formative human enamel (dental fluorosis), do not apply. Accidental swallowing of small amounts of correctly prepared solutions used during a treatment involve dosage so small that considerations of acute toxicity do not apply either.

The standardized methods of therapy which have resulted from these trials are set forth in Chapter 12. Despite occasional claims of greater success, caries reductions have seldom exceeded 40 percent under research conditions and are probably much less in service situations. This fact, coupled with the expense and professional time needed, has made it obvious that topical therapy cannot even closely approximate the cost efficiency of water fluoridation where the latter is possible.

DENTAL BENEFITS

Our first evidence of the dental benefits of water fluoridation came from the endemic low-fluoride areas. Typically, the caries findings were reported in numbers of DMF teeth, and reductions in caries approximated 60 percent. At least three other measures of interest are available, however, from the data assembled in this series of studies. Arnold calculated in 1943 that fluoridation to a level of 1 part per million decreases the number of missing permanent first molars by three-fourths, prevents all but about 5 percent of caries in the proximal surfaces of the four upper incisors, and increases six times the number of children age 12–14 who will show no caries experience.[28]

In subsequent years Russell and Elvove and Englander et al. demonstrated that similar benefits attended *adult* populations in an area of continuous residence.[29,30] Figs. 57 and 58 show differences between the native adults of Boulder, Colorado, where the water is essentially fluoride-free, and Colorado Springs, Colorado,

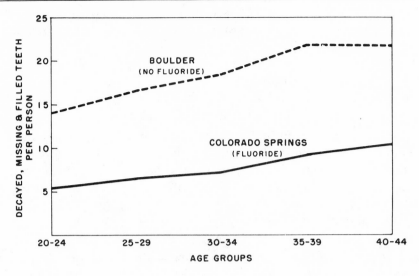

Figure 57. Decayed, missing, and filled teeth per adult in fluoride and nonfluoride communities. [Public Health Service, National Institute of Dental Research.]

where the water contained 2.5 parts per million of fluoride. Reductions in DMF permanent teeth in the latter community are seen to maintain a level approximately 60 percent lower than in the former community, and permanent-tooth mortality is likewise seen to run at a level approximately one-fifth as high.

Three pilot fluoridation studies were started in 1945: Grand Rapids, Michigan, with Muskegon as a control; Newburgh, New York, with Kingston as a control; and Brantford, Ontario. Each was designed to be a 10-year study, but after 5 years it became so apparent that the trial cities would duplicate the experience seen in cities of similar natural fluoride concentration that the U.S. Public Health Service gave its endorsement, stating that "communities desiring to fluoridate their communal water supply should be strongly encouraged to do so."[31] Since that time an increasing number of communities have recorded their experiences.

Table 38 summarizes studies in 14 communities where records of dental-caries experience are available at both the beginning and the end of a 10-year period of fluoridation. One should note that reductions of about 50 percent are the most commonly seen. Where the youngest ages at which caries of the permanent teeth can be studied are the only ones reported (ages 6 through 8), however, the reductions are invariably larger. Since the older children in the 10-year communities had some of their teeth formed before the fluoride was introduced, and since the most important effect of fluoridation appears to be upon the formation of tooth structure before teeth erupt into the mouth, it is obvious that the older children in these communities have received incomplete benefits. The younger children, however, show results which clearly approximate findings in the endemic fluoride areas.

Certain studies of periods longer than 10 years are available. A report from Grand Rapids, Michigan, after 15 years of fluoridation shows total caries experience to have been lowered by 50 to 63 percent in children 12 to 14 and 48 to 50 percent in those 15 or 16 years of age.[32] Fig. 59 shows the dental-caries experience in terms of decayed, missing, and filled teeth (DMF) per child for Grand Rapids as compared with that in Aurora, Illinois, the best documented natural fluoride community.

Newburgh, New York, after 15 years of fluoridation shows reduction of 70.1 percent in dental-caries experience as compared with the control city of Kingston among children 13 or 14 years of age, and reductions of 89.1 percent in number of missing teeth

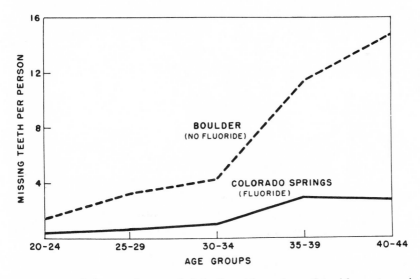

Figure 58. Missing teeth per adult in fluoride and nonfluoride communities. [Public Health Service, National Institute of Dental Research.]

Table 38. Reductions in decayed, missing, and filled permanent teeth among children in communities after 10 years of fluoridation.

Community	Age studied (yrs.)	Reduction (%)
Grand Junction, Colo.	6	94.0
New Britain, Conn.	6–16	44.6
District of Columbia	6	59.1
Evanston, Ill.	6	91.3
	7	64.6
	8	62.6
Fort Wayne, Ind.	6–10	50.0
Hopkinsville, Ky.	? (children)	56.0
Louisville, Ky.	1st 3 grades	62.1
Hagerstown, Md.	7, 9, 11, 13	57.0
Grand Rapids, Mich.	6	75.0
	7	63.0
	8	57.0
	9	50.0
	10	52.0
Newburgh, N.Y.	6–9	58.0
	10–12	57.0
	13–14	48.0
	16	41.0
Charlotte, N.C.	6–11	60.0
Chattanooga, Tenn.	6–14	70.8
Marshall, Texas	7–15	54.0
Brantford, Ont.	6	60.0
	7	67.0
	8	54.0
	9	46.0
	10	41.0
	11–13	44.0
	14–16	35.0

per child.[33] Reports from various states show large increases in totally caries-free teenagers after 15 or more years of fluoridation. In Philadelphia, caries-free 14-year-olds showed an increase from 4.2 to 23.0 percent; in Wisconsin, they went from 1.5 to 14.7 percent.

All these studies make it apparent that there is no longer any reason to doubt the fact that adjustment of a community water supply to optimum fluoride concentration produces results similar to those seen in the natural fluoride communities. The reductions are not as extensive in developed areas now, however, as they were a generation ago.

It is possible that water fluoridation also has a favorable effect on dental diseases and conditions other than dental caries. Russell has studied the severity of *periodontal disease* in fluoride and nonfluoride areas, and his findings suggest lower severity in the former.[34] The Russell and Elvove study on adults indicates a similar result.[29] The graph on missing teeth shows a widening difference between Boulder and Colorado Springs above age 34, when teeth are more commonly lost from periodontal disease than from caries. Ast, reporting findings from Newburgh, New York (fluoridated), and Kingston (control), states that 35 percent of the chil-

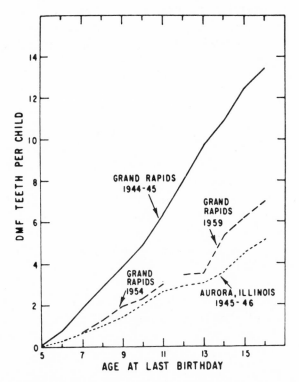

Figure 59. Dental caries in children after 10 and 15 years of fluoridation, Grand Rapids, Michigan, and Aurora, Illinois. [Copyright, American Dental Association. Reprinted by permission.]

dren in the former city and only 13 percent in the latter had normal *occlusion*.[35] The definition of normal occlusion in this instance is a rigid one, even minor deviations from an ideal occlusion being considered abnormal.

These varied benefits from water fluoridation are impressive. Beyond them, Arnold's analysis of the endemic areas shows that reductions in DMF teeth may actually underestimate reductions in man-hours needed for dental care.[28] Proximal lesions of dental caries are inhibited considerably more than pit-and-fissure occlusal lesions and the former take far more time to restore, especially on posterior teeth.

The question is often raised of the value to a fetus of fluoride supplements taken by a mother during pregnancy. The few studies available on this matter seem to give conflicting evidence. Some report later reductions of caries in the deciduous teeth and others do not. There is reason to doubt the ability of brief elevations of fluoride blood level to send appreciable amounts of fluoride across the placental barrier.

MECHANICS OF FLUORIDATION

The adjustment of fluoride concentration in a communal water supply presents a mechanical problem familiar to most waterworks engineers. The feeding machinery used to add fluoride resembles closely, or may be identical with, the machinery used for adding other chemicals. The knowledge of inorganic chemistry needed for manipulation of the chemicals and monitoring of the resulting water lies within the training of any competent waterworks engineer, and the Environmental Protection Agency has developed a specific manual of instructions.[36]

Feeding machinery used for adding fluoride is of two general types, (1) solution feeders, where a hand or mechanically prepared saturated solution of fluoride is fed into the water main at a carefully controlled rate, and (2) dry feeders, where solid material is fed into a dissolving tank at a measured rate by automatic machinery and the resulting concentrated solution is carried to the water main in a volume of water which is sufficient to assure that none of the solid material remains undissolved.

The solution feeders are of two types. The first, most useful in small communities, involves placing a powder such as a sodium fluoride in a vat and letting water remain on top of it until saturation has occurred. The saturated solution is then drawn off at a known rate into the main conduit, while another vat is filled to start a new saturation process. Two vats can be used alternately. The second method involves liquid delivered by tank trucks at known concentration and stored as a fluid in large tanks. Electrically controlled machinery then injects the fluid into the water main. This method is now becoming more popular than solid feeding for large cities. Solid feeding got off to an earlier start for cities, however, because of the initial work with sodium fluoride.

A number of different *fluorine compounds* will supply useful quantities of fluoride ion. Table 39 shows those compounds that are in most common use.[37] Dissociated fluoride ion is the active ingredient in all instances; results are similar regardless of the compound used.

Sodium fluoride was the material used in the original pilot programs started in 1945, but considerations of cost are now shifting the balance in favor of sodium silicofluoride. Fluosilicic acid is used where ease of diluting a material already in liquid form outweighs cost considerations, but its corrosive nature requires careful supervision. Experimental work is now being conducted with fluorspar (calcium fluoride), a material costing only about one-third as much as sodium silicofluoride but difficult to dissolve.

Fig. 60 illustrates a typical volumetric dry feeder with hopper above, electrically operated feeding device in the center, and solution tank below. The measurement machinery may operate to deliver either a measured volume or a measured weight of dry

Table 39. Sources of fluoride ion and their utilization in United States, 1960.

Chemical	Population served
Sodium silicofluoride	25,092,573
Sodium fluoride	5,360,543
Fluosilicic acid (hydrofluosilicic acid)	10,626,715
Ammonium fluosilicate	66,367
Calcium fluoride	7,296
Others, and adjusted natural fluoride	1,047,621

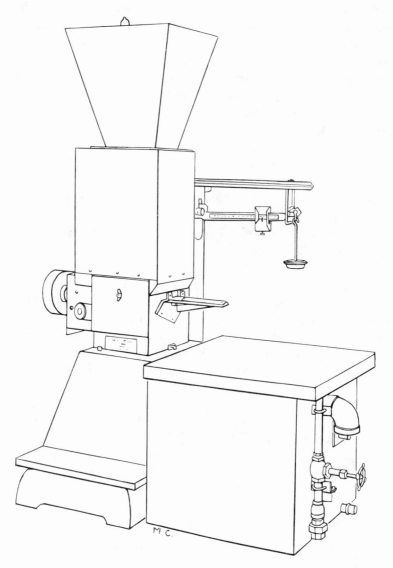

Figure 60. Volumetric fluoridator. [Wallace and Tiernan, Inc.]

chemical within a given time interval. The former type is simpler, less expensive, and probably more commonly used. It is very easy to have the hopper attached by a canvas mesh to the rest of the machine and suspended from a balance in such a way that the hopper can be weighed at any time, thus determining the weight of powder which has been discharged since previous weighing. This device, shown in Fig. 60, permits both volumetric and gravimetric control in one machine.

Fig. 61 shows a typical scheme for water treatment in an urban area of approximately 70,000 population. Fluoridation of the water treated in this plant is merely the final step in a long chain of operations which includes use of charcoal, alum, gaseous chlorine, and Calgon (a corrosion-control agent), as well as other chemicals on occasion. The dry feeder used to add sodium silicofluoride, though operating in a different part of the water-filtration cycle, stands in this plant alongside similar dry feeders used for adding alum and charcoal. No extra personnel has been added to the staff of the plant, either to operate the fluoride machinery or to monitor the water after fluoridation. Sacks of fluoride are stored on the second floor of the building and an enclosure has been made around the chute which leads into the fluoride hopper in order to limit the tracking of powder around the area where the sacks of fluoride are opened. There is a hood right over the opening of the chute with exhaust-ventilation machinery to carry away from the operator any dust which may arise during the dumping of sacks into the chute. If ventilation machinery were not available, it would be absolutely essential for the operator to wear a dust mask at this stage of the process.

In designing a water fluoridation installation it is important to apply the fluoride at a point where the risk of losing it in subsequent treatment is at a minimum. Alum-coagulation and activated-carbon treatment at low pH values are both processes which tend to remove a small amount of fluoride. The addition of fluoride, therefore, should occur after these processes have been completed, though not necessarily after filtration. Fluoridation, of course, need not occur at the water-filtration plant. Local pumping stations are equally suitable localities. Thus if one filtration plant serves several communities but each community has its own local pumping station, fluoridation is possible for an individual community in the system without involving the others.

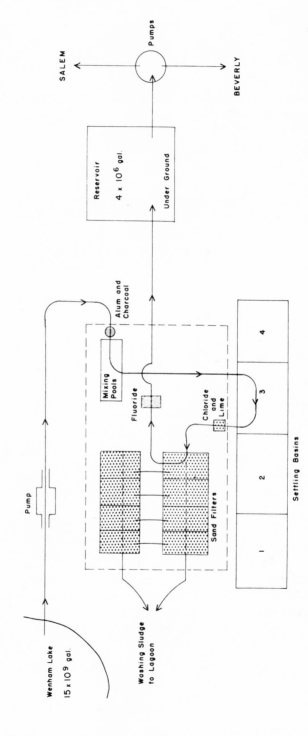

Figure 61. Sequence of water-treatment procedures in Salem-Beverly water filtration plant, North Beverly, Massachusetts.

Fluoride Concentration

The concentration of fluoride in treated water is a matter needing careful consideration. Evidence has been given for the use of a concentration of 1.0 part per million (1.0 milligram per liter) of fluoride ion. This is the concentration produced in most of the fluoridation installations throughout the United States today, and is also the concentration recommended by the U.S. Public Health Service. Most of the work on water fluoridation, however, has been done in the north central area of the United States, where average water consumption per person may not necessarily equal that in other parts of the country. Total fluoride dosage per day is the ultimate measure which must be used if dental caries is to be reduced without objectionable dental fluorosis being caused in the process. In hot climates, where water consumption is greater per person per day, the concentration of fluoride must be less in order to produce the optimum intake of 1 to 1.5 milligrams per person per day. Maier considers that 10 percent incidence of endemic fluorosis is the maximum which can be tolerated. Fluorosis at this level in the population would be entirely of the mildest variety, with no darkening of teeth and merely those slight whitish enamel opacities which are so difficult to distinguish from the early signs of caries. Such opacities occur in a manner and to an extent which is not in the least objectionable.

For practical purposes the U.S. Public Health Service sets up the standards for fluoride to which water-supply systems used by carriers and others subject to federal quarantine regulations must conform. Table 40 gives optimum fluoride concentrations for certain ranges of annual average maximum daily air temperatures.[38] A regulation of the Environmental Protection Agency of March 17, 1986, sets a top limit of 4 milligrams per liter for naturally fluoridated water supplies only.

Variability in individual water consumption is frequently cited as a reason for expecting pathologic effects among residents of fluoridated communities. It is true that individual water consumption does vary. Detailed studies are few. One by Galagan et al. shows a standard deviation so great that it is obvious that some children are drinking more than the average amount of water for their ages and body weights, and others drinking less.[39] Another

Table 40. Fluoride levels recommended for cool and warm climates.

Annual avg. maximum daily air temperatures[a]	Recommended control limits F concentrations in parts per million		
	Lower	Optimum	Upper
50.0–53.7	0.9	1.2	1.7
53.8–58.3	.8	1.1	1.5
58.4–63.8	.8	1.0	1.3
63.9–70.6	.7	0.9	1.2
70.7–79.2	.7	.8	1.0
79.3–90.5	.6	.7	0.8

a. Based on temperature data obtained for a minimum of 5 years.

study by Walker and his associates of some 800 children in widely separated areas throughout the United States shows small variability.[40] Nevertheless, the important fact is that populations available for study both in natural fluoride and in fluoridated areas are large enough so that all degrees of variability may be expected to have occurred. The fact that *no* true mottling (fluorosis above the mild level) or other signs of fluoride toxicity have been demonstrated in these areas is impressive evidence that variability in individual water drinking is unimportant.

Monitoring

Although small hourly variations in concentrations are of little consequence where the safety factors are as great as they are with water fluoridation, regular monitoring of water supplies is essential even at the smallest installation. State health departments usually have requirements for such monitoring. Four methods for monitoring are available:

1. Hourly check of the weight of chemical fed into the hopper. Dry feeders, if well maintained and adjusted, should be accurate well within 5 percent, and this is actually a greater degree of accuracy than exists with any of the chemical tests so far devised.

2. Colorimetric chemical testing through addition of zirconium-alizarin reagent, the result to be compared with standard color samples. Methods of this sort include the Scott-Sanchis, the Megregian-Maier, and the SPADNS. Accuracy is to within approx-

imately 0.1 to 0.2 parts per million of fluoride. Testing is usually done once or twice daily upon the effluent water.

3. Less frequent colorimetric testing is advisable (perhaps at weekly intervals) upon water at various parts of the distribution system, both near to and distant from the point of fluoride addition.

4. Continuous electronic measuring and controlling of fluoride concentration in water is available. The addition of small quantities of fluoride ion to the water supply produces extremely small changes in the electroconductivity of that water, and measurement of the change in conductivity will disclose the concentration of fluoride provided no other change has occurred in the water between the point at which conductivity is first and last recorded.

Fig. 62 shows such an installation at the Salem-Beverly (Massachusetts) water-filtration plant. The conductivity difference recorder is an electronic device with a pen which makes a continuous record upon a revolving disk. Differences in conductivity, expressed originally in electrical units, are later translated into parts

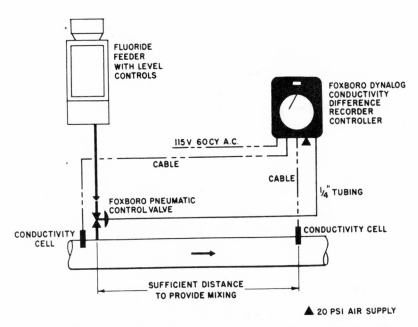

Figure 62. Diagram of fluoride concentration recorder installation. [Courtesy, Foxboro Company.]

per million of fluoride. Variations in concentration beyond a pre-determined range activate machinery which will turn off or restart the fluoride feeder.

For portable use, a simple electrode (Orion) is available, giving direct readings of fluoride concentration. The electrode sensing element is a lanthanum fluoride single-crystal membrane which separates an internal filling solution from the sample solution. This single crystal is an ionic conductor for fluoride ion, and fluoride ion alone.

Long-term average errors in adding fluoride to water supplies are completely avoidable in view of the large quantities of chemical involved, and even short-term variations can be controlled with a high degree of precision. In almost 3,000 tests of processed water over a 10-year period in Grand Rapids, Michigan, over 99 percent of the test findings were between 0.8 and 1.2 parts per million. Other cities have shown similar results.

Once fluoridation facilities are in operation, the measurements of concentration need careful and continuous monitoring. The chief risk in cases of careless operation is underexposure to the point of loss of benefit. Significant overexposure cannot exist without the purchase and introduction of large amounts of unneeded chemicals. Health or water departments have various ranges of concentration above and below optimal that they consider accept-able, and percentages of total time during which failure of com-pliance can be tolerated. These matters are easily computed at a given installation. Kuthy et al., in a study of 249 Illinois water supplies, identified four community or staffing characteristics they found significant in relation to compliance: source of water supply, operator turnover, classification of operator, and commu-nity size.[41] In general, the better levels of compliance were associ-ated with surface water supplies, low chief operator turnover in a 5-year period, high operator classification, and large community size.

ECONOMICS OF FLUORIDATION

The operating cost of supplementary fluoride added to a water supply usually runs from 20 to 50 cents per person per year. Where there is one filtration plant or other favorable location for addition, the lower figure is likely. Higher costs accompany multiple points for addition and other engineering problems. Installation costs often approximate 1 year's cost of operation but can run higher. The highest to come to my attention so far is in the city of Newton, Massachusetts, and even here it averages out to less than $1.50 per person in the community.

Opponents of water fluoridation have claimed that tablets for individual dosage could be bought in bulk and dispensed free at about 15 cents per person per year, and that this method of fluoride supplementation therefore compares favorably with water fluoridation. The estimate is incorrect in that costs of dispensing and packaging the material, arranging for individual prescription to each consumer, and distribution and monitoring of supplies—all of them necessary costs—have been omitted. More common estimates of the cost of properly dispensed and packaged fluoride tablets or drops approximate 1 cent per day, or $3.65 per person per year. Even here, the costs of prescription and distribution are neglected, as well as the psychological barriers to consistent long-term use of such supplements. Tablets are safe and effective for school classroom use when properly supervised. The costs of supervision are such, however, that community or school water fluoridation, when possible, is more cost-effective.

The known dental benefits of water fluoridation permit an estimation of the money value to the public of the healthy teeth that now will not require restorative dental treatment. One study in the Newburgh-Kingston series shows the cost of initial dental care to have been reduced by fluoridation from $32.38 to $14.16 among children 12 to 13 years of age, and yearly maintenance costs lowered from $11.00 to $5.90.[42] An estimate made by the writer in which the total cost of all restorative dentistry needed through the age of 16 on permanent teeth of children in Cambridge, Massachusetts, was compared with a similar estimate for Danvers, Massachusetts. The Cambridge estimate was based on the dental-decay rate found in the prefluoridation survey of 1959, and the Danvers estimate on rates after 8 years of fluoridation. The saving in cost was $303 per person. Several studies of cost savings such as these have led to cost-benefit ratios where 1 dollar spent on fluoridation is compared with the dollar value of savings in children's dentistry. These ratios have run all the way from 35 to 60, though they are smaller today. This matter is discussed in detail in Chapter 19.

The decreasing need for dental treatment among the young

people in a fluoridated community does not necessarily mean a diminution in demand for dental treatment in the community, since it has been brought out elsewhere that only a small fraction of needed dental treatment is now rendered in most parts of this country. The result of water fluoridation is actually a facilitation of extension of dental care to a much larger proportion of the population than now receives it, and better completion of maintenance care. Where adults who formerly lost all their teeth at an early age now keep and restore part of their natural dentition, demand for dental care should even increase per person. Dentists in fluoridated communities have been shown to remain fully occupied, but with older patients.[43,44]

Opponents of fluoridation occasionally claim that fluorides even at 1 part per million will corrode pipes, or will cause accumulation of fluoride in the iron or calcium carbonate tubercles that occasionally form within water pipes for other reasons. The first claim is chemically illogical and unsupported by any complaint from water departments in areas of both natural fluoride and fluoridation. It has also been chemically tested by the Massachusetts Department of Public Health and found to be without basis.[45] Accumulation of fluoride in tubercles is equally unimportant in view of the obvious difficulty of getting the fluoride back into solution. The point has been investigated carefully in many large cities, however, and the results of these studies have shown conclusively that fluoride residuals can be maintained satisfactorily. In San Francisco, for instance, an average of 640 tests taken throughout the system over a 1-year period showed a variation of only 0.04 part per million from the average dose actually added to the water plus its natural fluoride content.[46]

LEGAL AND POLITICAL ACTION

Fluoridation of a communal water supply is obviously a governmental problem requiring whatever authorization and control may be in effect in the area concerned. In a democratic country it is obviously the will of the people that must ultimately decide whether fluoridation will take place or not. Political action should ordinarily be undertaken at the level of government where the control of the communal water supply rests, though several states have passed mandatory fluoridation laws for communities over certain sizes. Two main methods are available at the local level: executive decision by elected or appointed officials, and referendum.

The issue of education is one which may often determine the wisdom of a given approach to the enactment of fluoride legislation in a community. Fluoridation is a complicated issue upon which to inform the great mass of a voting population. Scientific facts are easily distorted, emotions are easily aroused, as by the use of such terms as "rat poison." Judgmental evaluation on the part of a voter does not operate as reliably on a scientific problem as it does upon the choice of candidate who can be seen and heard as a person. The very mass of material necessary to an understanding of the fluoridation issue makes it inevitable that many voters who have attempted such an understanding will go to the polls with incomplete knowledge. Such knowledge may prove inadequate to stimulate affirmative votes, or may actually backfire by transforming uninformed proponents into semi-informed opponents. For these reasons referenda on fluoridation represent an inefficient use of the democratic process and in general are to be discouraged. Where inevitable, they should be preceded by a good educational campaign.

A much more informed decision can be obtained if a community is willing to entrust the fluoridation decision to a group of delegated or appointed officials, as it entrusts so many other issues of a complex scientific or legal nature. A city council, a health department, or a city water board is not only a small group to educate, but also one with specialized experience which permits the understanding of the fluoridation issue far more quickly than would be the case in an unselected group—and with responsibility for more detailed study.

The legal validity of water fluoridation has been thoroughly tested in the United States during the past decades, and has been invariably confirmed. The National Institute of Municipal Law Officers made an exhaustive study of water fluoridation and published a report upon the matter in 1952. Among the conclusions reached by this group were:

Fluoridation is not an unconstitutional invasion of the right of religious freedom.

Fluoridation is a constitutionally permissible exercise of the municipal police power.

Fluoridation to the recommended concentration will not create municipal tort liability.

Neither fluoridation nor the use of municipally fluoridated water in food manufacturing is precluded by the Federal Food, Drug, and Cosmetic Act.[47]

The reasoning behind these statements deserves some examination.

Water fluoridation has been opposed frequently as "compulsory mass medication." The contention has been that majorities do not have the right to compel minorities to ingest "medicine" without their consent. Actually, neither the word "compulsory" nor the phrase "mass medication" is applicable to water fluoridation. Nonfluoride bottled water is available for purchase quite easily in most large communities, and in rural areas citizens can dig their own wells. The fluoridation of a communal water supply through municipal action is, therefore, in no sense compulsion. No citizen is ordered not to drink whatever water he pleases in the sense that he would be ordered not to drive on the left-hand side of the street. Neither is fluoridation "medication." Medication is the cure of a disease; water fluoridation is for prevention, and for nutrition of healthy tooth structure.

In the eyes of the National Institute of Municipal Law Officers there is a "very close analogy" to fluoridation to be found in the compulsory food-enrichment laws. At the time of their report the enrichment of flour and bread was voluntary in 22 states, mandatory by local law in 26 states and 3 territories. It is incorrect and irrelevant to call fluoridation compulsion merely because it imposes a financial penalty upon minorities which wish to avoid it. Majorities are always taxing minorities to finance public improvements. A particularly clearcut example lies in school taxes, which parents are in no way able to escape if they wish to send their children to private school and which people with no children must also pay.

The First Amendment to the Constitution guarantees the right to religious freedom, but this right is not beyond interference by a state or municipality. The religious guarantees of the First Amendment embrace two concepts—freedom to believe and freedom to act. "The first is absolute, but in the nature of things the second cannot be. Conduct remains subject to regulations for the protection of society."[48] The National Institute of Municipal Law Officers report cites various examples in which a distinction has been made on such matters. Polygamy may be conceived of as a religious duty, but the state may also punish it as a crime. During the Prohibition era the federal government had authority to limit the quantity of wine that could be used for sacramental purposes. Courts have been especially reluctant to interfere with measures for the welfare of children on the grounds that they conflict with religious freedom.

Many lawsuits have arisen on the subject of water fluoridation. Of these, six reached the U.S. Supreme Court, but all were denied review. Fifteen or more have been settled at state level. In every instance the validity of water fluoridation was upheld.[49]

The setting of standards for monitoring of fluoridated water is a common function for a state health department, but state legislation on the initiation of water fluoridation is rare. Several states now require fluoridation, either in any approved water supply or in the water supplies of communities over a certain minimum population. Connecticut was the first state to enact such legislation; Minnesota, Illinois, and Delaware have followed suit. Kentucky and Michigan have regulations of a similar general import. There are three or four states that require referendum by the local community before the initiation of fluoridation.

COMMUNITY ACTION

The recommendation of water fluoridation as a public health measure has thrown dentists into a situation entirely new to them. In the first place, fluoridation is the first preventive measure they have been called upon to implement at the community rather than the individual level. In the second place, it has evoked an emotional opposition of an intensity seldom seen even in the field of public health. With all its embarrassments, the situation has its good points. It makes the dentist a part of his community in a sense that he never has been before. It has made for him a host of new friends in the field of public health and medicine. It has compelled him to study the social background for the acceptance of public health measures. This latter matter has been more thoroughly dealt with in Chapter 10. Finally, it has involved him in the practical political tactics by which community consent to a public health measure may be obtained.

The American Dental Association has put out advice on the subjects of methods and media.[50] Chief among its recommendations is the formation of a citizens' committee to include a wide representation of leaders of opinion and professional people in the community. As part of this committee, and beyond it, must be a strong group of lay people willing to work and to raise money for expenses. The parents of young children are among the best people to look for here.

The citizens' committee operates fully as effectively through personal contact with members of the community as it does through arranging the intelligent use of mass media such as newspaper and radio. One point, however, has become increasingly clear. The public can hardly be expected to take more than a lukewarm interest if fluoridation is presented as a single issue. Far more interest is likely to be aroused if the primary emphasis of the campaign is upon dental health in the broad sense. The citizens' committee can therefore concern itself with the whole problem of dental health at the community level, with particular interest in the school dental health education program. This not only will permit the urging of water fluoridation in a broader, more logical setting, but also will give the committee other constructive objectives in case temporary blocks are thrown in the path of the fluoridation issue.

Voluminous literature, both professional and lay, now exists on all aspects of the fluoridation question. Some of the best scientific sources are listed among the references for this chapter. Any community group desiring to initiate water fluoridation would do well to scan current printed accounts of the "fluoridation fights" reported in their part of the country at the time. Citizens' groups in large cities have put out some excellent literature on matters both factual and strategic. Some of the literature of the American Dental Association provides answers to criticisms made by the opponents of water fluoridation.[51] The U.S. Public Health Service provides various publications of value to the health professional.

For dentists and dental hygienists entering a fluoridation controversy, a few "do's" and "don'ts" are in order:

DO prepare yourselves on detailed facts concerning the benefits and safety of fluoridation, including the findings, localities, and authors of important studies on these matters.

DO learn something about the water supply of your community. Learn about or survey the dental status of the community through school-based samples (not just dental patients) and publicize your findings.

DO select opportunities for public statements which permit your audience to listen to reason without undue interruption. You, in turn, must also listen to their reasons.

DO clear your appearances or writings with your local dental society. Codes of ethics usually require this, and the society will also wish to help you.

DO maintain dignity and reserve sufficient to protect your status as a professional in the field.

DON'T engage in formal debate unless forced to by circumstances. The rules of debate give emotion a status equal to that of reason, assume equal "facts" on both sides of an issue, and give opponents of the issue that last word.

DON'T ridicule opponents of fluoridation. Fanatics often lead them, supplying irrelevant or false information, but the majority will usually be, and should always be assumed to be, sincere.

DON'T lose your "cool."

DON'T give up. Time is on your side.

Endorsement and Use of Fluoridation

Many national organizations in the health field have had reason to study and influence the adoption or nonadoption of a public measure such as water fluoridation. Each organization will study the measure from its own point of view and then express an opinion which is to be taken in the light of its own experience. Thus the endorsement of the American Dental Association, first given in 1950, carries most weight in the field of dental benefits, though of course this association has studied other aspects of the problem as well. The American Medical Association endorsed water fluoridation in December 1951 and again, after reviews of subsequent evidence, in

December 1957 and December 1974. In all instances their endorsement has carried greatest weight in the field of systemic safety. The American Waterworks Association endorsement carries greatest weight in the field of engineering. The U.S. Public Health Service, first endorsing fluoridation in 1945, did so on a multidisciplinary basis supported by the best first-hand dental epidemiological work in the country. The World Health Organization unanimously adopted a resolution in 1969 encouraging fluoridation.[52]

Many lay organizations, studying the matter from a well-rounded but not expert point of view, have given endorsements which should carry great public force. Among these are the American Legion, the Child Study Association of America, the American School Health Association, and the American Federation of Labor and Congress of Industrial Organizations.

As of the end of 1980 it was estimated by the U.S. Public Health Service that, not including communities with natural fluoride, 106,170,000 people in 8,278 communities were receiving controlled fluoridation. The greatest utilization has occurred in the larger communities. New York, Chicago, Philadelphia, Baltimore, Cleveland, Detroit, Washington, D.C., St. Louis, Milwaukee, Boston, and San Francisco all fluoridate. More than 10 million people also use natural fluoridation.

Table 41, provided by the Canadian Dental Association in 1983, gives a worldwide picture of fluoridation in 32 different countries. The size of the country varies all the way from Hong Kong to the United States; the total of almost 250 million people is what counts. Percentage proportions of populations vary widely. Ireland, one of the few countries where fluoridation is compulsory, shows only 48 percent compliance, perhaps because large segments of the population are not on community water supplies. Australia, on a voluntary basis, shows 65 percent compliance; New Zealand, 54 percent. The United States shows 53 percent compliance; Canada, 35 percent. Sweden, a high caries state in times past, is unlisted, since fluoridation is illegal there.

School Fluoridation

Where community water supplies are not fluoridated or where, as in rural areas, none exist, the larger public schools can have a water supply fluoridated to 4 or 5 parts per million. A limited daytime exposure to this concentration of fluoride is estimated to

Table 41. Countries reported to be large users of fluoridation.

Country	As of	Serving	First adjusted	Information source
Argentina	Dec. 1980	1,150,000	1969	Pan Am. Health Org.
Aruba-Curacao	Dec. 1980	0,200,000	1968	Pan Am. Health Org.
Australia	Dec. 1982	9,950,000	1956	Aust. Dept. Health
Brazil	Dec. 1980	19,500,000	1953	Pan Am. Health Org.
Canada (est.)	Dec. 1980	8,800,000	1945	Cdn. Dent. Assn.
Chile	Dec. 1980	4,100,000	1953	Pan Am. Health Org.
Colombia	Dec. 1980	8,470,000	1953	Pan Am. Health Org.
Costa Rica	Dec. 1980	0,650,000	1976	Pan Am. Health Org.
Cuba	Dec. 1980	0,100,000	1974	Pan Am. Health Org.
Czechoslovakia	Oct. 1980	2,500,000	1956	F.D.I. letter
Dominican Republic	Dec. 1980	0,300,000	—	Pan Am. Health Org.
Ecuador	Dec. 1980	1,300,000	1961	Pan Am. Health Org.
El Salvador	Dec. 1980	0,210,000	—	Pan Am. Health Org.
German Dem. Rep.	Dec. 1975	1,200,000	1952	28th World Health Assembly
Guatemala	Dec. 1980	0,700,000	1961	Pan Am. Health Org.
Hong Kong	Dec. 1974	3,900,000	1961	Fed. Dentaire Int.
Ireland	Apr. 1978	1,700,000	1964	Fed. Dentaire Int.
Israel	Apr. 1978	0,200,000	1977	Fed. Dentaire Int.
Malaysia	Oct. 1978	6,600,000	1966	Asst. Dir. Dent. Ser.
Mexico	Dec. 1980	4,700,000	1960	Pan Am. Health Org.
New Zealand	July 1979	1,740,000	1954	New Zealand Dent. Assembly
Nicaragua	Dec. 1980	0,260,000	(Natural F)	Pan Am. Health Org.
Panama	Dec. 1980	0,600,000	1950	Pan Am. Health Org.
Paraguay	Dec. 1980	0,500,000	1961	Pan Am. Health Org.
Poland	Dec. 1974	2,300,000	1967	28th World Health Assembly
Singapore	Dec. 1974	2,200,000	1958	Fed. Dentaire Int.
Switzerland	Apr. 1978	0,200,000	1972	Fed. Dentaire Int.
UK	Sept. 1982	5,500,000	1955	Fluoridation Soc.
USA (est.)	Dec. 1980	123,000,000	1945	US Fluor. Census (est.)
USSR (est.)	Dec. 1974	30,000,000	1960	Eur. Org. for Promotion of Water Fluor.
Venezuela	Dec. 1980	1,200,000	1952	Pan Am. Health Org.
Yugoslavia	Oct. 1980	3,000,000	(Natural F)	F.D.I. letter
		246.7 million		

give school children approximately the same total dosage as they would receive from 1 part per million in a 24-hour day. A carefully documented 12-year U.S. Public Health Service study of such an installation showed a 39 percent reduction in DMF teeth for continuously exposed children.[53] Thirteen states now have one or more fluoridated school water supplies. These serve over 124,000 children in almost 400 schools (1977).[54]

Other Sources of Systemic Fluoride

The supplementation of fluoride by tablets or drops on the part of residents of unfluoridated areas is taken up in Chapter 12.

The addition of fluoride to various foodstuffs follows essentially the same pattern as that involved in the use of tablets or drops. One small-scale study has been made in which homogenized milk was fortified with a dose of 1 milligram of fluoride, in the form of sodium fluoride, per half-pint container. Reductions in dental caries that appeared to approximate those of water fluoridation were obtained after a period of 4½ years.[55] Fluoridated salt and milk have been used in Switzerland with somewhat less success.[56] All these methods involve problems of supervision and cost that put them out of the level of practicality of community water fluoridation. They are to be considered, however, where community fluoridation is impossible.

Municipal Defluoridation

Communities which find themselves unable to obtain a natural water supply with less than 3 parts per million of fluoride will wish to reduce this concentration in order to reduce dental fluorosis in children's teeth. The U.S. Public Health Service has designed and acquired experience in the use of defluoridation machinery.[57] Calcined (activated) alumina is most commonly used as an absorbing agent. Installation of equipment and an alumina bed cost approximately $15,000 in 1963, and operating costs ran about $52 per million gallons of treated water. Costs such as these are believed to be within the resources of many communities using high-fluoride water, though only 11 plants designed for fluoride removal were operating in 1963.

CHAPTER 17

Delivery of Dental Care

SOCRATES, in defining the ideal state, gives as a prerequisite that men should divide labor, certain men becoming expert in certain fields, others in other fields, and all working as a team for the common good. This philosophy was in line with, and perhaps back of, much of the advance in the structuring of society we associate with the Golden Age of Greece. Socrates specifically mentions the profession of medicine. In these days, when the sum total of human knowledge is so much greater, the division of labor has proceeded much further, leading not only to professional specialties in the field of medicine but also to various types of auxiliary personnel. Between these individuals and groups there must be teamwork.

The need to apply in one area more knowledge than can be possessed by one person is not the only reason for teamwork. Some tasks actually require more than two hands. Other tasks are more quickly or better performed if one worker confines himself to part of the task, leaving other parts to other workers. Repetition without shift of attention makes for speed and accuracy. It is this philosophy which has produced the assembly lines in modern industry. A final reason for division of labor lies in the different levels of knowledge attainable within one field by persons of differing aptitude and opportunity for training. Certain parts of a task require top-level skill and knowledge. In dentistry these are the so-called "professional services." Other parts of the task require less skill and knowledge. These may safely and advantageously be delegated to auxiliary personnel. Society benefits from this sort of division of labor in that training time for professional personnel can be conserved. Those who do receive "full" training can make their best services available to a larger segment of the population if they have assistance on the more routine phases of their work, and the assistants may actually perform technical tasks better than the professional person could.

Since large tasks, and particularly communitywide tasks, are those where division of labor and teamwork are most needed, teamwork has become one of the prime characteristics of public health work. This chapter will consider how dental public health teams are organized for the delivery of care: the types of personnel available, and how they are arranged into working groups. Techniques for executive control have been discussed in Chapter 11. For convenience here, we shall first examine the organization of teams involving the dentist and his auxiliaries, then the organization of delivery teams among professionals, dental and otherwise.

DENTISTS AND THEIR AUXILIARIES

The numbers and types of auxiliary personnel now available to the dental profession are set forth in Chapter 13, with some indication of the combinations in which these auxiliaries are used. It is brought out there that dentists still outnumber their professionally trained auxiliaries. But since auxiliaries at all levels of training are important parts of the dental team, the various types are considered here, with more detailed attention to the duties of each as part of such a team.

Dental Assistant

The employment of general-purpose dental assistants, usually women, dates back to the middle of the nineteenth century when fixed dental offices began to replace itinerant dental practices. Since that time the variety of duties which dental assistants may perform has steadily increased. The Expert Committee on Auxiliary Dental Personnel of the World Health Organization, surveying current utilization of dental assistants, lists these duties:

1. Reception of the patient.
2. Preparation of the patient for any treatment he or she may need.
3. Preparation and provision of all necessary facilities, such as mouthwashes, napkins, receivers.
4. Sterilization, care, and preparation of instruments.
5. Preparation and mixing of restorative materials, including both filling and impression materials.
6. Care of the patient after treatment until he or she leaves, including clearing away of instruments and preparation of instruments for reuse.
7. Preparation of the surgery for the next patient.
8. Presentation of documents to the surgeon for his completion, and filing of these.
9. Assistance with x-ray work and the processing and mounting of x-rays.
10. Instruction of the patient, where necessary, in the correct use of the toothbrush.
11. Aftercare of persons who have had general anesthetics.[1]

There is still great variability in the utilization of dental assistants from office to office. Some dental assistants are in fact merely receptionists with the added duty of sterilizing instruments and replacing them in a cabinet. Other dental assistants, relieved of receptionist duties, stay constantly at the chair side. They anticipate the dentist's needs for instruments and materials, operate his coolant and suction systems for him, place cotton rolls, and take a large part in every dental operation which is performed. Because of this variability in function, it is difficult to lay down rules concerning the training and duties of an assistant. It is difficult also to predict her effect upon the efficiency of a dental office.

The Chair-side Dental Assistant. Broad statistical studies have been made upon the average number of patients treated by dentists using and not using assistants. Klein found in 1944 that the addition of one dental assistant increased the number of patients treated by a dentist by 33 percent if he were using one chair and by 62 percent if he were using two chairs.[2] Later studies made by the U.S. Public Health Service in Richmond, Indiana, show that a dentist can double his output with the help of one full-time and one half-time assistant.[3] Increases of this sort depend upon standardized operative techniques which use a minimum number of instruments, and careful indoctrination of the assistant to anticipate the operator's needs. Since instruments can be passed to him, the dentist may remain seated, and thus operate under less physical and mental strain. Quality of service and control of patient are both improved under such a system. Appointment periods also may be shorter per unit accomplishment, with less testing of the patient's endurance, particularly important in the handling of young children. The clinic set-up of the Public Health Service in Richmond involved two chairs per dentist so that he would not have to wait while patients were seated and unseated. Each dentist had a chair-side assistant trained to work with him as an individual, and each two or three dentists shared a roving assistant who seated patients and sterilized instruments, cared for handpieces, and mixed cement and amalgam. The chair-side assistant passed instruments and filling materials to the dentist. Fig. 63 shows the clinic arrangement schematically. Teamwork of this sort needs careful planning, and there must also be flexibility between the two dental assistants, one assuming the duties of the other instantly if routine is disturbed by some unexpected occurrence. The ratio of dentists to dental hygienists may easily change, particularly in clinics dealing with classes of low-caries children.

Since the pioneer work of the Public Health Service at Richmond, considerable sophistication has taken place in the utilization of dental assistants within currently accepted patterns of dental operating.[4] The term *four-handed dentistry* is now given to the art of seating both the dentist and the dental assistant in such a way that both are within easy reach of the patient's mouth. The patient is in a fully supine position. Newly designed dental equipment and carefully planned trays containing instruments for the operations scheduled for a given session permit the assistant to hand the

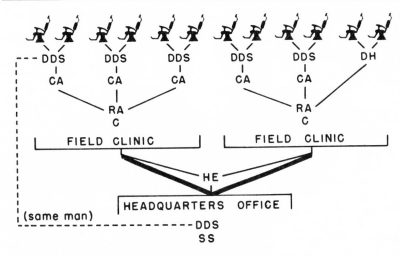

Figure 63. Schematic deployment of U.S. Public Health Service dental team in Richmond, Indiana, 1946–1951. *DDS*-dentist (one also is director); *CA*-chair-side assistant; *RA*-roving assistant; *C*-clerk (also acts as roving assistant); *HE*-health educator, working in advance of operators; *DH*-dental hygienist; *SS*-secretary-stenographer.

dentist a particular instrument at the moment he needs it. She also performs additional auxiliary tasks such as retraction or aspiration. This enables the dentist to keep his hands and his eyes in the field of operation. He can thus work with less fatigue and greater efficiency than was possible with even the most well-developed chair-side assisting of two decades ago. Not all operations, of course, lend themselves to such systematization, but the routinely performed tasks constituting the major part of dental practice can usually be adapted to four-handed methods.

Additional light upon the efficiency of the dental assistant is given by the American Dental Association's 1965 *Survey of Dental Practice*.[5] This survey shows the mean number of patients per independent dentist to increase in almost direct arithmetic proportion to the number of employees in the dentist's office. Since some three-fourths of the reported employees are dental assistants, this finding reflects primarily the efficacy of the assistant. Dentists with no employees care for a mean number of 876 patients per year. Dentists with 1 full-time employee care for a mean number of 1,235 patients per year. Those with 2 full-time employees care for a mean of 1,382 patients per year, and those with 4 or more employees care for 2,372 patients.

The training of the dental assistant varies with her expected duties. Some dentists who do not expect too much detailed work from their assistants prefer to train them themselves on the job. Many training courses exist, however, most of them extending over a period of 1 year and some for as long as 2 years. Courses of this nature involved business procedures, filing, typing, record keeping, chair-side and dental-laboratory procedures, and even first aid. Certification examinations are given by the American Dental Assistants' Association for graduates of ADA-approved courses. The ADA listed 94 approved programs for dental assistants in its 1968 *Directory*. Subsequent directories have not listed these programs.

Dental assistants can be trained informally by dental researchers and teachers for certain unusual tasks. Thus in a Harvard preventive dentistry research project in a Boston suburb, mothers of school children were taught to supervise fluoride rinse programs and even to apply sealants. For sealants the training program was six weeks long, with the trainees divided into two groups: sealant aides and assistant aides. Four-handed techniques were based on a carefully prepared manual, and a good quality result was obtained.[6]

Expanded-Function Dental Auxiliaries

For some time now, with the New Zealand dental nurse plan as an example, experimental efforts have been made to train dental auxiliaries to perform operations of a limited nature in the mouths of patients. Dental assistants have been chosen for these trials, and the duties have involved those procedures which were generally agreed to be *reversible*—that is, they could be either corrected or redone without undue harm to the patient's health. The assistants would not prepare cavities or make decisions as to pulp protection after caries had been excavated, as do the New Zealand dental nurses, but would work alongside the dentist and take over routine restorative procedures as soon as the cavity preparation and base had been completed. Assistants with such duties are called *expanded duty or function dental auxiliaries* (EDDAs or EFDAs).

In Alabama, a group of dental assistants was trained, over a 2-year period, in such a way as to receive basic instruction in dental science to approximately the level of the dental hygienist, and then instruction to perform the following operations:

1. Placing and removing rubber dams.
2. Placing and removing temporary restorations.
3. Placing and removing matrix bands.
4. Condensing and carving amalgam restorations in previously prepared teeth.
5. Placing of silicate and acrylic restorations in previously prepared teeth.
6. Applying the final finish and polish to the previously listed restorations.

After a period of clinical trial the work performed by these women was compared with that of senior dental students at the University of Alabama School of Dentistry, and the ability of the women to do work as good as or better than that of the dental students was clearly demonstrated.[7,8]

At Louisville, Kentucky, the U.S. Public Health Service has taken similarly trained dental assistants and placed them in a specially designed dental clinic so that one dentist was in charge of four auxiliaries and had access, in addition, to roving assistants and clerks to perform non-chair-side duties. Oval operating facilities have been designed with sterilizing and supply arrangements in the center accessible by a passageway. There are eight alcoves on the perimeter, each with a dental chair facing outward. In each alcove is full equipment for a modern dental operatory, often experimental equipment. Two dentists man each such "wheel." In a given alcove the expanded-duty dental auxiliary, the EFDA, seats a patient, performs initial inspection, and then, with x-rays available (taken in another room), calls for the dentist on a very carefully prearranged appointment schedule. The dentist examines the patient, performs diagnosis, and specifies a plan for treatment. At that session or a later session, the dentist gives local anesthesia and prepares a group of cavities, perhaps on a quadrant basis, inserting pulp-protection and cement bases. The EFDA helps him in a four-handed relationship. Thus the assistant sees and participates in all initial decisions and operations upon the case and is recognized by the patient as a responsible member of the operating team. The dentist then moves on to the next alcove while the assistant moves to the patient's right-hand side and completes the restorations. If problems arise, the dentist is only a few feet away and can be called back for consultation. A team spirit pervades this setting, which produces good patient cooperation as well as efficient operative dentistry. Certain procedures in the prosthetic field are made the subject for similar team action, on a separate day of the week when no operative dentistry is done.[9]

Since the Louisville program offered comprehensive dental care to a fairly average adult population, it is interesting to note the distribution of the dentists' chair-time by procedure category, first in the baseline period and afterward in the experimental period. Fig. 64 shows this distribution. It will be noted that 43 percent of the operating time of the dentist during his baseline period was taken over by the expanded-duty auxiliary in the experimental period. Operative dentistry is seen to be the largest component of this chair-time. The other categories, making up 29 percent of the total, include crown and bridge, denture prosthesis, oral surgery, endodontics, and pedodontics. It is an oversimplification, however, to place all the auxiliary duties together after the dentist's

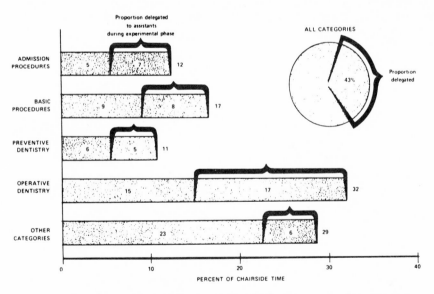

Figure 64. Distribution of dentist's chair-side time by procedure category and proportion of time delegated to assistants during experimental phase, Louisville program.

duties. The two are usually interspersed in such a way as to complicate description.

The first large-scale service application of the expanded-duty principle has been made in Philadelphia. Four of the dental clinics of the Philadelphia Department of Public Health have been rebuilt so that one dentist can work with three EFDAs, or, as they are called there, "technotherapists." David A. Soricelli, then Director of the Division of Dental Health, has reported, on the basis of 5 months' evaluation, that the average technotherapist produced work that is approximately 50 percent "superior" or better, 7 percent "needing improvement," and the remainder in various ranges of satisfactory.[10] Since each technotherapist takes a load at least equal to that of an average dentist, Soricelli estimates that the output of a dentist is increased by three or four times when working in this situation.

There seems little doubt about the economic advantage to the private dentist of the use of expanded-duty auxiliaries. Redig et al. studied three private dental offices in California for a period of 1 year, each office using one or two EFDAs on a full-time basis, and found that the net incomes in these offices increased by 44, 38, and 26 percent, respectively.[11] Integration of the EFDAs into conventional private-office practice was not easy, but results in terms of production and patient acceptance were good. Chapko et al. have studied the time saved per operation through the use of EFDAs performing the list of tasks permitted them in Washington state.[12] Of the dentists studied, 31 percent delegated infiltration injections to hygienists at an average saving of 3.66 minutes each time; 66 percent delegated the insertion of temporary fillings or crowns to an assistant with an average saving of 16.10 minutes each time. Twenty-five different tasks in all were delegated, with an average saving of 6.41 minutes each time performed.

All dentists, especially those in public health work, now need to know how to manage personnel and how to plan delegation of treatment functions with proper sequence and timing. Standardization of operative techniques is important, as is an understanding of quality-appraisal techniques. The techniques of four-handed dentistry are probably valuable, but Soricelli finds them too dependent upon the long-term accurate coordination of two individuals to be valuable where the dentist is working with a number of different EFDAs.[13] Modification of traditional four-handed dentistry techniques is an important aspect of team dental care.

Increasing experience in the use of EFDA teams has produced some interesting observations in the field of human relations. At Louisville, careful studies demonstrate that the dentist, because of his freedom from technical work when the patient is incommunicado, actually has more time than before to develop personal contacts with his patients.[14] Whether or not he does so seems to vary with the individual dentist. Some dentists are careful to develop personal contacts. Others tend to become monopolized by coordination duties, but there is never any doubt about the dentist's professional control of the patient's case. In Philadelphia, Soricelli reports a tendency for patients to concentrate on their personal relationships with the EFDAs (technotherapists) rather than with the dentists.[13] The patients seem entirely happy with this arrangement.

Both Campbell and Soricelli report the need to guard against the absence of an operator, and against monotony, by arranging for rotation of duties.[13,14] A trained EFDA will handle appointment work part of the time or will shift from operative to prosthetic, x-ray, or other phases of chair-side work, to provide a change of pace. There should always, if possible, be one more EFDA scheduled for a given session than the number that are to be engaged in actual operative work.

The American Dental Association and other professional groups are recognizing the validity of teamwork arrangements of this nature and are encouraging such further experimentation and service programs as will be permitted by liberalized state dental-practice acts. State licensing boards in more than 40 states have now passed statutes or regulations permitting varying degrees of expanded duties for auxiliaries.[15]

Some question exists as to whether the EFDAs of the future should be taken from the ranks of dental assistants or dental hygienists. There is a lot to be said for the development of one senior, all-inclusive auxiliary in the dental profession to match the registered nurse in the field of medicine. The dental hygienist, with an educational program far above that planned for any other dental auxiliary except the New Zealand–type dental nurse, is on her way to becoming such a senior auxiliary in the Western Hemisphere. To exclude her from the field of caries treatment may reduce the interest and the satisfaction of her job. It also forces on young persons at the outset a choice as to whether they will undertake training to help the dentist on caries or periodontal disease—one disease but not the other. A decision of this sort is difficult for an untrained person to make, and may easily impede recruitment.

In the field of training, firm curricular patterns have not yet emerged, but the U.S. Department of Health, Education, and Welfare had been encouraging university programs through TEAM (Training for Expanded-Duty Auxiliary Management) grants to dental schools. In many locations it was possible for dental schools to combine facilities with community colleges, junior colleges, and other institutions that had special programs in paramedical subjects.

In 1973, 17 dental schools had TEAM grant programs in progress. The U.S. Army had 22 EFDA teams in actual operation. The Indian Health Service had 200 or more EFDAs in service, some in sophisticated teams and others performing extended duties only occasionally. Fifty more were being trained annually. State and local governments were moving more slowly. Only Philadelphia and Puerto Rico had EFDA clinics in service. Further experience in service settings is still needed, together with cost-benefit analysis (Chapter 19).

Dental Laboratory Technician

Second in numbers but first chronologically among the professionally trained auxiliaries in the dental field come the laboratory technicians. This group has little impact in the fields of preventive dentistry and dental care for young children, but affects in a very important way the efficiency of dental treatment for older patients. Current estimates place the number of laboratory technicians in the United States at approximately 45,000, less than half of these being employed by dentists in private offices.

Apprenticeship has traditionally been the means of recruiting people for this field. Originally, apprenticeship was carried out in the dental office, the dentist teaching the technician and retaining him in the office later as an employee. Under these conditions the quality of the training varied with the ability of the dentist, but more important, perhaps, the relation between dentist and technician always remained close. The chance that the technician would perform unauthorized and hazardous procedures in the human mouth in the absence of the dentist was reduced to a minimum. Two facts, however, have operated to disturb this relation. First, only a very few dentists have enough prosthetic work to delegate to justify the employment of a full-time technician. Thus, technicians have tended to work for a number of dentists, and in the course of this have set up their own quarters. Second, the procedures involved in dental prosthetic work are often such as to profit by division of labor. One technician becomes an excellent porcelain worker, another an expert gold worker, and so on. Much of the plaster work and simpler plastic work can be delegated to the apprentices in the laboratory. Here is a reason for the grouping of technicians, an obvious impossibility in the average private dental office. These two factors have fostered the development of commercial laboratories in independent quarters.

Schools for dental laboratory technicians now exist with curricula covering as much as 2 years. The World Health Organization Expert Committee considers 3 years of training to be probably desirable, if possible.[1] Accreditation machinery for dental laboratories now exists in the United States, supervised by the American Dental Association. The Association itself accredits training programs in dental laboratory technology. Forty-nine accredited programs were listed by the U.S. Bureau of Health Manpower in 1980.[16]

There are now some 5,000 commercial laboratories in the United States, employing the large majority of all technicians. These laboratories, representing as they do the lifetime careers of a large group of people, have tended to become independent in action as well as in location. On the credit side, they have pioneered many advances in prosthetic dentistry, chiefly in the field of dental materials and their utilization. On the debit side, an occasional laboratory usurps the field of the dental practitioner. A dental chair is installed in the laboratory, served perhaps on a part-time basis by a dentist employed by the laboratory, but at other times available to the technicians who will carry out all phases of prosthetic treatment for a patient, contrary to dental-practice laws. Where violations of this sort exist, the dentist is often as much at fault as the technician. It is a continuing challenge to the dental profession to maintain professional leadership and realistic business practices in this field.

In a quantitative sense, the value of the laboratory technician is indicated by the American Dental Association's recent estimate that 70.4 percent of the dollar value of all dental laboratory work was done in commercial laboratories. Utilization of dental laboratories did not vary much region by region throughout the United States, though it was lowest in the Northwest and in the Central states. The American Dental Association also reports a tendency for dentists with a small amount of laboratory work to send it all to commercial laboratories, whereas dentists with a large amount of laboratory work tend to do more of it in their own offices.

In some states in the United States, technicians fabricating full and sometimes partial dentures are allowed to carry the entire process through from impressions onward in direct relationship with the patient. These technicians are called *denturists*. The American Dental Association has firmly opposed denturists in the United States on the ground that patients were endangered by lack of supervision and care from anyone but a fully qualified dentist. No end-result studies have come to my attention to substantiate this claim, however, and in the United States fabricators of limbs and other prostheses are commonly allowed to deal directly with the patient, as do pharmacists following a doctor's prescription. Prosthetic adjustments may or may not require further consultation with the doctor. Maine in 1977 passed a limited denturist bill, permitting technicians licensed and examined by the Maine State Board of Dentistry to fabricate full dentures under the direct supervision of a dentist.

Consumers, in contrast, have often favored denturism. Oregon, in 1978 passed the first state legislation permitting it, on the basis of an affirmative referendum. In August 1985, the American Association of Retired Persons urged its members to support similar legislation in other states. One of their staff members argued that "denturists work directly with patients from start to finish. They provide more personalized service, more follow-up, and post-delivery care than most dentists are willing to provide."[17] Cost effectiveness was also considered to be a factor.

Dental Hygienist

The development of the dental hygienist as a professionally trained auxiliary in the dental office has been outlined in Chapter 3. Dental hygiene is the only auxiliary dental service in the United States which involves direct contact with patients, and as such it has become a subject for state licensure. Licensing procedures for hygienists now exist in all states. The importance of the dental hygienist in a public health dental program was recognized from the start by Dr. Fones, but in spite of this nine out of ten dental hygienists now practicing in the United States are employed in private offices. In either location they have considerable impact on the quality of preventive dentistry and upon the volume of dental care rendered. The Bureau of Health Manpower lists almost 150 schools for dental hygienists, all of them either part of, or in some way affiliated with, an accredited college or university.[16] The standard curriculum is 2 years in length, though 1 year is thought appropriate by the WHO for countries wishing to train hygienists to enter their governmental health services.[1] The output of the schools in the United States approximates 4,000 per year, and it is estimated that about 32,000 hygienists are in active practice full or part time throughout the country. Few exist now in other countries.

The usual functions of the dental hygienist are cleaning of mouths and teeth, with particular attention to calculus and stains; topical application of fluorides, sealants, and other prophylactic solutions; screening or preliminary examination of patients as individuals or in groups, such as schoolchildren or industrial employees, in order that they may be referred to dentists for treatment; instruction in oral hygiene; and resource work in the field of dental health education. Actual classroom teaching is possible where additional training in education has been received. In a public health program the hygienist goes where dentists cannot, and presents a point of view much closer to that of the children with whom she is usually working than could the dentist. Her exact function in a dental public health program will be discussed later. It has been estimated that the amount of dental care provided in the United States might be expanded by 25 percent if a maximum number of hygienists were employed by dentists.

Hygienists in the United States are clearly looking for expanded duties, for more representation on professional boards, and for relaxed supervision. During 1984 legislation was introduced on these matters in 11 states. Alaska now permits hygienists to administer local anesthetics and expand their activity in other ways. Washington permits certain expanded functions under general supervision. Similar bills died or were defeated in 5 other states.

Limited Dental Practice by Auxiliaries

The range of operations performed by the dental hygienist upon the dental patient is so narrow that it hardly merits the two years of training usually required for certification. Workers in countries other than the United States, however, have assumed limited roles in the practice of dentistry under various circumstances, and, since they increase the manpower available where opportunities for dental education are limited, the role of such auxiliaries should be examined with care.

Perhaps the most familiar example of dental practice by auxiliaries has existed in Germany until recently. The fully educated group of dentists in this country have been and are termed *Zahnärzte,* while a numerous independent group termed *Dentisten,* trained primarily by apprenticeship, have shared the practice of dentistry in practically all phases except exodontia and oral surgery. To a system such as this the term "two-level dentistry" has been applied. The contrast in education between the two groups is startling, yet legal differentiation between the responsibilities of the two groups has been almost lacking. Public opinion, to be sure, allowed some differentiation between the skill of the *Zahnärzte* and the *Dentisten,* but low-quality work on the part of the *Dentisten* became so widespread that this group of practitioners was done away with in 1955.

A more carefully thought out program for limited practice of dentistry by auxiliaries is that found in New Zealand. In this country, young women are given a 2-year training course at a Dominion Training School for Dental Nurses, at the successful completion of which they are taken into government service as full-time dental nurses in the school system. Each dental nurse then becomes responsible for 500 or more children, for whom she is expected to provide dental care at 6-month intervals. Her duties include dental examination, dental health education, cleaning of teeth, cavity preparation, the placement of cement bases and amalgam, silicate, synthetic porcelain, and cement fillings, the capping of exposed pulps, and the extraction of primary and permanent teeth, using local anesthesia. Her curriculum gives the dental nurse an even larger number of hours devoted to oral diagnosis and to operative dentistry than is commonly seen among dental schools in the United States. Her educational duties include instruction not only of individuals but of groups such as school classes, teachers, and parent-teacher associations. For this work she is given instruction in teaching and in public speaking.

The work of the dental nurse is performed under the general supervision of a district principal dental officer, who delegates certain of his responsibilities to a dental nurse inspector. There are some 13 districts in New Zealand; each principal dental officer has some 100 nurses under his supervision. The principal dental officer visits the school dental clinic perhaps once every 6 weeks, the dental nurse inspector perhaps twice as often. Definite rules are laid down for the referral of patients requiring treatment beyond the scope of the dental nurse. Liaison between the government dental service and the public is maintained by a school dental clinic committee comprised of key people in the school system, the local dental profession, and such community groups as the parent-teacher association.

Levels of Supervision

A distinction needs to be drawn between *direct* and *general* supervision. Direct supervision is uniformly interpreted to mean that the supervisor (dentist) should be on the premises where the auxiliary is at work, though not necessarily in the same operatory. Frequent inspection of work is assumed, though not specifically required, as is the availability of the supervisor to answer detailed questions arising in the work of the auxiliary. EFDAs customarily work under direct supervision, since they share operations with a dentist, until the dentist moves to other operations for other patients at adjoining chairs.

General supervision is of importance when the dental team must perform part or all of its work at a location where the dentist cannot easily be present and is not actually needed. Thus, the dental hygienist can act as a scout for the dental team at a school or nursing home or do sealant work, without taking the time of a dentist. Careful, specific protocols, preferably written, and suitable training are needed for such assignments. The supervising dentist should monitor the work from time to time, but only often enough to ensure consistently good quality. Chapter 19 describes an instance where the cost per child of a sealant program was more than doubled and its availability decreased by the insistence that a dentist always be present while the hygienist-assistant team did the work.

General supervision is the method used in New Zealand and to a somewhat lesser extent in Australia, where the supervisor is in fairly close direct contact with 1 or 2 of his therapists in his central clinic, but not with 6 or 8 more. General supervision, implying trust from above and full contact between auxiliary and patient, appears to conduce to much better morale, particularly among experienced auxiliaries, than does direct supervision, where the supervisor is on the premises and checks results frequently. Direct supervision is also usually associated with a system whereby the dentist performs *all* examination of patients. This greatly increases the cost, scheduling, and general complexity of the service. It decreases flexibility. An officer of the New Zealand Dental Association told me once, "If you want to sabotage your program, insist that a dentist screen every case."

In New Zealand, the dental nurse plan celebrated its fiftieth anniversary in 1971. It now achieves utilization of dental services approaching 98 percent for the child population up to age 13, on a half-yearly maintenance status. The Department of Public Health is no longer seeking to expand its nurse corps but is actually cutting down the number of new dental nurses to be graduated each year. In 1972 a corps of 1,350 nurses could be maintained by the graduation of 200 new nurses per year. In 1984 that number had dropped to 30.[18] The corps of nurses on duty still numbered 1,300. This change appeared to result from an increase in job satisfaction, leading to increased career life. New Zealand nurses on the average are now spending almost 11 years apiece in service, many of them coming back to work after their children are old enough to be away from home.

Above age 13, adolescent children to age 18 are cared for at government expense in private offices, thus easing the transition to private care in the adult years.

The quality of dental care in New Zealand has been appraised by U.S. examining teams on several occasions and found to be excellent.[19,20,21] The World Health Organization, contrasting decayed, missing, and filled teeth among 13–14-year-old children in 5 different countries found the New Zealanders (Canterbury) to have the second highest total DMF tooth count but the lowest counts of decayed and missing teeth (Fig. 65).[22] This result reflects at least three factors: the assignment of dental nurses to no more children than they can maintain adequately per year, the good quality of the care, and the logistic advantage of bringing dental care to the children in clinics which are parts of the schools in which they normally congregate. Cost savings are also part of the picture, as discussed in Chapter 19.

Starting in 1966, Australian states have adapted the New Zealand plan to rapidly growing programs using so-called dental therapists. Tasmania, South Australia, and Western Australia have operating services, while New South Wales, Victoria, and Queensland have schools just beginning to graduate therapists. In South Australia, with a population of less than 2 million people, 2 training schools were in operation in 1977, and 69 school-based clinics.[18] The regional dental officers here supervise only 8 to 10 therapists and have operatories of their own where they perform operations beyond the usual scope of the therapists.

The New Zealand plan has spread to many other countries: England (London), Malaysia, and a number of other Southeast Asian countries, and in the Western Hemisphere, to Canada (Saskatchewan and other provinces), and to several Latin American countries. The United States has not yet become involved (1985).

The World Health Organization has now published a study of dental care delivery systems by dentists in 12 regional areas, based on data collected between 1973 and 1981. Extremely careful data collection has produced a clear picture of dental practice in Australia, New Zealand, Norway, West Germany, and Japan (these countries studied in 1973), and now Canada, East Germany, Ireland, Poland, and the eastern United States.[23] Although nonmetropolitan areas adjacent to principal cities are studied, the

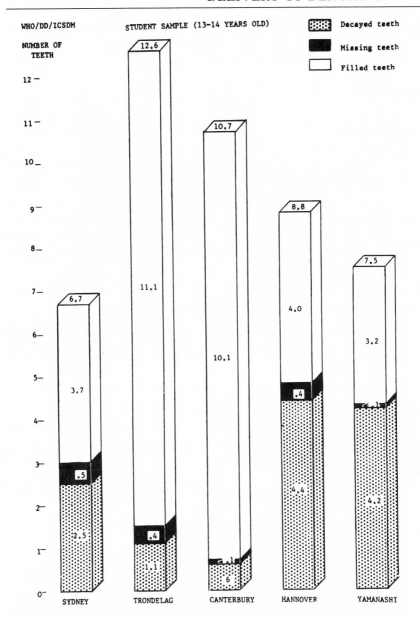

Figure 65. Oral-health status (presumably caries) of children aged 13–14 in areas of Australia, Norway, New Zealand (Canterbury), West Germany, and Japan, 1973–1974. [From World Health Organization/United States Public Health Service Collaborative Study, "The International Collaborative Study of Dental Manpower Systems."]

findings cannot be generalized to include either areas where sufficient providers were not available or parts of large countries other than the cities listed. Behavioral science material is included to a large extent, but the effects of water fluoridation and climate upon caries incidence are not considered. Caries and other oral needs figures are given for ages 8–9, 13–14, and 35–44.

The delivery systems had a number of predominant characteristics. Private practice with self-employment and direct payment was found in Australia, Canada, and the United States. Private practice with self-employment and indirect payment (insurance) was found in West Germany and Japan. Mixed private and public practice with mixed employment status and payment method was found in Ireland, New Zealand, and Norway. Public practice with salaried dentists and indirect payment (taxes) was found in East Germany and Poland.

Among the more interesting findings of the study are those for New Zealand and Norway, each country having a cold, damp climate and an extraordinarily high incidence of caries. Both countries have achieved outstandingly high filled-tooth ratios (F/DMF) among children 13–14 years old (see Figure 65), but by very different delivery systems. New Zealand (Canterbury) has a dentist-population ratio of 1:4330 in the nonmetropolitan area and an average of 1.27 operating auxiliaries per dentist. Norway (Trondelag) has a nonmetropolitan ratio of 1:1950 and no operating auxiliaries.

New Auxiliary Types

New techniques call into being new types of auxiliary personnel. In Sweden, with no community fluoridation programs to turn to, fluoride rinse programs have become widespread. Here, the supervisors of mouth rinse programs are called dental nurses. They are actually trained dental assistants with approximately one month's additional instruction in mouth rinse supervision and the simpler forms of dental health education. They are full-time government employees under general supervision only, going from school to school organizing rinses and, where the classroom teachers desire, giving basic dental health instruction.

Some countries have an acute dentist shortage and have no facilities for training dentists. Here, unusual measures must be taken to provide even the most rudimentary dental care for the population. The Expert Committee on Auxiliary Dental Personnel of the World Health Organization suggests two new types of dental auxiliary for such situations: the dental licentiate and the dental aide.[1]

The *dental licentiate* should be a semi-independent operator trained for not less than 2 calendar years to perform dental prophylaxis, cavity preparation and fillings of primary and permanent teeth, extractions under local anesthesia, drainage of dental abscesses, treatment of the most prevalent diseases of supporting tissue of the teeth, and the early recognition of more serious dental conditions. These people, presumably men, might be responsible to a fully trained dentist-in-chief at the national level, or, perhaps more realistically, to the chief of a regional or local health service. Supervision and control would probably be remote, as their service would probably occur in rural or frontier areas. Measures should be taken to increase the duration of their training and their educational requirements above the bare minimum as soon as possible.

The *dental aides* are conceived to be persons of even briefer training who would perform functions somewhat similar to those of the medical corpsmen now seen in military service. Their duties would include elementary first-aid procedures for the relief of pain, including extraction of teeth under local anesthesia, the control of hemorrhage, and the recognition of dental disease important enough to justify transportation of the patient to a center where proper dental care is available. The dental aides would operate only within a salaried health organization and be under such supervision as was possible under the circumstances: the closer the better, particularly at first. The teaching of sterilization procedures to the dental aides is regarded as of great importance. Formal training might last for from 4 to 6 months, followed by a period of field training under direct and constant supervision. The need for dental aides will probably disappear as soon as a sufficient number of dental licentiates or fully qualified dentists become available.

Frontier Auxiliaries

In developed countries with dentists in the urban centers, the number of areas too distant from public or private dental offices for the inhabitants to receive regular comprehensive care—or even emergency pain relief—remains distressingly large. Capable lay people, in particular nurses and former dental assistants, can provide a valuable service in these areas with a minimum of training. Simple dental prophylaxis can be performed, basic dental health education can be provided, dental first-aid can be rendered in cases with pain, and patients can be referred for the long trip to the nearest dentist more intelligently than would be possible by untrained people. Fluoride rinse programs can be organized under certain circumstances; simple denture repairs can be performed.

In 1981 I reported on a one-week training program for such "frontier auxiliaries" in Alaskan communities 40 or more miles from the nearest dentist.[24] The principal topics covered were:

1. Categories and functions of recognized dentists and dental auxiliaries. Situations requiring reference to these persons, either on an emergency basis or on a convenient trip to the city.

2. Dental anatomy, including names of teeth and tooth surfaces, and eruption times. Impacted teeth and some indication of whether they would be likely to cause trouble. Malocclusion and some indication of its severity and whether it would be likely to diminish as the child grew older.

3. Simplified outline of the caries process. Indications for sedation or temporary filling of troublesome cavities. Palliative measures for apical abscess: drainage, sedation, antibiotics to use in cooperation with the nurse, and necessity for eventual reference to a dentist for endodontic treatment or extraction.

4. Periodontal diseases in outline: gingivitis, chronic destructive disease, pericoronitis, and Vincent's infection. Indications for palliative treatment.

5. Prevention of dental disease. Toothbrushing, dentifrices, nutrition (a few basic concepts), and fluoride measures with emphasis on rinse programs.

6. Outline of the process of dental prophylaxis, with emphasis

on the opportunity thus afforded for recognition of early disease, including malignant or premalignant conditions.

7. Dentures, with indications for replacement, relining, or repair. Simple methods for temporary reline or relief of sore spots.

8. Basic list of the most useful textbooks, instruments, and medicaments. Care and sterilization of instruments.

9. Importance of learning the limitations of the auxiliaries (even dentists have their limitations, for the field of dentistry is now so large that no one person knows it all).

Two years later, case reports from two of the communities showed that a large variety of simple dental problems had been solved and intelligent references had been made to urban dentists for elective work or for prompt treatment after subsidence of acute infection.[25]

In Nyanga, Africa, the American Friends Service Committee reports a program where a physician trained a team of 4 local health workers to provide preventive and primary care, including extraction of teeth, to nearly 12,000 people who previously had little or no access to health care.

ORGANIZATION

Dentistry, like all other health fields, has become vastly more specialized in the past century and the effect is the more bewildering to an outsider because dentistry is a specialty of medicine to begin with. Specialization within dentistry has by now outstripped teamwork among professionals to the extent that one of the major complaints of the public is that the various specialists do not get together enough, and the patient, therefore, is left without adequate orientation. Teamwork can be a real help in coordinating the services of such diverse operators as the general dentist, the orthodontist, the oral surgeon, the pedodontist, and the physician. Each should know what the other is doing and be prepared to help him do it. Such teamwork becomes easiest when these practitioners are gathered under one roof. Group practice is the result.

Group Practice

The term *group practice* is most often applied to small numbers of practitioners responsible only to themselves, but the principles of organization used by these people are equally applicable to larger clinics, whether they are independent or are operated by a more all-inclusive agency such as an industry or a government. Some description of the small, independent group practice will therefore be of interest as a means of understanding those larger groups which have come to dominate so much of our professional life.

Most modern group practices differ from the old master-apprentice system in that the doctors concerned are more or less equal. They may be partners or they may be employees of a small organization run either by themselves or by a consumer cooperative of the people they serve. All the doctors have a more or less equal voice in management of the group when it comes to professional standards and ethics. Diversity of skills also sets the modern group practice apart from that arrangement, more common in the past and still frequently seen, whereby one senior practitioner trains a number of associates, most of them presumably being in his own field.

There must be at least one general dentist in each group, but the group will fail in one of its most important aspects if there are not specialists as well. These may be full specialists with limited practice or they may be "semispecialists." By a semispecialist is meant a general dentist with a special interest, special experience, and perhaps even full specialized training in a given dental specialty, but with no desire to limit his practice exclusively to that specialty. Many such dentists already exist, particularly in urban centers. They attract patients who have problems predominantly in the area of specialization but who also want a general dentist for periodic recall, preventive service, and referral to other specialists, if needed. Endodontics, periodontics, prosthodontics, and even, occasionally, oral surgery are handled in this manner. A group practice offers an ideal location for such dentists, since easy interchange of cases with dentists in other fields of concentration is available.

A fully developed group practice will naturally have one or two dental hygienists and a dental laboratory staffed by one or more technicians. Occasionally it may include a health educator, who may or may not be a hygienist, and who devotes full time to the indoctrination of new patients in plaque control and other features of home care, and to detailed explanations of many dental procedures, such as endodontics, where the dentist may wish to save time for more direct treatment during his appointment with the patient.

Dentists are included in many large group practices covering all the major phases of comprehensive medical care. As prepayment plans become increasingly associated with the larger organizations, it is likely that the number of all-inclusive groups will increase.

Group practice involves a number of organizational problems. Most groups form by merger of solo practices, but the process is not complete until full partnership has been arranged, with a unified system of bookkeeping and records for the group and financial equality through salary after a fairly short trial period. As the group gets larger, a nondentist business manager will usually be hired, and at least two students of the subject feel that ownership and management of real estate should be located outside the group.[25] The group eventually becomes more than the sum of its members. It develops a group image and group integration, in which individualities merge and consultation and peer review become natural. Patients, though often associated primarily with one dentist, accept a multiple dentist-patient relationship when they realize that the group operates as a team. The patients have a further advantage in continuity of care if their original dentist leaves the group.

A multitude of details require careful organization in group practice, but almost all of these problems are also present in the more mature solo practices. There should probably be one senior person in the group to act as chairman at meetings of the partners and as "communications officer" between times, but voting equality between all the partners is still both possible and desirable.

To justify all the complexities of group practice, there are important advantages. For the *patient,* they are:

1. *Quality of care.* The availability of several operators with different skills makes consultations quick and easy. The daily contacts between the operators—some of them specialists—work as an informal peer-review system to improve the knowledge and perspective of each operator. Referral among operators, where necessary, is easy for the patient, and no one operator is tempted to go beyond his field of competence.

2. *Continuity of care.* The patient's records are available to other members of the group if the regular dentist is unavailable.

3. *Convenience.* The "shopping-center concept" makes it easier for several different services to be rendered to a given patient, or to members of a family, all in one place. Billing and recall procedures are also simplified.

4. *Economy.* The centralization of reception, billing, purchasing, instrument sterilization, and other services may reduce overhead costs below those found in comparable solo offices. Informal specialist consultations may sometimes be available without charge where little time and communicative effort are involved. Cost-benefit analysis is beginning to measure these economics convincingly, in terms of cost to the patient per year (see Chapter 19). In terms of productivity, there are a number of studies indicating that the more auxiliaries a dentist uses, the higher his personal income and productivity, as mentioned earlier. Thus in 1975 the American Dental Association reported an average solo dentist with no employees to be making a median net income of $15,500, while a dentist with six or more employees was making $50,000.[27] Gross income varied more sharply. The use of expanded-duty dental auxiliaries has been specifically reported to have increased productivity as well as net income per dentist in a California study of private offices.[28] While use of dental auxiliaries is not per se the same as group practice among dentists themselves, good auxiliary utilization appears far more common in group practices than in solo practices. Reductions in cost to the patient might be possible; whether they have actually resulted, in our present inflationary era, is another matter.

5. *Security.* The reputation of a group is usually additive to the reputation of the individual dentist. The patient feels more secure knowing that good specialized care and good continuity of care are within his reach.

For the *dentist,* the advantages of group practice fall under the same headings. He can improve his own performance more easily than he could alone. He has associates to cover for him if emergencies or vacations threaten the continuity of his patient commitments. He has the convenience of a laboratory in the building, and a number of other services more reliably run than might be possible in a solo office. And the financial outlook is definitely a better one; he can serve more patients per year, and even with more auxiliary salaries to pay or share, he can still earn a higher income. Financing of equipment charges or insurance coverage also become easier. He gains security, particularly at the beginning of his career when the sponsorship of a group gives a young dentist a quicker start in practice. This security can also be important at other times, as in the case of disability.

Disadvantages of course exist. Personality conflicts, some of them associated with loss of individuality, may plague the members of a group. The location and the business procedures of the group may not please all members. Some patients may find bigness itself a disadvantage and fear being shuttled back and forth from one operator to another. But these problems are often correctible, and group practice does not mean the elimination of solo practice. There will still be solo offices for those dentists and patients who cannot adapt well to a group.

From the public health standpoint, group practice is advantageous in that it permits a given number of dentists to serve a greater number of patients per year without loss of quality. Also, groups can sometimes locate successfully in areas where solo offices would be culturally less acceptable (Chapter 10).

Group practices among dentists alone are understandably less common than among physicians, but in 1982 over 42 percent of the participants in the American Dental Association survey of dental practice were partners in practice, employed by other dentists, or sharing some items of office overhead.[5] This compares with a figure of under 4 percent of the dentists in the 1950 survey of dental practice similarly employed.[29] The increase in group practice over a 30-year period is striking.

Part-time Practice

It is becoming increasingly common for dentists to divide their time between offices, either private or public. The private offices may be either solo or group in nature. The public offices may be university health centers, school-based dental clinics, or neighborhood health centers. In these cases communication with professional colleagues or simply a change of pace is usually found to be more rewarding than any financial advantage. Physicians get the same advantages from their hospital appointments, in addition to providing bed care for their patients. Oral surgeons always need hospital connections, as do an increasing variety of dentists in certain situations. Dental school teachers derive advantages from part-time appointments, as do dentists in public health programs.

The Closed-Panel Concept

Group practices are frequently called closed-panel practices. This term derives from the efforts consumer groups or industries have frequently made to arrange group purchase of dental care for their members or employees from a limited number of dentists. These organizations hope thus to obtain not only better-quality care, through the selection of superior practitioners, but also some control over prices. Unfortunately, such closed panels have occasionally been ill-selected and have produced highly visible examples of poor quality, cut-rate dentistry. For a number of years now, the American Dental Association has been opposed in principle to closed-panel systems because of such abuses and because of the limitation upon choice of dentist that such systems impose. Gradually, however, it has become recognized that many dental closed panels can actually be superior in the care they render.

The term *closed-panel* includes a wide variety of dental care programs that have, almost of necessity, been administered by a limited-personnel selection system. Lindahl has identified the several types of programs.[30] They can be summarized as follows:

1. So-called open panels in which beneficiaries are provided with diagnosis or treatment planning or both at designated facilities or offices and then referred for treatment to dentists in the community.

2. An "open-closed" panel arrangement in which a consumer group arranges with a fairly large number of private practitioners to accept their beneficiaries at agreed upon fees-for-service.

3. Dental group practices, which in addition to their fee-for-service patients may contract with consumer groups.

4. Clinics or mobile dental units serving indigent schoolchildren, university students, or other special population groups.

5. Neighborhood health centers for the residents of defined areas, of whatever funding, public or private.

6. The health maintenance organizations which feature prominently in health proposals by the federal government.[30]

It is true that in all these systems a limited number of dentists are involved, but it is incorrect to state that patients cannot seek care from family dentists or dentists outside the panel. Patients can and frequently do seek such care, either within or beyond the scope of the service offered by the closed panel. In doing so patients may sacrifice some of the financial benefits for which they are eligible.

There is a strong consumer desire to choose dental care programs as well as dentists. Reporting for the Council on Dental Care Programs and the Council on Dental Health of the American Dental Association, Lindahl recommends that "it would be much more realistic and practical if the dental profession vigorously advocated dual choice of plan for consumers eligible for dental benefits."[30]

Newcomers in this spectrum of dental care delivery systems are the *preferred provider organizations* (PPO) and *contract provider organizations* (CPO). Essentially these are groups of dentists who offer, in the spirit of cost containment, a guaranteed maximum fee scale or benefit package of a competitive nature. They advertise, and make contracts with consumer groups. They usually charge their participants a membership fee and may limit the number of members. They may be managed by a nonprofessional agency, such as an insurance company. The quality of care offered by participating dentists may or may not be a matter of concern. Among the benefits offered by the larger PPOs are practice management consulting, corporate identity, relocation services, referral services between providers, and marketing services. The PPO and CPO concept has caused sharp controversy within the dental profession, centered chiefly on the management powers exercised by nondentists.

The decision between an open-panel and a group-practice program must often rest upon cultural factors. The "culture of poverty" has been mentioned in Chapter 13, indicating that there is an economic and psychological difficulty in getting lower-income families away from their residence areas and into private dental offices which operate upon fairly exact appointment systems. In such circumstances the people are far more easily assimilated into institutions such as health centers and settlement houses which have been built in their own vicinity and with their own particular needs in mind. Closed-panel or group-practice dental services are usually easiest to arrange in these situations. For serving school-children, small school-based clinics—almost by definition closed-panel ones—have no equal in bringing about high utilization of a public dental care program. New Zealand and Australia rely entirely on school-based clinics for their excellent results. The United States, in its concentration upon private practice, has down-graded such clinics. It is time for government service to be given a higher priority here, and for the quality of public clinics to be raised.

Neighborhood Health Centers

When disadvantaged people group together in deteriorated or ghetto areas where private medical and dental practitioners are not to be found in adequate numbers, unusual steps must be taken to provide them with health services. Neighborhood health centers are a modern attempt to do this. Similar centers are often needed in isolated rural areas.

City or even neighborhood health centers have been known for several generations. Usually, they have housed the offices of the local health departments and of certain closely allied community voluntary health agencies. Certain specialized services have been rendered in these health centers, dental care often being one of them. Auditoriums and other facilities have been provided for community health-educational gatherings. In the past, however, these centers were located more for civic dignity and the convenience of the professional staffs than for their accessibility to low-income groups. The present-day concept is to put the neighborhood health center right where the low-income people live, in a place that will seem homelike to them. Certain services must be provided in homes, and good primary medical and dental care must be provided in the center. The center should act as a referring agency to sources of specialized care or hospitalization. It must be a place where people are known as individuals and as families; and the various phases of their health care should be coordinated on a continuing basis. A legal mechanism now exists for justifying these qualifications: the "certificate of need" now required by some state-level comprehensive health-planning agencies.

The constituent elements of poverty—inadequate and improper diet, decayed housing that lacks the most primitive sanitary facilities, ignorance about personal hygiene—coalesce to create a disease-ridden environment. Such a situation, in the view of the Office of Economic Opportunity, has prevented the poor person from taking advantage of educational and training opportunities that might equip him for work or, once equipped, from seeking and keeping steady employment.[31] Thus, the neighborhood health center has a real function in vocational rehabilitation. It also has an unusual opportunity to train and employ local people. By employing local people, the center becomes more personalized. The community takes greater pride in the place, and better liaison with the community is established by the management of the health center. Community health advisory committees are an additional mechanism frequently used to improve liaison.

Supportive services offered by a neighborhood health center usually include public health nurses, social workers, and home counselors. The "nurse practitioner" is coming into service now, performing an expanded list of duties that were seldom delegated to nurses in urban areas, though they have often been so delegated in frontier areas. Health education is provided in the neighborhood center in connection with medical and dental visits. The center also serves as a focus for the health programs in the local schools and throughout the community.

In the field of community dentistry, dental-hygiene teachers, with offices and often with certain duties in the health center, can go to elementary and even high schools for purposes of classroom teaching, individual dental screening, and referral of children to sources of dental care. Oxman et al. have described a classroom curriculum giving varied approaches to the problem of dental health and dental care for children all the way from kindergarten through grade 12.[32] Dunning and Sanzi have documented the changes in community dental status that can occur in an interval as short as 3 years.[33] These changes include an increase in the filled component of the DMF tooth counts, a shift from emergency-treatment toward maintenance-treatment classification upon dental screening, and, in one limited area, an actual reduction in incidence of new caries. Fourth- and fifth-year surveys, following the above report, show a continuation of the same trend. On a different level, the center can serve for training and sensitization of dental students and dental auxiliary students from nearby dental schools. The center can also serve as a recruitment area for health professionals from minority groups.

The delivery of dental care at a neighborhood health center should approximate that of a well-developed group practice in method, even though the financing may be different. The center is an ideal location for the use of expanded-duty dental auxiliaries. Busing programs can bring dental patients to the center, thus eliminating many of the problems of supervising children as they are taken through city streets from school to the clinic, and assuring a smaller proportion of failed appointments than would be the case otherwise.[34]

While neighborhood health centers now attract more attention than school-based dental clinics in the United States, the reverse is true in Australia and New Zealand. There, the health services for children are firmly established in school-based clinics, with a utilization rate far surpassing most American school dental services.[35] Adult dental services, using these school-based facilities, are planned, at least in Australia. The Advisory Committee on Dental Health to the U.S. Department of Health, Education, and Welfare has recommended careful study and evaluation of all aspects of a school-based children's dental care program (Chapter 20).[36]

Health Maintenance Organizations

In current proposals for national health insurance, increasing attention is devoted to the restructuring of delivery systems for medical and dental care. Most prominent among the suggestions made is that of the health maintenance organization (HMO). Essentially this is either a large private group practice or a neighborhood health center, offering comprehensive care in all the major health areas including disease prevention, and with the concept of prepayment built in. It is conceived as a meeting-ground for advanced programs in the delivery of care and in the financing of care. Some federal legislation has already been passed to aid the financing of such organizations. More legislation may be expected.

The U.S. Department of Health and Human Services maintains

that a health maintenance organization is based upon four principles: "(1) It is an *organized system* of health care which accepts the responsibility to provide or otherwise assure the delivery of (2) an agreed upon set of *comprehensive health maintenance and treatment services for* (3) a voluntary *enrolled group* of persons in a geographical area and (4) is reimbursed through a prenegotiated and *fixed periodic payment* made by or on behalf of each person or family unit enrolled in the plan."[35] The first two of these principles imply patterns in the delivery of health care that are more or less familiar, but should be modernized, as by the increased use of dental auxiliaries with expanded functions. The innovation lies in the third and fourth principles, which postulate an enrolled group under periodic prepayment or *capitation*. Prepayment for individuals already exists to varying degrees in such programs as those of Blue Shield, the dental service corporations, and various other insurance carriers (Chapter 18). Prepayment of services for individuals will become universal under national health insurance. Why then the emphasis upon enrolled groups? It is easy to realize the increased health care benefits that accrue to the consumers of well-organized health services through group enrollment in recall systems that facilitate preventive health care procedures. Clerical procedures also become more efficient, in part through the planning of capitation fees or annual premiums based on actuarial experience. It is also easy to realize the desire of financiers to eliminate the adverse selection of cases that usually accompanies individual enrollment and to avail themselves of the funds that result from underutilization, which is more common in groups than in individual memberships.

The difficulty arises when an individual must become part of a group whether he wishes to or not, losing benefits if he makes other arrangements for health care, or by chance finds himself a member of two groups. It is perfectly possible for a working man and his family to be drawn into more than one HMO—one connected with the breadwinner's occupation and another with the geographical area in which the family lives. How are groups to be stratified so that they do not overlap one another or leave serious gaps? Industrial employees and their dependents have been the most attractive prospects for HMO enrollment, but geographical areas are much easier to separate one from another, and afford the opportunity to merge the unemployed and indigent segments of a population with the wage-earners. Some means must be found in the near future to straighten out these conflicts and permit individuals to enter and leave easily any given HMO.

There can be no denying the value of the pioneer work being done by the small number of health maintenance organizations now in existence. They are experimenting with methods for delivering health care in both middle-income and low-income areas. They are building a data base from which larger-scale prepayment plans can be reliably designed. They are providing experience in the contrasting of fee-for-service payment, fee-per-visit payment, and yearly capitation payment. No one of these is perfect, yet each has advantages, as yet inadequately documented. Among the best-known examples of privately managed health maintenance organizations are the Kaiser Foundation Health Plan; the Health Insurance Plan of Greater New York; the Group Health Cooperative of Puget Sound, Washington; the Group Health Association of Washington, D.C.; the Harvard Community Health Plan of Boston; and the San Joaquin Medical Care Foundation of California.

Certain situations seem better suited to HMO development than others. Colleges are in this category. Yale has pioneered in an urban setting. Clemson University, in South Carolina, is planning an HMO in a rural area.[37] Located in the foothills of the Blue Ridge Mountains, Clemson is the intellectual center of a community of 16,000 to 18,000 people served by only four private physicians. The University, with a student body of 8,000, has two full-time general physicians and a psychiatrist. A real opportunity for leadership exists here, and dentistry should be a part of it.

Cronkhite gives a checklist of problems confronting those who would organize HMOs:

1. Risk sharing is necessary during the early stages of development.

2. Exceptional efforts will be needed to reach low-income and unemployed people and people who live in areas with inadequate health manpower.

3. The financing of an HMO by government requires careful thought on the provision of adequate rewards to providers for efficient service, and for reserve funds for expansion of the HMO.

4. Evaluation of service must include attention to cost, consumer satisfaction, and outcome.

5. The HMO must be "marketed" in order to reach its assigned group. The traditional modesty of professional ethics must surrender to the need for informing the public as to services offered.

6. Financial incentives and other satisfactions to consumers and providers should be equalized in order to assure continuing success.[38]

These problems give some indication of why the HMO concept has been slow to take hold. In September 1978 there were 203 HMOs reported in the United States, 69 of which were qualified to receive federal aid.[39] Only 21 of these, however, were identified as providing "comprehensive" dental services. The difficulties of applying insurance methods to comprehensive dentistry are examined in Chapter 18.

The minimum dental care required for government support has been oral prophylaxis and topical fluoride treatment for children through age 11. It would be easy to design a package of preventive and emergency dental care for all ages beyond this one, for which a modest capitation fee could be charged within the main membership premium of an HMO. Fluoride therapy could be expanded to all relevant age groups and coupled with brief dental health education. Screening of patients and referral for further care could be included. Temporary fillings and minor denture adjustments could be combined with a variety of first-aid procedures for the relief of acute pain. Extractions would not be included. The temptation exists to call this package primary dental care, but that term is at present used in dentistry for a simple form of comprehensive care. An application of the package, minus fluoride treatment, to emergency cases in a naval shipyard during World War II is described in Chapter 21.

Since 1978, the development of HMOs has taken on speed. For example, the Harvard Community Health Plan, which then had a membership of about 80,000, rose to a membership of over 200,000 by the end of 1985. Even then it found itself in competition with several other thriving HMOs, all together serving over 800,000 members in the Boston area. The scope of the Harvard plan has increased to the point of covering heart and liver transplants.

The main Harvard Community Plan membership premium in 1985 did not cover comprehensive dental care. Prepayment did cover oral surgery, a preventive dental health plan for children under eleven, and dental care for patients undergoing radiation therapy. Plans were under way for a pilot program to cover comprehensive care for an initial group of some 5,000 members. Tertiary dental care items such as metal-on-porcelain restorations were to be handled on a copayment basis. Comprehensive dental care on a fee-for-service basis has existed in the plan since 1972, and the plan now operates 4 clinics with a total staff of some 85 dentists and auxiliaries.

Mobile Dental Clinics

In rural areas, or even in cities, mobile clinics are often useful. They have long been used in frontier and rural areas, and in cities too there is a great saving in patient transportation time if a dental truck or trailer can be parked in a schoolyard for purposes of screening, preventive care, or even comprehensive dental care. The city of Baltimore has recently invested in several such trucks. A representative design for a mobile dental clinic is shown in Fig. 66. Two dental operatories are included at either end of a 29-foot trailer. Access to the trailer is by a set of folding steps at the center, leading into a reception area. At the back of the reception area is a darkroom accessible from either operatory. Trailers of this sort can be built to use community electricity, water, and waste facilities or to provide their own through batteries and tanks. A trailer is usually more economical than a truck with its own power, since a power unit is not immobilized when the trailer is stationed in any one place for a length of time. Either method, however, is much more expensive than the use of portable equipment. Facilities for renting power units are available in most areas.

Portable Equipment

Large advances have been made in the design of portable dental equipment for a variety of community uses. Dentists can visit home-bound patients for extraction, denture, or other simple work with no more than a few pounds of instruments packed in light zippered overnight bags. This implies foreknowledge of the operations to be performed. It is surprising how much elementary care can be rendered to a patient sitting semiupright in a modern hospital bed or upright in a wheelchair.

An intermediate kit for visits to a group of patients—in a nurs-

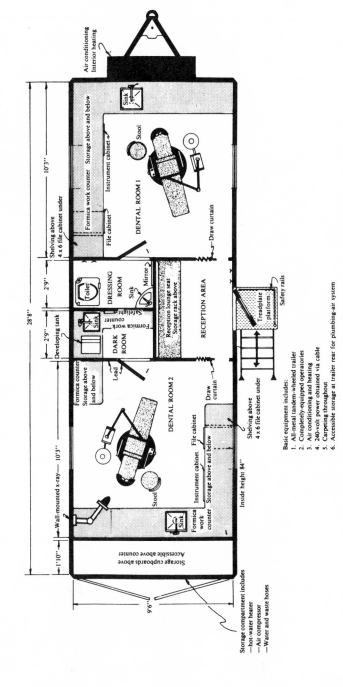

Figure 66. Typical dental trailer. [Courtesy, Medical Coaches, Inc., Oneonta, New York.]

ing home, for instance—would include an instrument case much like those used by dental students of a generation ago, plus a high-torque electric dental engine in a carrying case. The electric engine is combined in at least one commercially available unit with an amalgamator, an operating light, a pulp tester, and an electrically heated wax spatula. The unit can be powered either by house current or by batteries.

When extended comprehensive dental care is to be rendered in locations where a trailer is not available or cannot penetrate because of a lack of suitable roads, a combination of portable modules can supply what amounts to a complete dental operatory. One such assembly includes a chair, stool, light unit, compressor, and a unit with an air handpiece, air and water syringe, saliva ejector, evacuator, and waste system. These items, in four containers, total only about 300 pounds; the largest item, the chair, weighs 160 pounds. Instruments and supplies require additional containers, but all could be handled in a station wagon or a jeep. A smaller assembly, designed for missionary use in underdeveloped areas, involves an upholstered folding chair weighing approximately 50 pounds, a 35-pound self-contained dental unit operating on compressed air, and a small portable air compressor.

The province of Saskatchewan, Canada, makes use of an ingenious combination of fixed and portable equipment as part of a new New Zealand–type dental nurse plan. The Director, M. H. Lewis, describes his arrangements as follows:

There are approximately 15,000 children eligible for dental care this year in Saskatchewan. These children are scattered over a vast area of country and are frequently bused up to 20 miles to the closest elementary school. Saskatchewan has a declining school population and therefore most schools have an empty classroom or similar space which may be adapted for use as a dental clinic. To call these areas a dental clinic is perhaps misleading. The area is partitioned off from the rest of the school; improved lighting and increased numbers of power plugs are installed and a kitchen type sink unit with cupboards above is added.

An air compressor is placed in the furnace room with an air line with a quick connect run to the clinic area. The dental chair has a post-mounted light and is left in the clinic. The unit is an "Adec" mobile type unit which carries its own water system and high volume evacuation with waste collection. It also has a three-way syringe and a high and low speed handpiece. This unit weighs less than 40 pounds and is carried by the dental nurse from school to school. In many schools in the province there are less than 30 children enrolled in the Program and so dental nurses, for the first two or three years, will be doing a great deal of travel, from one school to another. In the larger centres a dental nurse might be established full time in one clinic, but for most of the province dental nurses will travel up to 50 miles from their headquarters to schools in their particular area.[40]

In these various ways, the delivery of dental care can be extended to a wide range of persons not within reach of a typical private dental office.

Functions of Public Clinics

The improved new school-based or other public clinics of the future may be expected to perform twelve functions. First, they will bring comprehensive dental care to people of all ages in dentist-deprived areas. These areas exist both in the ghettos of the inner cities and in sparsely inhabited rural areas. Dentists do not often set up private offices in either place. It is not uncommon to find dentist population ratios of from 5,000 to 8,000 persons per dentist there, in contrast to the ratio of less than 2,000 per dentist that is typical of the country as a whole. The low-income people in these areas are commonly without the means or the money for transportation to private offices in other areas. There are often no facilities to care for other children while the mother takes one child to the dentist. The public school system, however, must and does deal with these problems. Voluntary school busing services are already in existence in both ghetto and rural areas and have been shown to improve markedly the utilization of neighborhood health center dental clinics. When the clinics themselves are located in these schools, the result will be just so much better.

Second, school-based or other dental clinics of the future may be culturally more acceptable than private offices to certain population groups (Chapter 10).

Third, school-based clinics will facilitate classroom and chair-side dental health education during the childhood and early adolescent periods. They can circulate educational material to the entire enrolled population. The staff dental hygiene teachers they have today, and the dental nurses or therapists they could have in days to come, can educate groups in the classroom and also talk to the individual children at chair-side when children are called in for inspection or treatment. They can also deal with parents, seeking their cooperation in home care. This leads to better immediate utilization and to an increased demand for private dental care in later adolescence and adulthood.

Fourth, such clinics will provide an opportunity for cost-sharing programs. These are now seen from time to time in college or neighborhood health services. Certain basic items of dental care can be provided at government expense or through private prepayment, while other, more sophisticated, items of care are available at the patient's own expense, either in the clinic or in a private office.

Fifth, well-run clinics commonly generate the demand for more dental service than they can provide. Where this occurs, the clinics refer the extra patients to private practice. Thus, private dentists in middle- or upper-income areas are more likely to gain than to lose practice through the wise operation of local school-based dental clinics.

Sixth, school-based and other clinics give an excellent opportunity for the use of dental hygienists, and of extended duty dental auxiliaries, dental nurses, and therapists. A variety of employment systems can be built into these clinics, permitting either the direct supervision of auxiliaries by a dentist who is constantly present or the general supervision of auxiliaries in neighboring clinics by a supervising dentist located in the central clinic of the area.

Seventh, public clinics offer part- or full-time employment to young dentists starting, or about to start, a practice, and to older dentists desiring a "change of pace" from private practice. Within the past decade there has been an encouraging rise in the salaries paid to clinic dentists. So long as this trend continues the dental profession need not feel that the existence of public clinics in or near private practice areas will prove an economic threat to the image of dentistry. The greatest development of public clinics, however, should logically occur in areas poorly served by private practice.

Eighth, it is important to realize that public clinics can take a great variety of forms. At one extreme we have the one-nurse school-based dental clinics of New Zealand, bringing both dental health teaching and dental care to rural areas. At the other extreme we have the large "technotherapist" clinics of the city of Philadelphia, each employing several dentists in a well-defined relationship with a much larger number of auxiliaries of various types. All sorts of intergrades are possible. It is important that this country *not* seek one single ideal design for the school-based clinic, but experiment with a variety of formats, several of which are likely to prove successful in differing specific situations.

Ninth, the use of public dental clinics can substantially reduce the cost of dental care through the use of auxiliaries, both by reducing the cost of the training of personnel and by reducing the cost of clinic operations (Chapter 19).

Tenth, to the extent that public clinics employ groups of dentists and paradental personnel, they are natural settings for peer review, both informal and formal. The informal peer review occurs whenever staff members discuss their cases with each other or call each other into consultation. Some leadership is needed here, so that standards will go up, not down—but it can be handled on a friendly rather than an authoritarian basis. Formal peer review is also easier in a public clinic than in a private office. A chain of command exists wherever there is a public or third-party employer. The employer, though not privileged to supersede the professional standards of properly qualified staff members, does have a right to issue guidelines on output, and can sometimes even order disciplinary action. Again, good leadership is necessary. Where pride in a public service has been built up, peer-review procedures can be welcomed, even if arranged by the central authority.[13]

Eleventh, a further advantage to a clinic is the close coordination of medical and dental services there, with consultation on medical-dental problems on a somewhat easier basis than in private practice, except perhaps in the larger group practice.

Twelfth, the final advantage of school-based dental clinics is their ability to provide adult service out of regular school hours. It has proved a matter of considerable concern to school authorities that their physical plants are in use perhaps only 30 percent of the time. Some cities and towns therefore have instituted "community school programs" by which various adult activities may occur out of hours upon school premises. President Lyndon B. Johnson is quoted as having said, "Tomorrow's school will be the center of community life, for the grown-ups as well as the children: 'a shopping center for human services.' It might have a community health clinic, a public library, a theater, and recreational facilities."

Public Relations Factors

While the list of advantages for the public-school-based or neighborhood clinic offers an undeniable challenge, the success of such a clinic depends largely upon good public relations. The originators of the clinic should seek the advice and cooperation of local dental groups and societies, to the extent that these groups know that the services of local dentists are recognized and valued. Local dentists can usually be taken onto advisory committees, or employed part-time for a change of pace. The need for the clinic as an addition to local private facilities must be made clear. This need will ordinarily be made apparent now by certificate-of-need regulations. The function of the clinic as a referral agency, to and from private practice, should be emphasized. Where a community health committee controls the clinic, as in some neighborhood situations, an ethical and responsible division of labor should be worked out between professional personnel and lay managers.

The clinic ideally should be sponsored by local government, as a school-based clinic is, or by some broad-based consumer or citizens' group. It should not "stake out" a geographical area in which it plans to serve all comers, and then publicize itself in this area, unless it has a clear community mandate, or unless the inhabitants are of defined low-income status—as in a housing development— or members of an open third-party payment plan. In other words, the clinic must really *be* public, not just a private enterprise competing irresponsibly with private practice. And it must be designed to serve well the population it claims to serve.

The United States has shown that it can develop public school systems of outstanding quality. It has brought good public education to practically the entire child population of the country. There is no reason why this system should not be expanded to include health—and particularly dental—care for American schoolchildren. We must make our school dental clinics respectable and respected. We must develop them in numbers logically related to the loads they are expected to carry. More than that, we must make them pioneers in the development of new systems for the delivery of dental care that will reach a much larger proportion of our whole population than has ever been reached in the past. These clinics must be objects of pride, not slipshod charity. To achieve such status they must be well-equipped and be staffed by groups that have a strong sense of loyalty, both to their professions—hence good relations with "organized dentistry"—and to the consumer groups they serve.

A final word of caution is needed about the speed with which the development of a school-based delivery system may be expected to produce major changes in utilization of dental care. It is reported to have taken the New Zealand school dental service program more than 20 years of operation before 50 percent of the eligible children were receiving regular dental care and 35 years before 95 percent of eligible children were enrolled.

CHAPTER 18

Payment for Dental Care

THIS CHAPTER will deal with group-arranged methods of payment for dental health programs, such as have arisen in recent years. These methods either help the participant to share catastrophic risks with other people, help him to spread his own health bills over a long period of time, or help to channel financial aid to him from an outside source. There are three main methods by which this is done: insurance, prepayment, and budget postpayment. The methods overlap somewhat under ordinary conditions, and in large tax-supported plans they actually merge. Prepayment is, in a sense, a form of insurance and also involves budgeting. Each method, however, justifies individual consideration. These methods need to be examined for their separate characteristics and also for their adaptation to the needs of administering agencies. Major differences emerge according to whether a given plan is operated by the government, as with Medicaid, by the profession, as with dental-service corporation plans, by the consumer, as with labor union plans, or by private commercial carriers. It is increasingly common, moreover, for agencies to arrange financing from multiple sources and for individual consumers to do the same.

INSURANCE

The use of insurance to help spread the financial burden attendant upon death or severe accident is of long standing. Much more recent is the effort to apply this same principle to current medical and dental expenses. There are three aspects to an event which make it particularly attractive for insurance coverage: (1) unpredictability for the individual, (2) predicability among large numbers of individuals, and (3) a financial burden of catastrophic size if payment falls due all at one time. An individual has little reason to insure against a predictable condition; he can either save up for it, or budget it on an installment plan. For this reason, insurance programs covering items more or less predictable to an individual, such as dental care, usually deal only with groups of policyholders rather than with individuals. Mass predictability is of extreme importance to the insurance underwriter, since wide fluctuations in the frequency or unit cost of the insured condition might easily saddle him with obligations he could not fulfill. The size of the group needed to give predictability, of course, will vary from situation to situation. One hundred cases may be enough to produce a reliable average in one instance, and 10,000 may be needed in another. Finally, the event must be of catastrophic size in order to induce an individual to pay a premium which will include the necessary costs of insurance administration. Fire and theft insurance give good examples of these characteristics, and in the dental field, malpractice insurance does.

Insurance underwriters, to protect themselves, have three more requirements: (4) the event must be infrequent enough to permit reasonable premiums to build up a good reserve fund; (5) the plan must include enough people over a wide enough area that localized disasters such as epidemics will not produce demands involving a high proportion of policyholders all at one time; and (6) the existence of insurance should not of itself increase demand for service unduly. Demands for unnecessary medical attention might thus constitute a hazard to an improperly controlled medical insurance plan. Unnecessarily high limits on liability policies, again, tend to produce unduly high claims.

Insurance is always more expensive than direct payment, because of the cost of selling and administering it. The insurance company, of course, must maintain a reserve fund in order to cover the variations between the in-flow of premium money and the out-go to cover claims. This reserve fund is invested at least in part, and produces income that will defray part of the operating costs of the company. But this reserve fund needs personnel to manage it, and, had it remained in the hands of the policyholders, it would have produced income for them. This loss of income for the policyholder because of advance payment is one of the hidden costs of insurance.

It is easy to see under these conditions why the worst catastrophic events, such as death and severe accidents, were the first to be insured. The cost of hospitalization and of surgical care for specific conditions came next, because such bills can mount up in a way which is entirely beyond the ability of the individual to predict: very heavily in some years, very little or not at all in others.

Most employed Americans now have private health insurance by virtue of their employment status, but there are marked differences in proportion covered according to income level. In 1974, 91 percent of white persons under 65 with incomes of $10,000 or more a year had hospital insurance, but only 28 percent of blacks with income under $5,000 were covered. Less than 40 percent of the "working poor" are reported to have any kind of insurance.[1]

The current Blue Cross-Blue Shield policies concern themselves almost exclusively with infrequent events. Unlimited medical and surgical care for frequent events is not available through voluntary insurance in this country, since self-supporting insurance plans would be put out of business by such liberality unless exorbitant premiums were charged. Compulsory health insurance can handle such a load, as in Great Britain, but only through partial tax support and through salaries to the physicians on a capitation basis (so much money per person per year). This subjects the physicians to demands for unlimited service while offering them limited compensation—a system which can be fairly administered only after a careful study of actual demand.

One of the most recent comers in the health insurance field is also one of the best examples of "pure" insurance. This is *major medical* insurance, specifically designed to cover catastrophic illness. Policies of this sort are based upon the total cost of illness, not upon specific indemnities or fees per operation. They have very high top limits, but premiums are kept under control by a system of deductions which exclude the first payments for episodes of illness up to a certain sum, usually around $2,000. Policies of this sort have done much to spread the burden of the long episodes of chronic illness, seen particularly among older patients.

Dental care has been perhaps the last of the health services to receive attention. The incidence of dental disease is far more predictable on the part of the individual than is the incidence of most of his other complaints. It is true that major prosthetic work presents a financial hurdle which is occasionally very hard to surmount and which may come unpredictably. The average intelligent person, however, has followed his dental condition over the years sufficiently to know approximately when full dentures or large partial restorations will be needed. He is thus able to save up for them or include them in a postpayment budget plan. Routine medical bills themselves are less unpredictable to the individual than would be desirable in the ideal insurance situation. F. G. Dickinson, Director of the American Medical Association Bureau of Medical and Economic Research, has a word of warning on this point.[2] Referring to the fact that a given family will need the services of a physician three or four times a year, he says, "Any attempt to cover usual and minor expenses for medical care, then, actually violates this requirement of uncertainty of occurrence." He then calls attention to the fact that "the premium in such cases must be large enough to cover the cost of initial visits which the policyholder is almost certain to require each year, plus the cost of operating the plan, plus the necessary amount to build up their reserve to meet the occasional severe illness." The policyholder therefore is "actually paying more than he would pay if he dealt directly with his physician for these minor needs."

The only category of dental work lying clearly outside the range of individual predictability is oral surgery and such restorative procedures as follow in the wake of an *accident*. Here we have a situation which provides all the main inducements to insurance coverage. As a result, we have seen oral-surgery benefits included in Blue Shield policies and in many accident and health insurance plans for some years. As insurance underwriters gain experience in this type of coverage, a wider range of conditions is being included and such restrictive conditions as hospitalization during operation are gradually being liberalized. The *indemnity* principle still clings in this area, however. Companies agree not necessarily to reimburse the policyholder for the entire cost of correcting an injury or abnormality, but to pay a fixed sum of money which is usually based upon the minimum cost of correction under ideal circumstances. All insurance policies, of course, carry some sort of top limit, but the term "indemnity" is most commonly used where the payment per operation is set below, rather than above, the average fee usually charged for it. A scale of reimbursement per operation according to this system is known as a *table of allowances*.

Some plans distinguish between *service*-benefit members, who are not subject to an additional charge by a participating physician for services as defined, and *indemnity*-benefit members, who are entitled to receive the scheduled amounts as a credit toward the doctor's customary charge, the difference, if any, being the member's personal responsibility. Service-benefit membership in general is limited to low-income families. Both physicians and dentists generally prefer indemnity plans, because they interfere less with their traditional modes of practice and permit additional charges to be made. Consumer groups, however, usually resent such plans, since they never know how much of the cost of a given operation or illness their insurance will cover.

It is interesting at this point to note the extent to which dental service has been included in the Blue Cross-Blue Shield policies, which grew up so logically to help finance hospital and surgical care. A small list of surgical operations performed by the dentist is usually included in the Blue Shield contract (jaw fractures, impaction removals, and so on), and the dentist is to be reimbursed only if these operations are performed in a hospital, not in his office. The only relatively common operation, tooth extraction, is usually restricted by a proviso in the contract that no credit shall be allowed unless several (as for instance 7 or more) teeth are extracted at one time—a most infrequent occurrence. It is argued that if any of these restrictions were relaxed, the volume of dental care rendered would become so great that compensation at a proper level would bankrupt the program. The hospitalization restriction, however, is open to question at this point. Some borderline surgical cases may now be taken to the hospital at considerable expense to the plan which might well have been handled at the dental office at lesser cost if this restriction were relaxed.

Small claims upon an insurance policy cost almost as much to process as do large claims, and policies perform their function best if the small claims are minimized. A *deductible amount* is therefore defined by the U.S. Public Health Service as that portion of dental care expense which the insured must pay before the plan's benefits begin.[3] An example has been cited in the field of major medical insurance. Many dental care policies include deductible clauses. In general, the insurance companies like these clauses and the policyholders do not, the latter preferring what they call "first-dollar coverage." One great disadvantage in deductible clauses is that they inhibit preventive measures unless special provision is made to except these measures from the deductible arrangement. Catastrophe insurance policies are not very much concerned with prevention measures, but prepayment policies definitely are concerned.

Coinsurance is defined as an arrangement under which a carrier and the beneficiary are each liable for a share of the cost of dental services provided. For example, the dental plan may cover 80 percent of the cost of the particular service, and the beneficiary the balance.[3] Insurers and professional groups alike seem to approve of coinsurance clauses, since it keeps the policyholder interested, financially, in the amount of care he receives, and thus theoretically helps control overutilization of the policy. Coinsurance also helps keep premiums down.

The U.S. Public Health Service has published an excellent booklet entitled *Pre-paid Dental Care—A Glossary,* which includes definitions of many insurance terms and (for the benefit of the insurance people) dental terms most commonly mentioned in insurance policies.[3] Some terms are illustrated diagrammatically in Figure 67.

All forms of insurance, like prepayment, lend themselves to sharing of costs between employer and employee and to group purchase. To the extent that nontaxable fringe benefits thus come into existence and the individual can be aided in a subtle but

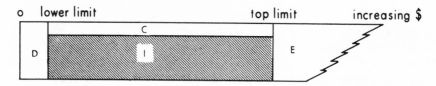

Figure 67. Diagrammatic presentation of hypothetical dental bill under third-party payment. *C*-coinsurance; *D*-deductible; *E*-excluded; *I*-insured.

systematic fashion, insurance plays a role in modern health care greater than might be expected from its merits as a financial device alone.

PREPAYMENT

Financial coverage for comprehensive dental care through prepayment is a problem very different from the "pure" insurance that has just been discussed. Most people learn before they are out of their teens whether they have caries-susceptible mouths or caries-resistant mouths. Most people require periodic dental care, and indeed, the best preventive dentistry is done on this basis, insuring that only the yearly increments of dental care will require treatment, rather than big backlogs of major restorative dentistry with attendant higher cost and damage to health. Thus the need for dental care is anything but infrequent. Dental bills, to be sure, seem high, but in good incremental practices with periodic recall systems catastrophic bills are very unlikely. The individuals most likely to wish to purchase comprehensive dental care coverage are just those caries-susceptible people who will produce the highest claims and bankrupt any insurance program unless the premiums are inordinately high. The formation of groups, therefore, becomes necessary in order to include some low-risk people with the high-risk people.

There are several inducements to the formation of groups for comprehensive dental care prepayment plans. Most important, perhaps, is the convenience of *group bargaining*. A labor union or other consumer group will usually have expert personnel in its management staff, better able to deal with banking and budgeting problems than the individual policyholder would be. "Band wagon psychology" plays a part in encouraging full enrollment. Bargaining is also facilitated by the fact that a labor group can negotiate a fringe benefit, not taxable either to the employer or to the employee.

The financing of a prepayment plan can often be done on an *expense-sharing basis,* the employer paying the basic cost of the policy while the individual employee pays a deductible item, a coinsurance percentage, and the excess over any predetermined maximum yearly limit. Fig. 67 illustrates this concept. The deductible item saves the insurance carrier the high cost of small claims that are better handled by direct payment than through a third party. The coinsurance not only helps reduce the financial burden on the underwriter by a given percentage, but maintains the interest of the patient in the size of the bill that is being run up. The maximum limit exempts the underwriter from unusually high claims, though as a matter of fact these high claims, because of their infrequency, are fairly easily covered by acceptably small additional premiums. The result is a sharing arrangement that permits a combining of the resources of the employer and the employee group. Employers and underwriters traditionally like these sharing arrangements, though labor unions and other consumer groups usually do not.

There are three other inducements to group programs for comprehensive dental care prepayment plans. The first of these is the extent to which such programs facilitate *preventive dentistry.* Periodic visits can be specified, and the best policies will exclude diagnostic and preventive procedures from any deductible item so as not to spoil the inducement toward this type of care.

The second inducement is *installment payment.* It is easy for an insurance underwriter or other fiscal agent to arrange installment payments just the way banks and loan companies do to assist in the financing of automobiles and refrigerators. The American public is used to this system, even if interest charges are involved. If the installments are made by deduction from payroll, the employee never sees them and does not come to count on the money involved. Labor union welfare funds are operated on this principle.

The third inducement is *underutilization.* In spite of the almost universal nature of dental disease, there always seem to be some people, even in the most educated groups, who neglect their teeth or regard them as expendable. These people are often included in consumer groups such as labor unions, and since they do not avail themselves of the care they are entitled to, it is easier for those who do want care to obtain it at a lower cost.

Over the years ground rules have evolved for the design and administration of dental prepayment plans. One of the best sets of such rules was formulated at a joint meeting of the Executive Council of the AFL-CIO and representatives of the American Dental Association on August 5, 1964, as follows:

1. Dental prepayment programs should make provision for insuring high-quality comprehensive dental care.

2. Where dental prepayment programs are organized, preference should be given to programs organized to serve groups within the entire community.

3. Regardless of the organizational structure of a prepaid dental-care program, the practice of dentistry is, of course, the exclusive prerogative of the dental profession; however, the provision of dental health services must also be the concern of the consumer and the public.

4. Freedom of choice for individuals under group programs should include not only free choice of dentist but free choice of plan or program as well. [This implies a choice between open-panel and closed-panel programs.]

5. Remuneration for professional services may be on a fee-for-service, per capita, salary, or other basis, depending upon the plan or program. Such remuneration should meet standards of adequacy in relation to the training and experience of the dentist and to the standards established by the dental profession.

6. Dental prepayment programs should provide for an effective mechanism to insure that the fee procedures stipulated in the contract between the subscribers and the providers of professional services are maintained.

7. Where funding limitations prevent consideration of a comprehensive prepayment program, deductibles and coinsurance should be considered, but the minimization of such features should be given high priority in future developments of the plan or program. High priority should be placed on comprehensive coverage for all patients, particularly children. [The exemption of preventive measures from deductible clauses might well have been mentioned at this point.]

8. Any contract between an organization offering dental prepayment plans and a group of consumers should provide means by which participants may receive the benefit of impartial review of grievances

which may arise out of services provided by the plan or its administration.

9. Provision should be made for public, consumer, and professional representation on the governing boards of dental prepayment and direct service organizations.

10. Dental health education should be part of dental prepayment programs and should be jointly planned and conducted by the dental profession and the consumer organizations involved.[4]

ACTUARIAL DATA

It is the essence of all prepayment dental care programs that an estimate be made in advance of the annual dental needs of the population to be served and the premium be charged on the basis of the cost of meeting these unexpected needs in that portion of the population which will actually *demand* them. Gross errors in any given year can be corrected in a future year by alteration of the premium scale or within the year itself by a draft upon a reserve fund. The plan may protect itself from an overload of extreme individual cases by limiting subscription to members of a preexisting group. Compilations of data on the cost of and the need for dental care locally are most important in the setting up of any prepayment program. Without such data an educated guess must be made and the sponsoring group must take the risk for any miscalculation that may occur during the first years of service. The organization of dental-survey data for actuarial purposes is well described in a Public Health Service booklet devoted to this subject.[5]

A word should be said here about preventive procedures in a program for comprehensive dental care. Dental health education is notably hard to include among services to which fees will be attached, yet time must be taken for proper instruction in oral hygiene, nutrition, and other relevant matters. The more formal plaque-control programs lend themselves fairly well to programs where fees are paid by the service, since the operations of plaque disclosure, toothbrush instruction, and the measurement of debris and calculus by the OHI-S (Oral Hygiene Index-Simplified) or other index are formalized enough to be easily recognizable as operations. Periodontists, whose patients face a visible threat, have made most use of the plaque control procedure, but general practitioners have lagged behind. In one plan in Utah where plaque control was offered, only 5 patients of the 6,000 enrollers used the plaque-control benefits.[6] The money paid for these benefits represented only 0.07 percent of the total for all phases of the program.

Community preventive programs, although their benefits to an individual policyholder are almost impossible to appraise, are much more easily handled where a group of policyholders live in a fluoridated community than where they live in a nonfluoridated one. The Connecticut General Life Insurance Company, for instance, has allowed a 12 percent credit on dependents' rates for dental plans in fluoridated areas.[7] A group policy involving dental care for children can thus be sold in such an area at 88 percent of the cost that would be charged elsewhere, though a variety of circumstances has usually prevented the full application of this discount. The rationale for such a discount is that, in areas such as Newburgh, New York, children have experienced a reduction of about 50 percent in bills for restorative dentistry as a result of prolonged fluoridation.[8]

FEES AND THEIR DETERMINATION

The exact method by which payment to the dentist is calculated is not a part of the general insurance principle and varies from time to time and from program to program. Most common at present is the *fee-for-service* basis, where a fee scale of charges per operation is constructed in accordance with prevailing local rates. Local and state dental societies have often conducted fee surveys in order to provide guidelines for sponsors of prepayment plans. The American Dental Association through its Bureau of Economic Research and Statistics is prepared to aid in the compilation and analysis of these surveys according to standardized techniques.

The fee scales per operation commonly seen today in the offices of American dentists reflect public acceptance as well as professional acceptance, but they are undesirable in that they often provide the dentist with a much greater compensation per chair hour for prosthetic service than for examination work and such preventive procedures as dental prophylaxis and periodontal care.

Inequities of this sort have led to a development of *relative-value fee scales,* based upon "intrinsic value" of certain operations. The American Dental Association Council on Dental Health and its Bureau of Economic Research and Statistics have developed such a scale.[9] It is based upon the judgments of a group of practitioners as to the following four characteristics in relation to an operation:

1. Knowledge: required content, understanding, judgment.
2. Skill: digital dexterity, experience, perceptual skills.
3. Effort: physical, mental, visual.
4. Responsibility: effect of error, correction of error.

Scales of this sort (and there are others) are always subjective to a certain extent, and do not necessarily represent the marketplace. They correct certain inequities, but they cannot be expected to last very long without adjustment. A theoretical disadvantage to a system of fee determination such as this is that it disregards the value of the service to the patient—not only the apparent value, but the true value in terms of disease prevention or control.

The entire question of a fee scale can be avoided, at least to the satisfaction of the dentist, by a system of *usual, customary, and reasonable fees* in which the insurance underwriter agrees to pay the dentist whatever he would "usually" charge his regular patients for a given operation, provided that charge is "customary" in his locale and "reasonable" in relation to other costs of living and in the view of the local dental society. To protect the underwriter, these usual fees must be specified in advance of the contract and must then be adhered to. Individual dentists must submit a "fee profile" for their most common operations, and they must revise this profile from time to time. The underwriter further protects himself from the occasional practitioner whose fees have been very high by specifying that the customary fee limit for a certain operation will be set at the mean value of such fees plus one standard deviation and rounded to the next higher dollar. These statistical constants are taken from a fee survey of a group of practitioners, to all of whom the plan is expected to apply. By this arrangement, some 90 percent of the charges of the dentists within a plan are paid without question. The dentist whose fees are higher will be reimbursed only to the agreed fee limit.

There are differing opinions as to whether this "usual, customary and reasonable" system will raise or lower costs for the consumer. On the one hand, it is argued that if a group of dental practitioners in a given geographical area is surveyed in advance and a fee scale set to represent the average of that group, it will actually be the dentists with average or below-average fees who will take most of the insurance cases, so that these people will actually be paid more money at a fixed fee scale than they would be if they received their usual and customary fees. On the other hand, the psychological impetus to increase one's fees is very great whenever a virtually unlimited reimbursement policy seems in prospect. One representative of labor asserts that "the introduction of the 'usual and customary fee' concept has resulted in an increase in dental fees charged to our people."[10] The dentist, he says, "cannot expect to reap the benefit of organized mass pre-paid plans while retaining every bit of his previous freedom as an independent practitioner." Clear evidence to back either contention seems lacking at the moment.

Any system of fees per operation is criticized from time to time by members of various branches of health service. These people feel that a professional person should charge for services on a time or visit basis and not allow charges to become associated with "commodities" such as inlays, bridges, or dentures. The bookkeeping of a group-care program, too, they argue, is simpler where hours or visits are the unit for payment rather than fees from a complicated table of operations. In terms of motivation, fees per operation stimulate the dentist to good quantity production. The effect upon quality, however, can be adverse. In England, such fees are reported to have led to "scamping," to overtime work of poor quality, to unnecessary, expensive operations, and hence to the creation of dental estimate boards and dental supervisors.[11]

An unfortunate occurrence in fee-per-operation programs has been the tendency among some dentists to charge higher fees to insured patients than to uninsured individuals. Documentation of this tendency comes from a study by Kagabines and Douglass of fees reported by comparable insured and uninsured groups between 1977 and 1983.[12] Fees rose for both groups in this period, but the rise was dramatically and statistically greater in the insured group.

Another fee system new to dentistry but old in the field of medical care is *capitation*. Essentially, capitation is the premium amount which must reach the provider of care annually to cover the cost of care for one average patient. In Britain, where physicians carry a large "list" of regular patients, the individual provider receives money from the National Health Service at a fixed amount per year for each patient who has asked to belong to his list. Individual dentists are unlikely to carry large enough lists of patients to make this system equitable, and in any case have resisted capitation strongly both in Britain and in the United States. Group practices, however, can afford to accept capitation contracts from consumer groups such as labor unions, and are finding it advantageous to do so.[13] Such contracts offer a unique opportunity to emphasize preventive procedures which are hard to measure in a system of fees per operation. Rosen et al., comparing the patient histories from three dentists some of whose patients were on capitation, some on fee-for-service, found that capitation cases were associated with improved preventive methods and fewer fillings.[14]

It has always been a toss-up whether fees-per-operation systems stimulate more energetic and thorough work than remuneration systems based on capitation. There are advocates on both sides of the fence. Naismith puts it well when he says that "both capitation and fee-for-service demand integrity and moral fiber of a dental group."[15]

DIVIDING THE FINANCIAL BURDEN

As mentioned earlier, the chance of sharing expenses for dental care is an important advantage to the prepayment method. Certain groups, such as employers, have a direct interest in the welfare of others. Other groups, such as labor unions, have a vested interest in the health of their own membership. The dental profession, insurance companies, and government all have an interest in the welfare of the public. All of these various groups can accomplish their objective best if they share the financial burden to a certain extent with the people who are insured. Often a tax advantage is involved. Money which is contributed toward a welfare fund by an employer has been taxable neither to the employer nor to the worker.

Subsidy from a noninsured party is best applied, of course, to the premium, which represents the per capita cost of the main contract. A financial item exists here which is relatively predictable for large groups. Employers find in this item an easy way to provide a fringe benefit for their employees. Government finds this the easiest benefit to provide to the public where public demand requires the use of tax funds to provide health care. Government, however, is more likely to restrict eligibility for, and scope of, service than to rely on deductible items and coinsurance.

The question of administrative cost, however, complicates any program where a third—or fourth—party steps in, either to bargain for the premium level or to share the cost. Thus an insurance program bargained for between a labor union and a commercial insurance company must add to the cost of dental care the salaries of the negotiators and the costs of record-keeping in both agencies, thereby raising the cost of care per insurance person.

THE BACKLOG

One reason for the slow growth of dental prepayment plans has been the backlog of accumulated dental needs among persons whose dental care has been unsystematic. These needs have occasionally been found to require as much as five times the dollar expenditure needed for early maintenance of these same persons after they have been brought "up to date." Early prepayment plans avoided this issue by requiring all new enrollees to be up to date when they entered the program. The deterrent effect upon enrollment was too great, however. A possible intermediate solution would be to spread initial costs over the first 3 years, with lower maintenance rates afterward for those who stayed on. Most modern programs, particularly those well-financed enough to take an early loss in the hope of later gains, absorb these initial costs without extra premium.

VARIATIONS IN PREPAYMENT PLANS

Basically, there are four types of sponsors of prepaid dental care in the United States today: (1) consumer groups, (2) the dental profession, (3) commercial carriers, and (4) the federal government. Industrial dental programs, considered to be the precursors of the true consumer plans, began during World War I, with the effort of industry to improve the efficiency of employees. Traditionally an examination and case-finding type of service, these programs were at first very paternalistic in their attitude and usually provided few direct services other than for the relief of pain. Although a few industrial programs have evolved into restorative programs of sorts, with the patient paying a reduced fee, they really cannot be considered to be prepayment plans.

The true consumer-founded prepayment groups, of which the Group Health Association, Inc., of Washington, D.C., is an excellent example, have not been widely successful, perhaps because of the severe financial impediments to the initiation of insured dental care programs. As a matter of fact, GHA required 7 years to evolve its dental program from a fee-for-service to a prepaid basis. It is interesting to note that this type of prepaid plan is very similar to the so-called Friendly Societies which were common in England around the end of the eighteenth century.

It seems quite natural that the most recent developments in the area of consumer group prepayment plans should have arisen at the union-management bargaining table. An early program of this type, known as the St. Louis Labor Health Institute, was founded in 1945, as a result of the establishment of a welfare fund in Local No. 688 of the International Teamsters' Union. The welfare fund, supported by contributions from management of a percentage of gross wages paid, became, in succeeding years, an acceptable substitute for wage increase in union-management bargaining. A full range of dental treatment was offered, including fixed bridges but excluding orthodontics. Utilization, low at first, increased until the Dental Department was at one time the largest single department in the Institute.

Organized dentistry's initial experience with dental prepayment came with the founding of Group Health Dental Insurance, Inc., by the First District Dental Society of New York in 1954. GHDI combined an indemnity plan for families of over $5,000 income with a service payment plan for families of under $5,000 income, with the dentist, in the latter case, accepting a reduced fee as payment in full.

About this same time the first dental service corporation, Washington Dental Service, came into existence. Although dental-service corporations are operated by state dental societies they do not provide direct services, as in the case of GHDI. Rather, they act as administrators and fiscal intermediaries in prepaid dental care plans which are, in turn, sponsored by labor unions, government agencies, employers, and similar interested groups.

Commercial carriers entered the field of prepaid dental care in the late 1940s, with a few scattered Blue Shield plans including oral-surgical procedures performed in hospitals and small indemnity payments for traumatic injuries to teeth. Comprehensive plans, however, were slow in developing until around 1960, when an accumulation of favorable experience resulted in considerable expansion of commercial plans. By 1976 they covered some 19 million persons, or over one-half of all persons participating in dental prepayment plans. It has been suggested that commercial plans, characteristically involving deductibles and coinsurance, have a tendency to inhibit the utilization of preventive services, which are usually not covered because of relatively low initial cost. Table 42 summarizes the sum total of third-party dental payment plans operating in the United States in 1966 and again in 1983. Note the amazing growth which has occurred over a 10-year period.

A new and controversial development in sponsorship is the appearance of many investor-owned for-profit (IOFP) hospitals, often in chains. Their rise has been favored by the existence of some not-for-profit (NFP) hospitals, poorly run by administrators of borderline competence. The IOFP hospitals have relied upon the American corporate image of efficiency, cleanliness, and success. Some have achieved these objectives, but subject to a charge, not yet clearly documented, of skimming off the better-paying pa-

Table 42. Approximate number of persons covered by third-party payment plans for dental care, 1966 and 1983.

Administrative mechanism	1966	1983
Commercial companies	900,000	71,100,000
Dental-service corporations	1,000,000	15,600,000
Blue Shield surgical	20,000	10,400,000
Other programs	1,200,000	6,000,000
Total	3,100,000	103,100,000

tients and operations, leaving others to the NFP hospitals. Other criticisms have included interference with quality of care through a differing doctor-patient relationship, and failures such as have been seen in the private management of railroad passenger service. Much further experience is needed in this area, and a pluralistic outcome could be the result, with both types of hospital management successful and working in concert.

GOVERNMENTAL PLANS

The role of the federal government in dental care has been that of provider of funds rather than services. Since the passage of the original Social Security Act in 1935 the government has furnished formula grants to states for the provision of dental care to certain categories of needy persons, that is, dependent children, crippled children, the blind, and so forth. More recently, project grants, made available by the Economic Opportunities Act of 1964, have provided funds for dental care for certain population groups, under such programs as the Neighborhood Health Centers and Head Start. With Title XIX of the Social Security Amendments of 1965 (Medicaid) came financial assistance for dental care for large segments of the American lower and middle classes.

All states by now have taken advantage of the provisions of Title XIX. Funds are made available to the states on a matching basis to provide, among other things, dental care for the medically indigent. Chapter 22 gives some general principles as to eligibility and priorities among the groups to be served, for state programs may be implemented piece by piece. Dental prepayment plans under Title XIX may operate either in an individual office setting (open panel) or in a clinic (closed panel), but the financing has often been different for these two settings.

In private offices, dentists are usually reimbursed on a fee-for-operation basis according to a scale arranged by the state administrative authority, in consultation with the dental society of the area. A "usual, customary, and reasonable" arrangement may also be made for the setting of fees. The indemnity principle, however, with permission for additional charges, is seldom if ever allowable. In a clinic setting, the concept of *reasonable cost* may govern reimbursement, just as it does in hospitals. The administrative agency for Title XIX may reimburse the clinic pro rata for those costs which relate to the serving of eligible patients under the plan. In practice this can be arranged by setting a scale of fees (usually considerably lower than private-practice fees) which, if applied to the yearly output of the clinic, will equal its cost. These fees are then applied per operation to those clinic patients eligible for the program, and bills for these services are sent to the Title XIX administrative agency. Dental schools and clinics operated by a variety of private or public agencies, including those operated by town or city governments, may receive reimbursement under this method. Patients have free choice of dentist under Title XIX, so that they need not attend clinics if they wish to go to private offices and can find practitioners willing to take them. In spite of this, many public clinics are surviving, particularly in poverty areas.

The open-ended nature of Title XIX necessitates measures to control the costs of care, particularly dental care. Aside from administrative measures related to the efficiency of the operation, the three basic ways to control costs involve limitation of *eligibility*, limitation of *scope* of service, and reduction of *fees*. Most adjustments are likely to be made by the first two of these methods, since reduction of fees below reasonable levels will force Title XIX back into the category of a charity program, like the old welfare dental services. A reduction in the quality of care might result from such a change, and a large number of dentists might be expected to withdraw from participation in the plan. Limitations upon the scope of service are likely to prove easiest. The mechanism of *prior approval* permits local discussion as to the authorization of operations which do not appear to be within the agreed limits of basic and essential dental services, but are valuable when special needs exist and funds permit.

Eligibility requirements for Medicaid vary greatly from state to state, and so also do the age groups receiving benefits. In recent years some 25 million persons were recipients, some 4 million of whom received dental care. Generally, children receive the largest share of Medicaid benefits; only 32 states offer care to adults. Political scandals, occasional fraud, and problems in the payment of dentists' claims have decreased Medicaid's usefulness, but over the years many low-income people have received care who would not have done so otherwise.

Apart from Medicaid grants for dental care, states in the past have received categorical grants for the support of fluoridation. With the advent of the Republican administration in 1981, some 40 federal categorical grants for health and social services were consolidated into four block grants to the states. In one of these blocks fluoridation was combined with several other categories of disease prevention and health care, and the money was given to the states with few strings attached. States have been able to decide how they will divide the money within the various programs in the group. Thus they have been able to support new and ongoing fluoridation programs, but they cannot become involved in the legislative contests for their initiation. This distribution of money to states has not affected the continuation of the section within the Center for Disease Control of the U.S. Public Health Service in Atlanta where information on the scientific aspects of fluoridation is available.

DENTAL SERVICE CORPORATIONS

The mechanism of the dental service corporation needs particular attention because it not only is a full-fledged financial mechanism for administration of prepaid care but goes further to express the concern of the dental profession for the quality of care. Dental service corporations are separate legal entities and distinct from their sponsoring dental societies; organizational policies are determined by members of the dental profession. Mitchell and Hoggard have ascribed five characteristics to a dental service corporation:

1. Professional sponsorship.
2. Nonprofit operation.
3. Participation permitted by all licensed dentists with the state.
4. Benefits provided on a service basis.
5. Freedom of choice allowed for both patient and dentist.[16]

Three of these characteristics need qualification at the present time.[17] First, the Delta Dental Plans Association and its affiliates are no longer "sponsored" by Dental Associations. Their organization policies are set by mixes of dentists and nondentists. Next, no mechanism which pretends to control quality can avoid the responsibility of debarring a member of the dental profession who consistently violates the rules of an agreement or provides poor-quality service. The Delta Plans, however, do what they can to influence quality through review of claims, reporting standards, use of regional consultants, random review of patient care, and program design to promote preventive care. Finally, the reference to benefits on a service basis may not always be true, although service-type programs seem indeed to be the major objectives of most dental service corporations. Schedules of allowances are mentioned by Mitchell and Hoggard as a possible payment mechanism for service corporations. These allowances place the program on an indemnity, not a service, basis, when they permit the dentist to charge to the patient any amount in excess of the listed allowance. This robs the policyholder of any exact knowledge of what services his policy usually covers in full.

The major concern of the dental profession in promoting dental service corporations appears to be the minimization of interference in the direct dentist-patient relationship by placing quality-control procedures in the hands of the profession itself. Evaluation of quality of care is discussed in Chapter 19. There is no doubt that dental service corporations do have an opportunity for quality control which is generally lacking in plans financed by commercial carriers. In commercial plans the patient can only maintain the quality of his care by changing dentists if he is dissatisfied. This opportunity for the maintenance of quality, Penchansky warns, is no more than a potential. "Whether service corporations will ever take steps to elevate standards is another question. Like Blue Shield organizations, which have made few attempts to influence the quality of medical services, dental service corporations may content themselves only with weeding out obviously substandard dental work."[18] Data do not exist that would prove or disprove the theory that higher quality of care accompanies professionally controlled prepayment plans.

Although dental service corporations have been organized and operate mostly at the state level, the need has grown clearer over the years for coordination and service at the national level. The National Association of Dental Service Plans came into being in June 1966, under auspices of the American Dental Association. Its first function was to facilitate the exchange of information among states. A more important function, however, was the creation of a vehicle through which individual dental service corporations could participate in the so-called multistate marketplace. A broad variety of interplan agreements has been projected, including agreements on such matters as nomenclature, benefit description, contract limitations and exclusions, rating considerations, and the development of a uniform dental claim form. The ultimate objective of the National Association of Dental Service Plans, now renamed Delta Dental Plans Association, has been the creation of a system of multistate dental service prepayment programs.

In 1983 there were 47 active state-level Delta Dental Plans, each with a number of intrastate programs. There were over 50 national (multistate) programs administered by Delta for large national corporations and other organizations. Of the 15 million persons served by Delta programs, 4 million were cared for through Medicaid, the Veterans' Administration, Bureau of Indian Health, the Office of Economic Opportunity, or state health agencies.[17] The Council on Dental Care Programs of the American Dental Association, working with the Delta Dental Plans Association, has worked to standardize and approve dental insurance claim forms, as shown in Fig. 68.

POSTPAYMENT

One of the oldest aids to the financing of dental care, and one avoiding many of the complexities of repayment, is postpayment. Postpayment involves nothing more than the spreading over a period of time of a lump sum of already existing indebtedness. Patients in private practice are constantly making use of bank loans to pay their dental bills without ever involving the dentist in the transaction. Dentists, too, wishing to aid patients, permit installment payment of bills for initial care, but in doing so they lose interest on the credit they have extended the patient and they take the risk of default in payment, as well.

Perhaps the first organized interest in postpayment was taken by banks. The first dental personal-loan plan of which we have knowledge was instituted by the National City Bank of New York in January 1929.[19] The Bank of America on the West Coast entered this field 2 months later, and made a strong drive for dental, medical, and hospital accounts. Business of this sort grew among

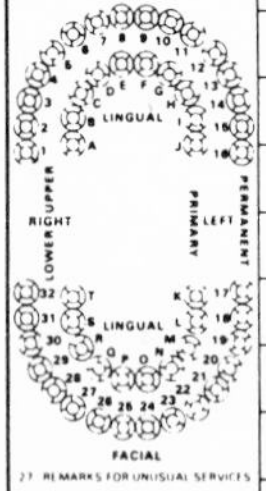

ATTENDING DENTIST'S STATEMENT
CHECK ONE
☐ DENTIST'S PRE-TREATMENT ESTIMATE*
☐ DENTIST'S STATEMENT OF ACTUAL SERVICES

Dental Service
of Massachusetts
P.O. BOX 2496
BOSTON, MA 02208

SHADED AREA DSC USE ONLY

1 PATIENT NAME | 2 RELATIONSHIP TO EMPLOYEE: SELF, SPOUSE, CHILD, STUDENT, HANDICAPPED | 3 SEX: M, F | 4 PATIENT BIRTHDATE: MO, DAY, YEAR | 5 IF FULL TIME STUDENT SCHOOL

6 EMPLOYEE SUBSCRIBER NAME FIRST INITIAL LAST | 7 EMPLOYER SUBSCRIBER I.D. NO | CITY

8 EMPLOYEE SUBSCRIBER MAILING ADDRESS | 9 EMPLOYER (COMPANY) NAME

CITY STATE ZIP

10 IS PATIENT COVERED BY ANOTHER DENTAL PLAN? | DENTAL PLAN NAME | UNION LOCAL | GROUP NO | NAME AND ADDRESS OF CARRIER

I have reviewed the following treatment plan. I authorize release of any information relating to this claim.

Signed (Patient, or parent if a minor) Date

FOR SERVICES OUTSIDE MASSACHUSETTS
Sign here for authorization to pay benefits to Dentist.
I hereby authorize payment directly to the Dentist named below of the Dental Service Benefits otherwise payable to me.

Signed (Patient, or parent if a minor) Date

11 DENTIST NAME
12 MAILING ADDRESS
CITY STATE ZIP
13 DENTIST SOC. SEC. OR T.I.N. | 14 DENTIST REGISTRATION NO | 15 DENTIST PHONE NO
16 FIRST VISIT DATE CURRENT SERIES | 17 PLACE OF TREATMENT: OFFICE, HOSP, ECF, OTHER | 18 RADIOGRAPHS OR MODELS ENCLOSED? NO, YES, HOW MANY?

19 IS TREATMENT RESULT OF OCCUPATIONAL ILLNESS OR INJURY? NO YES | IF YES, ENTER BRIEF DESCRIPTION AND DATES
20 IS TREATMENT RESULT OF AUTO ACCIDENT?
21 OTHER ACCIDENT?
22 ARE ANY SERVICES COVERED BY ANOTHER PLAN?
23 IF PROSTHESIS, IS THIS INITIAL PLACEMENT? | (IF NO, REASON FOR REPLACEMENT) | 24 DATE OF PRIOR PLACEMENT
25 IS TREATMENT FOR ORTHODONTICS? | IF SERVICES ALREADY COMMENCED ENTER | DATE APPLIANCES PLACED | MOS. TREATMENT REMAINING

26 EXAMINATION AND TREATMENT PLAN — LIST IN ORDER FROM TOOTH NO. 1 THROUGH TOOTH NO. 32 — USE CHARTING SYSTEM SHOWN

IDENTIFY MISSING TEETH WITH "X"
FACIAL / LINGUAL / RIGHT / LEFT / UPPER / LOWER / PRIMARY / PERMANENT / LINGUAL / FACIAL

TOOTH # OR LETTER	SURFACES	DESCRIPTION OF SERVICE (INCLUDING X-RAYS, PROPHYLAXIS, MATERIALS USED, ETC.)	DATE SERVICE PERFORMED MO	DAY	YR	PROCEDURE CODE NUMBER	DENTIST'S FEE	INTERNAL CODE	CREDIT TOWARD DENTIST'S FEE	LOCATION	UNIT	LINE ITEM
						0	00			1	01	1
						0	00			1	01	2
						0	00			1	01	3
						0	00			1	01	4
						0	00			1	01	5
						0	00			1	01	6
						0	00			1	01	7
						0	00			1	01	8
						0	00			1	01	9

27 REMARKS FOR UNUSUAL SERVICES

DENTIST'S STATEMENT: *I HEREBY CERTIFY THAT THE SERVICES LISTED HAVE BEEN OR WILL BE PROVIDED BY ME.*

TOTAL FEE ACTUALLY CHARGED ▶ 00 | DISP. CODE 1 | PAYEE CODE 1

Dentist's signature *Date*

CLAIMS FOR CROWNS, INLAYS AND ONLAYS SHOULD INCLUDE PREOPERATIVE XRAYS.

*PLEASE NOTE: PREDETERMINATION OF BENEFITS DOES NOT GUARANTEE PAYMENT.

Pre-Treatment Estimates are calculated based on current available benefits and patient's eligibility. Estimates are subject to modification based upon remaining benefits available and eligibility which applies at the time services are completed and a claim is submitted for payment.

REPORT DATE

MAIL THIS COPY TO: Dental Service of Massachusetts
P. O. BOX 2496, Boston, Mass. 02208

4017 (10-84) stock no. 260230
Form Approved by the Council on Dental Care Programs of the A.D.A. 1975

Administered by **Blue Cross** of Massachusetts

DENTAL SERVICE CLAIMS COPY

Figure 68. Dental claim form approved by American Dental Association.

the banks, but it was not until 1935 that the first dental society plan was established in recognition of the profession's interest in promoting and helping control personal loans for dental care. The first dental society postpayment plan of which we have detailed knowledge resulted from cooperation in 1941 between the Detroit District Dental Society and the Detroit Bank and Trust Company.[20] A few years later the California State Dental Association and the Los Angeles County Dental Society entered independently into successful arrangements with the Bank of America. The Los Angeles County plan in the first 6½ years of its existence purchased $20,865,846 worth of notes from dentists, covering 78,838 cases.[21] This business has now been taken over by the major credit card companies. Many dentists accept payment through such agencies as Visa and MasterCard, where loans are available. The interest of organized dentistry in the credit control offered by society-sponsored programs and the interest of banks in the quality control offered by such programs has passed into other areas, notably insurance and prepayment.

COMBINATIONS OF AGENCIES

The foregoing material indicates the variety of parties or agencies that may have an interest in a group prepayment plan. Each is likely to have special expertise and special interest to contribute to the plan. Suppose a labor group wants comprehensive dental care coverage. It turns to the state dental service corporation (Delta affiliate) for a professionally designed and monitored program. The dental service corporation, in turn, has found the actuarial and business details of the program beyond its competence and has engaged Blue Cross-Blue Shield or some other agency as an operating agent. Here we have not three-party involvement but five-party involvement. The union, the service corporation, and the operating agency are all interposed between the dentist and his patient—and all need money to operate. A sixth party exists if Medicaid pays the bill for a medically indigent group member. The same situation is found in the commercial insurance programs, though here only four or five parties are commonly involved.

Only large-scale programing, with extension of dental benefits to large groups of patients hitherto unmotivated to seek care, can justify such overhead costs. Employer subsidy for altruistic, public relations, or tax-saving reasons, and underutilization by portions of the eligible groups can operate to defray part of these costs. The result is fully justified if (1) people are served who would not otherwise receive care, and (2) attractive new jobs are provided to the community.

When a health maintenance organization clinic has arisen, or a dental group practice has contracted with an underwriting organization to provide care, still another party may enter the picture. It is an open question, however, as to whether this arrangement will add to or subtract from overhead costs. Cost-benefit analyses have been made in a number of situations, comparing a group practice or a clinic with neighboring private dental offices, and results have favored first one party then the other, or have proved about equal. Sociological considerations, such as the existence of a ghetto where private practice does not flourish, or unusual professional initiative, where an exceptional leader draws together an effective group practice, usually determine the outcome.

CHAPTER 19

Evaluating the Quality of Dental Care

DENTISTS HAVE traditionally demanded the right to appraise the quality of the work they do. Most of their standards have been drawn from their leaders in the technical and therapeutic fields of dentistry, from their own experience in private practice, and from the reactions of their individual patients, who were not expected to know much of the scientific background of the work they were receiving. Dentists have worked as individuals, resenting comments of either a critical or an authoritative nature from others. Their measure of success has lain in the technical or clinical outcome of their treatment of individual cases.

Two factors in the area of public health work have operated to require a broader viewpoint: the advent of third-party agents concerned with payment through either private or government group care programs, and the growing recognition that the "consumers" of care may be responsible agents in the planning of group care plans. The dentist must now expect not only to have the quality of his work for an individual patient appraised by his peers but also to have to tailor his treatment plans to the needs and financial resources of the group or groups to which his patients belong. Administrators of dental care programs must look not only at the quality of the completed restorations in their program but also at the extent to which the eligible group as a whole receives the scope of care designed for it. This brings access into the picture. Even with programs confined to primary nonrestorative care, the quality of the program is poor if the entire target population cannot be served. Quality is rightly considered as the upper segment of a dichotomy, where some attribute is better than something else. Any care, even the simplest, is better than no care.

PROBLEMS IN LARGE PUBLIC PROGRAMS

The practical objectives of the director of a large publicly funded dental care program are well illustrated by Bellin.[1] As Health Commissioner in New York City, he considered his responsibility to lie in four areas:

1. Assessing the quality of health care in accordance with standards stipulated by the Health Department.
2. Ascertaining the overutilization or underutilization of services either performed by the practitioner or received by the patient.
3. Identifying fraud.
4. Educating practitioners and recipients in the appropriate use of publicly funded health care programs.

Bellin postulated that "fraud and overutilization should be subject to penalty. All other irregularities call for education."

The area of *fraud* is a particularly difficult one to define. Bellin's first finding in this area was a discrepancy between claimed operations and operations observed to be completed. He invited allegedly erring practitioners to the central Medicaid office to discuss apparent irregularities. Only after such discussion was a determination made as to whether the discrepancies resulted from honest error or from fraud. Even then, apparent falsification of records was termed "alleged fraud," in the absence of court trial. Bellin reports 74 cases of alleged fraud among 425 health practitioners of various sorts who were studied because of their apparent deviations from their claims—the proportion is a disgraceful 17.5 percent.

Overutilization was an acute problem in Bellin's mind because of his responsibility for cost containment in hospitals. His budget was constantly threatened by competing institutions, all eager to have the latest expensive equipment and many of them overbuilt. Many were keeping patients longer than necessary and delivering care less skilled than the average for which the hospital was equipped. Overutilization of dental care was less of a problem, though the need for good preventive and diagnostic services had to be balanced against the temptation to run up large claims for not-really-necessary radiographs and for preventive procedures of questionable benefit in relation to costs.

The study of *underutilization* was a complex one, requiring a lot more than a glance at the extent of health-education measures and an assumption that demand for care was going to be a fixed quantity. A great many social and economic factors underlie the response a given population group may be expected to make to a program offered it, as is brought out in Chapter 13.

The *quality* of a health program is viewed somewhat differently from the dentist by the average patient or consumer. Angevine, representing the Consumers' Federation of America, has given a careful analysis of this view.[2] While insisting that dentists or physicians be "competent," her main emphasis is upon comprehensive coverage of the unmet medical needs of the public. Thus she states that "consumers also believe that the medical profession can vastly improve the quality of care through more widespread use of semi-professionals." This does not imply that the semi-professionals will do better work than the full professionals; rather it implies that if they do work that is *as* good, and for a larger segment of the population, the quality of the whole program will be elevated.

In 1971, an attempt to combine the viewpoints of dentist, director, and consumer was made at a workshop held in Asilomar, California.[3] The following aspects of quality were considered:

Program goals. The plan should have clearly defined goals as to how far it might go in providing primary or comprehensive oral-health care for a specific population.

Scope of services. The plan should list specific services within the

areas of prevention, diagnosis, correction of defects, and maintenance of oral health. Where necessary, priority scales should be set
up.

Availability of care. The plan should provide sufficient facilities,
manpower (including auxiliaries), and operating funds to furnish
the specified scope of care to the highest proportion of the eligible
population that can be expected to demand it.

Accessibility of care. This term refers to the ability of the consumer
to enter the delivery system. The factors to be considered are
convenience of location, culture, economics, communication, hours
of operation, and transportation and outreach services.

Acceptability of the program. Policymaking within the program
should provide for careful appraisal of patient satisfaction, including adjustment of grievances. Consumers should be included on
the planning and advisory boards. The measurement of satisfaction can be difficult. First is the evaluation of the care itself. This
can be a two-dimensional matter, concerned with measuring either
latent hostility or resentment to specific incidents, or measuring
the general image of the health providers.[4] Second is the evaluation of outcome. This involves, as in full denture service, both the
quality of the product by objective standards and the adaptability
of the patient to the product. High levels of accessibility and acceptability may be expected to increase both demand and utilization.

Eligibility requirements. The duration of eligibility should be as
long as possible, to permit maintenance care beyond the initial
treatment series. Age, family inclusion, and location of residence
are important. Conversion from one group to another or to individual coverage is also a problem.

Continuity of care. Provision should be made for continuity of
care as long as the patient is eligible, and with the same dentist if
possible.

Appropriateness and technical quality of care. In addition to being of
satisfactory technical quality, it is important that the level of care
be adjusted to the patient's prospect of getting lasting benefit from
it. Thus elaborate periodontal treatment is inadvisable for a patient unable or unlikely to maintain good home care afterward.
The consumer has a right to informed consent, and also a responsibility to perform his share of the treatment program.

Efficiency of program administration. This covers such matters as personnel and fiscal administration, records, internal communications, and so on. Chapter 11 deals with these matters.

Efficiency of patient care. The dentists must be able to work efficiently at those tasks, and preferably only those, which require their professional skill. Auxiliaries should be available where appropriate; and facilities, schedules, patient transportation, and so on, should be organized to minimize lost time.

Outcome and measurement of program status. The outcome of care for individual patients must be measured, as well as the progress of the program toward its overall objectives. If optimum care is rendered to some people while zero care is rendered to the rest of the eligible population, zero quality is the result for these latter people. In such circumstances it has been aptly said that "the best is the enemy of the good."

APPRAISAL TECHNIQUES

The various parameters for study can be investigated from several points of view. One is Schonfeld's, involving targets of differing magnitudes:

1. Specific activity, procedure, service, or task
2. Oral cavity
3. Person
4. Group—e.g., family, program recipients, or community.[5]

Each of these four levels requires consideration along four dimensions: technical, logistical, organizational, and financial.

Donabedian's approach is a functional one, with simpler dimensions:

1. Structure: physical facilities and equipment, administrative organization and qualifications of personnel.
2. Process: the quality by recognized professional standards of the activities of health workers in the management of patients.
3. Outcomes: the end results in terms of health and of patient satisfaction.[6]

In terms of technical methodology for the care of individual patients, Peterson's categories are the most practical.[7] He describes observational studies, end-result studies, and record-review studies.

Observational studies are those carried on during actual delivery of care. They are extremely difficult except in a setting such as a dental school. They do, however, give the observer an opportunity to understand not only the end result of the work, but the thoroughness of many intermediate processes that cannot be adequately inspected later, such as caries removal. They also provide an opportunity to study the psychological approach of the dentist or dental student and many other intangible matters that make up good dental care.

End-result studies are easier to institute in the dental field than in many others, because the finished restorations and the results of surgery are available for inspection. Some of the earliest careful work of this nature was performed by Gruebbel and Fulton in appraising the work of New Zealand dental nurses.[8,9] Both investigators used clinical investigations of completed cases and studies of bite-wing x-rays to pick up unfilled carious lesions, poorly contoured gingival margins of restorations, and other defects in operative dentistry. Neither method gives accurate appraisal of the thoroughness of caries removal, of the exact form of the original cavity, or of the correctness of the form of restoration used. Neither study was matched by an adequate control study among American dentists of the period, and, indeed, such control studies with matching populations, examiners, and techniques have been almost impossible to find in the literature since then. Ideal end results have repeatedly been described in textbooks as a standard for comparison, but average end results have almost never been documented on a large scale.

Record-review studies are commonly called *postaudits*. As itemized bills for dental service accumulate, following either the practitioner's interpretation of general rules or the prior approval of his program by institutional consultants, data accumulates on the dental treatment patterns that prevail in a given community or age group under a given set of payment rules. Deviations from these treatment patterns are quickly recognized. The reasons for these deviations are many, ranging from unusual interpretation of obscurely worded rules, to a desire for more thorough work than the rules seem to call for, and finally to a selfish desire to build up a big claim. Common events involve duplicate charges for a single operation, the pyramiding of fees for separate billing of operations that are supposed to be done as a unit (such as separate fillings on one tooth billed in excess of the maximum for one tooth), and billing for services restricted from the program. The Massachusetts Department of Public Welfare recognizes that "in most instances these violations are the result of inadequate knowledge of the regulations or clerical error; nonetheless, those dentists whose patterns of billing practice are in flagrant violation of the regulations have exposed themselves to both civil and criminal prosecution."[10]

The term *audit* usually applies to claim forms, which are studied for internal consistency and conformity to regulations, and to develop profile patterns for dental operators. Pre- and postoperative radiographs can be used for similar purposes, and also in connection with end-result studies of the patients themselves. Friedman has carried the audit process beyond cost containment into improvement of care, using x-rays, a preauthorization review of treatment plans, and a postoperative review, and a computer analysis to develop normal operating profiles for providers.[11] In a year and a half, over 10 million dollars' worth of claims were audited, and a preauthorization saving of 6 percent ($643,548.00) was realized, representing almost the entire cost of administering the program. The quality of care was improved, not only because additional needed services were suggested, even though they were more costly to the program, but also because more than 1,000 of the cases had involved gross misdiagnoses, ranging all the way from missed cavities to plans for unnecessary full dentures where teeth could be saved.

The use of the *profile pattern* needs some clarification at this point. It is a list of the frequencies of authorized operations performed by a given operator within a given time period. The value of the profile pattern depends upon the assumption that a certain degree of uniformity in dental needs exists among patients of certain ages in certain localities and cultural groups. Comparisons of information require continual updating of information. The statistical section of the Dental Estimates Board in Great Britain has been collecting data since it was established in 1948. Because the Board has some 30 years of experience, the comparison of a dentist's pattern of treatment with the national and regional values has become quite accurate. Additionally, every dentist has his pattern of treatment analyzed and compared to the regional average once every two years for two variables—(1) frequency distribution and (2) ratio of fillings to extractions. The frequency distribution demands that mean values be calculated for all of the services that a practitioner has provided for his patients in specific categories for a given period of time, and that these values be used for comparative purposes.[12] A high number of fillings in proportion to extractions indicates a practice of good restorative value, but allowance must be made for the difficulty of achieving such a ratio in an area of high accumulations of unmet dental needs.

The British system works well because it carries government authority, is large, and is standardized in recording procedures. It needs sensitive handling, however, since valid reasons often exist for an individual dentist to differ from the general pattern. Such deviations are carefully investigated.

The term "profile," in a different sense, is used by health insurance agencies to designate the record of the usual fees charged for covered procedures by an individual provider (dentist) during a specified period of time.

PEER REVIEW

Observational and end-result studies, almost by definition, need to be carried out by a person with training equal to that of the provider of care: his peer. Criteria for evaluation may be left to the judgment of the examiner, and hence be implicit and usually subjective, or may be spelled out carefully in advance, and hence be explicit and objective. For audit studies, peers must lay down the rules explicitly, but auxiliaries with or without computer aid may do the actual work.

An important factor in peer review is the authority back of it and the acceptability of that authority to the provider. In America, with its tradition of private practice, leadership is more important than law in determining acceptability. Voluntary peer review is therefore the choice of dentists or dental societies whenever possible. The financial interest and the group responsibility of third-party agencies in modern health care programming, however, demands positive control such as cannot usually be obtained without some degree of authority.

Much difficulty can be avoided if authority can be made secondary to leadership and if good habits of communication can be set up. A good example of leadership is reported by Soricelli.[13] He notes that dentists employed by the Philadelphia Health Department participate in a program whereby a selected group of children whose cases they have "completed" are examined twice yearly by a professor of pedodontics, operative dentistry, or other appropriate department from a local dental school. Appraisal is informal and accompanied by constructive comments. Soricelli states, "Today every man on our staff boasts of our method of evaluation and proclaims the results proudly. Each one admits . . . that the system has made him a better dentist."

In the area of comnmunication, group practice has fostered informal discussion of cases between dentists and their auxiliaries, as described in Chapter 17. Dental internships, by definition, are accompanied by teaching programs. Dental educators are now planning to extend peer-review procedures in predoctoral teaching programs, so that a student by assignment will appraise the work of a fellow student and discuss it with him before the instructor steps in and has the final say. At the graduate level, continuing education courses are becoming increasingly common, offered by dental societies and such national dental organizations as the American College of Dentists and the Academy of General Dentistry. Participation in these courses and in all the organized activities of dental societies will help keep dentists up to date in a manner that is educationally stimulating and financially and socially rewarding. Again the question of compulsion arises. In most states continuing education is voluntary, but an increasing number of states require some evidence of it as a condition for the annual renewal of a dental license and more states yet are considering such a requirement. Several state-level societies require evidence of continuing education for the renewal of membership.

Both the medical and dental professions have long considered it both a prerogative and a responsibility to police their own ranks. The growth of third-party payment programs has given rise to the need for review of claims, usually by professionals in the employment of the paying agency. The response of organized medicine and dentistry has been to develop *professional review committees* within their own ranks and to offer the services of these review committees both to the third-party agencies and to the practitioners who may be working for insured patients. Within the scope of activity laid down for them, these peer-review committees are achieving a useful purpose. Most states have now established dental review committees at the component or local level.

The more well-developed of the state professional review committees have published detailed guidelines for review committee activity, based upon American Dental Association policy.[14] The functions of the committees are "to determine the relevancy of the usual, customary, and reasonable fees and of treatment procedures to the terms of the contract." The functions are not to include "setting fees, determining practice, or interfering with the dentist-patient relationship." Consultants are to be employed as needed.

The influence these committees may have upon the quality of dental care is limited by the definition of their duties. One state in its peer-review procedure manual defined quality as being based upon "the averages of both the profession at large and the community—and on a rather broad cross section of the dental population."[14] This manual anticipates that most cases coming up for review will involve judgment and require an answer to the following questions:

a) Should the case be done, or have been done as planned?
b) Were the services rendered as reported?
c) Were the services performed necessary and desirable?
d) Are the services rendered acceptable under the terms of the insurance coverage?
e) Is there any overutilization of dental service?[15]

The manual emphasizes, however, that the review committees have only an advisory function and are without authority to discipline any practitioner. No patient should be examined without permission from the responsible dentist. The report of the actions of the component review committee should be concise. "No editorializing, philosophy, or prejudicial remarks are to be included." The committee should not review cases that are presently in litigation, should not set fees, and should not permit conflicts of interest among its members. Rules for procedure include submission of cases first to the chairman of the state professional review committee, with referral later to district professional review committees. Hearings are to be held before decisions are made. Appeals are possible from the district recommendation back to the state professional review committee.

Professional review committees could easily improve the communications and education of the profession, the public, and the third-party carriers. What will happen when patients present deep-seated complaints about quality is another matter. The patient has recourse to consultation with a disinterested dentist or to the law courts, however, and a malpractice suit may continue to be the ultimate answer in these new third-party payment situations, as it has been in the past for private practice.

Ethical restraints upon peer review have been a serious matter within the dental profession in years past. As late as 1972, the American Dental Association's Principles of Ethics stated that "the dentist has the obligation of not referring disparagingly, orally or in writing to the services of another dentist to a member of the public."[16] The section where this statement appeared was headed "Unjust Criticism." A revision was made of this section in late 1973, and it now reads, "The dentist has an obligation to report to the appropriate agency of his component or constituent dental society instances of gross and continual faulty treatment by another dentist."[17] Even the title of the section was changed. It now reads "Justifiable Criticism and Expert Testimony." Expert testimony, when essential to judicial or administrative action, has always been permitted.

Beyond the review committee level, physicians have formalized the review process by creating foundations for medical care. These are autonomous corporations sponsored and organized by a local (state or county) medical society and concerned with the quality and cost of medical care. They are formed for the same reasons as the tissue or pathology committees that have long existed in hospitals, combined with a desire to provide physicians in individual practice with a group-practice setting in which they may participate in capitation programs and meet requirements for peer review of professional service. In many ways the foundations resemble the state-level dental service corporations now becoming common, but the emphasis is more upon review than upon pre-payment, because prepayment in the medical field already exists through so many channels.

Foundations for medical care are of two major types.[18] *Claims-review* foundations restrict themselves to peer-review activities, reviewing payment claims that fall outside established norms and are referred by fiscal intermediaries. *Comprehensive* foundations, however, set minimum benefit packages, and process all patient-service payment claims for peer review when appropriate. Significant cost reductions in patient care have been demonstrated in the comprehensive foundations. Additional savings have been realized when hospital certification has also been undertaken. Some comprehensive foundations have assumed a portion of the underwriting risk for a defined population and have provided comprehensive health services for a fixed annual sum per person, thus approximating the concept of a health maintenance organization.[19]

SPECIFIC MEASUREMENTS

The actual means for appraising dental health status, as described in Chapter 14, form the basis of much of the information used to determine the overall quality of a dental program. Has susceptibility to dental disease decreased? The DMF tooth or surface counts taken before and after a given length of time, usually measured in terms of years, will help to answer this question. Has restorative dental care reached the eligible groups as a whole? An upward change in filled teeth as a proportion of total DMF teeth (F/DMF) will be valuable here. Decreases in the proportion of decayed or missing teeth are part of the story too. Special situations, however, call for careful study of underlying factors. An example is found in the World Health Organization study of five countries referred to in Chapter 17. In that study the New Zealand children were reported to have the highest proportion of filled teeth and the lowest proportion of decayed or missing teeth (see Fig. 65). Studies of adults aged 35 to 44 in the same countries, by contrast, have shown that New Zealand adults have the highest proportion of missing teeth, though the proportion of decayed teeth is still the lowest.[20] What had happened? Investigation disclosed that when these adults were children New Zealand had one of the highest susceptibilities to dental caries in the world, while the dental care program only reached about one-third of the child population.[21] The adults of the next generation, having had the full benefit of the current dental care program for children, should show a much smaller proportion of missing teeth.

In 1976 the Dental Research Unit of the Medical Research Council of New Zealand decided to study this question of missing teeth in depth. They found a negative attitude toward retention of natural teeth in a large portion of their sample, particularly among nonwhite groups, lower social and educational strata, people who did not receive care from the school dental service, and those without a regular dentist:

Denture-wearing complements total tooth loss. The number of edentulous persons without dentures was extremely small, which no doubt reflects a social or functional need. The large percentage of the population with full dentures, especially after age 45 years, is consistent with professional and lay attitudes to tooth extraction and the decision to move to the edentulous state. Most dentists (75 percent), according to their patients, favoured full mouth clearance when the question was discussed. It is also quite clear that when consulted, friends and relations overwhelmingly favoured such a course of action. According to the survey findings, the decision of the dentist in many of these instances cannot have been justified in terms of disease alone . . . Quite clearly, the individual considering the future of his or her natural dentition, appears to face both at the professional and lay level, little positive encouragement to retain natural teeth.[22]

For other dental conditions, such as periodontal disease and malocclusion, standard indices are also valuable. The advantage of widespread usage can be seen in periodontal disease, where Russell's Periodontal Index, though not necessarily a perfect index of the disease, has been used so widely throughout the world that there is strong pressure on new researchers to use the same index, so that their own results may be comparable.

In appraising the quality of restorations actually seen in the mouth, attempts have been to list explicit criteria in advance and then to apply them. Gruebbel and Fulton both did so.[8,9] The Philadelphia dental service reported by Soricelli started out that way.[13] Textbooks on operative dentistry describe ideal characteristics for restorations; Friedman also does so.[23] Specific characteristics like marginal ridges and contact points must be scored by subjective values such as "superior," "satisfactory," "needing improvement," or "unacceptable." The tendency in large programs, however, has been to average these comments and to apply one subjective value to the care rendered a given patient within a given period. End-result studies, as has been mentioned, can only measure the external characteristics of restoration. Caries removal, pulp protection, retention form, psychological handling of patients in the chair, and other characteristics as well can only be judged by inference. The use of one subjective value for one restoration or for one treatment program, therefore, has a good degree of logic.

Implementation of the production standards determined necessary in connection with all these various appraisal techniques is not a matter to be dealt with in detail here. Directors of programs and clinics will have a certain amount of authority, though there are limits to the extent to which they can *order* licensed practitioners to do this or that in areas where professional judgment must be accorded to the individual operator. Soricelli points out that in large city programs, district supervisors are necessary to get proper levels of productivity.

GOVERNMENT AGENCIES FOR QUALITY CONTROL

Any third party, whether private or governmental, that is responsible for financing and delivering dental care on a group basis must have authority over the providers to a certain extent. Professional personnel have technical and ethical standards which must be respected, but in matters such as scope of care, time per operation, and facilities to be furnished, the individual provider cannot be given complete freedom. Guidelines for teamwork must be laid down that are satisfactory to all three (or more) parties in advance—and implemented. Dental society programs, insurance programs, and labor union and other consumer-group programs thus all require some degree of authority to control overall quality. Foregoing material in this chapter has indicated some of the administrative mechanisms that can be used in the private sector. Government programs, almost by definition, need authority, and it is here that the most formal arrangements are found.

Local and Regional Government Agencies

New York State, to cite one example, has an enlightened but authoritative quality-control system. Cons describes this system as being based on prior approval of certain treatment items and posttreatment examination of patients.[24] The prior-approval mechanism operated through a team of local dental consultants who were given a one-week refresher course to insure uniform quality standards. In addition, a set of guidelines and a checksheet for local directors was developed. Posttreatment recall of patients was arranged on a semirandom basis, with a bias toward those cases with prior-approval treatment items or those for whom the providers' bills seemed to indicate a possible problem. During 1971, 43,672 patients were examined clinically throughout the state. Various recall methods were used, but letters were the most common. Cons considers the 23 percent of letter-recipients who kept their appointments to have been predominantly those with complaints, and hence not a representative sample of the whole. Treatment was analyzed by operator and by category, with the use of guidelines on such matters as morphology, occlusion, and polishing of restorative work.

Large cities and other similar population units could use a system such as this. Many variants are possible, of course. One already referred to is the Philadelphia plan reported by Soricelli.[13]

Another well-developed governmental system is that of the U.S. Indian Health Service.[25] Though the organization itself is national, it operates on a regional basis, and is therefore included at this point. Here an elaborate manual, with checksheets and guidelines, was prepared for the use of supervising dentists. The work on patients was divided between observed items (oral and radiographic examinations, prophylaxis, topical fluoride, patient management, and treatment process) and retrospect items (completion of records, quality of amalgam and other restorations, preextraction radiographs and evidence of completion of an extraction, suitability and sequence of treatment plan, and quality and timing of treatment to completion of case). The work of a whole service unit was then studied for adequacy of coverage of assigned population, proper distribution of services among preventive and treatment categories, and general appraisal of the oral health of the assigned population.

National Government Agencies

In the United States, where the fact-finding and preventive services of the Public Health Service have long been linked with appraisal of both public and private health care, two agencies offer services with a high potential for future development. The first of these agencies is the National Center for Health Statistics of the Department of Health and Human Services in Rockville, Maryland. For years it has collected information on illness, accidental injuries, disability, use of hospital, medical, dental, and other services, and other health-related topics. Its reports have covered such topics as health manpower, selected dental findings in adults, and dental visits, with time interval since last visit.[26,27,28] In a wider field, it has studied survey- and data-evaluation methods, birth, marriage, and death statistics, and many related subjects. Rutstein sees in this agency the potential for a guidance and research component in a national program for control of quality of health care.[29] This component would measure, follow, and interpret accomplishments and failures of health care programs—region by region—and lay out courses for subsequent programs. It would run continuous and extensive surveys. It would work toward continual improvement of facilities and health care delivery systems for the nation and its individual citizens.

The second agency is the Center for Disease Control in Atlanta, Georgia. This agency could collaborate with the statistical center in relating survey data to basic laboratory and clinical research activities, both in medical and dental schools and in teaching hospitals. Norms could be set up for diseases and causes of death, above which an early-warning system could signal developing epidemics. The relation of these findings to the quality of health care, however, would become the direct responsibility of other agencies, both governmental and voluntary.

More directly related to everyday control are the mechanisms coming into being for use with Medicare and Medicaid programs. In October 1972, the President signed P.L. 92-603 into law, creating *professional standards review organizations* (PSROs). PSROs involve groups of physicians in specified local areas as determined by the Secretary of Health and Human Services. All physicians in the area, whether or not they are members of medical societies, will have their work for government-covered patients reviewed. This review will involve, at present, only Medicare, Medicaid, and some welfare patients, but it is clear that a national health insurance act would lead to inclusion of all patients under this umbrella. Medical care foundations—or better, health care foundations—will usually be awarded government contracts to perform PSRO functions. The country has already been divided into areas and many contracts have been awarded.

The duties of a PSRO have been spelled out in the law (P.L. 92-603) as follows:

1. It must establish norms of diagnosis and treatment of disease (but not cost).

2. These norms must include accepted lengths of hospital stay and provide for review of each hospitalized patient under certain conditions.

3. Profiles must be established for each doctor, institution, and patient, including such items as claims submitted, services rendered, and drugs prescribed.

4. Supervision of ambulatory care is optional.

The fourth duty is what opens the way for the eventual inclusion of dentistry, if and when dental care becomes an important part either of Medicare or of a national health insurance program. As of 1985, with reduced federal funding, the activity of PSROs became limited to the monitoring of days of hospital inpatient care. Dentistry has never really been included.

Several major problems are likely to confront the health profession in the development of PSROs. In the first place, areas will be hard to designate. Standards do vary, as do norms of therapy and lengths of stay, between university teaching hospitals and smaller community hospitals. Similar differences may be expected to exist between city and rural practitioners in both medicine and dentistry.

Welch is concerned that medical practitioners will be in a vulnerable position, since the great bulk of available computer hardware and expertise is in the hands of the Social Security Administration or third-party carriers.[30] He is also concerned that the cost of the entire system may run as high as $1 billion, with a concomitant drain not only on national tax funds but on medical manpower.

Another question is *confidentiality*. The law indicates that the utmost effort will be made to maintain confidentiality. However, when individual profiles of doctors and of patients are required, it is hard to believe that these profiles will remain unavailable to the press. On the other hand, it is not reasonable to expect any utilization committee to identify a fraudulent prescriber or recipient of excessive amounts of drugs if all material remains anonymous. Where do psychiatric diagnoses fit in this picture? Finally, "What is the place of computers—those machines of eternal memory, with no conscience and no forgiveness?"[30]

Mainly, Welch is concerned about the relationship between PSROs and their constituent practitioners and institutions. It will be hard for PSROs to stand up against the pressures that surround them, and the physicans serving these organizations will be in a difficult position, caught between their professionally organized colleagues and the politically organized public.

In countries other than the United States, a wide variety of mechanisms for appraisal of quality exist, description of which would be beyond the scope of this book. But one country, Great Britain, has had such long experience in the field of quality control, and has had the mechanism so well described, that brief consideration is appropriate here.

Three agencies in Great Britain share the responsibility for administration of the General Dental Service there: a group of local executive councils (163 in 1974), appointed by the Department of Health and Social Security and operating through local dental service committees; the Dental Estimates Board, with offices in Eastbourne, England and Edinburgh, Scotland; and two National Health Service Tribunals, one for England and one for Scotland, responsible for deciding whether or not a dentist should be permitted to remain on the executive council list.[31]

It is the duty of the service committee to investigate cases in which a dentist is alleged to be in breach of his terms of service. Proceedings commence on complaint from a patient or on the initiative of the local executive council or the Dental Estimates Board. The majority of cases begin with the latter agency, but executive councils settle many of the disputes without recourse to service committee proceedings.

The Dental Estimates Board has two main functions: (1) routine sanctioning of estimates and authorization of payment of fees, and (2) the compiling of statistics. The latter work involves detection of fraud and malpractice.[31]

The Statistical Section at Eastbourne has had the task of analyzing 4 percent of the incoming dental estimates. One out of every 25 claims received by the Board has been selected randomly and used to identify those practitioners who are to be subjected to the statistical analysis. This analysis serves to establish a dentist's pattern of treatment in specific categories of services that patients of a certain age or sex may be receiving, such as one-, two-, or three-surface restorations of silver amalgam, extractions, prophylaxes, or the topical application of fluorides, to name only a few of the measures used. This information then is compared to the national and regional averages. If a practitioner should deviate from the regional average by a statistically significant degree, his dental treatment is statistically analyzed more carefully, or patients are recalled so that the completed treatment may be examined.[12]

COST ANALYSIS

One feature of the quality of a dental care program, and an aspect intimately related to its ability to achieve its goals, is the cost. There are several ways in which costs may be related to the feasibility of a program. Costs can be compared with the benefits to be realized by the program. This is cost-benefit analysis.

Costs may also be compared between two or more means of achieving a given goal. This is cost-effectiveness analysis. Where a change in proportionate risk occurs in a field where dollar estimates are particularly meaningless, the process can be called risk-benefit analysis. Finally, in a practical sense, the dollar cost of a program may be compared to the revenue it may bring in. This is revenue-cost analysis, and is all too commonly necessary in the dental field, where programs are so often expected to pay for themselves.

In its purest form, *cost-benefit analysis* involves the dollar measurement of a benefit in comparison to the cost of securing that benefit. This can seldom be done with full accuracy, because so many of the benefits of health are intangible or at least not easily reduced to dollars. In this category would be the sense of physical and mental well-being implied by the term "health" and increases in life span. Reductions in time lost from work can sometimes be appraised, but more often not. The best we can usually do is to set the cost of a preventive procedure against the cost of care if the preventive procedure had not existed and the disease or disorder had developed.

The *cost-benefit ratio* is expressed in dollars, or other monetary units, and takes the form of a ratio obtained by dividing the benefit by the cost of achieving it. The formula, where only the cost of caring for a disease is measurable and other benefits are negligible, thus becomes:

$$\text{Cost-benefit ratio} = \frac{(\text{cost of care without program}) - (\text{cost of care with program})}{(\text{cost of program})}$$

This ratio can be simplified by carrying out the division indicated so that a single number results. Any ratio larger than 1 indicates that the program will at least pay its own way, while any program with a ratio less than 1 will lose money. No such number can be accepted without estimating intangibles. On the cost side are several disadvantages, which may range from toxic side-effects to mere impracticality. Thus, unsupervised fluoride tablet programs fail on a local scale because people abandon them even if the tablets are furnished free of charge. On the benefit side are such items as satisfaction, comfort, and increased life span. These intangibles are always subject to consumer evaluation, so a priority scale of health items, or health and nonhealth items, may often be at variance with monetary considerations. Statistical significance cannot always be determined with practical importance.

A number of studies now exist demonstrating the reductions in dental disease, and consequent savings in dental bills for children, following the fluoridation of a communal water supply and other means of fluoride therapy. Perhaps the best of these is the work of Ast et al. over a six-year period on the Newburgh-Kingston study in New York State.[32] Here the actual cost of incremental dental care for children of comparable ages (fillings and extractions only) in Newburgh, with fluoridated water, was found to be only about 50 percent of the cost in Kingston, where the water was not fluoridated. This is not a complete cost-benefit analysis, because the cost of the benefit—community fluoridation—has not been included in the comparison. Studies of the cost of fluoridation have been made, however, not only in Newburgh but in many other places, and could be used by approximation to change Ast's gross dollar benefits into net dollar benefits. But even without such a change, Ast's and other similar cost studies still have a large usefulness. In Greater Boston, actual figures for total annual dental restorative work among representative children in the area were compared with expected total annual restorative costs for the same children after applying surface-specific reduction factors from data for comparable fluoridation areas. Savings in dental bills, of the magnitude of $11 to $15 per year for a child under 19, were shown to be possible.[33,34] The cost of fluoridation was estimated at $0.30 per capita if applied to the entire population, and about $1 if applied only to the child population, as might be more logical in the early years of a fluoridation program. At $0.30, the ratios would rise a range of 35.7 to 49. At $1, the ratios would still be 10 and 14. In total dollars, the savings were estimated at about $7 million per year: a more understandable figure than any ratio.

One of the most thorough cost-benefit analyses of fluoridation is that by Berenholz in North Reading, Massachusetts.[35] Berenholz found in 1971 that $1 expended upon fluoridation would save $35 in dental bills for children under the age of 20. This is a cost-benefit ratio of 35. The study suffers because only estimated savings in dental bills are available in the North Reading area, but, in comparison, real fluoridation costs are available from an existing program, and the cost of replacing missing teeth with fixed bridgework (an obvious component of good restorative dentistry) has been included, as has not happened in some other studies. The cost of fluoridating the North Reading water has been projected over a 15-year period. The dollar savings in dental bills, moreover, might have been reduced by an estimated 25 percent, because the medical deduction on yearly income tax returns will supposedly be reduced for the low-income residents of North Reading when their dental bills have been reduced. More practically, the drop in childhood dental caries that has occurred since 1971 has reduced the benefits of fluoridation—though not to the extent of impracticality.

The studies cited so far have been based on age-specific costs of rendering dental care and have assumed a fully developed fluoridation program, but the mix of children (local-born versus immigrants to the area) and a number of other factors that might well be relevant—some quantifiable, others not—have been ignored. Some of these factors are:

1. Variations in dental benefits with changes in scope of care, local economic conditions, and so on.

2. Hidden costs of care, such as travel time, loss of working time (child or parent), and child care for siblings.

3. Intangible effects of reduced suffering and improved oral appearance and efficiency.

4. Differences in patient compliance with dental treatment recommendations and in length of recall period for treatment.

5. Variations in size of population and in cost of care in ensuing years.

Not all ratios need to be carried into dollars to be convincing. As a dental officer in the New York Naval Shipyard during World War II, I examined the working man-hours saved per day among civilian employees as a result of palliative emergency dental service.[36] Sixteen man-hours were saved as a result of some 40 minutes of care per day by the dentist, assisted by one hospital corpsman. The salaries of the various persons concerned may not have been exactly comparable, nor was the overhead in the shops versus that in the dental clinic, but the ratio of 16.0 to 0.7 is striking enough to obviate further analysis.

Cost-effectiveness analysis has been most useful in the dental field where different delivery systems were to be compared, each providing the same scope and quantity of care. The target in terms of care is a single item or group of items not necessarily measured in dollars; the comparison is made between the costs of different routes to that target. A considerable number of such studies are available, and more are constantly being made.

A good example of cost-effectiveness analysis is that of Field and Jong, studying the effect of patient busing in a neighborhood clinic.[37] They give figures from which a true ratio can be computed. The net value of the dental services provided during the busing program was increased to 23 percent, or $4.67, per dentist work-hour, and 25 percent, or $2.20, per hygienist work-hour. This study required the analysis of production during a busing period and during a controlled nonbusing period of similar length. The dollar value of the services performed was estimated for these periods according to the Medicaid fee scale, and a percentage comparison was made between the two sets of values. The proper proportion of the cost of bus operation ($0.80 per child per hour) was deducted from the dollar value of services rendered during the busing period to compute the net value of the savings. The cost-effectiveness ratio for the work of dentists in this program thus was:

$$\frac{\text{Saving}}{\text{Cost of saving}} = \frac{\$4.67}{.80} = 5.8$$

The same dental staff offered the same scope of service with or without the busing; the dollar value of their work increased because of a reduction in idle time. The value of each dentist-hour of service to the patients was not measured, but time was converted into dollars for the purpose of constructing a cost ratio.

Another example of cost-effectiveness analysis is found in the work of Calderone in a sealant program in the New Mexico Health and Environment Department.[38] In the 1981–82 school year five dental hygienist and dental assistant teams applied sealants in 24 New Mexico communities. The hygienists operated according to written procedures and protocols from the Chief of the Preventive Health Services Bureau, a dentist, and received periodic on-site monitoring by his staff dentists. This program served 3,272 children, sealed 15,281 teeth, and cost $24,235.26 with proper allowance for salaries, travel, maintenance, amortized equipment, and supplies. The cost per child was thus $7.41, and the cost per tooth was $1.59. In the next school year the program was expanded to serve 42 communities; 6,238 children were served, and 36,181 teeth were sealed at similar costs.

In the 1983–84 school year, following a ruling by the New Mexico Board of Dentistry, hygienists were forbidden to apply sealants except when a staff dentist was present on site.[39] As additional funds were not available, this caused the elimination of 17 communities and 2,095 children from the program. Applying the cost of a salaried dentist present in the remaining 25 communities, the cost of sealants per child thus became $18.90. If the saving merely involves the elimination of an unneeded dentist, the cost-effectiveness ratio thus becomes:

$$\frac{\$18.90}{7.41} = 2.6$$

An added consideration here was the fact that the diversion of staff dentists to supervision duties which did not increase production meant that 397 low-income children were dropped from an existing state dental treatment program.

Revenue-cost analysis has assumed importance in recent years because the reimbursements available from Medicaid dental programs have not only opened the question as to whether dental care for low-income people was best rendered in public clinics or in private offices, but have provided fee scales by which totals of operations performed could be compared.

Jong and Leverett have studied the cost of operating a children's dental clinic for a given period of time in a low-income area in the city of Boston, and have compared this with the cost of providing the same dental services in private offices at the current schedule of fees of the Massachusetts Medicaid Program.[40] The revenue-cost ratio would be only $0.78 in reimbursable costs for each dollar expended in the operation of the clinic. A serious source of error exists, however, in that the staff of the clinic were rendering such services as school health education, school dental screening, and education of parents—all of them nonquantifiable and not reimbursable under the Medicaid program. Another source of error is that the clinic may have been performing direct services that would be unavailable to the eligible population otherwise—even if the funds were provided for the purchase of such services—either because of a lack of available private dentists in the neighborhood, or because the dentists would not accept the patients, or the patients the dentists. Allukian and Moore, studying another Boston neighborhood health center serving patients of all ages, found a revenue-cost ratio of 0.99, even though it had been held down by similar unreimbursed services.[41] They concluded that a dental program for all ages could have a potential revenue equal to its cost from only those operations that were reimbursable in the Massachusetts Medicaid program.

The whole field of cost analysis is so beset by intangibles both within dental care programs and in the relationship of such programs to other health and welfare programs that educated guesswork is often better than inaccurate figuring. One writer has aptly stated that "one can view cost-benefit analysis as anything from an infallible means of reaching the new Utopia to a waste of resources in attempting to measure the unmeasurable."[42] Nevertheless, we use the method and must attempt to perfect it.

CHAPTER 20

Community Dental Health Programs

IN PREVIOUS editions, this chapter was entitled "School Dental Health Programs." The sharp drop in childhood dental caries in the developed countries and elsewhere, however, has shifted the focus of local dental health programs from children to adults. In the adult field, the growth of the elderly population in America, coupled with their retention of more of their natural teeth, has given rise to that phase of care called geriatric dentistry. Care for the low-income people of all ages in a given community thus presents a public health problem which requires help from public sources. In urban areas where dentists are within easy access and Medicaid operates successfully, special care facilities may not be needed. In rural areas and urban ghetto areas, clinic facilities probably are needed for the functions outlined in Chapter 17. These clinics may logically be located in either public school buildings or neighborhood health centers.

In the United States, the usefulness of public school buildings for people of all ages has become common. The buildings are there and are equipped for a number of educational, recreational, or service projects out of normal school hours. In South Australia, where there are many school dental clinics equipped for a broad range of primary dental services, adult "pensioners" are often cared for. This could well occur in the United States.

SCHOOL PROGRAMS

In rural or urban target areas, where a high caries rate among children may be coupled with low family income, operative dental care may be needed at government expense, together with group preventive measures such as fluoride rinse programs, sealant application, or supervised fluoride tablet supplementation. It is important to set these programs in their proper place in the broad field of school health. It is out of keeping with sound theory in health education to emphasize one program to the exclusion of other efforts to provide for a child's welfare, and a public health dentist must not allow himself to be placed in a position of urging such a procedure. To do so, moreover, is to lose the cooperation of valuable colleagues in the fields of medicine, nursing, and nutrition.

There are three main divisions now recognized in the field of school health. All three divisions are to a certain extent the problem of the entire public health and educational team, including dental personnel, but the problem of school health is seen more clearly if these divisions are recognized as separate functional entities. The definitions agreed upon by the Committee on Terminology of the American Association for Health, Physical Education, and Recreation are:

School Health Services are procedures established: (*a*) to appraise the health status of pupils and school personnel; (*b*) to counsel pupils, parents, and others concerning appraisal findings; (*c*) to encourage the correction of remediable defects; (*d*) to assist in the identification and education of handicapped children; (*e*) to help prevent and control disease; and (*f*) to provide emergency service for injury or sudden sickness.

School Health Education is the process of providing learning experiences for the purpose of influencing knowledge, attitudes, or conduct relating to individual and community health.

Healthful School Living designates the provision of a safe and healthful environment, the organization of a healthful school day, and the establishment of interpersonal relationships favorable to emotional, social, and physical health.[1]

School health services, of course, include the more obvious procedures involving the use of medical and dental personnel. The starting point for school health service is *health appraisal,* which has been defined as "the process of determining the total health status of the child through such means as health histories, teacher and nurse observations, screening tests, and medical, dental, and psychological examinations."[2] It is inherent in this definition that medical and dental examinations are an important part, but by no means all, of the process called health appraisal. Teachers and nurses, in fact, have far more contact with schoolchildren than do physicians and dentists, and it is essential that the latter should indoctrinate the former in the detection of early physical defects in children.

Following appraisal comes *health counseling* and *follow-through.* Health counseling is defined as "the procedure by which nurses, teachers, physicians, guidance personnel, and others interpret to pupils and parents the nature and significance of the health problem and aid them in formulating a plan of action which will lead to solution of the problem."[1] The dental hygienist can be exceptionally valuable in this procedure. More will be said later on the subject of follow-through as it applies to dental care. The problems involved in securing correction of defects are much the same in both medicine and dentistry.

Two important aspects of the school health service, carried out mostly by the school nurse with the cooperation of the school physician or local health officer, are *emergency care* procedures and *communicable-disease control.* In each instance the nurse is likely to be the first person on the scene; she must know her responsibilities in relation to parents, private physicians, dentists, hospitals, and the health department. She must be quick to secure help when problems beyond her normal scope arise.

Health education, a large field in itself, is dealt with in Chapter 15. The term healthful school living involves a large variety of rather specific problems, ranging all the way from the physical fitness of school personnel to the administration of the school lunch program. Ventilation, water supply, and sewage disposal, sanitation in gymnasiums, locker rooms, and swimming pools, and elimination of communicable disease among school employees are common examples of the problems encountered. There is little in all this to concern the public health dentist except in connection with the *school lunch program*. There, to be sure, the dentist shares with the nutritionist and others the responsibility for seeing that a balanced meal, including the four basic food groups, is served to children, and that excessive refined carbohydrates are eliminated, both during the meal and in the vending machines for between-meal snacks.

A new addition to healthful school living has been school *fluoridation* of school water at an increased concentration where public water supplies are not available for community fluoridation. Horowitz et al. have tested such a program at 5 parts per million over a 12-year period with a caries reduction of 39 percent.[3] The U.S. Public Health Service as of February 1977 reports 383 schools in 13 states to be so fluoridated and to be serving over 124,000 children.[4]

School *health care* programs may be run either by the education department or by the health department. In favor of the former system are simpler administrative control and the fact that health services can more readily be made educational in character. In favor of the latter are the facts that medical services should be under medical supervision, school nursing services can and should be coordinated with community health nursing activities, and that the health department will in any case have to service all the private schools in the community. Since health department control is the more common in the United States, a typical organization chart for this system is shown in Fig. 69.[5]

COMMUNITY-WIDE PROGRAMS

In Chapter 13 dental services were arranged in a sequence such as a patient might experience them (Table 33). The preliminary services include dental health education, palliative emergency treatment, preventive measures, case finding through dental inspection

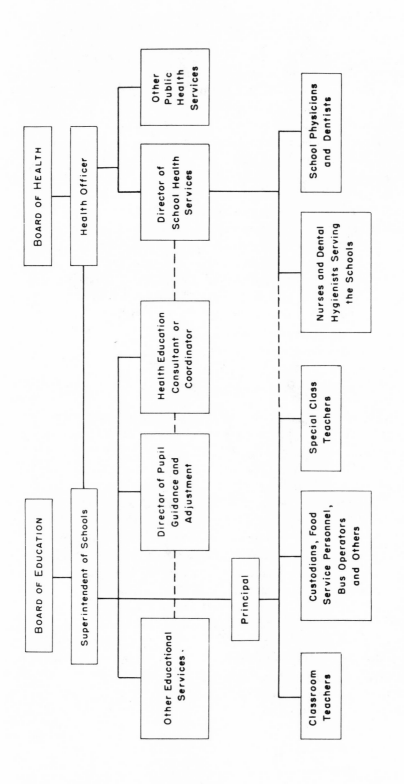

Figure 69. Administration of school health program where the services are operated by the department of health.

or other means, and referral to a source of treatment. These preliminary services are peculiarly appropriate to a dental public health program because they involve prevention and teamwork. Treatment services might or might not be part of a dental public health program, depending upon the claim of the population group on government aid. This pattern fits well in the field of school dental health service.

The actual services a community can provide in order to implement these objectives vary greatly with size of community, region, social need, and many other considerations. In general, however, important elements of the dental health program will include school-community organization, case finding, health education, specific preventive measures such as topical fluoride treatment, referral of defects, and follow-through, and, finally, dental care for the indigent or for such segments of the population as the people may wish. Interwoven with the program from the very beginning is the surveying of dental needs and services and the periodic evaluation of the program. Surveying is dealt with in Chapter 14.

Community-School Relations

Dental health programs succeed, as do so many other enterprises, not because they are grafted onto a community by a group of experts, but because the community has come to want the program. Experts may help in the process of motivation, but the more the community does for itself the better. One of the first steps, therefore, in organizing a dental health program is the formation of a *community dental health council* or *advisory committee*. This group may be a committee affiliated with the community health council if such exists, or it may be an independent body of citizens. In any case it should include broad representation from parents, teachers, health officers, community leaders, and, of course, the dental profession. In order to achieve a broad community base, representation should include as many as possible of the following: the school superintendent; the director of public health; the director of school health, with other school physicians if desired; the director of dental health and one or more school dentists; representatives of the local medical and dental societies (the chairmen of their school health committees if such exist); the head school nurse;

a representative of the parent-teacher association; one or more elementary classroom teachers; a high school science teacher, the school nutritionist or dietitian; the school health coordinator or educator; the school dental hygienist or a representative hygienist from private practice; two or more leading laymen in the community, such as representatives of the service clubs (Kiwanis, Rotary, and so forth).

A large council of the sort just described is cumbersome, to be sure. It will be difficult to secure a meeting time when all members can be present. Nevertheless, those members who are not present at any given meeting are available for consultation, and they serve as much to communicate the objectives of the dental health program to the groups they represent as they do to assist in the planning of the program. Detailed planning, of course, will rest with the dental health director, or with small committees which may be formed to accomplish special objectives. A survey committee will probably be one of the first such committees needed.

The first task of the council is the appraisal and publicizing of the dental needs of the community. Unless needs are found to exist—and are made to be felt throughout the community—no worthwhile program will come into being. Needs must be defined, and the danger of not meeting the needs be properly spelled out. In this way, not only does dental health achieve its true importance, but it becomes part of a broad health endeavor and therefore of greater community interest. After the dental program is fully under way, the council will have less to do than at first, yet constant educational publicity, reevaluation, and reinterpretation of the program will give the council a continuing reason for active existence.

Dental Case Finding

In a target area where a major proportion of the school population are expected to be affected by some degree of dental caries, the question of whether a system of dental inspections or examinations shall be part of a school dental health program becomes a matter for debate. The term *case finding,* as used in medicine, implies an intensive effort to find early cases of serious disease or physical defects in a population, the majority of which may be expected to be healthy. The three important arguments in favor of dental inspection are:

1. Every child, unless shown to the contrary, is likely to consider that he is one of the 5 percent "immune" in his class. The positive findings of dental inspection, therefore, give him far greater motivation to seek dental care than he would have had otherwise.

2. Dental inspection is an opportunity for *individual health education*. It is a fact-finding experience, not only for the child, but for school personnel as well, and it gives an opportunity to build a positive attitude in the child toward the dentist and dental care.

3. A system of dental inspections provide *baseline information* upon dental needs so that a sound dental health program may be organized. It also provides material for the periodic evaluation of that program.

In areas where dental disease constitutes an important problem among children, the proponents of dental case finding are likely to win the argument. It then becomes necessary to set up a program of screening, inspection, or examination which can be carried out year after year without undue strain upon personnel involved and without the inhibition of other phases of the dental program. Dentists, dental hygienists, or dental therapists should be employed to do the screening. Dental assistants or trained lay people should be available as recorders. The type of examination or inspection to be used will determine the personnel needed.

The American Dental Association classification of four types of examination, referred to in Chapter 14, must be reconsidered here, since this system differs somewhat when applied year after year for the service function of motivating children to seek dental care.[6] Type 1, *complete dental examination with all aids*, is obviously unsuited to case finding in entire school populations because of the expense and time involved. Moreover, the dentist responsible for treatment will wish to make his own final examination in order to construct a logical treatment plan.

Type 2, *limited examination using mouth mirror and explorer, bitewing x-rays, and, if necessary, periapical x-rays*, is adapted to school dental health programs on a continuing basis, but not for all children every year. In mouths with uncomplicated dental disease, this examination may well suffice as a basis for treatment without further review, since it is seldom subject to the danger of false negative findings which are found in Types 3 and 4. One situation in which the Type 2 examination fits particularly well is that where it has been decided to give schoolchildren fairly thorough health examinations every 2 or 3 years and none in between. The National Committee on School Health Policies gives a philosophy for intermittent medical examinations which applies in many respects to dental examinations:

During the school years students should have a minimum of four medical examinations, one at the time of entrance to the school, one in the intermediate grades, one at the beginning of adolescence, and one before leaving school. Pupils who have serious defects or abnormalities, who have suffered from serious or repeated illnesses, or who engage in vigorous athletic programs require more frequent examinations. The physician is the best judge of the need for repeated examinations and of the frequency with which they should be given. Additional examination, even annual examinations, may be arranged if money, time and personnel permit. But the quality of medical procedure should not be sacrificed to a desire for frequent and complete coverage of the school. Medical examinations should be sufficiently painstaking and comprehensive to command medical respect, sufficiently informative to guide school personnel in the proper counseling of students, and sufficiently personalized to form a desirable educational experience.[7]

To apply this concept to dental programs, a recommended procedure would be Type 2 examinations carefully performed for all children in grades 1, 4 or 5, 7 or 8, and 11 or 12. Reports would be obtained from the family dentist or dental clinic in intermediate years.

Because of the usefulness of bite-wing x-rays and their value when transmitted without comment to the private dentist, they should be used at all four of the major health examinations if possible. If this proves too difficult, peaks of efficiency for bite-wings have been pointed out at ages 6 and again at 17 (Chapter 14). This suggests the advisability of their use in either the first or second grade and in either the eleventh or twelfth grade.

Type 3, *inspection using mouth mirror and explorer and adequate illumination,* lends itself very well to school procedures and can be performed either by a dentist or by a dental hygienist. The inspection requires review later, no matter who has done the work, since proximal caries can often be detected in its early stages only by x-ray. Type 3 inspection, however, identifies major dental needs in most instances, and can be made the vehicle for excellent individual health education. It can be performed on school premises with portable equipment if necessary, and the hygienist can combine it with dental prophylaxis or with topical fluoride treatment. When carefully performed, it is worthy of choice for the dental phases of the four major health examinations just mentioned.

Type 4, *screening using tongue depressor and available illumination,* is dental case finding at its quickest, but at its lowest efficiency; yet the procedure is needed sometimes where dental personnel are not available to do a better job and where school physicians or school nurses are called upon to identify the most serious cases of dental disease. A grave danger exists that children who do not seem to have dental defects by tongue-depressor screening will consider their mouths to be healthy and will therefore not seek adequate dental examination. Type 4 screening, therefore, should be avoided wherever possible. Where used, it should be accompanied by a careful statement of the danger of false negative findings.

Referral for Dental Care

In areas where a government program does not supply full dental care to all schoolchildren, referral of some or all of these children to private dentists is an important part of the school dental health program. Where dental inspection or examination has been carried out at the school, it may or may not prove desirable to send exact findings to the dentist who will render treatment. Some dentists appreciate detailed information, since it gives them a head start on their own examination procedures. Others resent detailed findings, since they fear their own plan of treatment may be prejudiced thereby. A decision on this point can well be made by the dental health council or advisory committee. If findings are to be transmitted, it is a cardinal rule that reporting be *confined to a description of the conditions* that are found, and should not in any way involve recommendation for treatment. Thus certain tooth surfaces can be marked with a symbol meaning "apparently defective," leaving the private dentist to determine the magnitude of the defect and whether or not and how it shall be treated. Similarly with x-rays, if radiolucent areas are seen either in the crowns or in the periapical areas surrounding teeth, the pictures can be transmitted to the private dentist, perhaps with an arrow drawn in the direction of the radiolucency. The child can be told, "Here is a dark spot on one of your teeth. It probably means that the tooth needs attention. Your dentist will decide exactly what is wrong and what should be done about it." In this way inspection or examination findings can be made to serve as a strong motivating force toward the seeking of treatment, and yet need not prejudice the ability of the private dentist to plan his own method of treatment.

The mere issuance of referral slips to children following dental inspection will be of little value if steps are not taken to make it plain that the school is interested in how many defects really get corrected. Part of this interest can be expressed through health-education programs, already discussed, but it is equally important that individual children should be expected to return the report or certificate forms which have been issued to them, and should receive praise or help, in accordance with the information these forms contain. All this requires a good follow-up system. In practice, one person should be in charge of this system in each school, since what is everybody's business soon becomes nobody's business. The dental hygienist is the logical person to conduct a follow-up system if she is a member of the school health team; otherwise the dental assistant or the school nurse can work very effectively. Classroom teachers may do most of the actual work, connecting it with their health teaching, but it is important that someone from the school health service coordinate the efforts of the various teachers and make such additional contacts as may be necessary with the parents of the children.

Where certificates or reports are not returned promptly, there are various follow-up devices which can be used. The American Dental Association in its booklet *A Preventive Dental Health Program for Schools* covers this matter in some detail.[8] Experience shows the two most important questions to get answered are whether the child really is under dental supervision and the date of the last visit to the dentist.

If a conference on the part of some school official with the parents indicates that the child is unable to obtain dental treatment from a private practitioner at family expense, the family should be helped to obtain Medicaid (Title XIX) if eligible and if this is available, or be directed to a source of public treatment: the school dental clinic or elsewhere.

In a practical way, a school or neighborhood health center can link a public program with local private offices in the matter of dental referrals. Chapter 17 mentions a health center in a low-income residential area in Boston where dental hygiene teachers fanned out into census tracts surrounding the center.[9] They gave what classroom dental health education they could, but their major activity was dental screening in elementary and junior high schools and case referral. Where circumstances permitted, they referred children to private dentists; where circumstances were unfavorable, they referred children to the health center. Through records kept over a 5-year period, they demonstrated a real drop in emergency case referrals, a rise in the filled-tooth ratio (F/DMF), and a perceptible increase in community awareness of the importance of dental health.

In a rural setting, dental health education, dental prophylaxis, medical and dental histories, nutritional counseling, fluoride treatments, and referral to area dentists have been provided by a pair of trailers operating out of the University of Southern Illinois School of Technical Careers Program in Dental Hygiene at Carbondale.[10] The trailers were staffed by a dentist, two registered hygienists, and (in rotation) five dental hygiene students. Classroom instruction was also provided. Small towns were visited within a 50-mile radius of Carbondale, and senior citizens as well as schoolchildren were served. This program has provided not only a valuable service to local rural areas but also excellent education in dental public health for the hygiene students.

Excuses from School for Treatment

The National Education Association recommends that children should be excused to keep office appointments with the physician or dentist during school hours.[11] Most school superintendents will actually give such excuses. There are two good reasons for such a procedure. First, experience appears to show that the child is a more cooperative patient when medical and dental services are provided during the early or middle part of the day. Second, physicians and dentists can provide better service when the entire day is available for services to children and they do not have to crowd their child patients into afterschool hours and Saturdays.

Abuses of the school excuse system can often be avoided if simple excuse forms are printed with space for the date and hour of the appointment, the signature of a school official, signature of parents, and signature of dentist finally, to assure that the appointment was actually kept.

CARE IN STRESS AREAS

In most communities there are schoolchildren who cannot afford dental care in accordance with their needs and with the recommendations which are made to them. It is usual for such communities to make some effort to provide dental care for disadvantaged children, whether through a school dental clinic, a health-center dental clinic, or perhaps some other clinic maintained by a voluntary organization. Communities may equally logically arrange for dental care in private dental offices, either at state and federal expense (Medicaid, where available), or at local expense.

In a country which has led the way in periodic-maintenance dental care, the sad fact is that less than half of the child population gets such care, and that half undoubtedly includes much less than half of the lower-income segment. The cost of the care itself is only part of the story. Private dental offices are commonly located in the upper-middle-class areas or suburbs of our larger cities. Inhabitants of the inner-city ghettos and of rural areas find these offices hard to reach because of the expenses involved and the time used in transportation. Loss of income for working parents who must escort children to these offices is an additional factor. Moreover, the offices are often culturally incompatible. If utilization of periodic dental care by such disadvantaged children is to rise significantly above present levels, this *care must be brought to them* where they normally congregate—the schools—or to neighborhood health centers near their homes or schools. Good-quality government management of such services seems the most logical solution.

In New Zealand, where government dental nurses render the care up to age 13, and have their own clinics on the school premises, comprehensive care has reached virtually the entire school-age population.[12] In Sweden, dentists care for the children chiefly in district dental health clinics, not more than 10 kilometers from the schools, though some school clinics do exist. Busing occurs where necessary. The system is school-based, however, in that the schools appear to take full responsibility for recall schedules, which are arranged within school hours. Utilization rates for the whole country are 51 percent at ages 3 to 5, 77 percent at age 6, 95 percent at the school ages of 7 to 16, and 38 percent at ages 17 to 19.[13] The common denominator between these two successful programs is that they are both school-based, but before discussing physical facilities, the question of entry into similar programs in the United States must be considered on an age basis.

Primary dental care, including some operative work, at government expense is a costly proposition. Cost-efficiency is essential. Dentists cannot be paid salaries commensurate with their training to do work that can safely be delegated to auxiliaries under general supervision. The Australian and Saskatchewan programs, using dental therapists who number no more than 10 to a supervisor, have great attraction here. It is to be hoped that an increasing number of states will authorize such programs for stress areas.

INCREMENTAL CARE

The concept of incremental care at the earliest available age has been common to dental services for schoolchildren in the United States for at least two generations.[14] Treatment programs are "gotten off the ground" by taking the youngest available group the first year and carrying it forward in subsequent years as far as funds permit, each year adding a new class of children at the next earliest available age until an entire child population is being served to as high an age as available resources permit. In economic terms, this program is supposed to avoid high expenditures for initial dental care. In terms of dental health, it is supposed to confine dental disease to small yearly increments, thus reducing loss of teeth; and it is supposed to inculcate a habit of periodic return to the dental office in subsequent years. The trouble with the concept is that with the financing which has been customary in the United States, and probably also because of dental manpower limitations, the program usually terminates about the fourth grade (age 10) and is almost never carried through the high school period. This concept of incremental care needs reexamination as the nation proposes to move into a long-term effort to serve children through ages as high as 18.

At this point a look should be taken at some controlling facts. The drop in childhood dental caries noted in Chapter 8 has seldom been documented beyond age 13, and incremental care programs may still face higher costs per child per year above that age level, in both average and stress areas. In most urban areas, the difference in hourly requirements per child per year may have disappeared between elementary and high school children.

Two other pieces of evidence are available regarding the heavy load of restorative service needed by teenagers.[15] One is the large increase in DMF surfaces per DMF tooth which has been found to occur during this period. Every practicing dentist is familiar with the shift from occlusal to proximo-occlusal restoration work which occurs as additional surfaces become involved in the teeth of his teen-age patients. This should and does lead to increased operating time per person per year as the age of the patients advances. The other piece of evidence relates to the actual increase in chair hours per year needed for dental maintenance care beyond the heavy load of initial care the first year a new patient is seen. In a study of 877 patient-years of dental maintenance care in Massachusetts, children 16 to 18 years of age were shown to require 38 percent more dentist time per year than children 9 to 11 years of age. This situation is illustrated in Fig. 70. The superior preventive effect of fluorides on proximal surfaces has undoubtedly eliminated most of this increase in chair-hours in developed areas, but it probably continues to exist in high-caries localities.

Four disadvantages to incremental care at earliest available age must now be mentioned. The first is attention to deciduous teeth. Few dentists will deny the importance of the deciduous teeth, but conversely, few will assign them a value as great as that of permanent dentition. Much laborious proximo-occlusal restorative work is performed upon deciduous molars at a time when their permanent successors have already started calcification and are the controlling factors in mandibular growth. Where priority decisions must be made the permanent teeth deserve top listing.

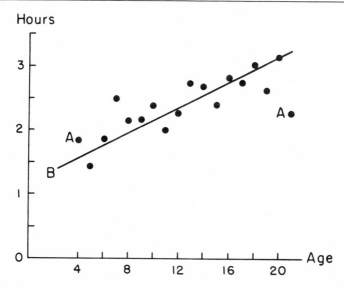

Figure 70. Chair hours per year needed for dental maintenance in Massachusetts, 1958. *A*-Sample of fewer than 18 observations; *B*-line computed from regression equation.

The second disadvantage in early-age incremental care lies in psychology, and in the changing patterns of modern family life. No longer do children move steadily from the habits taught them by their parents during childhood into similar adult habits of their own. One of the good features of teen-age rebellion is the responsibility young people feel for developing their own ways of life. Health habits and many other matters must therefore be taught directly to the teenagers. They must be reconvinced in terms of their own new motivation that teeth are worth keeping and that incremental care is the best way to assure this. Teenagers can be reached by reason much better than younger children. They have social motivation, not only in relation to their personal lives, but usually toward the community as a whole.

The third disadvantage relates to the increasing likelihood of interruption in children's dental health programs. In the social groups where systematic health care is easiest to attain, program breaks occur because of rising divorce rates and the increasing mobility of the average American family. Children are far more often involved in broken homes today and are more often moved with their families around the country in such a way as to interrupt programs for dental/maintenance care. Below these social strata there is a segment of the population with which practicing dentists have had little contact to date, where systematic recall habits will be difficult or impossible to induce. Faith cannot be pinned on a system which denies care to those children whose dental maintenance has been interrupted or whose background is deficient. These children may later become the best-motivated patients.

The fourth disadvantage is the inertia toward the seeking of private dental care found among dental patients who have received public care in early childhood. Lambert and Freeman, in a study of high school children in Brookline, Massachusetts, have observed that those children who received dental care on an incremental basis from the Brookline Health Department up through the fourth grade in school were in significantly poorer dental condition later on than were those children of a similar income level who had received care elsewhere.[16] The authors of this study conclude, "There is a sound basis to argue that given limited resources, young children should not be the sole focus of programs, but that teenagers should be given at least equal consideration."

If incremental care is to begin in the teenage period, inertia may still set in on termination of government aid. The children at this stage, however, will be nearer the end of their period of most rapid dental caries, and will have had a lot of valuable restorative work performed on their permanent teeth. If the successful program in New Zealand is followed, adolescent children 13 to 18 will be offered comprehensive care in private offices at government expense, thus bridging the gap to private care.

In view of all these facts, it is time to take a closer look at age variations in the need for dental care of the permanent teeth and patterns of motivation toward the utilization of dental care. Restorative efforts should be made available to those children who need care most and who are most likely to learn the lesson that is offered. Perhaps children should be received into the program on some individual estimate of their likelihood to continue periodic care. Perhaps certain incremental programs should be made available to high school or junior high groups, starting at age 12 or 13. Programs of this sort, of course, should be accompanied by preventive services for all ages and by efforts to save the first permanent molars of younger children, together with as much other restorative dentistry for other age groups as may be possible at the time. Sealants have an important function in this situation.

CLINIC VERSUS PRIVATE OFFICE

Practicing dentists commonly believe that communities would do best to pay them to treat public cases in their own offices rather than in a clinic. This is logical where transportation is available and the children and their families are educated to the appointment systems necessary in private offices. In disadvantaged and ghetto areas, however, people are often unable to afford transportation or child care and unaware of the value of time, hence unable to fit into a private practice routine. In such areas the dental care must come to the people, either in a school clinic or in a neighborhood clinic devoted to family care. Fig. 71 shows an example of the latter type. The clinics of the New Zealand and similar plans are located on school premises; the neighborhood clinics of Sweden (and many in the United States) are located as near the schools as possible, preferably within a mile. The functions of all clinics capable of providing comprehensive public dental care for children are discussed in depth in Chapter 17. Mobile clinics are occasionally preferable to fixed ones, and the Saskatchewan program in Canada has made imaginative use of rudimentary semiclinics in rural schools

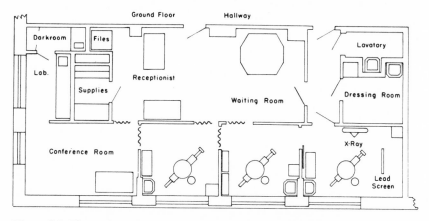

Figure 71. Floor plan of a typical neighborhood health center dental clinic. [Courtesy, Brookline, Massachusetts, Health Department.]

served on a rotating basis by dental therapists with portable instrument kits.

DENTAL AUXILIARIES

In both the teaching and the health care of all age groups dentists may be the leaders, but the backbone of the working staff is a corps of professionally trained auxiliaries employed on a full-time basis. In the field of dental health the professional groups best fitted to carry the load are the dental hygienists, the dental therapists, and the school nurses. The dental hygienists are specifically trained for dental health education, and wherever a school system is large enough to employ one or more hygienists they are the ideal persons to spark the dental program. They are at some slight disadvantage, however, in motivating people to seek dental care, not only because they are "interested parties" on account of their special training, but also because their viewpoint upon the whole spectrum of general health problems is not as broad as that of a school nurse. Hygienists are also hard to hire in small systems because employees of broader usefulness have to be hired first.

The school nurse, therefore, is always a person of importance in the conduct of the dental health program, and often the only auxiliary available. The functions of the dental hygienist and the school nurse in a dental health program are similar in many important respects in spite of differences in their training.

In order to picture the daily life of a dental hygienist, the Massachusetts Department of Public Health recently made a survey of the time devoted to certain specific activities by dental hygienists employed in state and local public health programs. Five types of activity were identified, with the range of percentage of dental hygienist's time devoted to each:

(1) Dental health education, 10–30 percent. This includes contact with public health nurses, teachers, parents, public health dentists, and private dentists. It also includes the placing of posters and distributing of mass media.

(2) Administration, 5–10 percent. This includes record keeping, compilation of reports, control of supplies, and other routine office duties.

(3) Technical activities, 40–75 percent. This includes dental inspec-

tion and referral of children, dental prophylaxis, and topical sodium fluoride therapy. Follow-up on dental care is also included.

(4) Community relations, 5–20 percent. These include activities with other agencies and organized local groups or committees.

(5) Internal administration, 7–12 percent. This covers time devoted to program planning, in-service training programs, staff conferences, and attendance at scientific meetings.[17]

Great variability may be expected within the pattern just described. Specifically, dental-hygiene teachers with advanced training in education may be employed by large school departments in such a way that all their time is devoted to resource and counseling work and to actual teaching.

The *school nurse*, in a broader sense, has duties very much like those described for the dental hygienist. Medical-screening work, counseling of children and parents, and resource work with the classroom teacher are all among their normal duties. Her technical activities lie largely in first-aid care and in the transporting of ill or injured children to homes or sources of treatment. Though she may lack the detailed knowledge of the dental hygienist in the field of dentistry, she is sometimes very much aware of the magnitude of the dental problem, and, if not, her interest can usually be aroused. She is fully able to take the essential steps such as urging dental care, oral hygiene, and better diet. Her interest in the dental program will vary with the other duties placed upon her, and with the extent to which the school dentist goes to her for help. Some school nurses take a deep personal interest in the dental program and can devote considerable time to it. One such nurse reports from her experience that "the nurse is usually the one to initiate special dental programs, exhibits, etc.," and she expresses the opinion that "the nurse must also see herself in the role of a sound informer and consultant for teachers needing up-to-date scientific material to draw upon for teaching, as well as for parents needing practical guidance."[18] She states with real pride that "the school dental health program provides a richer opportunity for motivating character and personality changes in students than any other phase of our health work." Her article closes with several case reports in which, through repeated conferences and other procedures, she secured dental care for children, with important improvements in their health and attitudes.

It is essential to the best utilization of both dental hygienists and school nurses that they not be asked to do too much routine clerical work. Dental assistants or lay volunteers can do much of the desk work needed in connection with follow-up procedures, record keeping, statistical reporting, and so on.

Lay assistants play an increasingly important part in preventive programs. One fluoride rinse program conducted in elementary schools in a Boston suburb has trained the mothers of local children to administer the fluoride at the classroom level. They were chosen because of their superior motivation and easy access to the school. The mothers were given a three-week training course and then kept under general supervision. They were paid in this program, but under other circumstances they might well be volunteers. Such assistants could also be used as aides in a sealant program in which a dentist or hygienist made the actual application, but a four-handed technique is the most effective one.

FLUORIDE THERAPY

In fluoridated communities and areas where the supply of private dentists is generous, fluoride therapy is of questionable value. Bohannan et al. in the National Preventive Dentistry Demonstration Program demonstrated questionable benefits and high costs for fluoride rinse programs and other forms of school-based preventive procedures.[19] In unfluoridated areas and areas where dentists are in short supply or absent, the story is different. Rinse programs, whose benefits average 30 percent in research programs, are popular.[20] They may show somewhat smaller benefits under service than in research settings, but they have a great educational advantage because of child participation, and they can on occasion be managed at far lower costs than Bohannan found. Thus, in Labrador the public health nurses supervise the rinses at no additional cost. The same can be true with supervised fluoride-tablet supplementation programs. Lay supervisors can be trained to administer either of these methods.

Neighborhood health centers are good sites for topical fluoride applications. Fluoride gel applied in trays seems the most effective of the various topical methods described in Chapter 12.

ORTHODONTIC TREATMENT

The demand for orthodontic treatment among lower-income schoolchildren is often a source of embarrassment to a school health program. The cost of orthodontic treatment is high in proportion to other health expenditures; hence the demands for assistance are frequent and for fairly large sums of money. From a public health point of view, however, orthodontic care is a low-priority item since so much of it is undertaken only for esthetic reasons. Dentists with Angle's classification in mind frequently name as malocclusion an alignment of teeth which, though theoretically abnormal, functions perfectly well and is only mildly unesthetic. Treatment of such cases is rightly considered to be a matter for private care. More appropriate to a public health dental program is the suggestion of the U.S. Public Health Service that only those cases be listed for orthodontic aid which cause speech defects, functional interference, or psychological handicaps.[21] The incidence of handicapping malocclusion is fortunately quite low, but the expense of treating each such case is high. Some of the problems of appraisal are discussed in Chapter 14.

Current approaches to the care of handicapping malocclusion lie through the use of federal funds for the aid of crippled children and for Medicaid (Title XIX). Access to these funds presents a complicated administrative problem, so that the few orthodontic care programs found in public school programs are in the largest cities or at the state level. Such programs are also better called "dental rehabilitation" programs than orthodontic programs, since, if a child deserves to be defined as crippled, dental care beyond the field of orthodontics may well be needed, such as plastic surgery and prosthodontic and speech-therapy services. Cases of this sort are often best handled in hospitals or special clinics where a combination of federal, state, local, and even private funding can divide the load.

PRESCHOOL PROGRAMS

Various surveys have emphasized that dental caries, in most United States communities, has become an important public health problem by the age of 3. A community dental health council, therefore, eager to begin its program of preventive dentistry at the real beginning, will wish to consider a preschool program. Preschool children can be reached through department of health baby clinics, nursery schools, day-care centers, kindergarten classes, and Project Head Start (described in Chapter 23). Administration of a preschool program is of course more easily centered in the health department than in the school department, but school dental clinics are sometimes available for use out of school hours if public health center clinics do not exist.

Evidence is accumulating that low economic status is associated with high dental caries in the preschool period and perhaps to a lesser extent in succeeding years (Chapter 8). Low-income children are likely to have had very little pediatric care or dietary supervision since birth, in spite of the existence of well-baby clinics. It is a common impression among private practitioners of dentistry that high-income children seldom need dental care before the age of 4, in sharp distinction to the reported recommendations from large public dental clinics that dental care for children in unfluoridated areas should begin at age 2.

Preschool dental health services can take many forms, but the easiest way to outline possibilities is to offer an example. Although fluoridation has now made this program unnecessary, Hartford, Connecticut, had a particularly well-designed preschool service, administered by the Hartford Health Department. This program offered three services:

1. A mail health education program involving letters to parents of children attaining their third birthday, with follow-up upon later occasions and letters to organizations caring for preschool children, such as nursery schools, day-care centers, and Sunday schools. This effort is supplemented by talks to professional and lay groups, the use of mass media, and demonstrations of preschool dental treatment in the health department's clinical facilities.

2. A preschool clinical program operated in conjunction with the Wellchild Conference of the Hartford Health Department. This involves individual dental health education, prophylaxis and examination, topical fluoride application, and finally, dental corrections. The first three of these items are cared for by a dental hygienist in a series of four visits per child. At the first visit the hygienist explains the purpose of early dental care and the value of topical fluoride in ad-

dition to giving the child a prophylaxis and a dental inspection. At the second visit she discusses the relation of nutrition to dental health and especially the harmful effects of sweets. At the third visit she gives instruction in tooth brushing and mouth hygiene, including instruction in the use of dental-floss silk. The fourth visit is used for review. If treatment needs are found, the child is then referred to one of the dentists in the restorative clinic to be treated as soon as the child is psychologically able to undergo treatment.

3. Children whose restorative dentistry has been completed are recalled routinely every 5 to 6 months for follow-up. As a final procedure, approximately 6 months after the child becomes ineligible for preschool service, the parents receive a dental reminder form stressing the need for continued periodic care through other channels.[22]

EVALUATION OF PROGRAMS

Many of the benefits of dental health programs will be intangible from the start. Other benefits may appear only after the school population is disbanded and measurement is therefore impossible. Some measurements, however, can be made if careful initial surveying of dental caries and other characteristics is matched by subsequent evaluation over a long enough period of years.

An example of such surveying and evaluation is available from the Askov Dental Demonstration in Minnesota, and is worth reporting here. Askov is a small farming community with a population mostly of Danish extraction. It showed very high dental caries in the initial surveys made in 1943 and 1946. During the period from January 1949 to September 1957, the Section on Dental Health of the Minnesota Department of Health supervised a demonstration school dental health program in Askov, including caries prevention and control, dental health education, and dental care. The Askov Dental Health Council acted as the governing body. All recognized methods for preventing dental caries were used in the demonstration, with the exception of communal water fluoridation, since until 1955 Askov had no communal water supply. Fluoridation was authorized for this water supply, but had not then been started. Dental care was rendered, for those who could not make other arrangements, by a group of five dentists from nearby communities employed by the Minnesota Department of Health. These dentists also gave topical fluoride treatments.

Detailed findings are available through a 10-year period.[23] They include a 28 percent reduction in dental caries in deciduous teeth of children 3 to 5 years old, a 34 percent reduction in caries in the permanent teeth of children 6 to 12 years old, and a 14 percent reduction in children 13 to 17 years old. Beyond these are improvements in filled-tooth ratios and many intangible benefits such as good health and dietary habits for the children to carry on to adult life. The cost of the program was greater and the caries reductions were smaller than are now occurring with water fluoridation in the same community—but fluoridation is by no means a substitute for such a program. Good health habits are valuable even for persons with resistant teeth, and dental care for the indigent is still needed in fluoridated areas.

Some of the clearest benefits of school dental health programs in a high-caries area are seen in a country like New Zealand, where almost the entire school-age population has received comprehensive dental care over a considerable number of years. Figure 65 in Chapter 17 shows the result in 1974 among 13- and 14-year-old children in an area of high caries susceptibility (Canterbury) where some 100 teeth had been filled for each tooth extracted.

GERIATRICS AND THE HANDICAPPED

Chapter 21 gives details on the care of the elderly, the housebound, and some categories of the handicapped. A community health center gives a good central point for the organization of programs for the benefit of these groups of the population.

Perhaps the most essential dental service of the center can be rendered by dental hygienists working under general supervision as scouts for the dental team. Given training as to the conditions they are to look for and a carefully-written protocol, they can visit nursing homes and private homes, giving health education, performing dental inspections and prophylaxes, and arranging case referrals where the services of dentists are required. To the extent that these cases can be referred to private dentists, specialized services, hospitals, or a variety of other community agencies, they can render a community service more valuable than any clinical service available at the center itself.

The blending of activities that go into a mature and successful local dental health program can only be indicated by detailed examples too lengthy for this text. A good source for such material is found in the Public Health Service publication *Selected Local Dental Health Programs.*[24]

Special Dental Health Programs

THIS CHAPTER deals with a number of types of dental health programs, most of them involving the same basic principles as those found in community health programs, but with enough special features to demand separate consideration. Important among these special fields is that of industrial dentistry; others are those of the college student, the chronically ill, the aged, and the handicapped. In addition, there is a brief consideration of the role of the dentist in time of disaster and the identification of the dead by means of the teeth.

INDUSTRIAL DENTISTRY

The reasoning by which certain institutions, such as central governments and local public school systems, have come to bear a responsibility in the field of health also applies to industry, with the added factor that, where industrial enterprises are conducted for profit, the cost of caring for illness or injury which results from the occupation of the worker constitutes a legitimate charge upon the receipts of the industry. In the United States, industry's responsibility for the care of occupational injuries, including dental injuries, is universally recognized, and in most states employer's liability insurance is compulsory. Beyond this, it is very common to find large industries conducting preplacement medical examinations. The objects of these examinations, according to the Council on Industrial Health of the American Medical Association, are:

(1) To measure the medical fitness of individuals to perform their duties without hazard to themselves or others.

(2) To assist individuals in the maintenance or improvement of their health.

(3) To detect the effects of harmful working conditions and advise corrective measures.

(4) To establish a record of the condition of the individual at the time of each examination.[1]

The Council further maintains that "The emphasis should be on the placement of individuals according to their ability and not simply selection of the physically perfect and rejection of all others. Unjust or questionable exclusion from work through improper application of the findings upon examination is against the public welfare and contrary to sound industrial health principles."[1] In continuing to describe what it considers a minimum medical examination, the Council includes examination of the teeth and mouth.

In conformity with these objectives it is natural for industry to take an interest in the prevention of nonoccupational as well as occupational disease, in health education, and often in the field of emergency nonoccupational medical care. As the labor unions enter the picture we find an interest arising in the full field of medical and dental care, usually through the medium of group purchase.

Aside from a few sporadic attempts to render the full scope of dental treatment in clinics on industrial premises, the development of industrial dentistry has followed public health lines. There has been emphasis upon postplacement dental examination, preventive measures, health education, and finally, referral to the private practitioner for any treatment other than that of an emergency nature. The first official recognition of industrial dentistry in the United States occurred in 1941 when the American Dental Association adopted a set of standards along these lines.[2] Since that time labor union interest in the group purchase of comprehensive medical and dental care and a realization that many industrial employees are in fact in need of aid in the financing of such care have compelled a modification of this attitude.

It is now obvious that group practices and clinics sponsored by employers, by employees, or jointly are with us to stay. Standards for their good conduct are being clarified. The problem is essentially one of nonoccupational disease. Attention will be given to industrial hazards later, but the substances involved are so commonly under control because of their danger to other parts of the body that the industrial dentist seldom has to worry about them. His problem is therefore essentially one of the recognition and prevention of the ordinary dental diseases and of palliative emergency treatment for the pain of these diseases. For the treatment of disease, the labor unions are frequent providers of dental health insurance.

Benefits

The need to convince employers of the value of industrial dental service has led to study of the benefits that might reasonably be expected to result. A discussion of these benefits not only gives ammunition to those who have the task of approaching industrial employers or employee groups but also clarifies the problem. The known benefits can be grouped under two main headings: reduction in industrial absenteeism and better dental health for the employee.

Reduction of Absenteeism. A study of common causes for industrial absenteeism has revealed several features differentiating absences for diseases of the teeth and mouth from absences for other causes.[3] The dental absences are a relatively small proportion of the total, but they assume an importance well beyond their frequency for three reasons: (1) the dental absences so listed are only those referred quite locally to the teeth and gums and do not include the more remote sequelae of dental infection; (2) they are usually associated with a need for corrective treatment beyond the mere abatement of acute symptoms; and (3) they are preventable to a surprising extent.

Data on absences for direct dental reasons are infrequently available. Puffer and Sebelius, studying five war production plants in 1945, found an annual frequency rate of dental absences of 47.3 per 1,000 persons.[4] Gafafer earlier reported annual numbers of dental absences of 17 per 1,000 among male and 37.8 per 1,000 among female public utility employees.[5] Each of these rates as Gafafer's is almost exactly 2 percent of the corresponding rate for all sickness absences. A study of claims for sick leave in the New York Naval Shipyard in 1943 showed 23 out of 1,200 to have been for dental reasons.[6] This again gives a rough 2 percent ratio. By 1979, Bailit et al. estimated that in a work force of just under 100 million in the United States, some 33 million work days were lost per year as a result of dental disease and treatment.[7] The workers lost some 3 billion dollars in wages as a result of these absences, exclusive of the cost of the dental care itself. The authors blamed most of this wage loss on the fact that most dentists then worked only within 9-to-5 business hours exclusive of weekends. Since that time the rapid growth of group dental practices associated with department stores or located near them in shopping malls has probably eased the situation. Most of these practices keep open until 9:30 P.M. on week days and work liberal business hours on Saturdays.

The first reason for giving more attention to dental absences than their frequency would suggest lies in the systematic damages that may result from dental infection (Chapter 13). Attempts at statistical measurement of the absenteeism resulting indirectly from dental disease have been unsuccessful for obvious reasons. We can only point to individual cases where dental treatment has brought relief from iritis, stiff neck, or the like.

The second reason for giving attention to dental absenteeism is that such absenteeism is almost invariably the sign of a need for corrective or restorative dental treatment. The situation is quite different from that of a minor respiratory infection, which may cause an even longer absence but leaves no need for treatment in its wake.

The third reason for interest in dental absences lies in their controllability. Data on this subject can be collected where palliative emergency dental service is available to industrial employees. In the New York Naval Shipyard a study was made of 633 civilian emergency visits to the dental dispensary.[6] Sixty percent of these visits involved disabling conditions which were relieved sufficiently for the worker to return to the job. Twenty-eight percent involved nondisabling conditions but ones which required consultation or simple care. Many of these cases might have required permission to seek outside dental care if service had not been available on the premises. Malingering was not a problem (and why should a malinger come to a dental office?). Only 12 percent involved disabling conditions not within the scope of the dental dispensary.

Emergency dental treatment is usually brief. The time required per case in the New York Naval Shipyard averaged 10 minutes. Each worker returned to work was saved an estimated 5.3 hours on the job, on the assumption that he would otherwise have left the Yard for the rest of the day. Actual savings were probably greater, since a number of the absences would have been for more than one day. More than nine out of ten of the conditions treated were nonoccupational. The few occupational conditions seen were the results of more or less unpredictable injuries, as from falls or from blows by heavy tools.

The four emergency dental cases seen per day at the New York Naval Shipyard in this period give an erroneously low estimate of the amount of such emergency treatment needed in a large working force. Naval authorities did not permit even the posting of an announcement of the dental service, and its existence was realized in only a few shops within the Yard. A much better estimate of the usual dental emergency load in industry is available from the Hood Rubber Company in Watertown, Massachusetts.[8] Here 5,600 employees in 1946 had access to one company dentist for emergency care, but there was no program of preventive dentistry. Fourteen to 20 emergency patients came to this dentist every day. They did not come until the pain was "pretty bad," and most of them were returned to work. Both here and at the New York Naval Shipyard it was felt that the majority of the workers, had they been forced to seek outside care for acute dental conditions, would not have received more than palliative care the first day from their own dentists. Definitive treatment would have had to be postponed.

It is interesting to turn these records for emergency visits into rates per 1,000 eligible persons per year. On this basis the New York Naval Shipyard emergencies were only 12 per 1,000 per year. The Hood Rubber Company emergencies approximated 610 per 1,000, a much more realistic estimate for heavy-industry plants at some distance from the homes of the workers. By contrast, white-collar establishments located in urban areas are likely to have much lower emergency rates. Harvard-Radcliffe University Health Services, serving some 28,000 eligible students, faculty, and staff, have reported about 120 emergencies per 1,000 persons per year. The Metropolitan Life Insurance Company in New York, which, in addition to emergency service has had a preventive program for home office employees based on case finding, health education, and reference to private practitioner for routine work, has treated about 60 emergency cases per 1,000 eligible workers per year.

Improved Dental Health. The lowered frequency of dental emergencies is only one of the manifestations of a general improvement in dental health which can occur when programs of preventive dentistry have been in effect for long periods of time among adults. Most of the best techniques of caries prevention, to be sure, require initiation during infancy or childhood. Yet a young person of 18 to 20 years of age, coming into industry even after a period of dental neglect, can still profit from dental prevention and care. At the Metropolitan Life Insurance Company, it was found in 1940 that, as a result of stimulation of the dental service, Home Office employees were receiving 1,705 fillings and crowns per 1,000 population per year as against 1,070 fillings and crowns in the highest-income group ($5,000 or more annual family income) reported by the Committee on Costs of Medical Care.[9] As a result of this and other forms of dental care, the Metropolitan employees were shown to have lost approximately five fewer teeth per person than this highest-income group, age for age, during the entire period of middle life from 35 to 65 years of age. This situation is shown graphically in Fig. 72. It was, however, demonstrated that the caries susceptibility of the Metropolitan group in terms of DMF teeth was no less than that of a sample of white persons throughout the United States of all income levels.

Even within this one company, improvements were found to have occurred since the inception of the program. The loss of teeth expressed as a proportion of the total DMF teeth (tooth

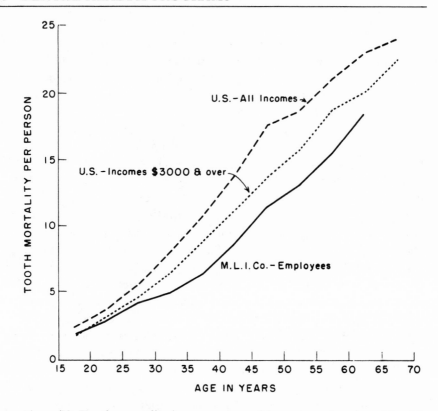

Figure 72. Tooth mortality in a company with a preventive dental health program and in the United States by income, 1942.

fatality) had dropped markedly during the entire period of middle life (ages 25 to 55) as compared with similar tooth-fatality rates among Metropolitan employees in the year 1927. These savings of teeth and reductions in dental emergencies represent large tangible benefits to the workers concerned, benefits which in most instances are productive of both good will and efficiency in the working force, as well as lowered absenteeism.

Frequency and Types of Service

Studies of the frequency of dental service in industry have been made from time to time and show in general about one large industrial concern in ten maintaining some sort of dental service for its employees.[10] The lists of firms from which these studies are constructed may often be biased, for those which have come to the writer's attention were of firms known to have medical programs or group insurance, factors indicative both of large size and of progressive attitude. A completely unselected list of firms might have shown smaller frequency. Companies of under 500 employees find considerable difficulty in maintaining a dental service and can seldom do so unless they are able to team up with other similar concerns. For these companies, group dental health insurance, as through one of the Delta plans, is the best and perhaps the only practical problem.

Health Education

Health education in connection with an industrial dental service might be expected to accomplish two objectives: first, stimulation to utilize the treatment services which are offered, and second, an increase in knowledge of preventive measures for dental disease. Industry does not offer a very favorable setting for generalized health education. The Health Education Unit at the Harvard School of Public Health, in a recent study of 25 plants, found a number of barriers to exist in the path of reception.[11] Activities fared best, however, that were an integral part of some type of medical or preventive service or were particularly appropriate to the needs of the plant or its workers. This indicates the advisability of focusing dental health education for an eligible group of industrial employees or their dependents upon use of an existing dental treatment service, and letting education on personal health habits assume a secondary role or be handled at chair side in connection with visits for treatment. The Harvard group also found that those media and methods which require little time, effort, or interruption of plant routine were more readily utilized in industry. These various findings give hints toward the efficient development of a phase of industrial dental service to which too little attention has so far been paid.

Industrial Hazards to the Teeth and Oral Structures

One of the major responsibilities of the industrial dentist is to minimize occupational hazards to the teeth and oral structures and to secure for the worker restoration of any damage which may have occurred from such sources. *Accidental injuries* to the teeth are probably the most common occurrence in this area. They are usually brought promptly to the dental office and because of the history of the accident there is seldom any doubt whether or not the events leading to it were of occupational origin. The dentist may have a role to play in the control of working situations conducive to facial injury, or in programs for use of the intraoral mouthguards described in Chapter 12.

More difficult to relate to occupation are a number of lesions of both the hard and soft structures of the mouth which may be caused over long periods of time by contact with various *abrasive, irritant,* or *cariogenic substances.* A good checklist of these substances should be at hand in any industrial dental clinic. Schour and Sarnat's careful summarization of the oral manifestations of occupational disease has been copied in various pamphlets and one of the most useful of their charts is adapted here as Table 43.[12] A more recent publication under a similar title is that of the U.S. Public Health Service in 1953, with abstracts of over 100 case reports and studies.[13] This pamphlet will probably be updated as additional information becomes available. The industrial dentist should take such a checklist as this to the industrial physician or perhaps to one of the production executives of the company in order to see how many of the substances listed may be found in use in any of the company operations. It is quite likely that certain of the substances will be found to be already under surveillance for medical reasons. The dentist can then perform a valuable service by watching constantly for early signs of oral damage.

Reference has already been made to workmen's compensation insurance. Dental injuries are compensable within this framework, and a variety of mechanisms are found in the different states as to disability rate, maximum benefit, and so forth. Morvay et al. provide a summary of regulations on this matter as of 1966.[14]

Hazards in the Dental Office

In the dentist's own office there are hazards worthy of the attention of the department of public health. Safety rules for dental radiography are discussed in Chapter 14. Matters of posture, psychological stress, and the like pose hazards of lesser degree. The American Dental Association lists an impressive number of chemical and physical hazards to be watched for in the dental office:

Electricity	Beryllium
Fire protection	Halogen containing organic
Gases	liquids
Liquids	Mercury
X-radiation	Nickel
Ultraviolet radiation	Nitrous oxide
Radio waves	Organic chemicals
Eye protection	Photographic chemicals
Noise	Pickling solutions
Infections	Plaster and other gypsum
Acid etch solutions	products[15]
Asbestos	

For each hazard there is a listing of sources and safety standards, followed by a practical series of do's and don'ts.

Health departments, particularly at the state level, have a responsibility for some of these problems. Thus in Massachusetts, and probably in many other states, the Division of Radiation Control requires a regulatory inspection of each new dental x-ray machine and reinspection perhaps every 5 or 6 years. Dentists are required to correct any defects found.

Administrative Problems

There are important differences in modus operandi between a community dental service and an industrial one. Dental examination will take more time per person among adults than it will among schoolchildren and more x-rays will probably be needed. The dental hygienist is an invaluable aid, as she is in a community dental health program, particularly since health education must depend even more heavily upon person-to-person communication than it does in a school system. Facilities for group education in industry are almost nonexistent, though mass media in the form of pamphlets have a certain usefulness. The personnel division of the industry can sometimes help to arrange schedules for initial and for periodic recall visits to the dental service. Referral of patients to private dentists for treatment not rendered on industrial premises is much the same as it is in the school dental health service. Other aspects of administration are covered in Chapter 11.

A common function of a state department of public health is the study of the various industries within the state to determine health

Table 43. Oral manifestations of occupational disease according to structure affected.

Structure affected	Etiologic agent	Manifestation
Tooth enamel and dentin	Dust	Staining
	Dust	Abrasion
	Prehension of instruments	Abrasion
	Acid	Decalcification
	Sugar	Caries
Supporting structures		
Gingivae	Dust, mercury compounds	Gingivitis
	Dust, heavy metals	Pigmentation
	Variations in atmospheric pressure, benzene	Hemorrhage
	Acid, mercurial compounds	Ulceration
Periodontal membrane	Mercurial compounds	Periodontitis
	Dust, flour	Calculus
Alveolar bone and jaws	As, Cr, Hg, P, Ra	Osteomyelitis and necrosis
	Fluorine	Sclerosis
Oral cavity		
Lips	Low humidity, dust	Dryness, fissure cheilitis, leukoplakia
	Aniline, carbon monoxide	Coloration of lips
	Tar	Carcinoma
Oral mucosa	Dust	Pigmentation
	Chemicals	Stomatitis
Tongue	Food tasting	Anesthesia, paresthesia
Salivary glands	Mercury compounds	Ulceration, ptyalism
	X-ray, radium	Xerostomia
	Increased intraoral pressure	Pneumatocele

needs. Only Pennsylvania, to the writer's knowledge, has so far attached a full-time dentist to its division of industrial hygiene, but other states may be expected to do this in the future. The objectives for such a person would be threefold: first, to determine the oral health of employees in the state's industries; second, to detect oral diseases of occupational origin; and third, to educate employees to the value of dental health.[16] His function should be that of consultant and advisor. Portable dental equipment will be of aid to the dentist, or to the dental hygienist if one is employed, in making implant surveys in various parts of the state. The greatest usefulness of consultants will be in plants that do not have their own dental health services. They may also determine the type of industry which should in general be urged to establish dental service. Thus, Aston in Pennsylvania found that the general condition of the mouths of workers employed in the heavy industries showed greater need for dental attention than those in lighter industry.[17]

COLLEGE DENTAL SERVICE

A closely related type of institutional dental health service is that rendered at colleges and other educational institutions. College dental health service involves almost the same administrative problems as those of industrial dentistry. There are two important differences, however—one psychological, the other relating to the scope of care which should be offered.

It is easy to imagine that the college student is uninterested in his dental health, but in the writer's experience this is not true. Away from home for the first time in many instances, the college student is working out his own plan for health service. He is therefore a most rewarding and receptive patient, with a mind which is more than usually alert. Dental health examinations should be linked with whatever system for physical examinations is in practice, and facilities for emergency dental service and reexamination should be available in addition. Restorative dentistry may be offered if circumstances make it advisable. The staff of the dental service should be selected with a view to interest in chair-side teaching as well as overall professional ability. College students ask searching questions and are entitled to answers on an adult plane.

Since so many college students are temporarily away from home and have family dentists who are in regular charge of their maintenance care, the college dental health service often has to assume the role of "substitute family dentist." Endodontic treatment for this reason becomes important. Suppose a pulp emergency arises which requires immediate treatment and the patient wishes to be made comfortable without prejudice to the restorative plans his family dentist may have for him. A few root-canal treatments may tide him over until he has a chance to get home on vacation, or complete endodontic treatment may be advisable. Consultation with the family dentist by mail or over long-distance telephone is often helpful upon this and other problems. The management of erupting and of impacted third molars, including the treatment of pericoronitis, is an important problem with the college student as with all young adults.

A college dental health service can engage very usefully in a small amount of restorative dentistry, though emphasis upon this phase of service should be secondary to emergency service, dental examination, and health education. Low-income or foreign students often find it difficult to make arrangements with a private practitioner and may deserve aid at reduced fees. The dean's office can be relied upon to help in the identification of worthy cases.

The American College Health Association, with headquarters currently at 15879 Crabbs Branch Way, Rockville, MD 20855, has a Dental Health Section which acts as a clearinghouse for information on designs and standards of college health services. The Association's two booklets on standards and on ethics are updated from time to time and contain valuable references to dentistry. They also have a leaflet for students on dental health.[18]

CARE FOR CHRONICALLY ILL AND AGED

It is increasingly obvious that the chronically ill and the aged require dental care of a type somewhat different from that rendered to normal ambulatory patients in the private office. It has been customary to treat these categories separately, but study will reveal that a great deal of overlapping exists between them. A child with cerebral palsy is usually called handicapped, but is certainly one of the chronically ill. The aged seldom require a specialized approach to dental care unless they are either chronically ill or handicapped.

This whole group of people, therefore, is essentially one, but within it are several different problems which require special attention. The largest of these is the problem of dental care for the home-bound.

The Homebound

The present-day dentist is oriented to office practice both by training and by routine. It is surprising, however, how much primary dental care can be rendered from a bag no larger than a physician carries on a house call. Modern hospital beds are easily tilted to angles much like those of the modern dental chair. The major problem, often a matter for persuasive action by the local dental society, is to develop a group of dentists willing to respond to house or nursing-home calls.

One of the important new developments in the field of chronic illnesses has been the development of home-care programs which will take the chronically ill patient out of a much-needed hospital bed and allow him to live at his own or a nursing home with proper assistance from the physician, the nurse, the caseworker, the dietitian, the occupational therapist, and other health workers. The dentist should be a member of this team.

The size of the problem is indicated by estimates that there is in the United States an increasing elderly population, now estimated as over 25 million, of whom some 5 percent are housed in institutions or other group quarters.[19] As of 1980, the U.S. Bureau of the Census estimates, 1.2 million persons 65 years of age or older were in nursing homes. Projecting to the turn of the century, the Bureau expects 2.2 million to be so located, or an 80 percent increase. Only recently have good studies appeared on the dental needs of chronically ill people domiciled away from large hospitals. In a survey of 855 residents of nursing homes, in Georgia covering an age range from 23 to over 99 years only 18.5 percent of these patients had received dental care within the past 5 years.[20] Among them were found 1,404 teeth that needed to be removed, 203 teeth to be filled, 511 new dentures to be made, and 363 existing dentures in need of replacement or repair. Seventy-seven percent of a similar group in Illinois were found to have some type of dental need, but only 41 percent had needs which were deemed capable of being treated.[21] A specific attempt was made in this instance to study prognosis. Prosthetic appliances were recommended only when the patient seemed to be physically and emotionally capable of using them. The American Dental Association, in a questionnaire survey of 2,966 nursing homes throughout the United States, found that 10.8 percent of the patients in these homes "wanted" dental care but were unable to get it.[22] This figure is undoubtedly an underestimate of the true situation, since it represents lay appraisal of dental needs in most instances, and many homes had had no dental examinations performed in the preceding year.

These figures emphasize the need for consideration of two points in making surveys of the dental needs of the aged: first, the aged are less adaptable and may therefore present poor prognosis, particularly in the efficient utilization of prosthetic appliances. Second, the masticatory needs of the aged are reduced. They need less food than active adults and have more time available in which to chew their food. They place smaller strains upon their dental apparatus and are often happy to be left alone with a situation which would be intolerable to a younger and more active person. These two facts are helpful since they reduce to more manageable size a problem which would otherwise appear colossal. The degenerative and pathological processes associated with old age, such as accelerated loss of teeth from periodontal disease and an increased need for operative treatment because of acute root caries, do indeed produce the increasing need for dental care which is mentioned in Chapter 13.

Kegeles, Lotzkar, and Andrews have developed some guidelines for the prediction of dental needs among residents of nursing homes as a result of pioneer experience in Kansas City, Missouri.[23] In their sample of 310 residents, 70 percent accepted care, and blacks accepted treatment more frequently than did whites. Persons under 75 years of age accepted more care than those older, and males accepted more care than females. Those who eventually accepted care responded to a questionnaire in such a way as to indicate they felt the need for care more; they practiced personal grooming more frequently, and, most obvious and also most important, they would accept care if offered. Care was also best rendered when convenient to the respondent, when no cost was involved, and when the work was seen as quick and easy.

The problem of organizing care programs for the homebound is complex. The *dental hygienist* is of great value as a scout, to chart the mouths of residents, make basic inquiries as to medical record, perform dental prophylaxis, help teach attendants to cleanse neglected dentures, and finally, to help the dentist organize a suitable but not overcomplicated operating kit to bring with him.

The question of *portable equipment* needs careful consideration. Portable dental engines, air compressors, and x-ray machines are now available. Dental students' portable cabinets usually suffice for those instruments which can be used easily at the bedside, though improvements are possible. One supply company has developed a two-container outfit for home use, each container weighing approximately 40 pounds.[24] One contains a portable high-speed dental engine, the other a compressor which can provide both compressed air and suction for surgical work. A simpler solution involves the use of a compact electric handpiece system with good torque and speeds up to 20,000 revolutions per minute. The problems encountered are by no means new. Much is to be learned from the methods presently used in frontier situations and in underdeveloped countries. More and more large nursing homes, however, are establishing a dental operatory to which patients can be brought if necessary in a wheelchair or even on a stretcher.

The financing of dental care for the chronically ill is also a difficult problem. Major long illness is usually disastrous to family finances, and the homebound therefore are more likely to need financial aid from community or government sources than are ambulatory patients. Means must be worked out for adequate reimbursement for the dentist, who will be taking more time per operation for these people than he would for patients who come to his own office. Title XIX offers a prospect, where available, as do federal crippled children's funds for young patients.

The home dental care problem is likely to increase in years to come owing to the increasing proportion of older people in the population. Since home dental care programs will probably involve a large number of part-time dentists and a good deal of organizational work among voluntary associations at the community level, it seems probable that organized dentistry will have an important part to play. State and district dental societies, through their councils on dental health, and the division of dental health of the state department of public health are probably the groups best suited to be of assistance.

Education for Geriatric Dentistry

There are a number of phases of the chronic-illness problem which suggest need for more adequate training of the dentist in both the undergraduate and the postgraduate years. Better basic training is needed on the nature of systematic diseases so that the dentist may drop his traditionally isolated attitude and be able to work smoothly as a member of the medical team. Included in this training should be an increased appreciation of the problems of the patient whose primary complaints lie outside the oral cavity and an understanding of how much dental treatment can be performed for a bedridden patient. All this involves more a shift of focus than any addition to the already overcrowded undergraduate dental curriculum. It means, in Galagan's words, "only that the environment in which the student renders a certain portion of his operative, prosthetic, and surgical requirements be changed from the dental clinic to the chronic-disease institution, and that the student changes from treating the otherwise well patient to treating the person suffering from some chronic illness."[25]

Teaching concerning the special treatment needs of the chronically ill and the elderly has developed most recently under the heading of geriatric dentistry. Predoctoral programs in a number of dental schools have involved lectures, seminars, and field trips to nursing homes or individual homes. In the best of these programs, dental students, accompanied by graduate students or instructors, perform screening and simple operations such as dental prophylaxis or denture adjustments.

Freedman and his associates at the University of Illinois describe a course in geriatric dentistry for third- and fourth-year students.[19] A series of five lectures is given in the third year; in the fourth year, through the Mayor's Office of Senior Citizens and Handicapped and the Chicago Visiting Nurses Association, visits are paid to nutrition sites, nursing homes, and individual homes. A portable x-ray unit and two Adec mini-ops permit a wide range of dental diagnosis and treatment. The twelve objectives for the course include attention to the changes in tissues with age, nutritional problems of aging, psychological components, social variables, the interdisciplinary nature of any provider team, the legal rights of patients, the issue of guardianship, and the many settings to which the dental team must go in order to reach geriatric patients.

Special dental techniques for the handling of patients with unusual handicaps can perhaps best be left for postgraduate training. Dental internships usually offer good opportunity for an appreciation of chronic disease. Since most general hospitals large enough to maintain dental interns are associated with some institution for the care of the chronically ill, arrangements can usually be made for the dental intern to spend some of his time in that institution.

THE PHYSICALLY AND MENTALLY HANDICAPPED

The preceding section has described dental care of a routine nature for patients who lack the ability to get to the dental office. Other handicaps, both physical and mental, alter the rendering of dental care without preventing visits to the dental office. Sometimes specialized techniques are required to do routine operations such as the placement of fillings. More often the problem involves the general management of the patient. These problems concern us here.

Cerebral palsy is a term covering a number of different conditions where the motor functions of the brain are affected. Spasticity is one of these conditions and involves hypercontractility of the muscles. When one muscle attempts to contract, its antagonist will also contract, resulting in a fixed position of the part. Athetosis is another, somewhat different, condition in which a series of involuntary muscular contractions are irregularly spaced and have no purpose. An athetoid patient trying to control himself may become very tense, which adds to the difficulty. Cerebral palsy patients are difficult to handle, first, because they cannot maintain good oral hygiene at home and need considerable assistance in this, second, because they are difficult to transport to the dental office (though most of them can be transported), and third, because they must be controlled and anesthetized more than usual in the dental chair in order that accurate restorative work may be performed. The last of these problems has given rise to a number of office procedures of help in the care of the handicapped and to the development of mouth rehabilitation under general anesthesia performed by specially trained pedodontists in a hospital environment. Sharry lists five techniques as of value in the office care of the cerebral palsy patient:

Premedication. Cautious use of barbiturates, probably in elixir form rather than capsule, proves helpful. This can often be arranged through the patient's parents before coming to the office. (Note: Adults are less affected by premedication and more muscular—hence more difficult to handle than children.)

Anesthesia. Local anesthesia can be used more often than would be considered necessary for dentistry for the average patient and will reduce the likelihood of convulsive movements. Where a large amount of restorative dentistry is needed for a difficult patient, rehabilitation under general anesthesia in a hospital should be considered. In using local anesthesia be very careful to have adequate finger rests and have the head of the patient immobilized against sudden movements.

Mouth props. Rubber or ratchet-type mouth props usually become covered with saliva and are difficult to maintain in place. A wedge of soft wood will often be of great assistance. Even with this precaution there is increased likelihood that the mouth will suddenly close and the operator should use buccal rather than occlusal finger rests. Props, rubber-dam clamps, and even cotton rolls should have lengths of dental floss attached to them to prevent involuntary swallowing.

Restraining measures. The patient is more easily maintained in place if the chair is tipped back. Webbing straps can be used to cross chest, arms, or legs. The head should be held by the assistant in such a way as not only to immobilize but to reassure the patient.

Aspirating equipment. Because cerebral palsy patients cannot easily reach the cuspidor or clear their mouths efficiently, good aspirating equipment should be available to collect saliva and other debris.[26]

The size of the cerebral palsy problem can be visualized from a recent estimate that there are 200,000 such children in this country.[27] The backlog of initial dental care in the group is larger than usual because of the difficulties involved in dental care and the recent devising of the special techniques just mentioned.

Another group often requiring similar care are the *retarded.* Though some of these patients are quiet and cooperative, many are spastic, athetoid, hyperactive, or subject to seizures. In some instances emotional problems tend to produce exaggerated reactions; there may also be abnormal fears and tensions. Some of the retarded may be on dilantin or other medication, resulting in considerable gingival hypertrophy or other abnormality.

An interesting example of a clinic designed to handle the physically handicapped and the retarded is the Joseph Samuels Dental Center at the Rhode Island Hospital, Providence, Rhode Island. A staff of a dozen or more dentists, some trained pedodontists and some trainees in this field, handle 7,000 or more noninstitutionalized patients per year in an outpatient setting. Most of the clinic is equipped for conventional dental operating with or without anesthesia. Upstairs there is a suite for general anesthesia, with trained anesthesiologists in attendance from the nearby hospital. General anesthesia is administered mostly for the purpose of diagnosis and the simpler forms of general dentistry. Many patients are completed at either the first or second such session. The more difficult cases are referred to the main hospital operating room for longer anesthesia and completion of more difficult operations.

The Orthodontics Department of the Samuels Dental Center has worked closely with the Orthopedic staff of the Rhode Island Hospital in treating children on whom the Milwaukee brace is utilized for the treatment of scoliosis. Research has indicated that this particular type of brace induces abnormal growth and development of the jaws and teeth of children, and proper orthodontic treatment is being provided to intercept the progress of such defects.

In addition to the dental care programs sponsored by the Samuels Dental Center, the facility is utilized as a teaching center. Both in-service education for staff personnel and training programs for the private dental practitioners of the state are features of this excellent dental facility. The Samuels Dental Center also participates in the education and training of dental auxiliary personnel.

Many disabled patients can profitably use a mouthpiece of some type to assist in the operation of electric wheelchairs, typewriters, and other devices.[28] An example is shown in Fig. 73. Included in this group are patients with cerebral palsy, poliomyelitis, and spinal nerve injuries. Mouthsplints without attachment are also valuable to prevent malocclusion in orthopedic patients who are under traction for long periods of time, or must wear the Milwaukee

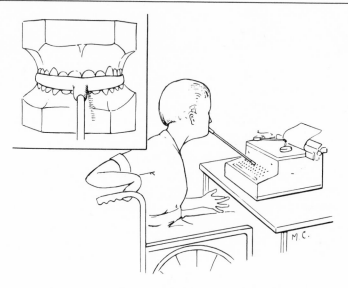

Figure 73. Mouthpiece fitted to teeth as a mechanical aid for handicapped individuals.

brace, with upward pressure on the mandible. These mouthpieces can be made of methyl methacrylate or other substances to fit accurately over both the patient's upper and lower teeth.

The *mentally ill* patient may also be difficult to treat because of inability to cooperate. The nature of the mental illness must be fully known, and suitable precautions taken. It is particularly important to have a dental assistant always present when handling mental patients in order to contradict hallucinations relating to improper conduct on the part of the operator. Dental treatment for some mental patients must be performed under general anesthesia. Large mental hospitals should normally have well-organized dental clinics, but the management of these clinics is not within the scope of this text.

In *epilepsy,* the dental concern is related chiefly to bruxism, and to the avoidance of removable bridges or dentures because of the chance of their becoming lodged in the throat during an epileptic seizure. The periodontal problem is also of importance in epilepsy, since dilantin is frequently used in therapy and can produce considerable gingival hyperplasia.

Arthritic patients are difficult to transport to the dental office, and sometimes need assistance on problems of mastication where movement of the temporo-mandibular joint is painful and the range of motion is limited. Because of the possibility that dental infection may be one of the causes for the arthritis, particular care should be used to remove oral foci of infection and a conservative attitude should be adopted toward endodontic treatment. Home hygiene can often be aided by use of the electric toothbrush.

Hemophilia, a hereditary disease found among males, calls for unusual precautions in the control of bleeding and also for cooperative planning with the family physician. Particular care should be taken to avoid minor hemorrhages as in the placement of matrix bands and in the course of dental prophylaxis. Caustic drugs should not be used. Hemostatic agents should be available in case of accident. Both local and general anesthesia have their dangers and should be avoided wherever possible. Local infiltration is the safest technique and only fine-gauge needles should be used. Endodontic treatment should be considered wherever possible in order to avoid extraction of teeth. If teeth must be removed, sockets should be packed with hemostatic agents and, if possible, not sutured. If gauze packing is to be used it should be coated with petrolatum to avoid incorporation in the clot.[26]

Patients with *cardiovascular diseases* need special handling in order to prevent bacteremia of dental origin. Any traumatic dental operation such as an extraction should receive antibiotic premedication, as with penicillin at a rate of 750 mg. per day, and continuation of the antibiotic for 2 or 3 days after operation. Consultation should always be held with the family physician on such cases. A history of rheumatic fever places the patient in this group.

The handling of the *tubercular* patient requires special consideration, not only because the removal of oral foci of infection is very important but because the dentist must protect himself from infection. He must consult with the physician in charge in order to know whether or not a case is in an active phase, and, if so, what precautions, such as masks, are necessary. Having done all he can to protect himself, however, he should move forward with courage in the treatment of the case just as do the other health workers who are needed.

Diabetes mellitus is another disease where control of oral foci of infection is particularly important. This disease also predisposes to periodontal disease, and dental prophylaxis should be carried out carefully as a preventive measure.

DISASTER PROGRAMS

Disasters always call for the utmost aid from the health professions and usually cast members of those professions in unaccustomed roles. Since World War II, the potentialities of thermonuclear warfare have made preparation for disaster necessary on a hitherto undreamed-of scale. Large cities will present the best targets for thermonuclear bombs, and hence the most difficult casualty problems. There would be traumatic injuries, burns, and radiation injuries in proportion to the intensity of the bomb, the distance from ground zero, and the protection individuals may have had. Radiation injuries will be slight from air bursts in favorable weather, but surface bursts can produce clouds of highly radioactive particles which can be carried great distances. Protection is therefore needed for massive fallout as well as from the immediate blast and radiation of the detonation itself.

With the recent escalation of the nuclear arms race, former civil defense precautions and emergency hospital facilities in any given area have become meaningless. Such dentists as survive must help ad hoc to the best of their ability.

Role of the Dentist

Dentists, because of their basic medical-science training and experience with handling patients often under conditions of pain, are qualified as a group of able assistants to physicians in providing emergency casualty care. Towle and Niiramen suggest that the dentist can provide assistance in any one of three ways: (1) he may provide direct emergency care through administration of anesthetics, parenteral therapy, or the treatment of wounds, burns, shocks, or radiation; (2) he may provide administrative assistance, perhaps by sorting and classifying casualties, by organizing groups for cooperation of effort, or by arranging for provision of needed facilities and supplies; (3) he may train others for casualty treatment. Before he is ready to undertake any of these roles, however, he must have practical training in casualty work himself.[29]

The initial course for any dentist to take in this area is *first aid*.

Local Red Cross chapters are usually prepared to organize such courses with medical or dental teachers. In the dental field, oral surgeons are usually better prepared than most to serve as instructors. Selected laypeople may also be useful, such as firefighters, rescue-squad personnel, or police. The best among these groups are those who have had combat-area experience. Each first-aid course, in addition to lecture and demonstration material, should provide personal observation of the handling of accident cases, in hospital emergency receiving wards, or even on the scene of accidents by riding the ambulance.

Advanced courses in casualty handling should be made available and be taken by as many dentists as possible. An example of such a course is that given at the U.S. Naval Dental School for naval dental officers. Here there are 30 hours of instruction, including lectures, demonstrations, films, and practical applications and first-aid procedures on available training aids. Trainee participation is stressed. The lectures in this course have included the subjects:

1. Basic structure of civil defense and its application to the Navy
2. Effects and potentialities of nuclear weapons
3. First-aid equipment supplies and their use
4. Categories of wounds, such as head and neck, chest, abdominal, and internal
5. Control of arterial and venous hemorrhage
6. Treatment of open and closed fractures
7. Management of maxillo-facial injuries
8. Emergency opening of closed airways
9. Burns
10. Shocks
11. Parenteral therapy
12. Medicaments
13. Bandaging and splinting
14. Resuscitation
15. Transportation of injured

The practical aids referred to for this course include facsimile arms, necks, abdomens, and so forth, for instruction in venipuncture, tracheotomy, clamping blood vessels, and such procedures.

Local dental societies can aid the civil defense authorities in mobilizing volunteer dental personnel and in promoting disaster training for at least a proportion of the available dental profession.

Identification of the Dead

The teeth are not only among the most resistant structures in the human body but are among the most distinctive because of the restorations and other identifying marks they carry. Where no previous dental record is available, the age, major facial characteristics, and some habits of the deceased can often be inferred from a study of the teeth. Age is told from the degree of formation, eruption, and wear of the teeth. The effects of habits are seen in notching of front teeth by bobby pins, abrasion and staining of teeth from pipe smoking, and so forth. The type and thoroughness of dental restorations often help determine the economic status and even the dentist of the deceased.

When the jaws of the deceased can be matched with good previous dental records, identification can be made with great precision. A listing of the location of decayed, missing and filled teeth (or, better, of surfaces) will usually produce a pattern so distinctive that chance duplication is most unlikely. Where previous dental x-rays or photographs can be matched with ones of the deceased from similar angles, so distinctive a pictorial pattern is often seen that duplication is unthinkable. The older the patient (unless edentulous) and the more recent the record or pictures, the better the chance of a reliable result. Sognnaes has presented in detail the wide variety of identification techniques now constituting the field of forensic stomatology.[30]

An indication of the importance of dental data for identification can be had from the experience following an airplane crash in 1975 in which 113 persons died.[31] Forty-two percent of the victims were identified by dental records alone: more than twice as many as were identified by fingerprints alone. The rest were identified by visual means, personal effects, or a combination of means.

The use of computer technology can speed immensely the identification of large groups of bodies. A computer-assisted postmortem identification program is now under test by the Army, using basic dental characteristics such as location of missing or filled teeth.[32] In a pilot test, the time for identifying a body from available dental records was reduced from 3 hours to 7 minutes, and accuracy was greatly improved.

Local or national registration of dental data is possible just as it is for fingerprints, though costs are greater. Location of decayed, missing, and filled teeth can be reduced to punched cards. Photographs can be taken of teeth in such a way as to show shapes of restorations, alignment of teeth, and so forth. The armed forces have pioneered in this direction for good reason. In default of large-scale registration of civilian data, dentists should be urged to record conditions of *all* the teeth of their patients (not only those teeth they have restored), and to keep the most recent x-ray surveys of their patients. State dental directors and state and local dental societies can encourage the accumulation of identification data in standardized form, and perhaps collect it in some central location.

CHAPTER 22

State Dental Health Programs

COMMUNITY AND specialized types of dental health programs have been described in earlier chapters as they would be conducted on the local level. These are the operating programs which make direct contact with the individual citizen. It is now time to consider the contributions that larger governmental units can make to the problem of dental health. To a certain extent, of course, state and even national dental health services may find themselves taking over local problems in rural areas that cannot help themselves. Large governmental units, however, have certain advantages over small ones, a fact which gives them peculiar functions of their own.

Large population groups with greater financial resources than local communities not only can command the services of experts but can also give financial assistance to local communities, either across the board or in such a way as to equalize the health services in the wealthy and the underprivileged areas. The experts can be used as consultants to local areas or as research workers on problems of general interest. Coordination is another function of the larger government unit. Uniform policies over large areas are sometimes of advantage in the health field. Control of communicable disease, for instance, depends very largely on such uniformity. Even in dental health service, uniformity pays dividends at times. Reliable work on the epidemiology of dental disease would be impossible if dental records could not be compared, one region with another. This accounts for the value of the concept of DMF teeth, so well understood now in many countries of the world. States often prove to be units of a convenient size for epidemiological study; they are large but not too large.

The development of state programs in the United States is of fairly recent origin. The first such program came into being in North Carolina in 1918, motivated largely by the need to help the large isolated and underprivileged rural populations of this state. Dental health services followed slowly in other states until 1935, when the passage of the Social Security Act made large sums of money available from the federal government to aid children's work. A rapid growth in dental programs then occurred, mostly within the framework of divisions of maternal and child health. As these dental programs became established and broadened their usefulness they worked their way up to separate division or bureau status.

Although North Carolina and a few other states and territories have always devoted a large amount of attention to direct dental care, most state dental health divisions have concentrated upon prevention, program development, education, and research. In the last few years, however, this traditional public health pattern has been sharply altered by the appearance of federally assisted dental care programs, chiefly under Title XIX of the Social Security Act (Medicaid). States must enact their own programs to utilize Title XIX. Although primary responsibility for the administration of Medicaid programs usually rests with the welfare department in a given state, health departments have so much to do with the standards of care rendered and the relationships of state government to the dental profession that the balance of activity in health department dental divisions has now shifted in this direction.

Some good reference material on state dental services is found in the Public Health Service publication entitled *Digest of State Den-*

tal Health Programs, revised 1965.[1] Table 44, taken from this booklet, lists and describes activities commonly engaged in by states, noting the number of states participating in each at that time. Even before the advent of Title XIX, dental care was prominently listed, although only 27 states at that time operated or supported care programs as against the 45 that promoted or offered consultation upon fluoridation.

DIRECT SERVICE

It has often been said in the United States that dental care was the responsibility first of the individual, then of the community, then of the state, then of the nation, in that order. This places the state third in the chain of responsibility, though state responsibility for direct service, where local communities cannot carry the load of care for the indigent, can often be shifted back again by giving state financial aid to the local programs. There are many states, however, where scattered rural populations or other situations make it imperative that the state render direct dental service. In these instances, preventive and emergency service should probably come first, and restorative service second, if at all.

Direct dental service can be carried out either through the assignment of state employees to local communities, using portable equipment, the use of permanent state clinics in fixed locations, or the use of a dental trailer owned and operated by the state. Many modern trailers such as the one shown in Fig. 66 provide facilities for mature dental practice. Permanent dental equipment can be fastened in place, and wall cabinets give an opportunity for the storage of a large selection of instruments. The dental health team usually operates in or alongside elementary schools in an attempt to create a well-rounded program such as is described in Chapter 20. Because of the brief stay which the team can make in a small community, however, certain phases of the program are apt to suffer, chiefly dental health education and the follow-up on dental referrals. A device for extending the program beyond the walls of the trailer (when one is used) is to employ two dental hygienists, one assigned to the trailer and one to work in the school with portable equipment. The hygienist in the school can devote more attention to dental health education than can the one in the trailer.

Table 44. Frequency of state health department participation in predominant areas of activity.

Activity	No. of states participating
Dental care	
Operates or supports dental care program for children	27
Provides financial assistance to local dental care programs	18
Operates or supports dental care program for special population groups, including the institutionalized	17
Provides orthodontic treatment or consultive services for cleft lip and palate program	9
Provides consultive services to care programs administered by local agencies and by other state health department units or other state agencies	9
Prevention and diagnosis	
Promotes and provides consultive services on fluoridation of communal water supplies	45
Conducts or supports topical fluoride application programs	27
Conducts or provides financial assistance to inspection and referral programs for children	27
Promotes or participates in programs of dietary practices for control of dental caries	18
Participates in surveillance of communal or private water supplies for fluoride content	11
Participates in surveillance of dental x-ray equipment	7
Participates in oral cancer detection programs	7
Dental health education of the public	
Presents lectures, participates in meetings, and provides consultation to professional and civic groups	33
Promotes dental health education in schools and provides consultation to teachers and school administrators	31
Prepares or distributes dental health educational materials	28
Participates in preparation or distribution of educational materials for classroom use	20
Participates in organized dental health educational programs for teachers and other professional groups	19
Public health education or teaching of health personnel	
Conducts or participates in courses in dental public health in dental, dental hygiene and dental assisting, or nursing schools	31

Table 44. (cont.) Frequency of state health department participation in predominant areas of activity.

Activity	No. of states participating
Provides orientation and in-service training for state and local health department personnel	30
Sponsors or promotes seminars, institutes, or workshops for dental, medical, nursing, or school personnel	18
Provides or participates in postgraduate and short courses in public health for practicing dentists	11
Provides field training for dental personnel	8
Program development	
Provides consultative services and technical assistance to other divisions of health department, other state agencies, and civic and professional groups	35
Provides consultation and assistance to local health departments in dental program development	26
Promotes participation of private dentists, local civic groups, and schools in state dental public health programs	10
Research and study projects	
Conducts or cooperates in surveys and evaluation studies related to use of fluorides	25
Conducts or participates in epidemiologic surveys or studies	16
Conducts studies of dental needs and resources, manpower, or cost	12
Participates in studies of radiation hazards from x-ray machines	11
Conducts surveys of dental needs of special population groups, including the institutionalized	9

She can also go ahead of the trailer, rounding up patients for the trailer dentist. Both hygienists can engage in case-finding activities, perform dental prophylaxis, and apply topical fluoride.

The *Digest of State Dental Health Programs* presents an interesting summary of dental health clinics and selected laboratory services operated by state health departments.[1] As of 1964, the various states, the District of Columbia, Guam, Puerto Rico, and the Virgin Islands operated 298 stationary and 78 mobile dental clinics. Over half of the stationary clinics were found in two localities—

Kentucky and Puerto Rico. Hawaii listed 34 of the mobile clinics, though it appeared the activities of these were limited to dental inspection, topical fluoride application, and referral work. Restorative work was confined to the 4 stationary clinics operated by that state. The other mobile clinics were widely scattered among 15 other states, presumably to reach only the most isolated rural populations. It is of interest that North Carolina then operated no clinics at all at the state level, but provided dental care to indigent schoolchildren by assignment of personnel and portable dental equipment to counties. All states but two offered water fluoride analysis as a laboratory service. Twenty-two states offered lactobacillus counts, and 19 offered oral biopsy.

Medicaid

Although the Medical Assistance program provided under Title XIX of the United States Social Security Act is national in origin and largely supported by federal funds, it is best listed as a state program, since states decide whether or not to enact it. By 1976 all states but one had done so.[2] Federal contributions to the program range from 50 to 83 percent, depending on the state average per capita income. Since each state determines eligibility and benefits, there are state-by-state differences as to who is eligible and for what benefits. Where Title XIX programs exist, they supplement the insurance program set up nationwide by Title XVIII (Medicare).

Dental services are included in the list of 15 types of health care which Title XIX may render, but not in the list of 5 mandatory services. The Act provides, however, that medical assistance "shall not be less in amount, duration, or scope, than the medical assistance made available to individuals receiving aid or assistance under any other such state plan." Thus states which have rendered dental care as a part of welfare programs in the past are committed to continue such care under Title XIX, at least to a similar extent. Dental services are defined by the Act as "any diagnostic, preventive, or corrective procedures administered by or under the supervision of a dentist in the practice of his profession."[3] This permits both general and specialized services without any restriction except such as may be made by states in order to conserve funds. Welfare departments in general will handle all financial aspects of the program, though health care standards and certain relationships with health care providers (that is, private dentists) may remain with the health department.

The patterns of eligibility for medical assistance programs are of interest. States must include in their programs from the beginning all persons who receive financial assistance from the federally aided public assistance programs for the aged, the blind, the disabled, and families with dependent children, including persons who may be actual residents of a state but who have not lived there long enough to satisfy certain state regulations which specify periods of time before welfare benefits are available. All children under 21 must be included who, except for a state age or school attendance requirement, would be eligible for assistance through the program to aid to families with dependent children.

As the Act was originally passed, there were no limitations upon states as to a maximum income they might declare eligible. Some states thus designated limits as high as $6,000 per year for a family of four. Later the Act was amended so that eligibility levels might not represent more than 150 percent of the amount allowed under the state's aid to families with dependent children program. Further reductions below that percentage have occurred since. The amendments also allow a state to establish different income levels for eligibility under Medicaid based on variations in the cost of housing between the urban and rural areas of the state. Local public welfare departments will determine eligibility on the basis of standards established by the state and on the basis of individual determinations with respect to the recipient's ability to pay for the cost of medical care.

As of June 1976, 12 states were offering dental services to people receiving federally supported financial assistance, and 22 more states were offering dental care also to people receiving state public assistance and such others as the aged, blind, or disabled who were financially eligible for medical care but not for financial assistance.[2] New York, California, and Massachusetts have for some years offered a wider scope of dental services than other states. Any increases in dental coverage since 1976 have been more than offset by the cutbacks of the recent federal administration.

Title XIX legislation applies equally to health care in private professional offices and in institutions. Freedom of choice of practitioner or program is optional with the states, but would presumably be permitted in most instances.

Determination of reimbursement for services rendered in private offices and in institutions will necessarily differ. In private offices, fees per operation or per visit are the rule. These may be from a schedule of specific fees in the private office or be "usual, customary, and reasonable" fees as described in Chapter 18. In institutions, the concept of "reasonable cost" prevails. An institution may divide the entire budget for its dental service according to the number and frequency of operations or other services performed during a given period, and then ask as reimbursement such a sum per operation as will represent both the cost and the relative value of the operation according to locally prevailing standards. Thus in one instance in Massachusetts the old state welfare fee scale for treatment in private dental offices was reduced by about 20 percent in order to produce a reimbursement level for the operations of a clinic which would approximate the actual cost of the services to that clinic. Locally operated clinics for indigent persons, ghetto populations, dental school patients, and the like may thus in many instances recover much of their costs through Title XIX.

In law, at least, as mentioned earlier, every state with a Medicaid program should provide children under 21 with comprehensive health care, including dental. Federal guidelines exist for an agency in each such state to provide early and periodic screening, diagnosis, and treatment (EPSDT) to all children eligible for Medicaid. Limitation of funds and manpower have hampered the implementation of this program in the dental field.

There is no space in a text such as this to attempt to describe the technicalities by which patients may become eligible for Medicaid benefits or dentists may proceed to secure reimbursement for the services they perform. These matters are specific not only to the states involved but also to local areas within states. Negotiations leading to the establishment of dental fees represent the marketplace just as do the negotiations for fees in private practice. In this instance the dental profession as represented by its dental society, state or local, becomes the supplier, and the government, with the taxpayer in the background, becomes the consumer.

Public health planners with prevention in mind originally hoped to see major expenditures under Title XIX devoted to children's care. A preliminary analysis in one state showed this to be the probable outcome.[4] Forty-five percent of the dental case load for a typical month, and 35 percent of the costs, concerned children 7 to 13 years of age. Since then, the decreasing needs of children and the increasing needs of adults and the elderly are causing a change of focus.

State-Operated Care

The rendering of care is often organized independently of the means for its payment. Thus the Association of State and Territorial Health Officers in 1982 reports 48 state health agencies directly operating 53 separate therapeutic and preventive dental programs.[5] The report deals only with the actual services provided, regardless of source of funding, and these vary widely. Almost all agencies provided preventive care, including prophylaxis, examination, and professionally applied fluoride. Restorative care to a varying extent and emergency treatment were provided by 34 state agencies.

Sealants were provided by 22 state agencies. Thirty-five agencies provided fluoride mouth rinse programs at 8,254 sites. Thirteen state agencies operated fluoride tablet programs; 11 had fluoridation of school water systems.

SOURCES OF AGENCY FUNDS

The variety of sources from which state agencies derive financial support is also large. From 1981 to 1982 the total dollars received increased 5 percent, but when adjusted for inflation, this figure meant a decrease of 2 percent. The Association of State and Territorial Health Officers tabulated the sources of funds, providing figures for both dollar amounts and percentages of the total, as shown in Table 45.[5]

In the face of rapidly rising costs, it is of interest to offer a provisional and perhaps incomplete listing of the ways in which costs can be controlled, some of which are entirely advantageous, whereas others involve to some extent a trade-off between dollars and quantity of service:

1. New facilities for health care may be planned with maximum efficiency and avoidance of duplication. (See Chapter 17).

2. The escalation of costs which might result from unbridled public demand for service of which there is an inadequate supply may be held in check by tying such costs to other costs more stable than medical, as for instance cost-of-living indices.

3. Auxiliary personnel may be used to maximum efficiency, with state laws adjusted to permit this. (See Chapter 17.)

4. Prevention may be used to best advantage (fluoridation, and other measures such as those discussed in Chapter 12).

5. Methods for assuring only the highest quality of care may be developed, along with complete honesty on the part of vendors regarding their charges and on the part of recipients as to their applications for eligibility. (These methods have been considered in some detail in Chapter 19.)

6. Income levels for eligibility can be controlled.

7. Scope of service may be controlled, concentrating health care on those basic operations which produce greatest health benefits for least cost. Prior approval may be required for items not necessarily to be eliminated.

8. Inefficiencies may be controlled in administration and communication.

EPIDEMIOLOGICAL SURVEYING

The state is a very good unit for epidemiological surveying. A small team of dentists, dental hygienists, and assistants, using proper sampling methods, can cover an entire state with reasonable ease and get detail enough that local variations are brought to light. Where the state team itself does not do the work it can aid local communities by the establishment of standards of measurement and perhaps supervision of survey work so that local surveys may become an accurate part of the state pattern. A state dental division can work with a university or other private agency—the agency supplying theoretical competence and specialized services, the state supplying official access to the population groups to be studied and financial aid, both for research and for service.

Most surveying will probably be for some specific purpose: the testing of some epidemiological principle or theory, the testing of

Table 45. Sources of funds for dental health programs of 48 state health agencies, fiscal year 1982.

Source of funds	Amount (millions of dollars)	Percent of total
Total	37.4	
State funds	22.5	60.3
Local funds	3.4	9.1
Fees and reimbursements	2.9	7.8
Other	0.2	0.5
Federal grant and contract funds	8.3	22.2
Centers for Disease Control	3.7	9.9
Fluoridation (PHSA, Sec. 317)	2.6	7.0
Preventive Health and Health Services Block Grant (PL 97-35)	1.1	2.9
Health Resources and Services Administration	4.3	11.5
Maternal & Child Health Services Block Grant (PL 97-35)	2.7	7.2
Maternal and Child Health (SSA, Title V)	1.5	4.0
Crippled Children (SSA, Title V)	0.1	0.3
Health Care Financing Administration (Title XIX, Medicaid)	0.1	0.3
Office of Human Development Services (Title XX)	0.1	0.3
Other federal	0.1	0.3

some caries-preventive measure or the evaluation of some local or regional dental service. A certain amount of surveying, however, is justified without specific purpose for the accumulation of *baseline data* on dental disease. Long-term (secular) trends in dental disease need to be measured, water fluoridation and other preventive dental programs need to be evaluated against previous baseline data, and problems for study occasionally arise which can be viewed properly only in retrospect. Cost-benefit and cost-effectiveness studies deserve high priority at the present time.

DEVELOPMENT AND RESIDENCY TRAINING

Program development work perhaps gives the state division of dental health its most congenial opportunity for usefulness. Here, the expert services of the state are brought to bear to determine priorities and to help local communities in problems of immediate interest to them. The division functions best in localities where it has been invited to assist, for advice is then likely to be taken and appreciated. Other localities should be approached with caution. Patterns for consultation and promotion work cannot be laid down in any set fashion.

With this approach to the development of new dental health programs comes an opportunity for residency training, which is of particular importance in view of the certification requirements of the American Board of Dental Public Health. Residents in this field can first be taken along for observation, then assigned various phases of the study and planning involved in the preparation of programs suited to state or local needs. The residents will report frequently to the state dental director or other training supervisor, and a chain of communication can be set up which will benefit the trainee, the division, and the local community.

Certain phases of epidemiological research fit well with a residency program. The trainee can assemble and analyze data under the guidance of a research sponsor, making a substantial contribution to epidemiological knowledge. Field trials of new preventive measures also make good training projects. State divisions of dental health can commonly offer a better residency program than would otherwise be possible, if they are in close contact with a university dental school. Such contact is fully as rewarding to the dental school as to the state division. Undergraduate as well as graduate dental students may find opportunities for useful experience, and helpful stipends, as summer apprentices or in some other capacity. It is to be hoped that the dearth of federal traineeship money which existed in the middle 1970s will be overcome, since residencies in dental public health pay big dividends in future preventive programs. Table 46 lists a number of methods by which dental personnel can serve the public through a state health department.

PERSONNEL AND ADMINISTRATION

There is no set pattern for the staffing of a state division of dental health. A full-time, properly trained public health dentist is, of course, necessary as director, and perhaps also a full-time dental hygienist or therapist, with public health and education training, as dental-hygiene coordinator. Beyond that, the pattern may vary widely. Additional dentists are advisable, particularly in large states, on either a full-time or a part-time basis, and an even larger staff of dental auxiliaries with experience and perhaps degrees in the field of education. Clerical staff will be needed, and, if direct service is rendered to patients, dental assistants as well. Administrative experience is important for a dental health director, as he must spend much of his time preparing budgets, obtaining and distributing grant funds, and consummating various financial arrangements, both state-federal and state-professional in nature. He must be able to function as a dental consultant in nondental public health organizations, both official and nonofficial. Particularly, he must work with the state dental society. This organization, through its trustees, and councils on dental health and dental care, is his best link with the dental profession. Through the society he can get support for his policies; through it his policies can be implemented in many instances; and through it, of course, the local dentists can influence his policies so that they will accord with local needs.

The size and composition of the typical state-level dental health team is worthy of study. Table 46 shows a typical distribution of personnel among various categories, not only in the primary unit

Table 46. Full-time equivalents of full-time and part-time employees engaged in dental health activities of state health departments, 1964.[a]

Employee category	Primary unit		Other units[b]		Total	
	Full-time	Part-time	Full-time	Part-time	Full-time	Part-time
Public health dentists	179	3.3	9.0	1.0	188.0	4.3
Clinical dentists	81	21.8	20.0	2.1	101.0	23.9
Dental hygienists	107	3.6	12.0	1.4	119.0	5.0
Dental assistants	74	3.5	15.0	0.2	89.0	3.7
Other	140	4.8	18.6	3.9	158.6	8.7
Total	581	37.0	74.6	8.6	655.6	45.6

a. A full-time equivalent represents 2,000 hours of service.
b. Organizational units of the state health department other than the dental health unit: mostly prisons, hospitals, and mental institutions.

but also in other dental care units operated by the state health departments, for the most part in prisons, hospitals, and mental institutions. The 179 full-time public health dentists were, of course, the core of this group. With them were important numbers of full-time dental hygienists and "other" personnel, presumably secretaries and clerks. The part-time personnel, however, must not be neglected, and they are probably underestimated by the process of listing them as full-time equivalents. The 21.8 full-time equivalents of clinical dentists actually represent 521 individuals. Of these, 200 in the state of Kentucky are not represented in the list of full-time equivalents, since an estimate of the number of man-hours they spent on dental health activities is unavailable. Part-time personnel present an administrative problem and a communications problem, but at their best they provide loyal and efficient service and a link with the private sector of the community, which is advantageous to all concerned.

A SAMPLE STATE ORGANIZATION

New York State, which offers an unusual breadth of activities, is an illustration not of an average program but of a top-level one. The organization of the whole New York Department of Health is described in Chapter 2. The organization chart of the Bureau of Dental Health is shown here in Fig. 74. Before recent federal cutbacks threw unusual tasks upon state governments, while at the same time producing cuts in ongoing state programs, the Bureau had a professional staff of 12 and a clerical staff of 8. A current listing of specific programs shows 11 ongoing ones and 24 proposed. The following subject areas are involved.[6]

Caries. The focus is upon prevention by the use of fluorides. Water fluoridation is promoted in interested communities. Funding is provided for the installation of equipment and for first-year supplies. Where fluoridation is not feasible, fluoride rinse programs are encouraged, and preschool populations are offered enrollment in a dietary fluoride supplementation program. A sealant program and intensive caries-control programs for underserved areas in the state are proposed.

Periodontal Disease. A statewide preventive program is proposed, with a network of dental hygienists at the regional level to work with institutional residents, industrial groups, and others. Pregnancy gingivitis will receive particular attention.

Malocclusion. The Physically Handicapped Children's (PHC) Orthodontic Program is currently providing corrective care for over 12,000 children annually. A statewide survey of orthodontic care delivery and its cost evaluation is planned.

Special Populations. Current programs include an oral health survey of the elderly, with emphasis on medically compromised dental patients and on the effect, if any, of fluoridated water on acute root caries. An assessment of adverse factors upon high-risk ethnic

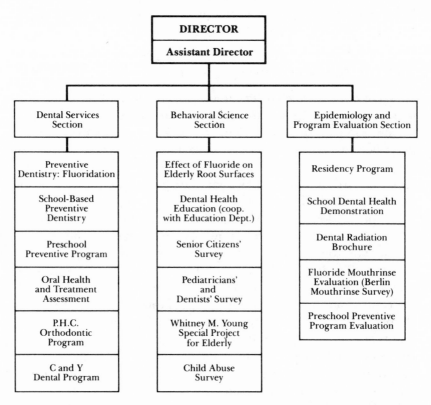

Figure 74. Organization chart of Bureau of Dental Health, State of New York Department of Health.

and minority groups, many of whom are underserved, is under way.

Injury. A survey of dentists' perceptions of child abuse is in process and a study of the long-term effects of craniofacial trauma has been designed. A program for preventing dental injuries to 8–10 year old boys, a high-risk group, is proposed.

Oral Cancer. Current screening programs for early cancer detection include free examination of high-risk elderly persons. An educational effort aimed at dental care providers and other health professionals dealing with high-risk populations is proposed.

Fear and Anxiety. A demonstration program has been designed to reduce fear and anxiety among young children attending a dental clinic for the first time.

Occupational Health. Educational programs are proposed for dental professionals on such hazards to themselves and their patients as mercury and nitrous oxide.

Service Delivery. Two programs are currently operating, one on the effect of fluoridation on dental practice in Newburgh and Kingston, and another on dental care for the elderly. In the latter area, a cost-effectiveness study is proposed.

Health Education. The New York State Residency Program in dental public health is ongoing, in affiliation with Harvard University. Another project involves the development of a dental radiation brochure, in cooperation with the state Office of Health Promotion. Curriculum development is under way for dental health instruction of school children from kindergarten to grade 12.

This overview of the functions of a state division of dental health has perhaps leaned too heavily on the current problems of the provision of dental care and its financial support. An impartial study of Table 44, however, both as to the program areas it presents and the frequency with which each is utilized throughout the United States, gives better perspective on the importance of preventive and educational projects within the state program. As the public dental care programs come under control, state dental health divisions can return their attention in greater proportion to these other activities.

State dental health activities do not occupy as important a place in total state public health programs as the importance of dental disease would appear to warrant. In 1964, during the pre-Medicaid era, for example, a total of only $8.5 million was spent in the entire United States for primary dental care units within state health departments, or an average of less than $200,000 per state. Similarly, the expenditure for dental health activities of only 6 cents per capita was a ridiculously small proportion of the per capita figure of $3.91 for all health activities. One can only hope that the public demand for dental care uncovered by Medicaid will turn the attention of health officials to a sensible approach to national health insurance dental services, and at the state level return attention to the important gains to be realized through prevention, not only in terms of health but in terms of taxpayer dollars.

CHAPTER 23

United States Federal Programs

IN SPITE of the concept mentioned in previous chapters that dental care is the responsibility of the individual, then of the community, the state, the nation, in that order, the United States federal government has been involved from its earliest years in dental care, as well as in the more conventional public health tasks of prevention, research, and health education. Until 1965, however, direct care was a minor enterprise restricted to certain designated wards of government, and the major efforts were in the areas of prevention and research. With the expansion of the Social Security Act to include medical care, however, and the development of large new grant systems for health care under various acts of the "New Society," federal health agencies have become deeply involved in the administration of care.

Owing to the current federal budgetary problems, it would not be reasonable to assume that the present trend will continue, with step-by-step increases in scope of care and extent of population served. Public demand for care will probably increase faster than public willingness to pay taxes for the care received, but the taxes may follow until an equilibrium is reached, much as has been the case with public school education throughout the country. Supplementing this trend will be (or should be) a strong effort among professional groups to maintain private initiative in the purchase of health care and a firm intent in government circles to concentrate as much tax money on prevention and research as may be needed for these enterprises, which are actually more valuable in terms of cost efficiency than an equal amount of money expended for health care.

DIRECT HEALTH CARE

Before 1965 the list of groups receiving federal health services in the United States had already become long. Members and veterans of the armed forces, American Indians, federal prisoners, isolated groups such as lepers and the relocated Japanese of World War II, as well as other groups whose work or life situation involved unusual health problems or hazards had been included. This last group includes the merchant seamen, who called the U.S. Public Health Service into being in 1798 but who ceased being eligible for care in 1981.[1]

The armed forces have developed large, well-organized health services with well-staffed dental services that have considerable autonomy. These dental activities have in general provided high-quality, comprehensive dental care and have gone further to engage in clinical research and in the training of health personnel at various levels. Basic research is also conducted by such agencies as the Armed Forces Institute of Pathology and the Office of Naval Research. The armed forces, which take for brief tours of duty approximately 15 percent of the 5,000 graduates of American dental schools, make a great indirect contribution toward public health training. Five thousand men and women serving in a military setting inevitably learn a great deal about public health teamwork, and in the larger military centers they find themselves under the guidance of expert professional leaders. Additionally, about 500 of the career armed services dentists are enrolled in postdoctoral specialty training (1984).[1]

The enactment of Titles XVIII and XIX of the Social Security Act in 1965 marked an important change in government approach to the rendering of health care. Title XVIII (Medicare) provides dental care only under certain specific medically related conditions, but represents the greatest political change in that an entire age group (65 and over) suddenly becomes eligible for extensive health care, regardless of income, hardship, or service to the national government. Title XIX (Medicaid) does, of course, permit extensive dental service, as has been mentioned in the previous chapter. In theory, Title XIX follows the old concept of providing care to needy groups, but these groups have been so widely extended that they merge to form an important fraction of the entire population. Title XIX has been described as a "state program," which it is in terms of administration. It is quite logically included in the federal Social Security Act, however, since the pressures upon states to participate in it are great and the care rendered through it will constantly be compared as to quality and scope with the care rendered by Title XVIII.

UNITED STATES PUBLIC HEALTH SERVICE

The department of the federal government most deeply concerned with health is, of course, the Department of Health and Human Services. The agency within the Department which has the greatest stake in dental health is the United States Public Health Service. The Service reports to the Department through the Assistant Secretary for Health and Surgeon General, and it includes a vast array of specialized health services devoted to specific health problems.

The major units of the U.S. Public Health Service are shown in Figs. 75 and 76. Within this framework, dentistry is found in a number of specific locations in the six operating agencies.[1] In the Office of the Assistant Secretary for Health and Surgeon General is the Chief Dental Officer, U.S. Public Health Service.

The major clinical dental activities within the U.S. Public Health Service reside in the Health Resources and Services Administration (HRSA). HRSA's Bureau of Health Care Delivery and Assistance (BHCDA) is comprised of:

1. The Maternal and Child Health Program (authorized by Title V of the Social Security Act), formerly the Children's Bureau, which manages the dental component of Project Head Start. (The overall responsibility for Project Head Start resides with the Administration of Children, Youth, and Families of the Office of Human Development Services). Additionally, the Maternal and Child Health Program provides funds for several demonstration projects, such as pit and fissure sealant application in a public health setting and dental services for developmentally disabled children.

2. The Community Health Center Program, employing 600 dentists in 300 locations. In 1984 it provided $81 million worth of dental services to 714,000 eligible indigent patients who resided in their service areas.

3. The National Health Service Corps, employing 200 dentists who work in dental health manpower shortage areas. In 1984 it provided comprehensive dental care to unserved and underserved individuals.

4. The Bureau of Prisons Medical Program, employing 55 dentists detailed to the Department of Justice to staff 47 federal correctional facilities. In 1984 it provided comprehensive dental services to the 38,000 federal prisoner population.

5. The U.S. Coast Guard Medical Program, employing 75 dentists detailed to the Department of Transportation to staff 32 clinics and six mobile units. In 1984 it provided comprehensive dental services to the 38,000 active duty personnel, their dependents, colocated active duty armed services personnel, and retired armed services individuals.[1]

The Indian Health Service (IHS) of HRSA is responsible for the delivery of comprehensive dental services to the 1 million American Indians and Alaskan natives who are members of federally recognized tribes. The Indian Health Service dental program, employing 275 dentists who staff 48 hospitals, 196 health centers, 24 mobile units, and 167 portable field sites, provided comprehensive dental services to more than 300,000 eligible patients in 1984.

Within HRSA, the responsibilities of the Bureau of Health Professions (BHPr) include: provision of dental expertise in planning, coordinating, and evaluating the nation's health manpower re-

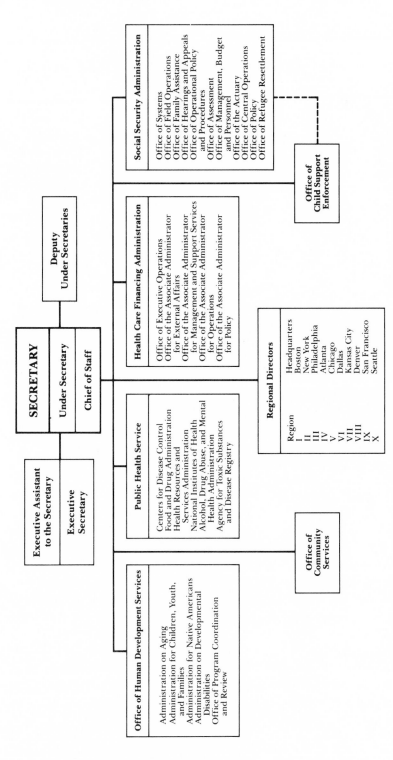

Figure 75. Major units within U.S. Department of Health and Human Services, January, 1984

sources and in assisting development and utilization; and support for the development, use, accreditation, and distribution of dental personnel. A significant program within these functions is the Dental General Practice Residency Program.

The Food and Drug Administration is responsible for ensuring the safety and efficacy of food, cosmetics, drugs, and medical devices in the United States. It contains three dental activities: the Dental Device Certification Panel, the Dental Product Advisory Committee, and the Bureau of Radiological Health, with a strong dental involvement.

The Centers for Disease Control contain the Dental Disease Prevention Activity. One of the functions of this office is to collect information on the safety, benefits, and other aspects of fluoridation and to assist states and municipalities with funds to support community water fluoridation. The agency is an excellent resource for the embattled promoters of fluoridation. The Dental Disease Prevention Activity is expanding its programing to include periodontal disease prevention.

Field trials and demonstrations constitute a large part of the research work of the U.S. Public Health Service. Outstanding examples were the fluoridation demonstration at Grand Rapids, Michigan, with Muskegon, Michigan, as a control city, and the test of methods for increasing the productivity of dentists through effective use of trained auxiliary personnel at Richmond, Indiana, and Woonsocket, Rhode Island. Research is also carried on in foreign countries, sometimes with the aid of funds paid for agricultural surpluses. Examples include the study of variations in the rate of oral calculus formation in India and the testing of the use of an insurance mechanism for comprehensive dental care in Israel.

The National Institutes of Health (NIH) are responsible for biomedical research and research training in the United States. One of the major units of the NIH is the National Institute of Dental Research (NIDR). This agency, with a 1985 annual budget of $100 million, is conducting and funding most of the important basic and clinical dental research worldwide. Its public health activities include behavioral science studies and clinical studies concerning the effectiveness of fluoride rinse programs, school water fluoridation in areas where community fluoridation is impossible or inoperative, and pit and fissure sealants.

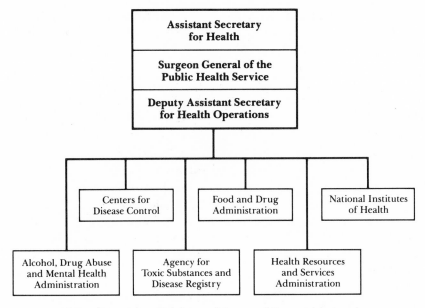

Figure 76. Major divisions of U.S. Public Health Service.

Within the Office of the Assistant Secretary for Health, the National Center for Health Statistics, through its Health Examination Survey and Health Interview Survey, is the source of most of the statistical publications in the United States concerning health, including dentistry. Most dental data are published in the Vital and Health Statistics Series 11. Each publication in the series addresses topics such as decayed, missing, filled Teeth Among Persons 1–74 Years, United States and Diet and Dental Health, A Study of Relationships, United States, 1971–74.

Last but not least are the ten Regional Offices of the U.S. Public Health Service. Each has a Dental Consultant whose responsibilities include implementing the functions of the major operating agencies within the specific Region. Personal communication through these consultants is of great assistance to dental educators, researchers, society officers, and young dentists wishing to enter government programs.

Within the Department of Health and Human Services, but outside the Public Health Service, are several important activities with dental components. The Health Care Financing Administration

(HCFA) manages the fiscal part of Medicare (Title XVIII) and the federal aspect of Medicaid (Title XIX). One full-time dentist is attached to the Health Care Financing Administration. An indication of the magnitude of the problem that the Health Care Financing administration faces is the extent of Medicaid expenditures in the fiscal year 1982: $34 billion (55% federal share, 45% states' share), of which dentistry accounted for $600 million.

Professional Review Organizations (PROs) have been set up in geographic areas to monitor the quality of care delivered in an institutional setting to patients for which Title V (Maternal and Child Health), Title XVIII (Medicare), and Title XIX (Medicaid) reimburse the providers. This concept may well be the forerunner of an expanded quality-of-care assessment system that will monitor all health services delivered in both institutional and ambulatory settings. The effect of such a system on the delivery of dental care cannot be emphasized too strongly.

NEW HEALTH-PLANNING AGENCIES

One of the more recent activities of the U.S. Department of Health and Human Services is health planning, with an emphasis on consumer participation. The Comprehensive Health Planning Act of 1966 (P.L. 89-749), more commonly called "Partnership for Health," set up a system of planning agencies at the local and state levels where over one-half of the members were to be consumers rather than providers of health care. This system was revised and extended by the National Health Planning and Resources Development Act of 1974 (P.L. 93-641). This Act set up more than 200 regional service areas across the country, each to be served by a *Health Systems Agency* (HSA), which must have from 51 to 60 percent of consumers on its governing board. By September 1976, 187 of these agencies had been established: 170 as private, nonprofit corporations, 15 as regional planning bodies, and 2 as units of local government.[2] Their functions are generally to prepare and implement plans for improved health services for area residents with objectives of increasing the accessibility, acceptability, continuity, and quality of health care; restraining increases in the cost of health care; and preventing unnecessary duplication of health resources.

P.L. 93-641 also mandates the formation of a State Health Planning and Development Agency (SHPDA) for each state. Each SHPDA is to be a unit of state government designated by the governor. The Agency has responsibility for conducting health planning for the state and implementing those parts of the state health plan and HSA plans that related to state government. It is to be advised by a State Health Coordinating Council (SHCC) which will contain representatives of the local HSAs within that state. Twenty-five SHCCs had been designated by September 1974, and funded by grants of almost $8 million.[2]

As part of its mandate to control unnecessary duplication, P.L. 93-641 requires states to set up a mechanism for processing *certificates of need* for new or expanded health facilities. About half the states had done so by 1975, using various administrative mechanisms. A typical process exists in Massachusetts, where the Department of Public Health has final authority to determine need for a facility, but does so in consultation with the local HSA and other recognized community agencies. The form of application is spelled out in state law; a public hearing is held if any registered group of 10 or more taxpayers requests it. All major construction plans are affected. The stated objective of the process is "the allocation of health care resources and the improvement of health care delivery systems such that adequate health care services are made reasonably available to every person within the Commonwealth at the lowest reasonable aggregate cost." The reference to "lowest . . . cost" implies the control of unnecessary duplication or high cost of facilities.

APPROACHES TO NATIONAL HEALTH INSURANCE

The subject of national health insurance in the United States has received growing attention in recent years. The examples quoted in Chapter 24 and others from other countries have provided background information. Medicare and Medicaid, of course, have been steps in this direction and now cover approximately 20 percent of the population. In 1982 the United States was spending an estimated 10.5 percent of its Gross National Product on health care ($322 billion) from all sources, public and private. This is a high percentage among the countries with which we might be compared. It must be remembered in this connection that neither the volume nor the cost of health care is necessarily correlated with actual health. Even though the United States may be devoting a high proportion of its Gross National Product toward health, the mortality and morbidity statistics from this country do not show similar preeminence. For example, some 15 other countries report longer average life expectancies, and a similar number report a lower infant mortality.

In the health insurance field, voluntary agencies have made substantial progress, thanks chiefly to the efforts of organized labor in cooperation with the organized dental profession. Both the payment systems and the delivery systems for health care can best be characterized as pluralistic. This, perhaps, is natural in a country where there are wide discrepancies in ethnic origin, cultural pattern, and economic level, and where private practice, largely free from the requirements of uniformity, has been the chief resource for the delivery of care. Chapter 18 gives a good indication of the pluralism and complexity of the health insurance efforts so far made in the United States. Much of this complexity arises from the restriction upon eligibility in each plan, with some persons eligible for several plans, some for none, and many abuses and embarrassments connected with the necessity for determining income levels of policyholders. Universal entitlement is needed.

The year 1971 saw some of the most constructive and variegated thought on the subject of national health insurance that has so far occurred in the United States. There is no need to describe all of the bills that have been placed before Congress during and since 1971. Four typical ones will do. The simplest of these was the American Medical Association's "Medicredit" bill (in 1974, S. 444; H.R. 2222). This bill was designed to provide hospital and medical care, including catastrophic coverage, to population groups not already covered by Medicare. A voluntary health insurance system would be federally financed, in whole for low-income groups and in part for all other persons. Certificates would be issued, redeemable for a percentage of the cost of approved basic coverage. For consumers paying an income tax, these certificates would be issued in proportion to a credit allowable on the tax. Certificates for all other persons would be financed through federal general revenues. The proposal did not seek to change the present health care delivery system—it was purely a financing proposal. No dental care was included in the original Medicredit bill, but a more recent modification of it has included comprehensive dental care for children between ages 2 and 6, as well as emergency care for everyone under 65 years of age.

The next simplest national health insurance proposal was made in 1971 under President Nixon's administration. Later entitled the Comprehensive Health Insurance Act of 1974, it had three separate programs: (1) an employee health insurance plan to be paid for mostly by the employer, (2) an assisted health insurance plan covering low-income persons and others not covered by the employee plan, and (3) an expanded Medicare plan covering persons age 65 and over. Private carriers were to be used. There was a $150 per person deductible item and 25 percent coinsurance. Benefits were fairly limited and the cost in billions was probably in single figures. "Comprehensive" dental care, with "comprehensive" largely undefined, was to extend up to age 13, free of deductible and coinsurance clauses. This bill would leave millions of persons outside of the various categories eligible for coverage. It would place an undue burden on small or marginal employers and upon low-income persons. If this appraisal is correct, the bill, while an economical start in the direction of national health insurance, would fall far short of achieving the comprehensive goals necessary in order to make a significant improvement in our health delivery system.

The most comprehensive bill that has been proposed is the Kennedy-Griffiths Bill, entitled the Health Security Act (in 1973 it was S. 3, H.R. 22). This proposal would cover all U.S. residents, recast the health delivery system, supply major federal resources for dental and medical education, and minimize if not eliminate state licensure systems for health professionals and allied auxiliaries. Nearly complete coverage of health services was specified, including dental services for children up to age 15, except for orthodontics. The only major exclusions were custodial care and workmen's compensation. Medicare would be abolished since all its benefits would be included. Fifty percent of the financing of the bill would be from federal general revenue, 36 percent from a 3.5

percent tax on employer payrolls, and the rest from employee contributions and taxes upon self-employed persons. The costs of the bill were estimated at between $40 billion and $80 billion a year, depending upon who made the estimate. Practitioners were to be reimbursed on a capitation basis through comprehensive health centers. No maximum benefits were specified, nor were deductible items, coinsurance, or waiting periods.

Fein considered this proposal to be sufficiently comprehensive to create a national system of health security.[3] He praised its first-dollar coverage without coinsurance or deductibles. He criticized the bill, however, for its failure to meet the responsibility that the taxpayers' dollars be spent wisely. It would fall short, he felt, if it were to behave merely as a conduit for collecting dollars from the public and passing them on to the providers. The administration's financing proposals would do better in that direction, as contained in the Comprehensive Health Insurance Act of 1974.

A later group of bills, taking form in 1974, has favored "catastrophic insurance," with coverage for medical bills above certain limits, such as 60 days in-hospital and/or a total cost of over $2,000. This would fill an important need, but would be inflationary since it would encourage the more expensive forms of medical treatment. Moreover, it would do nothing to control the delivery system, and only in rare instances would it cover dental care.

The new Mills-Kennedy Bill of 1974 showed a spirit of compromise in that it dropped back almost to the position of the then current administration bill and drastically limited the benefits found in the Kennedy-Griffiths Bill. The idea of all parties has recently seemed to be to find a wise starting point at an *acceptable* financial level, and work upward from this as soon as possible. The year 1975 saw 11 bills filed, covering a spectrum little changed from 1974. Definitive action has not taken place on any bill to date.

It is not the purpose of this book to enter into an economic analysis of the many financing problems involved in these various bills. One or two economic considerations are worth mention, however. Feldstein has studied carefully the effects of deductibles and coinsurance upon the probable future cost and availability of national dental health insurance coverage.[4,5] He feels that deductibles, though lowering the total cost of the program, would

exclude low-income people. Uniform copayment would also reduce slightly the total cost of a program, while a copayment schedule that varied with family income so as to exclude the
highest-income families completely from federal benefits would
drastically reduce the total cost. Dental prices would also be expected to rise less rapidly under the latter arrangement than
in more generous benefit programs. Feldstein estimates the
federal government costs for plans offering *comprehensive* dental
care to people of *all ages* in the United States, at 1970 price
levels, as:

No deductible, no coinsurance	$18 billion
No deductible, uniform 20% coinsurance	14 billion
No deductible, variable coinsurance	4 billion

Based upon an increase in the Consumer Price Index of 165 percent between 1970 and 1984, federal government costs for plans
offering comprehensive dental care to people of all ages in the
United States at 1984 price levels are estimated as:[1]

No deductible, no coinsurance	$48 billion
No deductible, uniform 20% coinsurance	37 billion
No deductible, variable coinsurance	11 billion

By variable coinsurance it is meant that no copayment would be
expected from families with incomes under $3,000, 100 percent
copayment (no federal aid) would be expected from families with
incomes over $15,000, and varying other percentages of copayment
from families with incomes in between. Feldstein does not estimate
the costs for plans offering less than a *full* scope of dental treatment by modern standards. A restricted list of operations would
naturally reduce costs. No changes, moreover, are considered in
delivery systems for dental care. In considering Feldstein's cost
estimates and comparing them with the contemporary total consumer expenditures of about $9 billion per year, one sees the
colossal cost of offering full coverage for full treatment for everyone. Even at this cost, full utilization is not assumed: Feldstein has
applied the price-elasticity concept to current demand levels only.
His variable coinsurance concept, while more reasonable in price,
is clearly not universal entitlement. It is merely an extension of
Medicaid, with all the eligibility problems continued. Any one of

his projections postulates a volume of dental care the American dental profession, as currently organized and restricted, could not deliver.

The question of whether federal control of the delivery system might diminish corruption and inflation is a difficult one. Hodgson feels that, "cleansed of the entrepreneurial temptations which the Administration's interpretation has allowed, the Health Maintenance Organization could develop into the key institution in a transformation of the economic structure of medicine which would diminish the conflict between the doctor's and the patient's interests. Probably the best hope of spreading the HMO system would be by linking it with a national health insurance system; and there are certainly ways in which this could be done."[6] This is an important concept for further study and further action.

NATIONAL PROGRAMS OF THE NEAR FUTURE

As legislative activity in the national health insurance field recommences with each new Congress, it is obvious that important compromises must be made if progress is actually to occur. The general principles of good financing and constructive change in the delivery system need not necessarily be abandoned, but limitations in scope of service will almost undoubtedly have to occur. Fein feels that pluralism in the delivery system not only should be maintained, but should be expanded by the creation of options that do not exist today.[3] But pluralism in the financing machinery, he feels, will lead to confusion and inequity. Our major need is to create universal coverage, not omitting those who are most vulnerable. Progressive taxes must be accepted by the public if national health insurance is to get anywhere. The public can remember, in accepting these taxes, that there is likely to be an equal reduction in private-sector health care expenditures.

In the dental field, limitations of scope of service are inevitable. None of the 1971 bills provided comprehensive dental care for persons of all ages, and indeed, there would be insufficient manpower to implement such a proposal. A package must be designed that the American dental profession can deliver. Here are some of the elements that have been proposed for such a package.

Emergency Care. It is a basic human-service postulate that people in actual pain should receive care first. Emergency dental care does not take very much time if it is confined to the relief of immediate pain. It also creates instant gratitude and a "teachable moment," when the patient can most easily be motivated to seek more definitive and preventive dental care. Any dentist can provide emergency care to a group much larger than he could possibly handle on a comprehensive basis. Those with experience in large public programs realize how difficult it is to make age distinctions among people in pain. Emergency care should, therefore, be available to all comers, with referral of the patient later to outside sources of care if comprehensive care is not available within the program. The American Dental Association endorses emergency care *for all,* as part of any national health insurance program, and I believe it can be delivered.[7]

The problem with emergency care, of course, is the difficulty in defining it and in preventing abuse of the category. During World War II, the dental officer for civilian personnel at the Brooklyn Naval Shipyard was not allowed to have any forceps, lest he fail to distinguish between an emergency and a routine extraction. Medicaid program administrators likewise have shied away from emergency dental treatment. The ill-will evoked by a medical care program that includes relief of pain in other parts of the body without relief of dental pain is so great, however, that I am convinced emergency dental care *must* be included. We must learn how to define it reasonably well, and must learn to live with a few unavoidable abuses.

Preventive Services. The best preventive service in the dental field at the moment is community water fluoridation. This measure may be assisted by certain general provisions of a national health insurance act, but it will not be accomplished through systems for delivering health care to individuals. The use of dietary fluoride supplements when appropriate, however, together with topical fluoride treatments, dental prophylaxis, toothbrush instruction, pit and fissure sealants, and the like, are widely applicable upon an individual basis.

It will probably prove difficult to reach an entire adult population with individual preventive measures, within the financial limitations of any health care bill. Children should receive first priority in the development of preventive services, partly because of their increased caries susceptibility, partly because they are more easily accessible, and partly because they are more teachable. Even among children, however, such items as topical fluoride treatments and dental prophylaxis require long periods of professional attention in proportion to the demonstrable results. Dental health education (toothbrush and dietary counseling), on the other hand, does not lend itself to accurate financing, either on a time basis or on an operation basis. A "word to the wise" delivered in almost no time at all may prove more valuable than a long harangue occupying a specified number of minutes. The practicality of including individual dental preventive services for any age group as reimbursable items in any national health insurance program, therefore, remains in doubt.

The matter should not be neglected, however. Sheiham, in his evaluation of the success of the British national dental care program, deplores the fact that "the amount spent on prevention is so small that figures for comparison are not available."[8] This imbalance, he says, depresses the morale of the profession, as it involves a departure from one of its best principles. Water fluoridation and topical fluoride therapy are recommended for inclusion in the British program.

In this country, we are doing pretty well on fluoridation, and could do better if the federal government provided additional funding for community programs as part of a national health insurance program. Topical fluoride therapy could be defined in a way to minimize abuse, and could probably be delegated to auxiliaries at prices below the current levels, since now the dentist himself is expected to do the work much of the time. This procedure could be part of a good national program—and could be delivered to large child population groups. Pit and fissure sealants appear to have the potential to supplement existing caries preventive modalities and are now being identified as a good public program targeted at specific population groups.

Comprehensive Care for Children. The American population is sufficiently transient and sufficiently forgetful that ideal incremental care cannot be maintained on any very perfect basis, even among children, and certainly not among adults. Comprehensive care must, therefore, be rendered, if it is to be rendered at all, without too rigid an insistence upon recent prior dental care. The dental prepayment plans now in operation have already discovered this fact. Schoen feels that a capitation system could be designed for the American population of all ages.[9] Capitation, he expects, will provide a much simpler financing mechanism than a fee-per-operation system and will cut down the overhead of the program. He may be right about this, but the dental profession to date has not been favorably inclined toward capitation fees in the rendering of comprehensive dental care. Schoen also feels that with predictable underutilization, and with ideal use of auxiliaries, comprehensive dental care could be supplied to the entire country on a national health insurance basis.[10] His assumptions are courageous, but difficult to substantiate.

The inclusion of dental care for children up to age 15 in several bills is to be applauded. This is in accordance with the recommendations of the American Dental Association. An eventual upward extension of age limits through age 17 would be desirable. There is little chance, however, that American taxpayers can tolerate or that the American dental profession can deliver the levels of care shown in Feldstein's estimates.

A Starting Point and a Financial Inducement. As a starting point, it is difficult to improve upon the recommendations of the Health, Education, and Welfare Advisory Committee on Dental Health that "the Department should propose and support a national health insurance proposal that includes at the outset a dental component that gives priority to preventive and therapeutic services for children and emergency dental care for all."[11]

The main reason for wishing to see dental care for children extended up through age 17 in the future proposals for national health insurance is to cover the teen-age period of most rapid tooth decay. To do this, a financial inducement might be offered to those states willing to cooperate by licensing dental therapists (dental nurses) in school-based clinics to prepare cavities as well as fill them. The substantial savings available through the use of these therapists in school-based dental clinics (Chapter 20) might be offered to these states to permit extension of dental care through age 17. States unwilling to license therapists to perform these services would be offered aid only for younger children.[12]

With these changes, it would appear that a package of dental care that the dental profession could adequately deliver might be offered to the American public at a price they could pay, and in a manner logistically efficient enough to promote high utilization.

CHAPTER 24

Foreign and International Programs

No OTHER country seems to have as large a network of national, state, and local organizations devoted to research and promotional work on the subject of dental disease as does the United States, but a number of other countries have far larger programs, per unit of population, for the financing and rendering of dental treatment. It is possible also that some of these countries do more for prevention than appears on the surface, particularly "secondary prevention" in connection with dental care programs for schoolchildren. Water fluoridation has started in many countries, but an even one-half of the millions of people receiving such water throughout the world are in the United States, as shown in Table 41.

DENTAL SERVICE IN DEVELOPED NATIONS

Great Britain has perhaps the best-known dental care program, since it is part of the compulsory health insurance plan. Upon its establishment in 1948, the National Health Service in Great Britain offered to all citizens the full range of dental care, an event which attracted worldwide attention. Subsequent efforts to bring an acceptable quality of care and some degree of economic justice out of a situation which suddenly offered the public more service than the dental profession was prepared to provide has been followed closely by students of public health practice.

Funding for the British National Health Service (NHS) has been from two principal sources: a tax on liquor and cigarettes and National Health Insurance premiums. The total expenditure for health service in Great Britain requires between 5 and 6 percent of the Gross National Product.[1] The NHS premiums are generally compulsory from the time of leaving school, with a flat rate for each individual worker and for each member of his family. Employers also contribute a sum roughly equivalent to each employee's contribution. In hardship cases, an individual receives aid drawn directly from tax monies. Ninety-seven percent of the population is considered to be covered by the insurance scheme.[2]

Though the physicians and dentists in certain government health services are employed on salary, most of the health care for the nation is provided by private practitioners. The physicians are paid on a capitation basis, the dentists on a fee-for-service basis. Originally, all NHS services were free, but coverage exclusions have now been made in certain areas, including dentistry.

Children and expectant and nursing mothers receive free dental care. Except for these groups, all other patients have to pay a certain sum per visit to their dentist for each treatment, the excess to be covered by National Health Insurance. Patients also pay 50 percent of the cost of dentures. This coinsurance mechanism has been shown to produce an immediate and dramatic decrease in the demand for dental care, and those most deterred by the charges are those people who for sociological reasons tend not to make full use of any of the state-provided services, such as education and welfare.[3] The list of dental operations authorized without specific approval has been fairly broad, including amalgam and silicate fillings, root-canal treatment, and acute periodontal treatment and denture repairs, but dentures themselves, gold work, bridges, definite periodontal treatment, and orthodontics all require prior approval by the Dental Estimates Board. Extractions require approval too: a wise encouragement to conserve teeth.[4]

In the course of long experience in paying dentists per operation for their work, the British have developed a very thorough postaudit system, described in some detail in Chapter 19. In a center at Eastbourne, England, 4 percent of all bills are checked constantly for correspondence to local dental treatment patterns. Every dentist receives an audit once in each 2-year period.

Statistical material developed by the Dental Estimates Board is translated into dental fees by a Dental Rates Group. In recent years fees have been adjusted in such a way that the practitioners in the National Health Service are, in effect, paid by the hour.[5] A dentist cannot earn the approval rate, however, unless he completes a certain quota of work. The system, therefore, contains its own built-in accelerator.[3] Severe inflation has tested the fairness of this system, since expenses for dentists have risen faster than income. In spite of these limitations, the majority of dentists have been shown to be strongly in favor of continuing under a system that seems to them to offer the "best possible treatment for the greater number of patients." In the field of prevention, only about 10 percent of the British population receives fluoridated water, although the children generally have shared the caries reduction mentioned in Chapter 8.[1]

The German National Health Insurance system, oldest in the world, was initiated by Bismarck in 1883. Reorganized in 1955, it is now administered by private physicians through the mechanism of sickness insurance contracts.[2] No qualified physician or dentist can constitutionally be barred from insurance practice. The financial aspects of the contracts are handled through sickness funds, with compulsory coverage for all workers whose incomes fall below a certain level, for most pensioners, and for many self-employed persons. All those who are financially able are permitted to take care of themselves. About 87 percent of the West German population is covered. About 11 percent participate in private insurance schemes.

Government claims are reimbursed on a fee-for-service basis, with payment routed through the vendor's own professional organization. Prosthetic and orthodontic services are not on the regular fee scale. Indemnities are paid by the government, with the rest of the bill paid by the patient. Information on the proportion of the Gross National Product now being devoted to health expenditures in West Germany seems not available, but it should appear to be less than 5 percent. Almost two-thirds of the dentistry done in Germany is done through social health insurance agencies.

Sweden has the highest income taxes in the world, averaging nearly 41 percent. Sweden also returns more of its Gross National Product to its citizens in the form of social welfare than any other country—more than 20 percent. The proportion of the Swedish Gross National Product spent on health in 1971 was 6.2 percent.[2]

Health insurance has been compulsory and universal in Sweden since 1955. It is administered by a special government agency in Stockholm—the Riksforsakringsverket (RFV), or State Insurance Board. The RFV receives its funds from three sources: (1) insurance fees paid by individuals, (2) fees paid by employers and calculated according to the individual employee's salary, and (3) limited amounts from the state treasury to cover the indigent. One hundred percent of the population is covered. More than 90 percent of all Swedish physicians and about 40 percent of the dentists are employed by the state, and they are paid according to a governmentally-determined fee-per-operation schedule. In-patient hospital care is free of charge, but out-patient treatment has been subject to small coinsurance payments since 1970. Private practitioners technically operate under the government fee schedule, although they may charge higher fees than the suggested amounts, and their patients are reimbursed 75 percent of the fee stipulated by the insurance program regardless of the actual charge. Dental care for children and pregnant women in rendered free of charge, but all other dental care is paid on a fee-for-service basis. Sweden's standing in international health statistics would indicate that the quality of Sweden's health care is high.

Dental service providing full dental care to schoolchildren of all ages appear to be quite common in Europe, whether locally or nationally managed. These services are paid for out of tax funds, and are frequently of high quality. Good examples are to be found in the Scandinavian countries and in Switzerland. Systems of this sort, with acceptance of service made voluntary, give an opportunity for incremental care and for preventive procedures. Sebelius, studying dental services in Oslo and Drammen, Norway, found over 90 percent acceptance.[6] In Oslo there were regulations that preschool children must enter the service at 3 years of age, or, if at a later age, with dental care completed. Young people 14 to 18 years of age were accepted only if they had received periodic dental service during the school years preceding. Indicative of the results obtained were findings for a group of 296 children 13 years of age in the two cities. The DMF count per child was 9.68 teeth, of which 8.55 had been filled. This gives a filled-tooth ratio of over 88 percent. These same children had lost only 6 permanent teeth per 100 children, including teeth indicated for extraction.

The children's dental service in Sweden has been mentioned in Chapter 20. The essential feature of it is that it is school-managed with service rendered in nearby district health clinics. Utilization of care here has reached 95 percent in the school ages 7 to 16.[7] Sweden is the only country in the world known to prohibit fluoridation on a national basis; nevertheless Swedish children have shared the caries reductions referred to in Chapter 8.

On the other side of the globe, New Zealand and South Australia are achieving virtually complete utilization of dental care among children by the use of dental nurses or therapists, as mentioned in Chapter 17. These school-based systems have undergone changes in the past 10 years. The New Zealand Dental Service has greatly reduced the number of dental nurses in training. Declining birth rates, changes in disease patterns, revisions of diagnostic criteria, and longer employment trends in women have all had an impact on the system. The South Australian School Dental Service has expanded rapidly to serve a high percentage of eligible South Australian children. This system is also responding with flexible programs to meet new trends. Both systems are examples of comprehensive programs of quality dental care that provide equal access to continuous care for all children.[8] The New Zealand program has been criticized because of the high rates of edentulism among adults, which are only now beginning to drop. The reasons for these rates are historical and cultural, and the responsibility for them rests with the adult consumers and with the dental profession, not with the children's program.

DENTAL SERVICE IN DEVELOPING NATIONS

It would be an impossible task to outline even the salient dental problems in the various developing countries of the world and the dental services that are arising to meet them. Remarks on a few typical areas, however, are of interest to show the lines of approach that are being used in developing nations where only one dentist is available to population groups of 10,000 or more. It must be realized from the start that figures such as those seen in Table 31 for numbers of dentists in countries throughout the world give a seriously oversimplified picture of the true situation. Where census figures seem reasonably valid and ratios are found such as that of one dentist to almost 70,000 people in India, the 9,000-odd dentists involved are registered personnel only and probably concentrated in the larger cities. Untrained or partially trained dental workers must exist in considerable numbers beyond this. On the other hand, where Brazil lists a ratio of one dentist to every 3,800 people, it is noted that no population estimate is available for the Brazilian jungles. This ratio, therefore, is not as good as it might appear at first sight.

In urban centers in countries such as these, one looks for good, modern dentistry and an intelligent start toward preventive measures, particularly water fluoridation. Thus, in China the 10,000 graduate dentists and 20,000 "less thoroughly trained" dentists are set in a country with a population of one billion. These dentists work in the urban areas, where they render modern care ranging from adequate to excellent in quality.[9] In the rural communes, even the health centers have no more than rudimentary facilities, sufficient at best for basic emergency care for acute conditions. The "barefoot doctors," however, were reported to be well-equipped and able to perform routine tooth extractions.

For rural or less developed areas, dental nurses, dental aids, or "assistant dental officers" are being trained in a number of localities. A recent study in New Zealand of the dental nurse program there records overseas students from Ghana, Sabah, Singapore, Sri Lanka, New Guinea, Borneo, and the Cook Islands in training under various scholarship plans.[10] Dental nurse plans similar to New Zealand's, already well developed in Tasmania, and South and Western Australia, are springing up in the other Australian states, in Indonesia, Canada, Latin America, and many other parts of the world. In the Fiji Islands of the South Pacific, natives become "assistant dental officers" after 3 years of training. Fuller stated that children in this area in 1964 got the best dental service, while adults were less served or understood.[11] People were not educated to pay for dental care, and the major efforts at such care came through government. Eight countries in the South Pacific area have fluoridation: the least developed countries have been the most receptive, perhaps because of the lack of available dental care.

In 1964 Karim reported an extensive dental service in Malaysia, with school and hospital clinics and two dental clinic boats giving priority to children 6 to 12 years of age for dental care.[11] Indigent adults also received attention. One hundred and fifty dentists were employed, and 175 dental nurses. In 1978, some 450 dentists and 600 dental nurses were reported in government service.

The situation in India deserves further comment, since sophisticated efforts are under way to improve dental health in the staggeringly larger population there. Dental educators in the 14 dental schools of this country have hoped to achieve a ratio of one dentist per 30,000 within the not-too-distant future, bettering by more than three times the ratio which existed in 1968.[12] One dentist to 4,000 is their ultimate ideal. Dental hygienists and mechanics are to be found, and it is planned to train them in increasing numbers under a 15-year plan. In 17 of the states of India a plan exists to provide one dentist and one dental hygienist for each 3,000 schoolchildren. There are dental research problems in India which are of particular interest. Dental-caries incidence is low. Excessive amounts of fluoride are often present in the water supply, and the Department of Public Health has a Fluorosis Committee investigating this. In contrast, high periodontal disease needs further study and is actually the nation's number-one dental health problem. A population of over 600,000,000 needs to be cared for on a very limited budget.

Another rapidly emerging nation is Saudi Arabia, visited in 1975 by the writer. With new wealth, this country was then in a position both to expand its somewhat limited public health dental program and to design a dental school (first in that area) as part of the new King Faisal University College of Medicine and Medical Sciences on their Gulf coast which is rapidly growing in population. The dental needs of the country, subject to much wider survey, seemed to be chiefly for periodontal preventive measures and treatment. A preliminary inspection of children's mouths in Riyadh indicated low incidence of caries, heavy calculus, incipient periodontal damage, and some dental fluorosis of natural origin. More prevalent caries was reported in rural areas. A nucleus of urban dental practitioners was supported by a few good dental clinics in large city hospitals, and one in the Aramco settlement in Dhahran managed by American personnel. The major need was for primary dental care in the rural areas, and a dental-therapist training program was envisioned at the new dental school to accompany training of dentists for team management and primary care.

In Latin America, dental-caries incidence appears generally to be high, and important efforts are under way to increase and improve the training of dentists and dental therapists there. The dentist-population ratios are generally better than those seen in Asia and Africa, but certain jungle populations remain unestimated, as has been noted. The population of Latin America is growing rapidly, though infant mortality is high. Large population groups are subsisting on an inadequate diet. Tooth loss is high among the young adult population, and preventive measures are being instituted only to a very limited extent as yet. A new Association of Latin American Dental Schools has recently been formed. Training of public health dentists at São Paulo is achieving considerable success, and a new International Center for Dental Epidemiology has been formed there in cooperation with the U.S. Public Health Dental Health Center in San Francisco.

A word should be said about the "dental ambassadors" serving in developing countries under a variety of different programs.[13] The United States Peace Corps has done excellent work. The People to People program, a private agency, has sent dentists, both for service and for teaching, to a variety of countries. Dentists participate in Project HOPE, which has operated a hospital ship serving underprivileged coastal areas in various parts of the world. There are many church-sponsored medical missions and private enterprises. The sum total of these philanthropic efforts is probably small in terms of direct service, but it is of distinct educational value and is an important expression of international good will. It involves a cultural exchange which will undoubtedly help developing nations to help themselves.

INTERNATIONAL DENTAL HEALTH

There is much that international associations or governmental groups can do in the broad field of public health. In a negative or defensive sense, communicable diseases, so easily transported across national borders, call urgently for international control. In a positive sense, "peace on earth, good will toward men" is a concept which calls for international exchange of information and cooperation on health problems of all sorts. The more developed countries are often in a position to help the less developed ones, if they will listen to expressions of need and not merely pontificate. Again, pooling of intellectual or physical resources may accomplish results in the study and control of disease which no one country could accomplish by itself. Thus conferences which bring together the medical scientists and public health people of various nations produce a spread of information impossible otherwise. Finally, through pooled financial resources, teams of public health researchers or public health educators can be sent to any corner of the world where their services will be of help.

Important efforts in the field of international health seem to have arisen only since the beginning of the twentieth century. In the Western hemisphere, the Pan-American Sanitary Bureau was organized in 1902. Worldwide, the International Office of Public Health, formed in 1907, started a growing stream of effort which was taken over by the Health Organization of the League of Nations in 1921 and by the World Health Organization in 1948. The constitution of the WHO affirms that health is "one of the fundamental rights of every human being, without distinction of race, religion, political belief, economic or social condition."[14] WHO's current work has developed under six main headings:

Health services: the identification of priority problems and the provision of assistance to countries in programing services.

Manpower development: promotion of the health team approach to service and assistance in the training of auxiliary personnel.

Family health: maternal and child health, nutrition, family planning, and the psychosocial health of the family.

Disease control: assistance in developing immunization and control programs for a wide range of problems from malaria and cancer to drug dependence and mental health.

Environmental health: sanitation, pollution control, industrial hygiene, and the like.

Coordination of biomedical research, with special emphasis upon tropical diseases.

Indicative of the areas where the World Health Organization can be of most help is India. Life expectancy there is hardly half of what it is in the United States, communicable diseases such as malaria, plague, cholera, typhoid, and dysentery still claim an enormous number of victims every year. Poverty, hunger, and disease are arrayed in force against the people, yet the population is increasing at a rapid rate because the birth rate, varying from 25 to 40 per thousand per year, exceeds the death rate. International aid can help in such a situation, not only by controlling disease but by improving the utilization of food supplies and encouraging birth control. Assistance from the WHO in controlling malaria has aroused public consciousness to new possibilities of settlement and cultivation of neglected areas, with a very substantial improvement in food supply. In order to accomplish results in a situation like this, barriers of nationalism, local interest, and prejudice, and of fancied superiority must be broken down. Brock Chisolm, Director-General of the WHO in 1951, tells the anecdote: "Once when I was indicating a certain degree of impatience with social development in a certain Communist country, a Russian made a remark that I have remembered. He said, 'You know, Dr. Chisolm, you would also have some difficulties if you had to live intimately even with your own great-grandparents.' "[15]

The World Health Organization belongs to the United Nations family of international agencies, but is largely independent because (1) it has its own governing body, the World Health Assembly, composed of representatives of all its own member states; (2) it has its own membership (165 member states and one associate member in 1985), nations that do not necessarily belong to the UN as well or to the other UN agencies; and (3) it has its own budget ($554 million, plus almost $437 million extra budgetary resources, for 1986–87), contributed directly by its own member states. The headquarters office of the WHO is in Geneva, but much of the work of the organization is carried on by regional offices in Africa (Brazzaville), the Americas (Washington), the Eastern Mediterranean (Alexandria), Europe (Copenhagen), Southeast Asia (New Delhi), and the Western Pacific (Manila).

Although the WHO sponsored research such as Fulton's study of the New Zealand dental nurse plan as early as 1950, its continuing dental health program did not start until June 1955 with the appointment of John W. Knutson, lent from the U.S. Public Health Service, as first Dental Health Officer.[16] The position of Chief Dental Officer is now a permanent one, in the Oral Health Unit, with headquarters in Geneva. The 1986–87 budget is expected to total $4,929,300, including extrabudgetary resources. The number of full-time-equivalent dental health staff posts is now 15:3 in the headquarters, 3 in the regional offices, and 9 in the field.[17]

In support of the Oral Health Unit there is a large advisory panel on dental health, and for particular problems expert committees are appointed to make reports. One of the most recent of such reports is Scientific Group Report No. 621, "Epidemiology, Etiology, and Prevention of Periodontal Diseases." Soon to appear is Expert Committee Report No. 713, "Prevention Methods and Programmes for Oral Diseases."

The dental activities within the WHO have so far consisted of research and consultation on an ad hoc basis. Among the subjects studied have been public health aspects of water fluoridation, the epidemiology of periodontal disease in India, dental health services for European children, and the uses of auxiliary dental personnel. The most extensive recent WHO study dealt with the delivery of dental care in local areas of ten different countries: Norway, West Germany, Australia, New Zealand, Japan, Canada, the German Democratic Republic, Ireland, Poland, and the U.S.A. Uniform statistical techniques were adopted to measure dental needs and the effects of dental care. Behavioral science was called upon to measure attitudes and cultural patterns in these contrasting countries. A comprehensive report has also appeared.[18]

Regional seminars and study groups, involving 20 to 45 participants each, have been held on different dental topics in different parts of the world. This method has much promise of future usefulness. The regional dental public health training program started in São Paulo, Brazil, in 1958, was largely assisted by the WHO.

An important activity, which only the WHO was really in a position to perform, has been the standardization in reporting of dental diseases and conditions throughout the world. An expert committee on dental health produced a technical report on this subject in 1962 which has already achieved great usefulness. The WHO's *Oral Health Surveys, Basic Methods* is about to appear in a third edition.

The World Health Organization has done a great deal to aid individuals who show potential for public health service in underdeveloped countries. To date, several hundred fellowships have been awarded for studies in dental health. It is interesting to note that the greatest number of these were granted to the Western Pacific region. Twelve Fellows were selected in 1967 by their respective governments to attend a WHO course for training teachers in child dental health at the Royal Dental College, Copenhagen. These Fellows represented Sri Lanka, Colombia, Egypt, Fiji, Greece, Guatemala, Hungary, Indonesia, Iran, Iraq, Nigeria, and Taiwan.[19]

Two other developments have taken place recently within the WHO. The first is the completion of data for 10 countries, described in Chapter 17. The other is the development of the WHO Epidemiological Data Bank. This bank embraces the entire world and is accumulating data on dental disease and the need for preventive and curative dental services and in the developing as well as the developed countries.

A look at the activities of the Pan American Health Organization, with a head office in Washington, D.C., gives a picture of the spectrum of activities possible at the regional level. Fig. 77 shows the location of other offices throughout the hemisphere.

Dental diseases, especially dental caries, are prevalent throughout populations of the Region. In particular, limited studies have revealed that 95 percent of schoolchildren suffer from these diseases. Preventive programs for dental caries are inadequate in scope and in the range of appropriate and preventive strategies employed. The extension of coverage of these programs is also constrained, not only by a shortage of professional dental personnel, who are inequitably distributed between rural and urban ar-

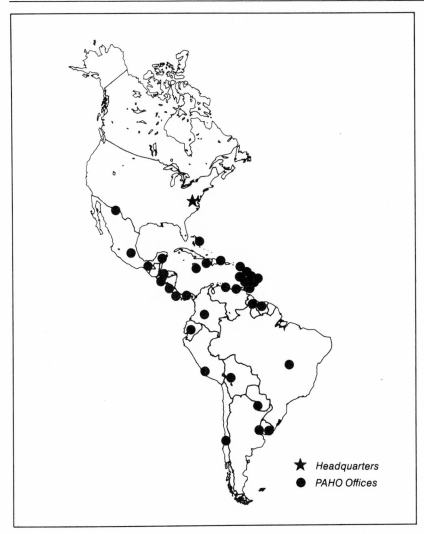

Figure 77. Headquarters and offices of Pan American Health Organization.

eas, but also by a lack of auxiliary dental personnel. There is thus a clear need for the intensive development of preventive dental services which utilize innovative, cost-effective, and appropriate strategies and technologies.[20]

The Regional Plan of Action has identified several areas for pursuing improved dental health status in the countries of the Region. Program activities in support of the countries in 1987 will focus on: (1) development of suitable methodology to evaluate program delivery and monitor population coverage and oral health status; (2) promotion of definition of principles and preparation of policies in dental health services, with emphasis on prevention and integration of such services with primary health care; (3) development of training strategies, curricula, manuals, and materials for personnel, with particular emphasis on auxiliary personnel; (4) preparation and implementation of plans, guidelines, and methodologies for the use of fluorides in cities with populations of 10,000 or more, and other techniques for preventive dental care; (5) encouragement of establishing programs for the population under 15 years of age, with emphasis on education in oral health and prevention and treatment of disease; (6) promotion of community and individual education and participation in preventive practices and oral hygiene; (7) development of guidelines for use of space and personnel in constructing dental facilities and for maintenance of dental equipment; (8) promotion of the development and application of appropriate technologies and simplified techniques; and (9) support of appropriate research in priority areas relating to the origins of dental disease, particularly in connection with the use of effective preventive agents or factors affecting oral hygiene status, and the development of simplified and readily applicable epidemiological techniques.[20]

The budget for the Oral Health program in 1986–87 is a little over one million dollars. A full-time dental officer is employed, and many specialty dental consultants are active in various fields.

The evolution of the WHO dental program may be expected to continue rapidly. Current publications should be watched for survey findings, methods of delivery of dental care, and other reports of interest—also for word of the administrative expansion of the program.

PART IV

The Future

CHAPTER 25

Conquest or Equilibrium?

ANY TREATISE on the principles of dental public health should logically conclude with a few words of speculation as to the goals this branch of health service may be expected to attain within the foreseeable future. Such goals should recognize the existing trends in the use of the teeth and in dental disease among human beings and also the end results of the efforts of the health professions in the advancement of science and in the application of science to human living habits. Can dental caries and peridontal disease be conquered with the same success as smallpox and yellow fever? If conquest is impossible, will man reach an equilibrium with these major dental diseases, preventing them in part, controlling them in part, so that his health and happiness will be essentially unimpaired? To define a plausible goal toward which to aim, three aspects of the situation must be studied: major trends in dental disease, variations in human culture and economic resources, and the professional resources necessary to provide appropriate care.

TRENDS AFFECTING DENTAL DISEASE

An examination of long-term trends in the prevalence of dental disease does not yield encouraging results. Dental caries appears to be a disease of civilization, increasing steadily in prevalence since earliest recorded times. Periodontal disease, much harder to trace, may have had a somewhat similar history. These trends, to be sure, are seen only among civilized societies, for only there have records been kept.

This rise in degenerative disease gives the appearance of being part of a long-term deemphasis of the human dentition. The evolution of the human skull has seen, in recent geologic epochs, a proportional diminution in the size of the jaws and teeth. As Gregory describes it, "The erect or semierect posture, together with the increasing use of the hands as such and the correlated swelling of the brain, has conditioned or is associated with . . . the reduction in size and retraction of the jaws and dentition beneath the overhanging nose and forehead, which is so characteristic of the higher races of man."[1] Human civilization is very brief in comparison with the geological epochs during which these changes have occurred.

It seems probable that man's success in preparing cooked food and in altering this environment has further diminished his need for an efficient dentition. This may have accelerated the reduction of the human dentition. A continuation of recent evolutionary processes, therefore, seems the logical thing to expect in the ages to come, our teeth becoming smaller and more alike, third molars disappearing, and the congenital absence of other teeth becoming more frequent. This process is called secondary polyisomerism, and other examples of it are known in the animal kingdom as adaptation to environmental change requires alteration of the physical characteristics of a species.[2] The evolutionary process, however, is not likely to rid us of all our teeth, though civilization has increased dental disease in recent centuries.

In contrast to the studies among civilized societies, a number of studies of the diets and dental conditions of "natural races" were made soon after the turn to the twentieth century. Pickerill, in 1912, cites a variety of dietary patterns among uncivilized races, accompanied by varying levels of dental caries. Even the highest of these caries levels are "incomparably lower than those prevailing among civilized races at the present time."[3] This contrast is shown in transition in Fig. 22, where the older Alaskan natives, as studied about 1960, are seen to have passed the years of rapid caries with a low incidence, while living on a native diet without the refined carbohydrates and other concomitants of civilization. The younger people actually had more DMF teeth than their elders.

Today large population groups throughout the world are in a slow transition from a native diet, to which they have been accustomed for centuries, to a civilized diet with Pepsi, Coca Cola, and the other "advantages" of civilization. These peoples show increasing caries. In the developed, heretofore called "civilized" countries, however, preventive measures have borne fruit, and caries among children is dropping. Are we headed toward an "endemic level" of dental caries, as Barmes has hypothecated?[4] Or do we face a multitude of cultural groupings in the world, some with stable low caries levels, some with rising levels in a newly developing environment, and others with caries apparently coming under control in a not-so-new developed environment?

Certain facts in relation to the nature of dental disease also need to be considered in estimating the future course of dental public health efforts. In the first place, both caries and periodontal disease are chronic, multifactorial diseases. This has raised the thought that their complete prevention will be elusive and difficult, as is proving to be the case with other chronic diseases.

CULTURAL TRENDS IN DENTAL DEMAND

Not only are there wide variations in the incidence of dental disease based on dietary environment, but there are also variations in attitudes toward dental care based on the cultural milieu. Primitive peoples sometimes attach aesthetic significance to the teeth, usually by decorating them, blackening them, or knocking them out. Natural teeth in ideal occlusion are not valued as highly in primitive as in developed countries, if for no other reason than that professional personnel are not available to keep them so. As dental care becomes possible, there are three levels at which it can be rendered. Relief of pain is the first objective, and removal of teeth is the easiest cure. This kind of care is called primary care in the narrowest sense. It is wanted almost universally and can be provided by auxiliary personnel, preferably trained.[5] Quality can be attained in primary care, for quality dentistry does not have to involve porcelain-on-metal restorations.

The next or secondary level of care has been known as "blood and vulcanite" dentistry. This level of care is found in developed countries where dietary or climatic factors have produced such a high incidence of caries that available dental care cannot keep up with it. Although people there have come to value the appearance of natural teeth and want efficient mastication, restorative dentists are either too few or too high-priced to be generally accessible. A culture based on the use of removable prostheses may develop among such people and may persist even after caries has been controlled, as in New Zealand. Again, this secondary type of dentistry can be rendered in good quality.

The top or tertiary level of dental care is based on the maximal preservation of natural teeth. A surprisingly large proportion of the American public want such care, can pay for it, and should be able to receive it, with all the specialized procedures now available. Here quality is indeed the major concern, and it must reach a high level of mechanical and aesthetic perfection, coupled with biological safety. Long training, good experience, and elaborate equipment have necessitated high charges for this care, but the charges are liable to vary over a wide range, depending on office location, personnel, overhead, and many other factors. Two of the most important attributes of quality in the health care field, however, are access and appropriateness. Tertiary care is not always at its best in these areas.

The organized dental profession has been stoutly opposed to what it calls "two-level dentistry." This attitude stems from the situation in Germany almost a century ago, when two dental groups, the *zahnärzten* (fully qualified dentists) and the *dentisten* (semi-trained operators), operated independently on different academic levels. If teamwork had resulted, with the zahnärzten in control, the result might have been very different, but teamwork did not result. The American Dental Association would like to provide all citizens with one level of high-quality comprehensive dental care, that is, tertiary care. This goal has never been attained, and it probably never can be. With the current emphasis on the work of the private sector and the curtailment of government aid, this goal seems farther away than ever. Actually we now have three or more levels of care in this country. We would do well to recognize this fact, as has occurred in the field of medicine in the designation of hospitals. Quality care must exist at all levels, with the emphasis on providing appropriate care for the largest possible number of people, coupled with sincere respect for the patient, and continuity of care. Tertiary care has no monopoly on quality.

TRENDS IN DENTAL CARE ADMINISTRATION

An ethical dilemma now arises which has been given careful attention in the medical area. Halberstam, addressing the issue of the expenditure of government funds for health care, states, "We realize that the ethic of the legislator and the ethic of the physician are not merely different but are, in fact, antithetical. The legislator's ethic . . . is the greatest good for the greatest number. The physician's ethic is the greatest good for the individual that he is charged with taking care of."[6] Hence the physician's emphasis is on kidney transplants, open-heart surgery, and the like, often at the expense of large-scale preventive measures which might make many of these operations unnecessary. The dentists who want government money to pay for Ceramco crowns and big bridges are thus on the physician's side of the fence. The public health dentists are on the legislator's side. Both are right, according to their own ethics.

In the United States, as in other developed countries, the drop in childhood dental caries has caused a major change in the delivery of dental care. No longer is incremental dental care for children a necessary prelude to adult care and the prevention of tooth loss in middle life. The DMF tooth counts among children have gone down a long way, but even more important, fluoridation and fluoride therapy have all but eliminated proximal caries, the restoration of which takes the greatest amount of time and skill on the part of the dentist. On the occlusal surfaces and other pit areas sealants are now proving valuable and can be applied by auxiliaries under the general supervision of a dentist. Preventive dentistry has thus taken most of the load of operative dentistry for children off the dentist and given him or her the opportunity to be a team leader with auxiliaries reaching a much larger segment of the child population than ever before.

In spite of this development, the tertiary dentists have plenty to keep them busy. The load of adult dental care is expected to increase, in the form of periodontal, endodontic, operative, and fixed prosthetic work. The reason for this increase is partly that people will be keeping more of their natural teeth into adult life and partly that there will be more people in the older age groups. It is the opinion of many of us in the field of dental care administration that there are *not* now too many dentists in the United States. Our fear is only that many of the dentists have been pricing themselves out of the market in the past few years.

Claims by dental organizations that *all* the public has access to comprehensive dental care are clearly false. Statistical figures for the United States in 1983 showed 15 percent of the population, or over 32 million people, to be at the poverty level.[7] This level meant that a single person had an annual income of just over $5000, and a family of 4 had just over $10,000. These people can hardly have spared enough money from major living expenses to go to private dentists for periodic prophylaxis, x-ray surveys, and operative dentistry.

Above the poverty level, a large number of people may be ready to seek private care if given a push. A good referral service from the public to the private sector may then increase the volume of private care and reduce the load on public programs.

Public dental services, which have been reduced in capacity by federal cutbacks in health care funding, can handle only a fraction of the remaining load. Changes in the delivery systems are needed to reduce the unit cost of services. Auxiliaries must be allowed to do all they safely can, and the supervising dentists in public programs must be given all possible freedom to make innovations in the use of auxiliaries, particularly hygienists and therapists. A mass of evidence exists that auxiliaries can perform many technical operations as well as, and sometimes better than, dentists. The dentists, however, are needed for their diagnostic skills and for the preparation and implementation of protocols for the work of auxiliaries.

The current expansion of dental assistant duties through the EFDA concept is valuable in fairly large group clinics, such as those pioneered by the city of Philadelphia. EFDA's, however, who can operate only alongside licensed dentists, should prove to be only a transitional group in the trend toward dental therapists or dental nurses. These auxiliaries, as in Australia or in Saskatchewan, Canada, can range far afield under adequate general supervision, handling large volumes of simple dental treatment and acting as scouts and recruiters for the practicing dentists, both public and private.

One of the important tasks in dental public health today is the search for and care of pocket areas of high caries incidence and dental neglect, as in urban low-income areas or rural areas. Surveys have shown that a very small percentage of children in a given group or area usually account for a very large percentage of the care needed. The finding that 20 percent of the children need 80 percent of the care is common.

Fears that public programs will undermine private practice should prove unfounded if proper communication and referral exist between the public and private sectors. A thorough workshop, with both sectors represented, which was held in New Zealand in 1978 to evaluate the dental nurse program, concluded that the efforts of the government, health department, provider organizations, and individuals would all be required if its objectives and targets were to be achieved.[8] The same is surely true in the United States.

FUTURE COURSES OF ACTION

Hanlon, in discussing "the past as a prologue to the future" in public health, points to three main channels into which effort can be directed: the consolidation of past successes, the remediation of the backlog of disabilities, and a truly vigorous, carefully planned attack upon both new problems and unsolved old problems.[9] These categories apply equally well to dental public health. The "consolidation of past successes," in practical terms, means the fuller use of the tools now available for the control of dental disease. Fluoridation, diet, tooth brushing, dental care—none of these measures are used as widely or as effectively as they could be. We must continue the old fight, perhaps with national health insurance to give universal entitlement for primary dental care and with new allies, such as the social scientists. The benefits of water fluoridation will not be as striking as they were at first, because fluoridation has already accomplished much of what was hoped of it. It still ranks, however, at the top of the list of preventive measures, where public water supplies can implement it, because of its low cost per person and its universal availability to low-income population groups. Modern bonding techniques, moreover, have allowed the "erasing" of any unsightly fluorosis which occasionally results in sound teeth from an overdosage of supplements.

In the field of restorative care, the lines between primary, secondary, and tertiary dental care are too sharp for most forms of clinical dentistry. The average general dentist will continue to provide all three kinds, with the emphasis on secondary and tertiary care in well-developed urban areas. Primary care in its narrowest sense (emergency care, prophylaxis, case finding, and health education) will continue to be a main function of public dental programs, though secondary care may be rendered in a number of areas.

It is important, however, that public and private dental programs learn to cooperate with and help each other—rather than opposing each other, as happens at times today. The case-finding activities of a public program have been shown to send practice into private offices, as in industry, where many wage earners are potential private patients, and in schools, where there is a mix of low-income and middle-income children.[10] The private sector can, and should, respond by allowing public programs to pioneer in making changes in the dental care delivery system, changes which in the end may turn out to be as useful in the private sector as in the public sector. Quality care has a quantitative component from the government point of view. We must not allow "the best," in Voltaire's phrase, to become "the enemy of the good."

The World Health Organization gives a good prescription for the future:

These problems suggest that different manpower structures and, more importantly, a different philosophy stressing health, not oral disease, is needed, using community sectors and providers together.

Some of the specific features of such an approach might be a change of emphasis away from schoolchildren to a more balanced distribution of prevention and treatment services to families and underserved groups. In populations that have, and will have, altered age distributions, consideration of high risk detection and care, surveillance of trends and examination of prevailing systems, manpower productivity and distribution have to be undertaken to meet the changing needs of the population.

Fundamental to these changes is the concept of primary health care, which must form the broad use of education and promotion of preventive behaviour; emphasis on prevention by providers and community sectors and utilization of low technology procedures delivered by such individuals as health auxiliaries, schoolteachers and health volunteers in a variety of places in the community: the community, the work place, the schools. When a base of such preventive services is secure, disease prevalence will diminish and a more rational and appropriate referral network and specialized dental manpower structures for more complex treatment problems can be organized. Development of uniform, reliable and valid techniques to measure changes in oral health risk and in unmet treatment needs surely represents a continuing and important challenge to dental research. Distribution of preventive and treatment services according to risks would then conserve resources, reduce costs and improve oral health for the entire population.[11]

RESEARCH

The attack upon new and unsolved problems must lie through research, both basic and applied. If the field of dentistry is compared with that of medicine as a whole, it would appear that the dental research effort has not yet reached its proper size. This is due in part to a lack of adequate funds for dental research and in part to the inability of the dental profession to make wise use of such funds. Skillful researchers with adequate training in the basic sciences are all too scarce in the field of dentistry. It is a responsibility of dental schools and also of dental public health programs to foster the training of such individuals, then put them to work. In practical terms, we need more and better departments of dental public health and preventive dentistry, or dental ecology, in dental schools, staffed by qualified full-time teachers.[12] We need more qualified full-time administrators in dental health programs, even down to the district or county level. Applied clinical research will then help dental public health to rise above the technical loads which now shackle it and to move forward on a more imaginative plane.

Recent progress in the prevention and control of disease permits the conclusion that workers in the field of dental public health do not need to accept failure as an important probability. The complete conquest of dental disease is also a difficult outcome to imagine. Even with acute infectious diseases, such as yellow fever and smallpox, continuous preventive programs and constant vigilance are needed, or else the occasional cases of these diseases that still occur will erupt into epidemics. Chronic disease is even harder to "conquer" than acute disease. If, therefore, the reasoning presented here appears to point more to a state of equilibrium between dental disease and dental care than to a complete conquest of dental disease, the matter should cause no surprise or discouragement. Human life is always more of an equilibrium than a finished fight. Equilibrium implies the challenge of new endeavors and also a satisfying proportion of success in old ones. It also implies *control,* a concept almost as satisfying as complete conquest.

In the meanwhile, the chance to make dental caries and periodontal disease as rare as smallpox does exist. Scientific advances may produce highly efficient preventive measures not incompatible with modern cultures; health education may secure virtually universal utilization of these measures; and long-range changes in the diseases themselves or in human resistance to them may reverse the upward trends of recent centuries. Without all three, the likelihood of full success is small.

In the field of dental care delivery, the great need now is for more teamwork. The diverse needs of world populations and the rapid scientific growth of professional dentistry have overshadowed the leadership of the superb clinical dentist keeping a tight rein upon his or her office staff. The licensed dentist must continue to be the leader, but of a more far-flung and responsible team than ever before. Dental public health is the special discipline for such leadership—to be built upon general dentistry with a quality approach to all levels of care from primary upward.

Whatever changes do occur, the chronic nature of the diseases dentists are dealing with will make the changes very slow. As Hanlon puts it, we must "remember that intelligent mankind is still very young and that the future will last a long time."[9] For the present, the hope of attaining a firm control of dental disease can lead us forward, and the possibility of a real conquest of such disease need not be dismissed.

REFERENCES

INDEX

REFERENCES

1. Public Health in Theory

1. C.-E. A. Winslow, "The untilled fields of public health," *Mod. Med. (Minneap.)* 2, 183–191 (1920).

2. American Dental Association Council on Dental Education, Annual Report, in *Transactions of the American Dental Association, 1976* (Chicago), p. 475.

3. J. E. Gordon, *The newer epidemiology: Tomorrow's horizons in public health* (Public Health Association of New York, New York, 1950).

4. B. D. Paul, *Health, culture, and community* (Russell Sage Foundation, New York, 1955).

5. M. Rader, *Ethics and society* (Holt, New York, 1950), chap. 6.

6. American Medical Association, *Principles of Ethics of the American Medical Association* (Amer. Med. Ass. Chicago, 1957; reprinted 1977), sec. 10.

7. J. C. Snyder, "Ethics and public health," sermon presented at Riverside Church, New York, N.Y., March 1, 1959.

8. M. Lerner, *America as a civilization* (Simon and Schuster, New York, 1957), p. 119.

9. D. F. Striffler, W. O. Young, and B. A. Burt, *Dentistry, dental practice, and the community* (Saunders, Philadelphia, ed., 3, 1983), chaps. 1 and 4.

10. H. C. Doben, Veteran's Administration, Washington, D.C., personal communication, 1957.

GENERAL READINGS

J. J. Hanlon, *Public health administration and practice* (Mosby, St. Louis, ed. 6, 1974), chaps. 1–4.

H. R. Leavell and E. G. Clark, *Preventive medicine for the doctor in his community* (McGraw-Hill, New York, ed. 3, 1965), chaps. 1 and 2.

2. Public Health in Practice

1. Association of State and Territorial Health Officials, National Public Health Program Reporting System, *Comprehensive NPHPRS report: Services, expenditures, and programs of state and territorial health agencies, fiscal year 1978,* ASTRO-NPHPRS Pub. No. 47 (Silver Spring, Maryland, Association of State and Territorial Health Officials, 1980).

2. World Health Organization, *Manual of the international statistical classification of diseases, injuries and causes of death* (2 vols., WHO, Geneva, 1977). Also obtainable from National Office of Vital Statistics, Washington, D.C.

3. S. Shapiro and J. Schachter, "Birth registration completeness, United States, 1950," *Publ. Hlth Rep. (Wash.)* 67, 513–524 (1952).

4. *Statistical abstract of the United States, 1976* (Government Printing Office, Washington, D.C., ed. 97).

5. W. G. Smillie, *Public health administration in the United States* (Macmillan, New York, ed. 3, 1949), p. 276.

6. National Organization of Public Health Nurses Committee on Nursing Administration, "Public health nursing responsibilities in a community health program," *Publ. Hlth Nursing 41,* 68–69 (1949).

7. J. J. Hanlon, *Public health administration and practice* (Mosby, St. Louis, ed. 6, 1974), Table 21-5, p. 402.

8. "Nation-wide inventory of sanitation needs," *Supp. 204, Publ. Hlth Rep. (Wash.),* (1948).

9. K. R. Boucot and D. A. Cooper, "A critical evaluation of mass roentgen surveys," *J. Amer. Med. Ass. 142,* 1255–1258 (1950).

10. F. Goldmann, "Multiple screening for chronic diseases," *Mass. Hlth J. 33,* 3–6 (1953). See also F. I. Tomson, "Multiphasic screening program in low-income areas," *Publ. Hlth Rep. (Wash.) 73,* 533–536 (1958).

11. Cooperative for American Remittances Everywhere, "CARE: A report to the people," *New York Times,* Feb. 10, 1957, sec. 10, p. 4.

GENERAL READINGS

J. J. Hanlon, *Public health administration and practice* (Mosby, St. Louis, ed. 6, 1974).

H. R. Leavell and E. G. Clark, *Preventive medicine for the doctor in his community* (McGraw-Hill, New York, ed. 3, 1965).

3. Milestones in Dental Public Health

1. J. A. Salzmann, *Principles and practice of public health dentistry* (Lee Stratford Co., Boston, 1937).

2. V. Guerini, *History of dentistry* (Lee and Febiger, Philadelphia, 1909).

3. American Dental Association, "Proceedings of Tenth Annual Meeting," *Dent. Cosmos 12,* 455–472 (1870).

4. M. L. Rhein, "Oral hygiene," *New Engl. J. Dent. 3,* 356–361 (1884).

5. W. D. Miller, "Agency of micro-organisms in decay of the human teeth," *Dent. Cosmos 25,* 1–12 (1883).

6. J. L. Williams, "Prevention of dental caries," *Dent. Items of Interest, 148–149* (1898).

7. W. G. Ebersole, "Report of work accomplished by the National Dental Association Oral Hygiene Committee," *Dent. Cosmos 53*, 333–339 (1911).

8. W. G. Ebersole, "History of the oral hygiene campaign as inaugurated by the Oral Hygiene Committee of the National Dental Association," *Dent. Cosmos 53*, 1386–1393 (1911).

9. C. M. Wright, "Plea for a sub-specialty in dentistry," *Int. Dent. J. 23*, 235–238 (1902).

10. Committee on Costs of Medical Care, Publ. 1, p. 14; Publ. 6, pp. 141–142; Publ. 9, pp. 265–266; Publ. 10, p. 46; Publ. 12, pp. 13–14 (Washington, D.C.).

11. W. J. Gies, *Dental education in the United States and Canada* (The Carnegie Foundation, New York, 1926).

12. J. A. Salzmann, "Effective provision of dental service to population groups," *J. Amer. Coll. Dent. 11*, 280–294 (1944).

13. World Health Organization coordinator, *Oral Health Care Systems* (Quintessence Publishing, London, 1985).

4. Biostatistics: Selection of Data

1. C. Bernard, *An introduction to the study of experimental medicine* (Macmillan, New York, 1927).

2. G. U. Yule and M. G. Kendall, *An introduction to the theory of statistics* (Hafner, New York, ed. 14, 1950), p. xvi.

3. J. B. Conant, *On understanding science* (Yale University Press, New Haven, 1947).

4. F. J. Orland et al., "Experimental caries in germfree rats inoculated with enterococci," *J. Amer. Dent. Ass. 50*, 259–272 (1955).

5. L. K. Frankel, "A consideration of evidences on oral sepsis in relation to systemic disease," *Dent. Cosmos 66*, 35–40 (1924).

6. T. P. Hyatt and A. J. Lotka, "How dental statistics are secured in the Metropolitan Life Insurance Co.," *J. Dent. Res. 9*, 411–455 (1929).

7. *Health of ferrous foundrymen in Illinois* (Public Health Publication No. 31; Federal Security Agency, Washington, D.C., 1950).

8. H. T. Dean et al., "Domestic water and dental caries, including certain aspects of oral *L. Acidophilus*," *Publ. Hlth Rep. (Wash.) 54*, 862–888 (1939).

9. E. R. Aston, "Dental study of employees of five lead plants," *Industr. Med. Surg. 21*, 17–20 (1952).

10. R. B. Robinson, "Incidence of periodontal disease in adult diabetics," *Harv. Dent. Alumni Bull. 14*, 17–23 (1954).

11. C. T. Messner et al., "Dental survey of school children, ages 6–14, made in 1933–1934 in 26 states," *U.S. Publ. Hlth Bull. (Wash.) 226* (1936).

12. H. T. Dean, F. A. Arnold, Jr., and E. Elvove, "Domestic water and dental caries. V." *Publ. Hlth Rep. (Wash.) 57*, 1155–1179 (1942).

13. Statistics Section, American Public Health Association, "On the use of sampling in the field of public health," *Amer. J. Publ. Hlth 44*, 719–740 (1954).

GENERAL READINGS

Clinical testing of dental caries preventives (American Dental Association, Chicago, 1955). Also in summary, *J. Amer. Dent. Ass. 54*, 275–283 (1957).

T. Colton, *Statistics in Medicine* (Little, Brown, Boston, 1975), chaps. 1–3.

G. A. Ferguson, *Statistical analysis in psychology and education* (McGraw-Hill, New York, ed. 2, 1966), chaps. 1 and 9.

5. Biostatistics: Appraisal of Variability

1. A. Bradford Hill, *Principles of medical statistics* (Oxford University Press, New York, ed. 8, rev., 1966), pp. 31–34.
2. American Dental Association Bureau of Economic Research and Statistics, "The 1971 survey of dental practice, II," *J. Amer. Dent. Ass. 84*, 397–402 (1972).
3. J. M. Dunning, "Variability of dental caries experience and its implication upon sample size," *J. Dent. Res. 29*, 541–548 (1950).
4. P. H. Forsham et al., "Clinical studies with pituitary adrenocorticotropin," *J. Clin. Endocr. 8*, 15–66 (1948); also A. G. Ship, personal communication, 1952.
5. W. D. Wellock, personal communication from Division of Dental Health, Massachusetts Department of Public Health, 1951.
6. R. A. Fisher, *Statistical methods for research workers* (Oliver and Boyd, London, ed. 10, 1946), chap. 5.
7. G. W. Snedecor, *Statistical methods* (Iowa State College Press, Ames, Iowa, ed. 4, 1946), chaps. 10 and 11.

GENERAL READINGS

T. Colton, *Statistics in medicine* (Little, Brown, Boston, 1975), chap. 4.
J. A. Weintraub, C. W. Douglass, and D. B. Gillings, *BIOSTATS: Data analysis for dental health care professionals* (Waban, Mass., CAVCO, Inc., 1984).

6. Biostatistics: Correlation and Other Tests

1. A. Bradford Hill, *Principles of medical statistics* (Oxford University Press, New York, ed. 8, 1966), chap. 10.
2. J. W. Knutson and W. D. Armstrong, "The effect of topically applied sodium fluoride on dental caries experience. II. Report of findings for the second study year." *Publ. Hlth Rep. (Wash.) 60*, 1085–1090 (1945).
3. J. R. Forrest, "The fluoridation of public water supplies. (*a*) The dental aspect," *Roy. Soc. Hlth J. 77*, 344–350 (1957).
4. S. Siegel, *Nonparametric statistics for the behavioral sciences* (McGraw-Hill, New York, 1956).
5. J. B. Conant, *On understanding science* (Yale University Press, New Haven, 1947), p. 24.

GENERAL READINGS

N. W. Chilton, *Design and analysis in dental and oral research* (Lippincott, Philadelphia, 1967), chaps. 8 and 14.
T. Colton, *Statistics in medicine* (Little, Brown, Boston), chaps. 6 and 7.

7. Epidemiology: General Principles

1. H. R. Leavell and E. G. Clark, *Preventive medicine for the doctor in his community* (McGraw-Hill, New York, ed. 3, 1965).

2. J. E. Gordon, "The newer epidemiology," in *Tomorrow's horizons in public health* (Public Health Association of New York City, 1950).

3. American Public Health Association, *Control of communicable diseases in man* (APHA, New York, ed. 8, 1955), p. 14.

4. J. E. Gordon, "Medical ecology and the public health," *Amer. J. Med. Sci. 235*, 337–359 (1958).

5. M. G. Candau, *Man's health in relation to the biosphere and its resources* (UNESCO House, Paris, 1968).

6. H. A. Schneider, "Strategic concepts in epidemiology," in *Biological foundations of health education* (Proceedings of the Eastern States Health Education Conference, April 1–2, 1948; Columbia University Press, New York, 1950), pp. 139–147.

7. E. Wellin, "Water boiling in a Peruvian town," in B. D. Paul, ed., *Health, culture, and community* (Russell Sage Foundation, New York, 1955).

8. C. E. Taylor and J. E. Gordon, "Synergism and antagonism in mass disease of man," *Amer. J. Med. Sci. 225*, 320–344 (1953).

9. R. E. Shank, "Nutrition in preventive medicine," in Leavell and Clark, chap. 6.

10. A. L. Russell, "A social factor associated with the severity of periodontal disease," *J. Dent. Res. 36*, 922–926 (1957).

11. Citizen's Board of Inquiry into Hunger and Malnutrition in the United States, *Hunger U.S.A.* (Boston Press, Boston, 1968).

12. H. D. Chadwick, "A review of the campaign to eradicate tuberculosis," *New Engl. J. Med. 223*, 1001–1005 (1940).

13. B. MacMahon, T. F. Pugh, and J. Ipsen, *Epidemiologic methods* (Little, Brown, Boston, 1960), chap. 4.

14. J. W. Knutson and W. D. Armstrong, "The effect of topically applied sodium fluoride on dental caries experience. II. Report of findings for second study year," *Publ. Hlth Rep. (Wash.) 60*, 1085–1090 (1945).

15. W. G. Smillie, *Public health administration in the United States* (Macmillan, New York, ed. 3, 1949), pp. 203–207.

GENERAL READINGS

A. M. Lilienfeld, *Foundations of epidemiology* (Oxford University Press, New York, 1976).

B. MacMahon and T. F. Pugh, *Epidemiology, principles and methods* (Little, Brown, Boston, 1970).

J. N. Morris, *Uses of epidemiology* (Williams and Wilkins, Baltimore, ed. 2, 1964).

8. Epidemiology: Dental Caries

1. W. D. Miller, "Asepsis and antisepsis in practice," *Dent. Cosmos 35*, 2–3 (1893).

2. A. Krikos, "The progress of decay in Greece from the most ancient times down to the present," *Trans. Amer. Dent. Soc. Europe* (1935).

3. R. F. Sognnaes, "Histological evidence of developmental lesions in teeth originating from paleolithic, prehistoric, and ancient man," *Amer. J. Path. 32*, 547–577 (1956).

4. R. F. Sognnaes, "A survey of dental caries in Greece," *N. Y. St. Dent. J. 15*, 15–21 (1949).

5. L. M. Waugh, "Discussion. Relationship between diet and dental caries," *J. Dent. Res. 11*, 570–571 (1931).

6. M. Mellanby, *Diet and the teeth: an experimental study. Part III. The effect of diet on dental structure and disease in man* (Medical Research Council, Special Report Series, No. 191, H. M. Stationery Office, London, 1934).

7. R. L. Glass, ed., "The First International Conference on the Declining Prevalence of Dental Caries," *J. Dent. Res. 61*, Special Issue (November 1982).

8. I. J. Möller, "Impact of oral diseases across cultures," *Int. Dent. J. 28*, 376–380 (1978).

9. F. J. Orland et al., "Experimental caries in germfree rats inoculated with enterococci," *J. Amer. Dent. Ass. 50*, 259–272 (1955).

10. R. J. Gibbons and J. van Houte, "Dental caries," in *Annual Review of Medicine 26* (Annual Reviews, Inc., Palo Alto, Cal., 1975), pp. 121–136. Last sentence confirmed by Gibbons, 1984.

11. R. W. Hyde, "Socio-economic aspects of dental caries," *New Engl. J. Med. 230*, 506–510 (1944); C. E. Scribner, personal communication, September 1958.

12. H. C. Mao, "Some observations on the dental conditions in Peiping, China," *J. Canad. Dent. Ass. 16*, 572–576 (1950); H. Klein and C. Palmer, *On the epidemiology of dental caries* (University of Pennsylvania Bicentennial Conference, University of Pennsylvania Press, Philadelphia, 1941).

13. U.S. Department of Health and Human Services, *The prevalence of dental caries in United States children, 1979–1980,* NIH Publication No. 82-2245 (1981), Tables 12 and 13.

14. American Dental Association Bureau of Economic Research and Statistics, "Survey of need for dental care, 1965. II. Dental needs according to sex and age of patients," *J. Amer. Dent. Ass. 76*, 1355–1365 (1968).

15. F. Hollander and J. M. Dunning, "A study by age and sex of the incidence of dental caries in over 12,000 persons," *J. Dent. Res. 18*, 43–60 (1939).

16. W. J. Pelton, E. H. Pennell, and A. Druzina, "Tooth morbidity experience for adults," *J. Amer. Dent. Ass. 49*, 439–445 (1954).

17. Committee on Community Dental Service, New York Tuberculosis and Health Association, *Health dentistry for the community* (University of Chicago Press, Chicago, 1935), p. 32.

18. J. M. Dunning and H. DeWilde, "Variations in the efficiency of bitewing roentgenograms as related to age of patient." *J. Amer. Dent. Ass. 52*, 138–148 (1956).

19. C. F. Bodecker, "Variations in the lesions and activity of dental caries," *J. Dent. Res. 16*, 51–58 (1937).

20. J. S. Stamm and D. W. Banting, "Abstract 405," *J. Dent. Res. 59*, Special Issue A (1980).

21. J. N. Mansbridge, "Heredity and dental caries," *J. Dent. Res. 38*, 337–347 (1959).

22. J. M. Dunning, "Measurement of short-term changes in dental caries associated with stress: Four case reports," *J. Prev. Dent. 6*, 291–295 (1980).

23. M. S. Burstone, "The psychosomatic aspects of dental problems," *J. Amer. Dent. Ass. 33*, 862–871 (1946); I. B. Hyams, "Personality factors and dental caries," *J. Canad. Dent. Ass. 14*, 473–474 (1948).

24. J. M. Dunning, R. W. Hyde, and P. J. Dalton, "Dental disease in psychiatric patients," *J. Dent. Res. 30*, 806–814 (1951).

25. J. D. Boyd, "Prevention of caries in late childhood and adolescence," *J. Amer. Dent. Ass. 30*, 670–680 (1943).

26. J. M. Dunning, "A comparison of dental caries on the buccal and proximal surfaces of premolar teeth," *J. Dent. Res. 20*, 195–201 (1941).

27. O. Backer-Dirks, "Longitudinal dental caries study in children 9–15 years of age," *Arch. Oral Biol. 6*, 94–108 (1961).

28. D. M. Hadjimarkos and C. A. Storvick, "Bilateral occurrence of dental caries. A study in Oregon State College freshman students," *Oral Surg. 3*, 1206–1209 (1950); and "Geographic variations of dental caries in Oregon, V," *Amer. J. Publ. Hlth 41*, 1052 (1951).

29. J. W. Knutson and W. D. Armstrong, "The effect of topically applied sodium fluoride on dental caries experience. II," *Publ. Hlth Rep. (Wash.) 60*, 1085–1090 (1945).

30. T. Jay, "Bacillus acidophilus and dental caries," *J. Amer. Dent. Ass. 16*, 230 (1929).

31. H. V. Jordan, H. R. Englander, and S. Lim, "The presence of potentially cariogenic streptococci in various population groups," prepublished abstract No. 370, 46th general meeting, International Association for Dental Research, *Program and Abstracts of Papers* (Int. Ass. Dent. Res., Chicago, 1968).

32. J. M. Dunning, "The influence of latitude and distance from seacoast on dental disease," *J. Dent. Res. 32*, 811–829 (1953).

33. C. T. Messner, W. M. Gafafer, F. C. Cady, and H. T. Dean, *Dental survey of school children, ages 6–14 years, made in 1933–34 in 26 states,* Public Health Bulletin No. 226.

34. B. R. East, "Some epidemiological aspects of tooth decay," *Amer. J. Publ. Hlth 32*, 1242–1250 (1942).

35. A. E. Nizel and B. G. Bibby, "Geographic variations in caries prevalence in soldiers," *J. Amer. Dent. Ass. 31*, 1619–1626 (1944).

36. R. H. Britten and G. St. J. Perott, "Summary of physical findings on men drafted in the world war," *Publ. Hlth Rep. (Wash.) 56*, 41–62 (1941).

37. R. A. Ferguson, "Some observations on diet and dental disease," *J. Amer. Dent. Ass. 22*, 392–401 (1935).

38. U.S. Department of Health and Human Services, *The prevalence of dental caries in United States children, 1979–1980,* NIH Publication No. 82-2245 (1981), p. 8.

39. T. Ockerse, *Dental caries, clinical and experimental investigations* (Department of Health, Pretoria, Union of South Africa, 1949).

40. N. H. Andrews, "A study of the dental status of male and female personnel, Royal Australian Air Force, 1939–45," *Aust. J. Dent. 52*, 12–24 (1948).

41. *Yearbook of the Commonwealth of Australia* (Commonwealth Bureau of Census and Statistics, No. 38, 1951), pp. 64 ff.

42. A. L. Russell, "World epidemiology and oral health," in S. J. Kreshover and F. J. McClure, eds., *Environmental Variables in Oral Disease* (American Association for the Advancement of Science, Washington, D.C., 1966), p. 26.

43. U.S. Department of Commerce, *Sunshine tables* (Weather Bureau Publications No. 805; reprinted 1944).

44. B. R. East, "Mean annual hours of sunshine and incidence of dental caries," *Amer. J. Publ. Hlth 29*, 777–780 (1939).

45. H. K. Stiebeling et al., *Family food consumption and dietary levels, five*

regions (Farm Series, U.S. Department of Agriculture Misc. Publ. 405, Table 50; Urban and Small Village Series, Misc. Publ. 452, Table 35).

46. U. S. Department of Agriculture, Agricultural Research Service, *Dietary levels of households in the United States, Spring, 1965, a preliminary report* (A.R.S. Report 62–17, Washington, D.C., January, 1968), Table 1.

47. A. Van Burkalow, "Fluorine in United States water supplies," *Geog. Rev. 36*, 177–193 (1946).

48. C. Röse, "Deficiency of mineral salts and degeneracy," *Dent. Cosmos 51*, 135–137 (1909). (Selected, translated.)

49. D. M. Hadjimarkos, "Micronutrient elements in relation to dental caries," *Borden's Rev. Nutr. Res. 27*, No. 3, 1–14 (1966).

50. T. G. Ludwig, W. B. Healy, and R. S. Malthus, "Dental caries prevalence in specific soil areas at Napier and Hastings," *Trans. Joint Mtg. Comm. IV and V* (Int. Soc. Soil Sci., New Zealand, 1962), p. 895.

51. D. E. Barmes, "Features of oral health care across cultures," *Int. Dent. J. 26*, 353–368 (1976).

52. J. T. Fulton, *Experiment in dental care* (World Health Organization Monograph No. 4, Geneva, 1951).

53. A. L. Russell, "The epidemiology of dental caries and periodontal diseases," in W. O. Young and D. F. Striffler, eds., *The dentist, his practice, and his community* (Saunders, Philadelphia, 1964), chap. 6.

54. American Dental Association Bureau of Economic Research and Statistics, "Survey of needs for dental care, 1965, V," *J. Amer. Dent. Ass. 74*, 789–792 (1967).

55. Z. M. Stadt et al., "Socio-economic status and dental caries experience of 3911 five-year-old natives of Contra Costa County, Cal.," *J. Publ. Hlth Dent. 27*, 2–6 (Winter, 1967); and L. F. Szwejda, "Observed differences in total caries experience among white children of various socio-economic groups," *Publ. Hlth Dent. 20*, 59–66 (1960).

56. U.S. Department of Health, Education, and Welfare, *Decayed, missing, and filled teeth in adults, United States, 1960–1962* (National Center for Health Statistics, Public Health Service Publ. No. 1000, Series 11, No. 23, Washington, D.C., 1967).

57. G. Toverud, "The influence of war and post-war conditions on the teeth of Norwegian school children," *Milbank Mem. Fd. Quart. 34*, 35 (1956–1957).

58. M. Mellanby and H. Mellanby, "The reduction in dental caries in 5-year-old London school children (1929–1947)," *Brit. Med. J. 2*, 409 (1948).

59. R. F. Sognnaes, "Analysis of wartime reduction of dental caries in European children," *Amer. J. Dis. Child. 75*, 792–821 (1948).

60. R. F. Sognnaes, "A possible role of food purification in the etiology of dental caries," *Science 106*, 448 (1947).

61. O. W. Kite, J. H. Shaw, and R. F. Sognnaes, "The prevention of experimental tooth decay by tube-feeding," *J. Nutr. 42*, 89–105 (1950).

62. R. L. Glass, ed., "The First International Conference on the Declining Prevalence of Dental Caries," *J. Dent. Res. 61*, 1301–1383, Special Issue (1982).

63. Ibid., p. 1350.

64. H. S. Horowitz, R. J. Meyers, S. B. Heifetz, M. S. Driscoll, and S.-H. Li, "Eight-year evaluation of a combined fluoride program in a non-fluoride area," *J. Amer. Dent. Ass. 109*, 575–578 (1984).

65. H. A. Zander, "Effect of a penicillin dentifrice on caries incidence in school children," *J. Amer. Dent. Ass. 40,* 569–574 (1950).

66. R. J. Gibbons, personal communication, December 11, 1984.

67. D. E. Barmes, "Indicators for oral health and their implications for developing countries," *Int. Dent. J. 33,* 60–66 (1983).

9. Epidemiology: Periodontal and Other Diseases

1. I. Glickman, *Clinical periodontology* (Saunders, Philadelphia, ed. 3, 1964), chaps. 20 and 30.

2. M. Brucker, "Studies of the incidence and cause of dental defects in children," *J. Dent. Res. 22,* 309–314 (1943).

3. M. Massler, I. Schour, and B. Chopra, "Occurrence of gingivitis in suburban Chicago schoolchildren," *J. Periodont. 21,* 146–164 (1950).

4. C. D. M. Day et al., "Periodontal disease: prevalence and incidence," *J. Periodont. 26,* 185–203 (1955).

5. W. A. Bossert and H. H. Marks, "Prevalence and characteristics of periodontal disease of 12,800 persons under periodic dental observation," *J. Amer. Dent. Ass. 52,* 429–442 (1956).

6. W. G. McIntosh, "Gingival and periodontal disease in children," *J. Canad. Dent. Ass. 20,* 12–16 (1954).

7. C. D. M. Day and K. L. Shourie, "Gingival disease in the Virgin Islands," *J. Amer. Dent. Ass. 40,* 175–185 (1950).

8. M. L. Ainsworth and M. Young, *Incidence of dental disease in children* (Med. Res. Council, Special Report Series, No. 97; H.M. Stationery Office, London, 1925).

9. G. Westin et al., *An investigation into questions of social hygiene in the counties of Vasterbotten and Norbotten, Sweden.* Parts II–IV, 1937.

10. I. Schour and M. Massler, "Gingival disease in postwar Italy (1945). I.," *J. Amer. Dental. Ass. 35,* 475–482 (1947).

11. J. Schwartz, "Teeth of the Masai," *J. Dent. Res. 25,* 17–20 (1946).

12. C. E. Dawson, "Dental defects and periodontal disease in Egypt, 1946–1947," *J. Dent. Res. 27,* 512–523 (1948).

13. C. D. M. Day and K. L. Shourie, "Incidence of periodontal disease in the Punjab," *Ind. J. Med. Res. 32,* 47–51 (1944).

14. C. D. M. Day and K. L. Shourie, "Hypertrophic gingivitis in Indian children and adolescents," *Ind. J. Med. Res. 35,* 261–280 (1947).

15. C. D. M. Day and K. L. Shourie, "A roentgenographic study of periodontal disease in India," *J. Amer. Dent. Ass. 39,* 572–588 (1949).

16. J. C. Greene, "Periodontal disease in India: Report of an epidemiological study," *J. Dent. Res. 39,* 302–312 (1960).

17. B. G. Anderson, "Hypertrophic gingivitis among Chinese," *Nat. Med. J. China 15,* 453–454 (1929).

18. F. W. Clements and R. M. Kirkpatrick, "Medical and dental survey of school and pre-school children of New South Wales," *Dent. J. Aust. 10,* 418–429 (1938).

19. T. D. Campbell, "Food, food values, and food habits of the Australian aborigines in relation to their dental condition," *Aust. J. Dent. 43,* 1–15 (1939).

20. S. F. Williams, "Dental service in Western Samoa," *N.Z. Dent. J. 35,* 115–131 (1939).

21. G. H. Davies, "Dental conditions among the Polynesians of Pukapuka (Danger Island)," *J. Dent. Res. 35,* 734–741 (1956).

22. G. Andrews and H. W. Krogh, "Permanent tooth mortality," *Dent. Progr. 1,* 130–134 (1961).

23. A. L. Russell, "Some epidemiological characteristics of periodontal disease in a series of urban populations," *J. Periodont. 28,* 286–293 (1957).

24. C. W. Douglass, D. Gillings, W. Sollecito, and M. Gammon, "National trends in the prevalence and severity of the periodontal diseases," *J. Amer. Dent. Ass. 107,* 403–412 (1983).

25. A. L. Russell, "World epidemiology and health," in S. J. Kreshover and F. J. McClure, ed., *Environmental variables in oral disease* (Amer. Ass. Adv. Sci., Washington, D.C., 1966), Pub. No. 81, pp. 27–35.

26. Glickman, chaps. 11 and 27.

27. Ibid., chap. 28.

28. C. M. Belting and O. P. Gupta, "Incidence of periodontal disease among persons with neuropsychiatric disorders," *J. Dent. Res. 39,* 744–745 (1960).

29. H. Löe, E. Theilade, and S. B. Jensen, "Experimental gingivitis in man," *J. Periodont. 36,* 177 (1965).

30. B. Rosling, S. Nyman, and J. Lindhe, "The effect of systematic plaque control on bone regeneration in infrabony pockets," *J. Clin. Periodont. 2,* 38 (1976).

31. M. G. Newman and S. S. Socransky, "Predominant cultivable microbiota in periodontosis," *J. Periodont. Res. 12,* 120 (1977).

32. S. S. Socransky, "Microbiology of periodontal disease: Present status and future considerations," *J. Periodont. 48,* 497–504 (1977).

33. F. J. Walters et al., *Oral manifestations of occupational origin* (Public Health Publ. No. 228, U.S. Department of Health, Education, and Welfare, Washington, D.C., 1953).

34. F. S. Mehta, M. K. Sanjana, B. C. Schroff, and R. H. Doctor, "Relative importance of the various causes of tooth loss," *All-India Dent. Ass. J. 30,* 211–221 (1958).

35. S. Loos, "Prevalence of parodontal (periodontal) disease: 3. Europe," *Int. Dent. J. 5,* 319–326 (1955).

36. Glickman, chap. 26.

37. A. L. Russell, "Fluoride domestic water and periodontal disease," *Amer. J. Publ. Hlth 47,* 688–694 (1957).

38. A. L. Russell and E. Elvove, "Domestic water and dental caries. VII. A study of fluoride-dental caries relationships in adult populations," *Publ. Hlth Rep. (Wash.) 56,* 1389–1401 (1951).

39. C. M. Benjamin, A. L. Russell, and R. D. Smiley, "Periodontal disease in rural children of 25 Indiana counties," *J. Periodont. 28,* 294–298 (1957).

40. A. F. Stammers, "Vincent's infection: Observations and conclusions regarding the etiology and treatment of 1017 cases," *Brit. Dent. J. 76,* 147–155, 171–177, 205–209 (1944).

41. D. B. Giddon, P. Goldhaber, and J. M. Dunning, "Prevalence of reported cases of acute necrotizing ulcerative gingivitis in a university population," *J. Periodont. 34,* 366–371 (1963).

42. American Dental Association Bureau of Economic Research and Statistics, "Survey of needs for dental care. II, 1965," *J. Amer. Dent. Ass. 73,* 1355–1365 (1966).

43. Glickman, chap. 31.

44. D. B. Ast, "Fluoride link to malocclusion," *Dent. Times 6,* 1 (Feb. 16, 1963); D. M. Erickson and F. W. Graziano, "Prevalence of malocclusion in seventh-grade children in two North Carolina cities," *J. Amer. Dent. Ass. 73,* 124–127 (1966).

45. W. J. Pelton et al., *The Epidemiology of Oral Health* (Harvard University Press, Cambridge, 1969), chap. 4.

46. J. D. Jago, "The epidemiology of dental occlusion: A critical appraisal," *J. Pub. Hlth Dent. 34,* 80–93 (1974).

47. J. C. Greene, "Epidemiology of congenital clefts of the lip and palate," *Pub. Hlth Rep. (Wash.) 78,* 589–602 (1963).

48. E. J. Curtis, F. C. Fraser, and D. Warburton, "Congenital cleft lip and palate," *Amer. J. Dis. Child. 102,* 853–857 (1961).

49. J. C. Greene, "Epidemiologic research, 1964–1967," *J. Amer. Dent. Ass. 76,* 1350–1356 (1968).

50. U.S. Department of Health, Education, and Welfare, Public Health Service, National Vital Statistics Division, *Monthly vital statistics report: Annual summary for the United States, 1962,* vol. 11 (Washington, D.C., 1963).

51. L. R. Cahn and D. P. Slaughter, *Oral cancer: A monograph for the dentist* (American Cancer Society, New York, 1962).

52. M. H. Merrill, *Cancer registration and survival in California* (California Tumor Registry, California Department of Public Health, Berkeley, 1963).

53. C. J. Smith, "Global epidemiology and aetiology of oral cancer," *Int. Dent. J. 23,* 82–93 (1973).

54. American Dental Association, "Leukoplakia: What the dentist should know about it. Part 2," *Dent. Abstr. 13,* 222–226 (1968).

55. Pelton et al., chap. 3.

GENERAL READING

J. D. Bader, ed., "Symposium on oral health status in the United States," *J. Dent. Educ. 49* (June 1985), Special Issue.

10. The Social Sciences

1. E. Wellin, "Water boiling in a Peruvian town," in B. D. Paul, ed., *Health, culture, and community* (Russell Sage Foundation, New York, 1955), pp. 71–103.

2. B. D. Paul, "Social science in public health," *Amer. J. Publ. Hlth 46,* 1390–1396 (1956).

3. B. D. Paul, "Medicine's third dimension," *J. Nat. Med. Ass. (N.Y.) 48,* 323–325 (1956).

4. A. Jong, *Patterns of dental health behavior of a segment of low-income families in an urban environment,* thesis for post-doctoral certificate, unpublished (Harvard School of Dental Medicine, Boston, 1968).

5. B. D. Paul, ed., *Health, culture and community* (Russell Sage Foundation, New York, 1955).

6. American Dental Association Bureau of Economic Research and Statistics, "A motivational study of dental care," *J. Amer. Dent. Ass. 56,* 434–443, 566–574, 745–751, 911–917 (1956).

7. C. Lambert, Jr., and H. E. Freeman, *The clinic habit* (College and University Press, New Haven, 1967).

8. A. H. Trithart, "Understanding the underprivileged child: Report of an experimental workshop," *J. Amer. Dent. Ass. 77*, 880–883 (1968).

9. Ad Hoc Advisory Committee on the President's Committee on Consumer Interests, recommendations presented to V. Knauer and transmitted to Health, Education, and Welfare Secretary E. L. Richardson, October 27, 1970.

10. T. W. Cutress et al., *Adult oral health and attitudes to dentistry in New Zealand* (Wellington, Dental Research Unit, Medical Research Council of New Zealand, 1979).

11. R. B. Jones, "The school-based dental care systems of New Zealand and South Australia: A decade of change," *J. Pub. Hlth Dent. 44*, 120–124 (1984).

12. S. N. Frankl, F. R. Shiere, and H. R. Fogels, "Should the parent remain with the child in the dental operatory?" *J. Dent. Child. 29*, 150–163 (1962).

13. R. Johnson and D. C. Baldwin, Jr., "Relationship of maternal anxiety to the behavior of young children undergoing dental extraction," *J. Dent. Res. 47*, 801–805 (1968).

14. D. C. Baldwin, Jr., "An investigation of psychological and behavioral responses to dental extraction in children," *J. Dent. Res. 45*, 1637–1651 (1966); and "Value of a waiting period in psychological preparation for dental extraction," *J. Dent. Res. 43*, 826–827 (abstract, 1964).

15. H. M. Wallace, V. Eisner, and S. Dooley, "Availability and usefulness of selected health and socio-economic data for community planning," *Amer. J. Publ. Hlth 57*, 762–771 (1967).

16. W. I. Wardwell, *Index of social need in 69 communities* (Greater Boston Community Survey, General Study No. 3, Boston, 1948).

17. J. M. Dunning, "Dental care in the greater Boston area," *New Engl. Dent. J. 11*, 10–14 (1949).

18. A. B. Hollingshead, *Two-factor index of social position* (A. B. Hollingshead, New Haven, 1957).

19. World Health Organization, *Oral Health Care Systems* (Quintessence Publishing, London, 1985).

20. R. A. Cowin, E. P. Rice, and W. M. Schmidt, "Social work in a child health clinic: A report of a demonstration," *Amer. J. Publ. Hlth 55*, 821–831 (1965).

21. B. Mausner and J. Mausner, "A study of the anti-scientific attitude," *Sci. Amer. 192*, 35–39 (1955); J. A. Hutchinson, "Small-town fluoridation fight," *Sc. Monthly*, 240–243 (November 1953).

22. W. A. Gamson, *Approaches to the study of fluoridation* (Document 13, mimeographed; Social Science Unit, Harvard School of Public Health, 1960).

23. B. D. Paul, "Synopsis of report on fluoridation," *Mass. Dent. Soc. J. 8*, 19–21 (1959).

24. T. Weaver, "Community and social structure: The case of fluoridation," lecture at Forsyth Dental Center, Boston (mimeographed, March 9, 1967).

25. J. J. Hanlon, *Public health administration and practice* (Mosby, St. Louis, ed. 6, 1974), p. 373.

GENERAL READINGS

N. D. Richards and L. K. Cohen, ed., *Social science and dentistry* (Fédération Dentaire Internationale, London, 1972), and Vol. II (1984).

B. D. Paul, ed., *Health, culture, and community* (Russell Sage Foundation, New York, 1955).

J. P. Kirscht et al., "A national study of health beliefs," *J. Hlth Hum. Behav.* 7 (1966).

A. Donabedian, *Aspects of medical care administration: Specifying requirements for health care* (Harvard University Press, Cambridge, 1973), chaps. 1 and 3.

11. Principles of Administration

1. M. E. Dimock, *The executive in action* (Harper, New York, 1945), p. 179.
2. Ibid., p. 215.
3. W. D. Scott, R. C. Clothier, S. B. Mathewson, and W. R. Spriegel, *Personnel management* (McGraw-Hill, New York, ed. 6, 1961), pp. 6–7.
4. A. R. Jonsen, "Effects on equitable access," National Academy of Sciences, Institute of Medicine, 1984 Annual Meeting, October 10, 1984.
5. Dimock, p. 155.
6. E. M. Allen, "Why are research grant applications disapproved?" *Science* *132*, 1532–1534 (1960).
7. C. N. Parkinson, *Parkinson's law* (Houghton Mifflin, Boston, 1957).
8. Scott et al., chap. 2.
9. Dimock, p. 252.
10. W. J. Pelton and J. M. Wisan, *Dentistry in public health* (Saunders, Philadelphia, ed. 2, 1955), p. 183.
11. J. J. Hanlon, *Public health administration and practice* (Mosby, St. Louis, ed. 6, 1974), pp. 215–217.
12. C. D. Flagle, W. H. Huggins, and R. H. Roy, *Operations research and systems engineering* (Johns Hopkins University Press, Baltimore, 1960).
13. M. F. Arnold et al., *Health program implementation through PERT*, Continuing Education Monographs No. 6 (Western Regional Office, American Public Health Association, San Francisco, 1966).
14. R. Nowjack-Raymer, "The role of the dental consultant in Project Headstart," presented at 113th Annual Meeting, American Public Health Association, Washington, D.C., November 20, 1985 (Abstract p. 154).
15. American Board of Dental Public Health, Inc., *Informational brochure* (1980).
16. U.S. Department of Health, Education, and Welfare, *Residency training in dental public health* (Dental Health Center, San Francisco, rev. ed., 1965).
17. E. H. Schell, *Technique of executive control* (McGraw-Hill, New York, ed. 8, 1957), chap. 2.
18. Dimock, p. 197.
19. C. I. Barnard, *The functions of the executive* (Harvard University Press, Cambridge, 1968), p. 165.
20. W. Osler, *Counsels and ideas* (H. Frowde, Oxford, ed. 4, 1908), p. 90.
21. Barnard, p. 273.

GENERAL READINGS

C. I. Barnard, *The functions of the executive* (Harvard University Press, Cambridge, 1938 and 1968 paperback).

M. E. Dimock, *The executive in action* (Harper, New York, 1945).

J. J. Hanlon, *Public health administration and practice* (Mosby, St. Louis, ed. 6, 1974), chaps. 10 and 11.

A. Donabedian, *Aspects of medical care administration: Specifying requirements for health care* (Harvard University Press, Cambridge, 1973), chaps. 2, 4, and 5.

E. H. Schell, *Technique of executive control* (McGraw-Hill, New York, ed. 8, 1957).

W. D. Scott, R. C. Clothier, S. B. Mathewson, and W. R. Spriegel, *Personnel management* (McGraw-Hill, New York, ed. 6, 1961), chaps. 1 and 2.

12. Preventive Dentistry

1. H. R. Leavell and E. G. Clark, *Preventive medicine for the doctor in his community* (McGraw-Hill, New York, ed. 3, 1965), chaps. 2 and 10.

2. R. F. Sognnaes, lecture at Harvard School of Dental Medicine, Jan. 7, 1959.

3. American Dental Association pamphlet, *Toothbrushing* (Chicago, 1957).

4. S. B. Finn et al., *Clinical pedodontics* (Saunders, Philadelphia, ed. 3, 1967), chaps. 27 and 28.

5. R. S. Manly and F. Brudevold, "Relative abrasiveness of natural and synthetic toothbrush bristles on cementum and dentin," *J. Amer. Dent. Ass. 55*, 779–780 (1957), and *Dent. Abstr. 3*, 200 (1958).

6. M. K. Hine, "The toothbrush," *Int. dent. J. 6*, 15–25 (1956).

7. American Dental Association pamphlet, *Don't be misled* (Chicago, 1955).

8. Council on Dental Therapeutics, American Dental Association, *Accepted dental remedies, 1966* (Amer. Dent. Ass., Chicago, 1965), p. 212.

9. L. S. Fosdick, "The reduction of the incidence of dental caries. I. Immediate toothbrushing with a neutral dentrifice," *J. Amer. Dent. Ass. 40*, 133–143 (1950).

10. A. J. Smith and D. F. Striffler, "The reported frequency of toothbrushing as related to the prevalence of dental caries in New Mexico," *J. Publ. Hlth Dent. 23*, 159–175 (Fall, 1963).

11. P. H. Keyes, "Research in dental caries," *J. Amer. Dent. Ass. 76*, 1357–1373 (1968).

12. C. Lundqvist, "Oral sugar clearance, its influence on dental caries activity," *Odont. Revy. 3*, suppl. 1 (1952), p. 107, Table 36.

13. J. F. Volker, "The effect of gum chewing on the teeth and supporting structures," *J. Amer. Dent. Ass. 36*, 23–27 (1948).

14. Lundqvist, reference 12, pp. 34–93.

15. R. L. Weiss and A. H. Trithart, "Between meal eating habits and dental caries experience in preschool children," *Amer. J. Publ. Hlth 50*, 1097–1104 (1960).

16. H. T. Knighton, "Effect of various foods and cleansing agents on elimination of artificially inoculated yeast from the mouth," *J. Amer. Dent. Ass. 29*, 2012–2018 (1942).

17. R. W. Bunting, "Diet and dental caries," *J. Amer. Dent. Ass. 22*, 114–122 (1935).

18. H. Becks and A. Jensen, "Dental prevention service," *J. Dent. Res. 27*, 737 (abstract) (1948).

19. D. F. Radusch, in. W. C. McBride, *Juvenile Dentistry* (Lea and Febiger, Philadelphia, 1952), p. 337.

20. L. Page and E. F. Phipard, *Essentials of an adequate diet—facts for nutrition programs* (U.S. Department of Agriculture, Agriculture Information Bulletin No. 160, Agricultural Research Service, Washington, D.C., 1956).

21. A. E. Nizel, *The science of nutrition and its application in clinical dentistry* (Saunders, Philadelphia, ed. 2, 1966).

22. J. C. Witschi, personal communication, November 28, 1984.

23. L. W. Hoover, ed., *Nutrient Data Bank Directory* (University of Missouri, Columbia, Mo., ed. 4, 1984).

24. Food and Nutrition Board, National Research Council, *Recommended dietary allowances* (Publ. 1146, ed. 8, rev., Washington, D.C., 1980).

25. Hyatt Study Club, *Prophylactic odontotomy* (Macmillan, New York, 1933).

26. W. A. Bossert, "Relation between the shape of the occlusal surfaces of molars and the prevalence of decay, I," *J. Dent. Res. 13*, 125–128 (1933), and "II," *16*, 63–67 (1937).

27. American Dental Association Council on Dental Materials, Instruments, and Equipment, "List of classified dental materials, instruments, and equipment," *J. Amer. Dent. Ass. 105*, 938 (1982).

28. Massachusetts Department of Public Health and Massachusetts Research Institute, Inc., *Pit and fissue sealants: A reference and training manual* (Massachusetts Department of Public Health and Massachusetts Research Institute, Inc., 1984), p. 24.

29. J. J. Calderone, personal communication, February 19, 1985.

30. Judy Jakush, "Pit and fissure sealant use: An issue explored," *J. Amer. Dent. Ass. 108*, 310–322 (1984).

31. D. C. Clark, J. W. Stamm, G. Robert, and C. Tessier, Results of a 32-month fluoride varnish study in Sherbrooke and Lac-Megantic, Canada. *J. Amer. Dent. Assn. 111*, 949–953 (1985).

32. J. W. Knutson, "Sodium fluoride solutions, technique for application to the teeth," *J. Amer. Dent. Ass. 36*, 37–39 (1948).

33. J. C. Muhler, "Topical treatment of the teeth with stannous fluoride— single application technique," *J. Dent. Child, 4th Quart.*, 306–309 (1958).

34. W. D. Wellock and F. Brudevold, "A study of acidulated fluoride solutions, II," *Arch. Oral, Biol. 8,* 179–182 (1963).

35. H. R. Englander et al., "Clinical anti-caries effect of repeated topical sodium fluoride application by mouthpieces," *J. Amer. Dent. Ass. 75*, 638–644 (1967).

36. H. S. Horowitz, "Effect of topically applied acidulated phosphate-fluoride on dental caries in Hawaiian school children," prepublished abstract No. 256, 46th general meeting. International Association for Dental Research, *Program and Abstracts of Papers* (Int. Ass. Dent. Res., Chicago, 1968).

37. H. S. Horowitz, "The prevention of dental caries by mouthrinsing with solutions of neutral sodium fluoride," *Int. Dent. J. 23*, 585–590 (1973).

38. L. W. Ripa, A. Levinson, and G. S. Leske, "Supervised weekly rinsing with a 0.2 percent neutral NaF solution: Results from a demonstration program after three school years," *J. Amer. Dent. Ass. 100*, 544–546 (1980).

39. S. B. Heifetz, R. Meyers, and A. Kingman, "A comparison of the anti-

caries effectiveness of daily and weekly rinsing with sodium fluoride solutions: Findings after two years," *Pediatr. Dent. 4*, 300–303 (1981).

40. J. G. Messer, "Pediatric dental health care within the Grenfell Regional Health Services," *Grenfell Clin. Quarterly 1*, 14–15 (1984).

41. J. M. Bentley, P. Cormier, and J. Oler, "The rural dental health program: The effect of a school-based dental health education program on children's utilization of dental services," *Amer. J. Pub. Hlth 73*, 500–505 (1983).

42. S. M. Sanzi-Schadel, "The switch from fluoride mouthrinse to tablets," presented at American Public Health Association session 3007, Anaheim, California, November 14, 1984.

43. American Dental Association, *Accepted dental therapeutics* (Chicago, ed. 40, 1984), p. 401.

44. L. Baumgartner, *Report to the Mayor on fluoridation for New York City* (New York City Department of Health, 1956).

45. F. P. Hadley, "A quantitative method for estimating *Bacillus acidophilus* in saliva," *J. Dent. Res. 13*, 415–428 (1933); B. E. Diamond, "A selective medium for lactobacilli counts from saliva," *J. Dent. Res. 29*, 8–13 (1950); M. Rogosa, J. A. Mitchell, and R. F. Wiseman, "Selective medium for isolation and enumeration of oral lactobacilli," *J. Dent. Res. 30*, 472 (1951).

46. M. D. Snyder et al., "Evaluation of laboratory tests for the estimation of caries activity," *J. Dent. Res. 35*, 342–343 (1956).

47. I. Glickman, *Clinical periodontology* (Saunders, Philadelphia, ed. 3, 1964), part 5; American Dental Association, *They're your teeth, you can keep them*, Pamphlet G22 (Amer. Dent. Ass., Chicago, 1968).

48. W. J. Charters, "Eliminating mouth infections with the toothbrush and other stimulating instruments," *Dent. Digest 38*, 130 (1932).

49. G. H. Curtis, C. M. McCall, Jr., and H. I. Overaa, "A clinical study of the effectiveness of the roll and Charters methods of brushing teeth," *J. Periodont. 28*, 277–280 (1957), and *Dent. Abstr. 3*, 198 (1958).

50. S. B. Finn, *Clinical Pedodontics* (Saunders, Philadelphia, ed. 3, 1967), chaps. 12 and 13.

51. T. K. Barber, "Prevention of malocclusion, and minor orthodontics" in R. C. Caldwell and R. E. Stallard, *A textbook of preventive dentistry* (Saunders, Philadelphia, 1977), chap. 20.

52. K. Rothman and A. Keller, "The effect of joint exposure to alcohol and tobacco on risk of cancer of the mouth and pharynx," *J. Chron. Dis. 25*, 711–716 (1972).

53. G. Shklar, I. Meyer, E. Cataldo, and R. Taylor, "Correlated study of oral cytology and histopathology," *Oral Sur. Oral Med. Oral Path. 25*, 61–69 (1968).

54. W. D. Heintz, "Mouth protectors: A progress report" (Bureau of Health Education), *J. Amer. Dent. Ass. 77*, 632–636 (1968).

55. Amer. Ass. of Public Health Dentistry, "A position paper of the Amer. Ass. of Public Health Dentistry," *J. Publ. Hlth Dent. 46*, 13–22 (1986).

56. J. Jakush and E. W. Mitchell, "Infection control in the dental office," *J. Amer. Dent. Ass. 112*, 458–468 (1986).

57. S. Silverman, Jr., "Infectious and sexually transmitted diseases," *J. Publ. Hlth Dent. 46*, 7–12 (1986).

58. American College of Dentists, "Report of Committee on Preventive Service, 1958," *Amer. Coll. Dent. Reporter 3*, 4 (1959).

13. Dental Needs and Resources

1. *Expert Committee on Auxiliary Dental Personnel report,* World Health Organization Technical Report No. 163 (Geneva, 1959).

2. J. M. Dunning, "The practical duties of frontier dental auxiliaries in Alaskan communities: A progress report," *J. Pub. Hlth Dent. 44,* 138–140 (1984).

3. T. W. Cutress et al., *Adult oral health and attitudes to dentistry in New Zealand, 1976* (Dental Research Unit, Medical Research Council of New Zealand, Wellington, 1979), p. 270.

4. L. W. Burket, "Studies of the apices of teeth. II. Results," *Yale J. Biol. Med. 9,* 347–358 (1937).

5. C. B. Favour, C. A. Janeway, J. G. Gibson, II, and F. A. Levin, "Progress in the treatment of sub-acute bacterial endocarditis," *New Engl. J. Med. 234,* 71–77 (1946).

6. American Heart Association, "Committee report on prevention of bacterial endocarditis," *Circulation 56(1),* 139A–143A (1977).

7. H. R. Leavell and E. G. Clark, *Preventive medicine for the doctor and his community* (McGraw-Hill, New York, ed. 3, 1965), p. 311.

8. American Dental Association Bureau of Economic Research and Statistics, "Survey of need for dental care, 1965," *J. Amer. Dent. Ass. 73,* 1128–1132, 1355–1365 (1966); *74,* 145–150, 489–492, 789–793, 1034–1035, 1291–1294, 1561–1562 (1967).

9. National Center for Health Statistics, E. S. Johnson, J. E. Kelly, and L. E. van Kirk, "Selected findings in adults by age, race, and sex, United States, 1960–62," *Vital and health statistics* (Series 11, No. 7, PHS Publ. No. 1000, PHS, 1965).

10. National Center for Health Statistics, J. E. Kelly, L. E. van Kirk, and C. C. Garst, "Decayed, missing, and filled teeth in adults, United States, 1960–62," *Vital and health statistics* (Series 11, No. 23, DHEW Publ. No. [HRA] 74-1278, PHS, 1973).

11. National Center for Health Statistics, C. R. Harvey, and J. E. Kelly, "Decayed, missing, and filed teeth among persons 1–74 years, United States, 1971–74," *Vital and health statistics* (Series 223, DHHS Publ. No. [PHS] 81-1673, PHS, August 1981).

12. C. W. Douglass and M. D. Gammon, "The epidemiology of dental caries and its impact on the operative dentistry curriculum," *J. Dent. Educ. 48,* 547–555 (1984).

13. D. E. Barmes, "Indicators for oral health and their implications for developing countries," *Int. Dent. J. 33,* 60–66 (1983).

14. C. W. Douglass, M. D. Gammon, D. B. Gillings, W. Sollecito, and D. Rundle, "Estimating the market for periodontal services in the United States," *J. Amer. Dent. Ass. 108,* 968–972 (1984).

15. J. E. Kelly and C. R. Harvey, "Basic data on dental examination findings of 1–74 years, United States, 1971–74," *Vital and health statistics* (Series 11, No. 214, Hyattsville, Md., National Center for Health Statistics, DHEW Publ. No. [PHS] 79-1662, 1979).

16. K. D. Nash, C. W. Douglass and J. Wilson, *Economies of scale and productivity in dental practices,* final report, Research Triangle Institute contract no. 231-75-0403, 1979, 151 pp.

17. U.S. Department of Health, Education, and Welfare, *Periodontal disease in adults,* Public Health Service Publ. No. 1000, Series 11, No. 12 (Washington, D.C., 1965), p. 10.

18. National Center for Health Statistics, "D, M, F teeth among youths 12–17, U.S.," *Vital and health statistics* (Series 11, No. 144, U.S. Department of Health, Education, and Welfare Publ. No. [HRA] 75-1626, Washington, D.C., 1974).

19. U.S. Department of Health, Education, and Welfare, "Dental visits," *Vital and health statistics* (Series 10, No. 76, Washington, D.C., 1969).

20. J. M. Dunning, S. R. Fishman, and R. E. Mecklenburg, "Dental manpower and education in 1966," *J. Publ. Hlth Dent. 27,* 174–192 (1967).

21. W. J. Pelton and Ruth Bothwell, "Forecast of dental service needs in the South," *Publ. Hlth rep. (Wash.) 73,* 15–21 (1958).

22. U.S. Bureau of the Census, *Statistical abstract of the United States, 1976* (Government Printing Office, Washington, D.C., 1984).

23. P. J. Feldstein, *Financing dental care: An economic analysis* (Heath, Lexington, Mass., 1973), chap. 2.

24. J. M. Dunning, ed., *Woodstock workshop in dental health education, 1966* (New England Council on Dental Health and Care, Boston, 1967).

25. American Dental Association Bureau of Economic Research and Statistics, *The 1975 survey of dental practice* (American Dental Association, Chicago, 1976).

26. American Dental Association, "Briefs," *ADA News,* January 7, 1985, p. 1.

27. American Dental Association Bureau of Economic and Behavioral Research, *1984–85 Dental Statistics Handbook* (American Dental Association, Chicago, 1984).

28. B. S. Hollinshead, "Preview of the survey of dentistry report," address to American Association of Dental Schools, Chicago, March 22, 1960.

29. *The world almanac and book of facts 1985* (Newspaper Enterprise Association, New York, 1984).

30. F. E. Law, "Dental care study project in fluoride and non-fluoride areas," Dental Health Memorandum to Public Health Service personnel, September 15, 1956.

31. H. A. Dunlevy and L. C. Niessen, "An economic analysis of the return on investment for a dental education," *J. Dent. Educ. 48,* 453–457 (1984).

32. T. D. Dublin, "The migration of physicians to the United States," *New Engl. J. Med. 286,* 870–876 (1972).

33. U.S. Department of Health, Education, and Welfare, *Health resources statistics, 1965* (Public Health Service Publ. No. 1509, Washington, D.C., 1967).

34. W. C. Allwright, R. J. S. Tickle, and S. Matsumiya, "Dentistry in Asian countries," *Int. Dent. J. 10,* 327–349 (1960).

35. H. Klein, "Dental needs versus dental manpower," *J. Amer. Dent. Ass. 31,* 263–266 (1944).

36. Commission on the Survey of Dentistry in the United States, *Dentistry in the United States: Status, needs, and recommendations* (American Council on Education, Washington, D.C., 1960).

37. D. F. Beck, *Dental care for adults under clinical conditions* (American College of Dentists, Lancaster, Pa., 1943).

38. G. E. Waterman and J. W. Knutson, "Studies on dental care services

for school children," *Publ. Hlth Rep. (Wash.) 68*, 583–589; *69*, 247–254 (1954).

39. J. M. Dunning and H. Klein, "Saving teeth among home office employees of the Metropolitan Life Insurance Company," *J. Amer. Dent. Ass. 31*, 1632–1642 (1944).

40. W. J. Pelton and J. M. Wisan, *Dentistry in public health* (Saunders, Philadelphia, ed. 2, 1955), p. 79.

41. D. A. Soricelli, "Methods of administrative control for the promotion of quality in dental programs," *Amer. J. Publ. Hlth 58*, 1723–1737 (1968).

42. J. J. Hanlon, *Public health administration and practice* (Mosby, St. Louis, ed. 6, 1974), p. 619.

43. H. R. Leavell and E. G. Clark, *Preventive medicine for the doctor in his community* (McGraw-Hill, New York, ed. 3, 1965), pp. 655–658.

44. P. Adler, "The incidence of dental caries in adolescents with different occlusion," *J. Dent. Res. 35*, 344–349 (1956).

45. M. Allukian, I. Kazmi, S. Foulds, and W. Horgan, "The unmet dental needs of the homeless in Boston," presented at 112th annual meeting of American Public Health Association, Anaheim, Calif., November 15, 1984.

14. Surveying

1. S. Shapiro et al., "Medical economics survey-methods study: design, data collection, and analytical plan," *Med. Care 14*, 893–912 (1976); K. H. Marquis et al., "The measurement of expenditures for out-patient physician and dental services: methodological findings from the health insurance study, *Med. Care 14*, 913–931 (1976).

2. U.S. Department of Health, Education, and Welfare, *Public health personnel in local health units* (Public Health Publ. No. 682, Washington, D.C., 1967).

3. H. M. Wallace, N. Eisner, and S. Dooley, "Availability and usefulness of selected health and socioeconomic data for community planning," *Amer. J. Pub. Hlth 57*, 762–771 (1967).

4. A. B. Hollingshead, *Two-factor index of social position* (A. B. Hollingshead, New Haven, 1957).

5. National Center for Health Statistics, *Health survey procedures: concepts, questionnaire development and definitions in the health interview survey* (Public Health Publ. No. 1000, Series 1, No. 2, Washington, D.C., 1964), p. 11.

6. F. C. Lindaman and M. A. Costa, "The voice of the community," *Amer. J. Pub. Hlth 62*, 1245–1248 (1972).

7. American Dental Association Bureau of Economic Research and Statistics, "Survey of patient-to-dentist travel," *J. Amer. Dent. Ass. 53*, 461–466 (1956).

8. World Health Organization, *Oral health surveys: basic methods* (World Health Organization, Geneva, ed. 2, 1977).

9. O. Backer-Dirks, "Post-eruptive changes in dental enamel," *J. Dent. Res. 45*, 503–511 (1966).

10. H. Klein, C. E. Palmer, and J. W. Knutson, "Studies on dental caries I. Dental status and dental needs of elementary school children," *Publ. Hlth Rep. (Wash.) 53*, 751–765 (1938); and H. Klein and C. E. Palmer, *Dental caries in American Indian children* (Public Health Bulletin No. 239, Government Printing Office, Washington, D.C., 1937).

11. H. Löe, "The gingival index, the plaque index, and the retention index systems," *J. Periodont., Part II 38*, 610–616 (1967).

12. C. D. M. Day and K. L. Schourie, "A roentgenographic survey of periodontal disease in India," *J. Amer. Dent. Ass. 39*, 572–588 (1949); I. M. Sheppard, "Alveolar resorption in diabetes mellitus," *Dent. Cosmos 78*, 1075–1079 (1936).

13. A. L. Russell, "A system of classification and scoring for prevalence surveys of periodontal disease," *J. Dent. Res. 35*, 350–359 (1956).

14. J. M. Dunning and L. B. Leach, "Gingival-bone count: Method for epidemiological study of periodontal disease," *J. Dent. Res. 39*, 506–513 (1960).

15. S. Schluger, R. A. Yuodelis, and R. C. Page, *Periodontal disease* (Lea and Febiger, Philadelphia, 1977), pp. 285–290.

16. S. P. Ramfjord, "Indices for prevalence and incidence of periodontal disease," *J. Periodont. 30*, 51–59 (1959).

17. J. Ainamo et al., "Development of the WHO Community Periodontal Index of Treatment Needs (CPITN)," *Int. Dent. J. 32*, 281–291 (1982).

18. J. C. Greene and J. R. Vermillion, "Oral hygiene index: A method for classifying oral hygiene status," *J. Amer. Dent. Ass. 61*, 172–179 (1960).

19. J. C. Greene and J. R. Vermillion, "The simplified oral hygiene index," *J. Amer. Dent. Ass. 68*, 7–13 (1964).

20. H. L. Draker, "Handicapping labio-lingual deviations: A proposed index for public health purposes," *Amer. J. Orthodont. 46*, 295–305 (1960).

21. J. A. Salzmann, "Malocclusion severity assessment," *Amer. J. Orthodont. 53*, 109–119 (1967).

22. R. M. Grainger, *Orthodontic treatment priority index* (Public Health Service Publ. No. 1000, Series 2, No. 25, U.S. Department of Health, Education, and Welfare, Washington, D.C., 1967).

23. J. P. Carlos, "Evaluation of indices of malocclusion," *Int. Dent. J. 20*, 606–617 (1970).

24. J. W. Knutson, "An index of the prevalence of dental caries in school children," *Publ. Hlth Rep. (Wash.) 59*, 253–263 (1944).

25. J. W. Knutson, "Epidemiological trend patterns of dental caries prevalence data," *J. Amer. Dent. Ass. 57*, 821–829 (1958).

26. H. R. Englander and D. A. Wallace, "Effects of naturally fluoridated water on dental caries in adults," *Publ. Hlth Rep. (Wash.) 77*, 887–893 (1962).

27. F. Hollander and J. M. Dunning, "A study by age and sex of the incidence of dental caries in over 12,000 persons," *J. Dent. Res. 18*, 43–60 (1939).

28. D. M. Hadjimarkos, "Bilateral occurrence of dental caries: A study in Oregon State College freshman students," *Oral Surg. 3*, 1206–1209 (1950).

29. J. W. Knutson and W. D. Armstrong, "The effect of topically applied sodium fluoride on dental caries experience. II," *Publ. Hlth Rep. (Wash.) 60*, 1085–1090 (1945).

30. American Dental Association, *Official policies of the American Dental Association on dental health programs* (American Dental Association, Chicago, 1957).

31. American Dental Association, *Current policies, adopted 1954–1975* (American Dental Association, Chicago, 1976), p. 136.

32. R. M. Grainger and A. H. Sellers, "The Welland district dental health program," *Canad. J. Hlth 43*, 415–425 (1952).

33. California State Department of Public Health, Division of Dental Health, *Dental caries survey: Who, why, how* (Sacramento, 1955), p. 11.

34. H. Klein and C. E. Palmer, "Studies on dental caries. X. A procedure for the recording and statistical processing of dental examination findings," *J. Dent. Res. 19*, 243–256 (1940).

35. A. O. Gruebbel, "A measurement of dental caries prevalence and treatment services for deciduous teeth," *J. Dent. Res. 23*, 163–168 (1944).

36. J. Doyle and H. S. Horowitz, "Influence of extracted teeth on DMF surface increments in clinical trials of caries preventives," *J. Dent. Res. 49*, 1417 (1970).

37. J. M. Dunning and H. De Wilde, "Variations in the efficiency of bitewing roentgenograms as related to age of patients," *J. Amer. Dent. Ass. 52*, 138–148 (1956).

38. J. M. Dunning and L. B. Leach, "Variations in the measurement of periodontal disease with the use of radiographs," *J. Dent. Res. 47*, 1149–1152 (1968). Also same title, prepublished abstract No. 144, 46th general meeting, International Association for Dental Research, *Program and Abstracts of Papers* (Int. Ass. Dent. Res., Chicago, 1968).

39. O. Backer-Dirks, J. Van Amerongen, and K. C. Winkler, "A reproducible method for caries evaluation," *J. Dent. Res. 30*, 346–359 (1951).

40. National Academy of Sciences, National Research Council, *The Biological effects of atomic radiation: A report to the public* (Washington, D.C., 1956).

41. National Council on Radiation Protection and Measurements, *Medical x-ray and gamma ray protection for energy up to 10 MeV: Equipment design and use* (NCRP Report No. 33, National Council on Radiation Protection and Measurements, Washington, D.C., 1968); and *Dental x-ray protection* (No. 35, 1970).

42. American Dental Association Council on Dental Materials and Devices, "Recommendations in radiographic practices," *J. Amer. Dent. Ass. 96*, 485–486 (1978). See also their recommendations for radiographic practices, *J. Amer. Dent. Assn. 109*, 764–65 (1984).

43. J. M. Dunning and H. Klein, "Saving teeth among home office employees of the Metropolitan Life Insurance Company," *J. Amer. Dent. Ass. 31*, 1632–1642 (1944).

44. J. M. Dunning and S. Sanzi, "Changes in dental care following dental health program in Boston schools," *J. Dent. Educ. 37*, 26–30 (1973).

45. J. M. Dunning, "Dental care in the greater Boston area," *New Engl. J. Dent. 2*, 10–14 (1949).

46. D. A. Soricelli, "Methods of administrative control for the promotion of quality in dental programs," *Amer. J. Publ. Hlth 58*, 1723–1737 (1968).

15. Dental Health Education

1. National Education Association, *Health education* (Washington, D.C., ed. 4, 1948).

2. M. A. C. Young, "Dental health education—whither?" *J. Amer. Dent. Ass. 66*, 821–824 (1963).

3. H. S. Horowitz, "Promotion of oral health and prevention of dental caries," *J. Amer. Dent. Ass. 103*, 141–143 (1981).

4. T. Albertini, J. Boffa, and N. A. Kaplis, "A dental health education

program in the open classroom: Report of a pilot study," *J. School Hlth 43*, 566–571 (1973).

5. I. L. Janis and S. Feshbach, "Effects of fear arousing communications," *J. Abnorm. Soc. Psych. 48*, 78–92 (1953).

6. K. Lewin, *Field theory in social science* (Harper, New York, 1951).

7. American Dental Association, *1983–84 catalog* (American Dental Association, Chicago, 1984).

8. D. B. Armstrong, Jr., "The dynamics of mass media, publicity, and advertising," in *Psychological dynamics of health education* (Columbia University Press, New York, 1951).

9. American Dental Association, *Learning about your oral health:* Level I, *Grades K–3;* Level II, *Grades 4–6;* Level III, *Grades 7–9;* Level IV, *Grades 10–12* (American Dental Association, Chicago, 1973).

10. American Dental Association, *A speaker's guide for dentists,* Pamphlet P13 (American Dental Association, Chicago, 1968).

11. D. B. Nyswander, *Solving school health problems* (Commonwealth Fund, New York, 1942), pp. 211, 220.

12. F. A. Stoll and J. L. Catherman, *Dental health education* (Lea and Febiger, Philadelphia, ed. 3, rev., 1967), p. 126.

13. J. M. Dunning, ed., *Woodstock workshop on dental health education, 1966* (New England Council on Dental Health and Care, Boston, 1967).

14. E. H. Kasey, "Curriculum planning in dental health: Problems, processes, and prospects," in *Woodstock workshop on dental health education, 1966* (New England Council on·Dental Health and Care, Boston, 1967).

15. J. M. Bentley, P. Cormier, and J. Oler, "The rural dental health program: The effect of a school-based dental health education program on children's utilization of dental services," *Amer. J. Publ. Hlth 73*, 500–505 (1983).

16. M. D. Hazen, B. J. Roberts, and M. A. C. Young, *Health education in the industrial setting* (Harvard School of Public Health Monograph, Boston, 1958).

17. F. C. Lindaman and M. A. Costa, "The voice of the community," *Amer. J. Publ. Hlth 62*, 1245-1248 (1972).

18. J. M. Dunning and H. Klein, "Saving teeth among home office employees of the Metropolitan Life Insurance Company," *J. Amer. Dent. Ass. 31*, 1632–1642 (1944).

19. R. M. Grainger and A. H. Sellers, "The Welland district dental health program," *Canad. J. Publ. Hlth 43*, 415–425 (1952), and *Dent. Abstr. 4*, 32 (1959).

20. W. A. Jordan, A. G. Neal, and F. E. Valento, "Practicing your dental health teaching in 1958," *Northwest Dent. 37*, 277–282 (1958).

21. J. B. Moosbruker and D. B. Giddon, "Effect of experience with aged, chronically ill, and handicapped patients on student attitudes," *J. Dent. Educ. 30*, 278–286 (1966).

GENERAL READINGS

M. Lantner and G. Bender, *Understanding dentistry* (Beacon Press, Boston, 1969).

F. A. Stoll and J. L. Catherman, *Dental health education* (Lea and Febiger, Philadelphia, ed. 5, rev., 1977).

W. O. Young and D. F. Striffler, ed., *Dentistry, dental practice, and the community* (Saunders, Philadelphia, ed. 3, 1983), chap. 15.

16. Water Fluoridation

Parts of this revised chapter have been reproduced with permission of the publisher from an article by the author, "Current status of fluoridation," *New Eng. J. Med. 272,* 30–34 and 84–88 (1965).

1. H. T. Dean et al., *Fluorine and dental health* (Amer. Ass. Adv. Sci. Washington, D.C. 1942), No. 19, p. 26.

2. H. S. Horowitz, W. S. Driscoll, R. J. Meyers, S. B. Heifetz, and A. Kingman, "A new method for assessing the prevalence of dental fluorosis: The tooth surface index of fluorosis," *J. Amer. Dent. Ass. 109,* 37–41 (1984).

3. H. T. Dean et al., "Domestic water and dental caries, including certain aspects of oral *L. Acidophilus,*" *Publ. Hlth Rep. (Wash.) 54,* 862–888 (1939).

4. H. T. Dean et al., "Domestic water and dental caries. II. A study of 2832 white children ages 12–14 in 8 suburban Chicago communities," *Publ. Hlth Rep. (Wash.) 56,* 761–792 (1941).

5. G. N. Jenkins, "Theories on mode of action of fluoride in reducing dental decay," *J. Dent. Res. 42,* 444–452 (1963); G. N. Jenkins, "The mechanism of action of fluoride in reducing caries incidence," *Int. Dent. J. 17,* 552–563 (1967).

6. R. F. Sognnaes et al., *The problem of providing optimal fluoride intake for prevention of dental caries* (National Research Council Publ. No. 294, Washington, D.C., 1953), p. 6.

7. H. C. Hodge, "Fluoride toxicology," in E. Newbrun, ed., *Fluorides and dental caries* (Charles C Thomas, Springfield, Ill., ed. 2, 1975), chaps. 7 and 8.

8. F. A. Smith, "Safety of water fluoridation," *J. Amer. Dent. Ass. 65,* 598–602 (1962).

9. U.S. Department of Health, Education, and Welfare, Public Health Service, F. J. McClure, "Physiological effects of fluoride," in *Fluoride drinking waters: Selection of Public Health Service papers on dental fluorosis and dental caries, physiological effects, analysis and chemistry of fluoride* (Government Printing Office, Washington, D. C., 1962).

10. J. R. Blayney, R. C. Bowers, and M. Zimmerman, "Evanston dental caries study no. 22: Study of fluoride deposition in bone," *J. Dent. Res. 41,* 1037–1044 (1962).

11. K. Roholm, *Fluorine intoxication: A clinical-hygienic study, with a review of the literature and some experimental investigations* (H. K. Lewis, London, 1937).

12. C. Rich and J. Ensinck, "Effect of sodium fluoride on calcium metabolism of human beings," *Nature (London) 191,* 184 (1961).

13. D. S. Bernstein et al., "Prevalence of osteoporosis in high- and low-fluoride areas of North Dakota," *J. Amer. Med. Ass. 198,* 499–504 (1966).

14. F. M. Parkins, "Fluoride therapy in osteoporotic lesions," *Ann. Otol. 83,* 624–634 (1974).

15. I. L. Hagen, M. Pasternack, and G. C. Scholz, "Waterborne fluorides and mortality," *Publ. Hlth Rep. (Wash.) 69,* 450–454 (1954); R. Doll and L. Kinlen, "Fluoridation of water and cancer mortality in the U.S.A.," *Lancet 1,* 1300–1302 (June 18, 1977).

16. J. D. Erickson, "Mortality in selected cities with fluoridated and non-fluoridated water supplies," *New Eng. J. Med. 298,* 1112–1116 (1978).

17. B. H. Cohen, A. M. Lilienfeld, and A. T. Sigler, "Some epidemiologic aspects of mongolism: A review," *Amer. J. Publ. Hlth 53*, 223–236 (1963).

18. H. L. Needleman, S. N. Puschel, and K. J. Rothman, "Fluoridation and the occurrence of Down's Syndrome," *N. Eng. J. Med. 291*, 821–823 (1974).

19. W. T. C. Berry, "Study of incidence of mongolism in relation to fluoride content of water," *Amer. J. Ment. Defic. 62*, 634–636 (1958).

20. A. L. Russell, "Dental fluorosis in Grand Rapids during seventeenth year of fluoridation," *J. Amer. Dent. Ass. 65*, 608–612 (1962).

21. R. J. McCloskey, "A technique for removal of fluorosis stains," *J. Amer. Dent. Assn. 109*, 63–64 (1984).

22. E. R. Zimmerman, "Fluoride and nonfluoride opacities," *Publ. Hlth Rep. (Wash.) 69*, 1115–1120 (1954).

23. Executive Committee, American Academy of Allergy, "A statement on the question of allergy to fluoride as used in the fluoridation of water supplies," *J. Allergies 47*, 347–348 (1971).

24. *Chronic Illness Newsletter 5*, No. 4, 1954.

25. H. B. Baldwin, "The toxic action of sodium fluoride," *J. Amer. Chem. Soc. 21*, 517 (1899).

26. C. R. Cox and D. B. Ast, "Water fluoridation: A sound public health practice," *J. Amer. Water Works Ass. 43*, 641 (1951).

27. National Academy of Sciences, *Recommended dietary allowances* (National Research Council Publ. No. 589, rev., Washington, D.C., 1958), p. 22.

28. F. A. Arnold, Jr., "Role of fluorides in preventive dentistry," *J. Amer. Dent. Ass. 30, 499*–508 (1943).

29. A. L. Russell and E. Elvove, "Domestic water and dental caries. VII. A study of fluoride-dental caries relationships in adult populations," *Publ. Hlth Rep. (Wash.) 56*, 1389–1401 (1951).

30. H. R. Englander et al., "Dental caries in adults who consumed fluoridated versus fluoride-deficient water," *J. Amer. Dent. Ass. 68*, 14–19 (1964).

31. *American Dental Association Newsletter*, June 1, 1950.

32. F. A. Arnold Jr., et al., "Fifteenth year of Grand Rapids fluoridation study," *J. Amer. Dent. Ass. 65*, 780–785 (1962).

33. G. W. Moore, "Water fluoridation practices," *Health News 37*, No. 4, 12–17, 19 (1960); *Dent. Abstr. (Chicago) 5*, 618 (1960).

34. A. L. Russell, "Domestic water and periodontal disease," *Amer. J. Publ. Hlth 47*, 688–694 (1957).

35. D. B. Ast, "Fluoride link to malocclusion," *Dent. Times 6*, 1 (February 16, 1963).

36. E. Bellack, *Fluoridation engineering manual* (U.S. Environmental Protection Agency, Water Supply Programs Division, Washington, D.C., 1972, reprinted by Department of Health and Human Services, Center for Disease Control, Atlanta, 1984).

37. F. J. Maier, *Manual of water fluoridation practice* (McGraw-Hill, New York, 1963), chap. 7.

38. U.S. Department of Health, Education, and Welfare, Public Health Service, *Public health drinking water standards* (Government Printing Office, Washington, D.C., 1962).

39. D. J. Galagan et al., "Climate and fluid intake," *Publ. Hlth Rep. (Wash.) 72*, 484–490 (1957).

40. J. S. Walker et al., "Water intake of normal children," *Science 140,* 890 (1963).

41. R. A. Kuthy, C. Naleway, and J.-A. Durkee, "Factors associated with maintenance of proper fluoride levels," *J. Amer. Dent. Ass. 110,* 511–513 (1985).

42. D. B. Ast, N. C. Cons, J. P. Carlos, and A. Maiwald, "Time and cost factors to provide regular periodic dental care in a fluoridated and nonfluoridated area," *Amer. J. Publ. Hlth 55,* 811–820 (1965).

43. B. L. Douglas, D. A. Wallace, M. Lerner, and S. B. Coppersmith, "Impact of water fluoridation on dental practice and dental manpower," *J. Amer. Dent. Ass. 84,* 355–367 (1972).

44. F. F. Bliss, "The future of private dental practice in the seventies," *Harvard Dent. Alum. Bull. 30,* 98–101, 117–118 (1970).

45. J. A. McCarthy, "Effect of fluoride on corrosion," *Sanitalk 7* (3), 2 (1959).

46. A. P. Black, "Feasibility of water fluoridation," *J. Amer. Dent. Ass. 65,* 588–594 (1962).

47. C. F. Rhyne and E. F. Mullin, Jr., *Fluoridation of municipal water supply: A review of the scientific and legal aspects* (Report 140, National Institute of Municipal Law Officers, Washington, D.C., 1952).

48. Cantwell v. Connecticut, 310 U.S. 296, 60 S. Ct. 900 84 L. ed. 1213 (1940).

49. R. Roemer, "Water fluoridation: Public health responsibility and the democratic process," *Amer. J. Publ. Hlth 55,* 1337–1348 (1965).

50. American Dental Association, *Fluoridation for your community and state* (American Dental Association, Chicago, 1977), catalog item 6–19.

51. American Dental Association, catalog item W120 (Chicago, 1983–84).

52. Director-General, World Health Organization, *Fluoridation and dental health* (Report A22/P and B/7, World Health Organization, Geneva, 1969), p. 8.

53. H. S. Horowitz, S. B. Heifetz, and F. E. Law, "Effect of school water fluoridation on dental caries: Final results in Elk Lake, Pa., after 12 years," *J. Amer. Dent. Ass. 84,* 832–838 (1972).

54. U. S. Department of Health, Education, and Welfare, Center for Disease Control, News Release 00-3040 (Atlanta, February 1977).

55. H. Kopel, "Fluoridated milk of value in preventing dental caries in children," *J. Dent. Child. 28,* 334 (1961).

56. T. M. Marthaler, "The value in caries prevention of other methods of increasing fluoride ingestion, apart from fluoridated water," *Int. Dent. J. 17,* 606–618 (1967).

57. F. J. Maier, *Manual of water fluoridation practice* (McGraw-Hill, New York, 1963), chap. 16.

17. Delivery of Dental Care

1. World Health Organization Expert Committee on Auxiliary Dental Personnel, *Report* (WHO Technical Report Series No. 163, Geneva, 1959).

2. H. Klein, "Civilian dentistry in war time," *J. Amer. Dent. Ass. 31,* 648–661 (1944).

3. G. E. Waterman, "Effective use of dental assistants," *Publ. Hlth Rep. (Wash.) 67*, 390–394 (1952).

4. G. E. Robinson, A. H. Wuehrmann, G. M. Sinnett, and E. J. McDevitt, "Four-handed dentistry: The whys and wherefores," *J. Amer. Dent. Ass. 77*, 573–579 (1968).

5. American Dental Association Bureau of Economic Research and Statistics, "The 1983 survey of dental practice" (Chicago, 1983).

6. L. Dogon, personal communication, July 2, 1985.

7. P. E. Hammons and H. C. Jamison, "New duties for dental auxiliaries: The Alabama experience," *Amer. J. Publ. Hlth 58*, 882–886 (1968).

8. P. E. Hammons and H. C. Jamison, "Expanded functions for dental auxiliaries," *J. Amer. Dent. Ass. 75*, 658–672 (1967).

9. Writer's observation, supplemented by statements from W. J. Simon, Director, Dental Clinical Development Center, U.S. Public Health Service, Louisville, Ky. (1967).

10. D. A. Soricelli, "Practical experience in peer review controlling quality in the delivery of dental care," *Amer. J. Publ. Hlth 61*, 2046–2056 (1971).

11. D. Redig, M. Snyder, G. Nevitt, and J. Tocchini, "Expanded duty dental auxiliaries in four private dental offices: the first year's experience," *J. Amer. Dent. Ass. 88*, 969–984 (1974).

12. M. K. Chapko et al. "Delegation of expanded functions to dental assistants and hygienists," *Amer. J. Publ. Hlth 75*, 61–65 (1985).

13. D. A. Soricelli, "Delegating duties in a local health department dental clinic," address to American Association of Public Health Dentists, Houston, Tex., Oct. 26, 1973.

14. E. Campbell, "An overview of TEAM concepts and developments," address to American Association of Public Health Dentists, Houston, Tex., Oct. 26, 1973.

15. U.S. Department of Health, Education, and Welfare, *Legal provisions on expanded functions for dental hygienists and assistants* (U.S. Department of Health, Education, and Welfare, Publ. No. [HRA] 75-21, ed. 2, rev. 1974).

16. U.S. Department of Health, Education, and Welfare, Bureau of Health Manpower, *Dental manpower fact book* (U.S. Department of Health, Education, and Welfare, Publ. No. [HRA] 79-14, 1979).

17. American Dental Association, "AARP calls for states to pass denturism legislation," *ADA News*, August 5, 1985, p. 12.

18. R. B. Jones, "The school-based dental care systems of New Zealand and South Australia: A decade of change," *J. Publ. Hlth Dent. 44*, 120–124 (1984).

19. J. T. Fulton, *Experiment in dental care* (World Health Organization Monograph No. 4, Geneva, 1951).

20. J. W. Friedman, "New Zealand School Dental Service, a lesson in radical conservatism," *J. Amer. Dent. Ass. 85*, 609–617 (1972).

21. D. Redig, F. Dewhirst, G. Nevitt, and M. Snyder, "Delivery of dental services in New Zealand and California," *J. So. Cal. Dent. Ass. 41*, 318–350 (1973).

22. D. E. Barmes, "Features of oral health care across cultures," *Int. Dent. J. 26*, 353–368 (1976).

23. World Health Organization Coordinator, *Oral Health Care Systems* (Quintessence Publishing, London, 1985).

24. J. M. Dunning, "An extended guest editorial. A new response to an old need: The frontier dental auxiliary," *J. Publ. Hlth Dent. 41*, 135–137 (1981).

25. J. M. Dunning, "The practical duties of frontier dental auxiliaries in Alaska communities: A progress report," *J. Publ. Hlth Dent. 44*, 138–140 (1984).

26. W. E. Marshall, "Leadership and management in group practice" in C. R. Jerge et al., ed., *Group practice and the future of dental care* (Lea and Febiger, Philadelphia, 1974), chap. 16.

27. American Dental Association Bureau of Economic Research and Statistics, *The 1975 survey of dental practice: Number of patients and patient visits* (American Dental Association, Chicago, 1976).

28. D. Redig et al., "Expanded duty dental auxiliaries in four private dental offices," *J. Amer. Dent. Ass. 88*, 969–984 (1974).

29. American Dental Association Bureau of Economic Research and Statistics, "The 1950 survey of the dental profession. II," *J. Amer. Dent. Ass. 41*, 376–382 (1950).

30. R. L. Lindahl, "A place for the closed panel," *J. Amer. Dent. Ass. 83*, 170–173 (1971).

31. E. M. Bishop and H. M. Christensen, "Dentists and the war on poverty: A discussion of neighborhood health centers," *J. Amer. Dent. Ass. 75*, 45–54 (1967).

32. J. Oxman, P. Hannigan, and J. M. Dunning, "A dental health teaching program for urban elementary and high schools," *J. Dent. Educ. 34*, 584–587 (1971).

33. J. M. Dunning and S. Sanzi, "Changes in dental care following a dental health teaching and screening program in Boston elementary and junior high schools," *J. Dent. Educ. 37*, 26–30 (1973).

34. H. M. Field and A. Jong, "Cost-effectiveness of bussing pupils to a dental clinic," *HSMA Hlth Rep. 86*, 222–228 (1971).

35. J. M. Dunning, "Deployment and control of dental auxiliaries in New Zealand and Australia," *J. Amer. Dent. Ass. 85*, 618–626 (1972).

36. U.S. Department of Health, Education, and Welfare, Health Services, and Mental Health Administration, *Health maintenance organizations: The concept and structure* (Rockville, Md., 1971).

37. J. E. Hair, "The relationship of HMO to the college and university health service in the rural setting," *J. Amer. Coll. Hlth Ass. 21*, 105–107 (1972).

38. Leonard W. Cronkhite, Jr., reacting as a "provider" to a series of papers by U.S. Department of Health, Education, and Welfare, Boston, June 10, 1971.

39. American Dental Association Council on Dental Care Programs, "Dental care in federally qualified HMOs," *J. Amer. Dent. Ass. 99*, 672–696 (1979).

40. M. H. Lewis, personal communication, Regina, Saskatchewan, Oct. 18, 1974.

GENERAL READINGS

M. Dickson, *Where there is no dentist* (Hesperian Foundation, Palo Alto, Cal., 1983).

C. R. Jerge et al., *Group practice and the future of dental care* (Lea and Febiger, Philadelphia, 1971).

U.S. Public Health Service, *Inclusion of dental health services in health maintenance and related organizations* (U.S. Department of Health, Education, and Welfare Publ. No. [HSA] 75-13018, 1974).

U.S. Public Health Service, *Group practice of dentistry* (U.S. Department of Health, Education, and Welfare Publ. No. [HRA] 77-8, 1977).

18. Payment for Dental Care

1. A. R. Somers and H. M. Somers, *Health and health care: Policies in perspective* (Aspen Systems Corp., Germantown, Md., 1977), p. 432.

2. F. G. Dickinson, "Fundamental requirements of insurance applied to voluntary medical prepayment plans," *J. Amer. Med. Ass. 133,* 483–484 (1947).

3. U.S. Department of Health, Education, and Welfare, *Pre-paid dental care: A glossary* (Public Health Service Publ. No. 679, Washington, D.C., 1965).

4. American Dental Association Council on Dental Health, "ADA and AFL-CIO set up principles for dental pre-payment," *Report on dental prepayment 1,* 1 (Aug. 1964).

5. R. D. Eilers, *Actuarial services for a dental service corporation* (Public Health Service Publication No. 1563, U.S. Department of Health, Education, and Welfare, Washington, D.C., 1967).

6. American Dental Association, Council on Dental Care Programs, "Dental prepayment," *J. Amer. Dent. Ass. 85,* 1185 (1972).

7. R. L. Gery, Connecticut General Life Insurance Co., personal communication, March 6, 1973.

8. D. B. Ast, "Time and cost factors to provide regular periodic dental care for children in a fluoridated and non-fluoridated area: Final report," *J. Amer. Dent. Ass. 80,* 770–776 (1970).

9. American Dental Association, Council on Dental Health, and Bureau of Economic Research and Statistics, "Study of relative values of dental services," *J. Amer. Dent. Ass. 76,* 117–122 (1968).

10. B. B. Berkov, "What labor wants," address to 18th National Dental Health Conference, American Dental Association, Chicago, April 17–19, 1967 (mimeographed).

11. H. Eckstein, *The English health service* (Harvard University Press, Cambridge, 1958), p. 203.

12. E. Kagabines and C. W. Douglass, "Assessing the relationship between dental insurance and the case mix and price of dental services provided," thesis in partial fulfillment of D.M.D. degree, Harvard School of Dental Medicine, 1985.

13. C. R. Jerge et al., ed., *Group practice and the future of dental care* (Lea and Febiger, Philadelphia, 1974), chap. 12.

14. H. M. Rosen, R. A. Sussman, and E. J. Sussman, "Capitation in dentistry: A quasi-experimental evaluation," *Med. Care 15,* 228–240 (1977).

15. R. Naismith, "Group practice and prepayment," address to 24th National Dental Health Conference, American Dental Association, Chicago, March 26–28, 1973.

16. G. E. Mitchell and F. M. Hoggard, Jr., *The dental service corporation: Organization and development* (Public Health Service Publ. No. 1274, U.S. Department of Health, Education, and Welfare, Washington, D.C., 1965).

17. Delta Dental Plans Association, personal letter from K. Smith, June 24, 1985.

18. R. Penchansky and B. M. Safford, "Prepayment for dental care: Need and effect," *Publ. Hlth Rep. (Wash.) 81,* 541–548 (1966).

19. C. E. Rutledge and J. G. Rooks, "Impact of budget payment on the business practices in the dental office," *J. Amer. Dent. Ass. 56,* 174–182 (1958).

20. E. J. Gesell, "Problems and responsibilities of the bank in the operation of a dental budget payment plan," *J. Amer. Dent. Ass. 56,* 171–174 (1958).

21. F. M. Silverman, *Postpayment plan progress* (Los Angeles County Dental Society, Los Angeles, 1956).

GENERAL READINGS, CHAPTERS 17–18

A. R. Somers and H. M. Somers, *Health and health care: Policies in perspective* (Aspen Systems Corp., Germantown, Md., 1977).

P. Penchansky, ed., *Health services administration: Policy cases and the case method* (Harvard University Press, Cambridge, 1968).

H. H. Avnet and M. K. Nikias, *Insured dental care: A research project report* (Group Health Dental Insurance, New York, N.Y., 1967).

G. E. Mitchell and F. M. Hoggard, Jr., *The dental service corporation: Organization and development* (Public Health Service Publ. No. 1274, U.S. Department of Health, Education, and Welfare, Washington, D.C., 1965).

19. Evaluating the Quality of Dental Care

1. L. E. Bellin, "Policing publicly funded health care for poor quality, overutilization, and fraud: The New York City Medicaid experience," *Amer. J. Pub. Health 60,* 811–820 (1970).

2. E. Angevine, "What organized consumers want in health care," address to 22nd National Dental Health Conference, American Dental Association, Chicago, Ill., April 26–28, 1971.

3. M. H. Schoen, ed., *The evaluation of the quality of dental care programs; Summary of a workshop, Asilomar, Cal.* (University of Connecticut School of Dental Medicine, Hartford, 1971).

4. A. Hengst and K. Roghmann, "Two dimensions in satisfaction with dental care," *Med. Care 16,* 202–213 (1978).

5. H. K. Schonfeld, "Evaluation of the quality of oral care systems," in W. E. Brown, ed., *Oral health dentistry and the American public* (University of Oklahoma Press, Norman, 1974), pp. 229–278.

6. A. Donabedian, *A guide to medical care administration: II, Medical care appraisal—quality and utilization* (American Public Health Association, Washington, D.C., 1973).

7. O. L. Peterson, "Medical care: Its social and organizational aspects," *New Eng. J. Med. 269,* 1239–1245 (1963).

8. A. O. Gruebbel, *A study of dental public health in New Zealand* (American Dental Association, Chicago, 1950), pp. 46–47.

9. J. Fulton, *Experiment in dental care,* World Health Organization, Monograph no. 4 (Geneva, 1951), pp. 34–43.

10. R. Petree, Director for Sanctions, Medical Assistance, Massachusetts Department of Public Welfare, letter to dental providers, Feb. 18, 1975.

11. J. W. Friedman, "PSROs in dentistry," *Amer. J. Publ. Health 65*, 1298–1303 (1975).

12. H. DeJong and J. M. Dunning, "Methods for evaluating the quality of programs for dental care," *J. Publ. Health Dent. 30*, 223–227 (1970).

13. D. A. Soricelli, "Methods of administrative control for the promotion of quality in dental programs," *Amer. J. Publ. Health 58*, 1723–1737 (1968).

14. American Dental Association, "Dental society review committees," in *American Dental Association current policies adopted, 1954–1975* (Chicago, 1976), pp. 85–86.

15. California Dental Association, Southern California Dental Association, *Peer review procedure manual* (California Dental Association, San Francisco; Southern California Dental Association, Los Angeles, 1970), p. B8.

16. American Dental Association, "A.D.A. principles of ethics with official advisory opinions as revised November 1972," *J. Amer. Dent. Ass. 86*, 60–64 (1973) (Section 8).

17. American Dental Association, "Changes in 'principles' obligates dentists to report grossly poor work of others," *ADA News 4*, 5 (Dec. 3, 1973).

18. R. H. Egdahl, "Foundations for medical care," *New Eng. J. Med. 288*, 491–498 (1973).

19. E. Brian, "Foundations for medical control of hospitalization: CHAP— a PSRO prototype," *New Eng. J. Med. 288*, 878–882 (1973).

20. Letter from L. K. Cohen, USPHS, containing unedited unpublished material from World Health Association studies, Dec. 6, 1976.

21. Letter from R. K. Logan, Director, Division of Health, New Zealand Department of Health, Wellington, Feb. 20, 1977.

22. T. W. Cutress et al., *Adult oral health and attitudes to dentistry in New Zealand, 1976* (Dental Research Unit, Medical Research Council of New Zealand, Wellington, 1979).

23. J. W. Friedman, *A guide for the evaluation of dental care* (School of Public Health, University of California, Los Angeles, 1972).

24. N. C. Cons, "The clinical examinations of Medicaid's patients in the state of New York," *J. Pub. Health Dent. 33*, 186–193 (1973).

25. U.S. Department of Health, Education, and Welfare, *Quality dental care evaluation system for the Indian Health Service* (Indian Health Service Dental Branch, Rockville, Md., 1972).

26. U.S. Department of Health, Education, and Welfare, National Center for Health Statistics, *Health manpower* (Public Health Service publ. No. 1000, Series 14, No. 1, Washington, D.C., 1968).

27. U.S. Department of Health, Education, and Welfare, National Center for Health Statistics, *Selected dental findings in adults by age, race, and sex* (Public Health Service Publ. No. 1000, Series 11, No. 7, Washington, D.C., 1965).

28. U.S. Department of Health, Education, and Welfare, National Center for Health Statistics, *Dental visits: Time interval since last visit* (Public Health Service Publ. No. [HSM] 72-1066, Series 10, No. 76, Washington, D.C., 1972).

29. D. D. Rutstein, "Quality control of medical care," *Technology Rev. 76* 35–71 (1974).

30. C. E. Welch, "Professional standards review organizations: Problems and prospects," *New Eng. J. Med. 289*, 291–295 (1973).

31. C. E. Renson, "The administration of dental services: The example of

Great Britain," chap. 7 in J. L. Slack, ed., *Dental Public Health* (J. Wright and Sons, Bristol, Eng., 1974), pp. 134–159.

32. D. B. Ast, N. C. Cons, S. T. Pollard, and J. Garfinkel, "Time and cost factors to provide regular periodic dental care for children in a fluoridated area: Final report," *J. Amer. Dent. Ass. 80*, 770–776 (1970).

33. G. Cusacq and R. L. Glass, "The projected financial savings in dental restorative treatment: The result of consuming fluoridated water," *J. Pub. Health Dent. 32*, 52–57 (1972).

34. M. Allukian, "Cost and benefits of fluoridation, Metropolitan District, Massachusetts," mimeographed report for joint Committee on Regional Fluoridation, Boston, 1973.

35. J. Berenholz, "Benefit-cost analysis of the North Reading water fluoridation system," master's thesis in business administration, Northeastern University, 1972.

36. J. M. Dunning, "Industrial dentistry at New York Naval Shipyard," *Naval Med. Bull. 46*, 1857–1864 (1946).

37. H. M. Field and A. Jong, "Cost-effectiveness of bussing pupils to a dental clinic," *HSMHA Hlth Rep. 86*, 222–228 (1971).

38. J. J. Calderone and L. A. Mueller, "The cost of sealant application in a state dental disease prevention program," *J. Publ. Hlth Dent. 43*, 249–254 (1983).

39. New Mexico Health and Environment Department, Memorandum to the Legislature, Jan. 13, 1985.

40. A. Jong and D. H. Leverett, "The operation of a community dental clinic in a health center: An evaluation," *J. Publ. Hlth Dent. 31*, 27–31 (1971).

41. M. Allukian and G. Moore, "Revenue-cost analysis of a neighborhood health center dental program," abstract 413-G in *Annual meeting program and abstracts* (American Public Health Association, San Francisco, Cal., 1973).

42. A. R. Prest and R. Turvey, "Cost-benefit analysis: A survey," *Econ. J. 75*, 683–735 (1965).

GENERAL READINGS

H. Allred, ed., *Assessment of the quality of dental care* (London Hospital Medical College, London El 2AD, 1977).

J. W. Friedman, *A guide to the evaluation of dental care* (School of Public Health, University of California, Los Angeles, 1972).

P. Milgrom, *Regulation and the quality of dental care* (Aspen Systems, Germantown, Md., 1978).

M. H. Schoen, ed., *The evaluation of the quality of dental care programs: Summary of a workshop, Asilomar, Cal.* (University of Connecticut School of Dental Medicine, Hartford, 1971).

20. Community Dental Health Programs

1. American Association for Health, Physical Education, and Recreation, "Report of the committee on terminology in school health education," *J. Amer. Ass. Hlth, Phys. Ed. and Recreation 22*, 7 (1951).

2. C. C. Wilson, ed., *School health services* (National Education Association, Washington, D.C., 1953).

3. H. S. Horowitz, S. B. Heifetz, and F. E. Law, "Effect of school water

fluoridation on dental caries: Final results in Elk Lake, Pa., after 12 years," *J. Amer. Dent. Assoc. 84,* 832–838 (1972).

4. U.S. Department of Health, Education, and Welfare, Center for Disease Control, "Release FL-90" (Atlanta, Feb. 1977).

5. C. C. Wilson, ed., *Health education* (National Education Association, Washington, D.C., ed. 4, 1958).

6. American Dental Association, *Official policies of the A.D.A. on dental health programs* (American Dental Association, Chicago, 1957).

7. National Committee on School Health Policies, *Suggested school health policies* (American Medical Association, Chicago, 1945).

8. American Dental Association, *A preventive dental health program for schools* (American Dental Association, Chicago, 1977).

9. J. Oxman, P. Hannigan, and J. M. Dunning, "A dental health teaching program for urban elementary and high schools," *J. Dent. Educ. 34,* 584–587 (1971); J. M. Dunning and S. Sanzi, "Changes in dental care following a dental health teaching and screening program in Boston elementary and junior high schools," *J. Dent. Educ. 37,* 26–30 (1973).

10. M. W. Paulk et al., "Dental health education is alive and well in rural southern Illinois," *Quintessence J. 10,* 33–35 (1980). See also reports in *Q.J. 1,* 31–36 (1982) and *Q. Internat. 12,* 1303–1305 (1984).

11. Wilson, pp. 127–128.

12. R. B. Jones, "The school-based dental care systems of New Zealand and South Australia: A decade of change," *J. Pub. Health Dent. 44,* 120–124 (1984).

13. Personal communication from L. E. Granath, Professor and Dean, Lunds Universitet Odontogiska Fakulteten, Sept. 15, 1977.

14. The material in this section is excerpted from J. M. Dunning, "A word of warning in incremental dental care," *New York J. Dent. 38,* 56–59 (1968), by permission of the publisher.

15. J. M. Dunning, "Chair time needed for dental maintenance care of children at different ages," *Mass. Dent. Soc. J. 8,* 16–20 (1959).

16. C. Lambert, Jr., and H. E. Freeman, *The clinic habit* (College and University Press, New Haven, 1967), p. 179.

17. B. D. Forsyth, "A plan for a state or local dental hygiene program," unpublished report to Harvard School of Public Health, May 1954.

18. E. S. Brown, "Contributions of the school nurse in a school dental program," *Amer. J. Publ. Hlth 40,* 984–987 (1950).

19. S. P. Klein, H. M. Bohannan, et al., "The cost and effectiveness of school-based preventive dental care," *Amer. J. Pub. Hlth 75,* 382–391 (1985).

20. J. P. Carlos, "Fluoride mouthrinses," in S.H.Y. Wei, ed., *Clinical uses of fluorides* (Lea and Febiger, Philadelphia, 1985), chap. 6.

21. U.S. Department of Health, Education, and Welfare, *Evaluation schedule* (Dental Health Service, U.S. Public Health Service, Washington, D.C., 1956).

22. L. F. Menczer, "Hartford's preschool dental program," *J. Amer. Dent. Ass. 52,* 698–702 (1956).

23. W. A. Jordan et al., "The Askov dental demonstration: A.D.A. ten-year study of a community dental health program, 1948–1958," *Northwest Dent. 38,* 445–465 (1959); editorial, "The Askov dental demonstration has come to a close: What did it prove?" *J. Amer. Dent. Ass. 61,* 112–113 (1960).

24. G. E. Mitchell, S. Sonken, and K. J. Connor, *Selected local dental health programs* (Public Health Service Publ. No. 1402, U.S. Department of Health, Education, and Welfare, Division of Dental Health, Washington, D.C., 1965).

GENERAL READINGS

American Dental Association, *A dental health program for schools* (American Dental Association, Chicago, 1978).

21. Special Dental Health Programs

1. Council on Industrial Health, American Medical Association, "Guiding principles of medical examinations in industry," *J. Amer. Med. Ass. 161*, 975–978 (1956).
2. Committee on Dental Economics, American Dental Association, "Essentials of an industrial dental service," *J. Amer. Dent. Ass. 29*, 299 (1942).
3. J. M. Dunning, "Dental aspects of industrial absenteeism," *Industr. Med. Surg. 21*, 431–432 (1952).
4. R. R. Puffer and C. L. Sebelius, "Absenteeism in Tennessee industrial plants caused by disease of the teeth and gums," *J. Amer. Dent. Ass. 33*, 1122–1131 (1946).
5. W. M. Gafafer, *Manual of industrial hygiene* (Saunders, Philadelphia, 1943), p. 427.
6. J. M. Dunning, "Industrial dentistry at New York Naval Shipyard," *Naval Med. Bull. 46*, 1857–1864 (1946).
7. H. L. Bailit et al., *Work loss and dental disease* (Robert Wood Johnson Foundation, Princeton, 1983).
8. H. J. Donigan, verbal report to author, March 15, 1946.
9. J. M. Dunning and H. Klein, "Saving teeth among home office employees of the Metropolitan Life Insurance Co.," *J. Amer. Dent. Ass. 31*, 1632–1642 (1944).
10. U.S. Department of Health, Education, and Welfare, *A digest of prepaid dental care plans, 1963* (Public Health Publ. No. 585, rev., Washington, D.C., 1963).
11. M. A. C. Young, *A study of health education programs in Massachusetts industries* (Harvard School of Public Health, Boston, 1957).
12. I. Schour and B. G. Sarnat, "Oral manifestations of occupational origin," *J. Amer. Med. Ass. 120*, 1197–1207 (1942).
13. U.S. Department of Health, Education, and Welfare, *Oral manifestations of occupational origin: An annotated bibliography* (Public Health Publ. No. 228, Washington, D.C., 1953).
14. L. S. Morvay, L. B. Kaban, and J. M. Dunning, "State compensation laws for dental and jaw injuries," *J. Occup. Med. 9*, 388–396 (1967).
15. American Dental Association, *The dentist's desk reference* (American Dental Association, Chicago, ed. 2, 1983).
16. E. R. Aston, "The industrial dental program in Pennsylvania," *Penn. Dent. J. 18*, 3–6 (1951).
17. E. R. Aston, "A report of dental health studies in 19 selected industries," *Industr. Med. Surg. 20*, 74–78 (1951).

18. American College Health Association, *Recommended standards and practices for a college health program* and *Don't let your teeth be false to you* (American College Health Association, Evanston, Ill., 1977).

19. K. A. Freedman et al., "Geriatric dentistry in the predoctoral curriculum," *J. Dent. Educ. 49,* 300–305 (1985).

20. J. E. Chrietzberg, F. D. Lewis, and J. B. Carrol, "Surveys of dental conditions in the nursing homes in Fulton county," *J. Georgia Dent. Ass. 31,* 15–19 (1958); *Dent. Abstr. (Chicago) 3,* 346–347 (1958).

21. R. L. Hass, "Dental Findings of nursing home residents in Northeast Illinois," *Bull. Amer. Ass. Publ. Hlth Dent. 19,* 19–23 (1959).

22. American Dental Association, Council on Dental Health, "Dental care: Views from the nursing homes," *J. Amer. Dent. Ass. 77,* 117–120 (1968).

23. S. S. Kegeles, S. Lotzkar, and L. W. Andrews, "Predicting the acceptance of dental care by residents of nursing homes," *J. Publ. Hlth Dent. 26,* 290–302 (1966).

24. S. Lotzkar, "Experiences in providing home dental care for chronically ill persons," in *Proceedings of the First National Conference of the Joint Council to Improve the Health Care of the Aged* (Joint Council, Chicago, 1959), pp. 158–160.

25. D. J. Galagan, "Development of dental health care programs for persons with chronic illness," *J. Amer. Dent. Ass. 53,* 686–693 (1956).

26. J. J. Sharry et al., "Treatment of the handicapped child," in S. B. Finn, ed., *Clinical pedodontics* (Saunders, Philadelphia, ed. 2, 1962), chap. 19.

27. American Public Health Association, *Services for children with cerebral palsy: A guide for public health personnel* (Amer. Publ. Hlth Ass., New York, 1967).

28. A. J. Cloran et al., "Oral telescoping orthosis: An aid to functional rehabilitation of quadriplegic patients," *J. Amer. Dent. Ass. 100,* 876–879 (1980).

29. H. J. Towle and J. V. Niiranen, "Dentistry: An aid in disaster," *J. Amer. Dent. Ass. 55,* 22–32 (1957).

30. R. J. Sognnaes, "Forensic stomatology," *N. Eng. J. Med. 296,* 79–85, 149–153 and 197–203 (1977).

31. H. S. Glazer and D. Sadowsky, "The need for forensic odontology: Eastern Airlines flight 66," *N.Y. Dent. J. 43,* 341–344 (1977), and *Dent. Abstr. 23,* 70–71 (1978).

32. American Dental Association, "Computer speeds identification of victims," *ADA News,* August 5, 1985, p. 13.

GENERAL READING

U.S. Senate Special Committee on Aging, *Aging America,* PL3377 (584) (Washington, D.C., 1984).

22. State Dental Health Programs

1. U.S. Department of Health, Education, and Welfare, *Digest of state dental health programs* (Public Health Service Publ. No. 889, rev., Washington, D.C., 1965).

2. U.S. Department of Health, Education, and Welfare, *Medicaid services by state* (Social Rehabilitation Service Bulletin 24601, Washington, D.C., June 1, 1976).

3. U.S. Department of Health, Education, and Welfare, *Questions and answers on the medical assistance program* (Welfare Administration, Bureau of Family Services, U.S. Department of Health, Education, and Welfare, Washington, D.C., 1966, mimeographed).

4. Massachusetts Department of Public Health, Division of Dental Health, "Preliminary study of medical assistance dental services," March 1968, unpublished.

5. Association of State and Territorial Health Officers Foundation, *Public health agencies, 1982, vol. 2: Services and activities* (ASTHO, Kensington, Md., 1984).

6. T. Rebich, Director, Bureau of Dental Health, State of New York, Department of Health, personal communications, July 19 and August 1, 1985.

23. United States Federal Programs

1. R. M. Lawrence, Regional Consultant U.S.P.H.S., personal communication, July 2, 1985.

2. U.S. Department of Health, Education, and Welfare, "Status of HSAs and state health planning agencies," *Pub. Hlth Rep. 91,* 483 (1976).

3. R. Fein, statement before Subcommittee on Health, U.S. Senate Labor and Public Welfare Committee, mimeographed (Washington, D.C., Feb. 23, 1971).

4. P. J. Feldstein, *Financing dental care: An economic analysis* (Heath, Lexington, Mass., 1973), chap. 6.

5. P. J. Feldstein, "Funding and payment of dental care: An analysis of alternatives," in W. E. Brown, ed., *Oral health, dentistry, and the American public* (University of Oklahoma Press, Norman, 1974), pp. 193–227.

6. G. Hodgson, "The politics of American health care," *Atlantic Monthly 232,* 45–61 (Oct. 1973).

7. American Dental Association, "Congress is told ADA's position," *ADA News,* May 20, 1974, p. 1.

8. A. Sheiham, "An evaluation of the success of dental care in the United Kingdom," *Brit. Dent. J. 135,* 271–279 (1973).

9. M. H. Schoen, "Capitation payment to dental group practice: Methodology and effect on the delivery of dental care," address to Dental Health Section, American Public Health Association, Nov. 14, 1972 (Abstract 324 D).

10. M. H. Schoen, "Dental care as an essential component in national health insurance," address to Dental Health Section, American Public Health Association, Nov. 16, 1972 (Abstract 503 A).

11. Advisory Committee on Dental Health to U.S. Department of Health, Education, and Welfare, "Report and recommendations," *J. Amer. Dent. Assoc. 87,* 101–123 (1973).

12. U.S. House Ways and Means Committee, *National health insurance: Hearings* (Washington, D.C., 1974), vol. 3, pp. 1240–1257, statement of J. W. Friedman and J. M. Dunning, May 10.

GENERAL READINGS

Committee on Ways and Means, U.S. House of Representatives, *National health insurance resource book* (U.S. Government Printing Office, Washington, D.C., 20402, rev. 1976).

A. R. Somers and H. M. Somers, *Health and health care: Policies in perspective* (Aspen Systems, Germantown, Md., 1977).

24. Foreign and International Programs

1. J. E. Fogarty International Center, *The British National Health Service,* U.S. Public Health Service Pub. No. (NIH) 77-1205 (1976).

2. "Four lessons in universal health insurance from abroad: Western Europe," *Perspective (Blue Cross) 7,* no. 2, 1–11 (1972).

3. J. N. Peacock, "The financing of dental care service by the public sector: The British National Health Service," *Int. Dent. J. 20,* 249–253 (1970).

4. Adapted from National Health Service, England and Wales, *Statutory instrument no. 1329* (1970).

5. N. DeJong and J. M. Dunning, "Methods for evaluating the quality of programs for dental care," *J. Pub. Hlth Dent. 30,* 223–227 (1970).

6. C. L. Sebelius, "Trends in preventive dentistry in United States and Scandinavia," *J. Amer. Coll. Dent. 19,* 313–320 (1951–52).

7. Personal communication from L. E. Granath, Professor and Dean, Lunds Universitet Odontologiska Faculteten, Sept. 15, 1977.

8. R. B. Jones, "The school-based dental care systems of New Zealand and South Australia: A decade of change," *J. Pub. Hlth Dent. 44,* 120–124 (1984).

9. J. M. Dunning, Impression upon visit to five major Chinese cities, October 1980.

10. J. M. Gonzalez, *The New Zealand dental nurse: Forty-four years of service* (Department of Health, San Juan, Puerto Rico, 1967, mimeographed).

11. J. F. Fuller and M. Karim, remarks on Western Pacific area at joint meeting on public dental-health services worldwide, sponsored by American Dental Association, Fédération Dentaire Internationale, and American Association of Public Health Dentists, San Francisco, Nov. 6, 1964.

12. N. N. Bery, remarks on Southeast Asia at joint meeting on public dental-health services worldwide, sponsored by American Dental Association, Fédération Dentaire Internationale, and American Association of Public Health Dentists, San Francisco, Nov. 6, 1964.

13. T. M. Check and H. V. Day, "Dental ambassadors," *J. Amer. Dent. Ass. 75,* 90–94 (1967).

14. World Health Organization notes, *F.D.I. Newsletter 91,* in *Quint Internat. Dent. Digest 6,* 16–17 (July 1975).

15. B. Chisholm, "International health. No. 2. The role of W.H.O., past, present, and future," *Amer. J. Publ. Hlth 41,* 1460–1463 (1951).

16. J. T. Fulton, *Experiment in dental care* (World Health Organization Monograph No. 4, Geneva, 1951).

17. D. E. Barmes, personal communication, April 24, 1985.

18. World Health Organization coordinator, *Oral Health Care Systems* (Quintessence Publishing, London, 1985).

19. Fédération Dentaire Internationale, "World Health Organization," *F.D.I. Newsletter,* no. 63, 5–6 (July 1968).

20. World Health Organization, Pan American Health Organization, personal communication from Elizabeth A. Henning, August 6, 1985.

25. Conquest or Equilibrium?

1. W. K. Gregory, *The origin and evolution of the human dentition* (Williams and Wilkins, Baltimore, 1922), p. 411.

2. W. K. Gregory, "Polyisomerism and anisomerism in cranial and dental evolution among vertebrates," *Proc. Nat. Acad. Sci. U.S. 20*, 1–9 (1934).

3. H. P. Pickerill, *The prevention of dental caries and oral sepsis* (Bailliere, Tyndal, and Cox, London, 1912), p. 264.

4. D. E. Barmes, "Indicators for oral health and implications for developing countries," *Int. Dent. J. 33*, 60–66 (1983).

5. *Expert Committee on Auxiliary Dental Personnel Report* (World Health Organization Technical Report No. 163, Geneva, 1959).

6. M. J. Halberstam, "Professionalism and health care," in Institute of Medicine, *Ethics of health care* (National Academy of Science, Washington, D.C., 1974), p. 248.

7. *The world almanac and book of facts, 1985*, poverty by family status, sex, and race (Newspaper Enterprise Association, New York, 1985), p. 255.

8. Editorial, "The workshop report," *New Zealand Dent. J. 75* (340):77–79, 1979.

9. J. J. Hanlon, *Public health administration and practice* (Mosby, St. Louis, ed. 6, 1974), chap. 41.

10. J. M. Dunning and H. Klein, "Saving teeth—(at) the Metropolitan Life Insurance Co.," *J. Amer. Dent. Ass. 31*, 1632–1642 (1944); J. M. Dunning and S. Sanzi, "Changes in dental care following a dental health teaching and screening program," *J. Dent. Educ. 37*, 26–30 (1973).

11. World Health Organization coordinator, *Oral Health Care Systems* (Quintessence Publishing, London, 1985).

12. Psychologists use the term *ecology* to refer to the problems of the human community. In keeping with this practice several dental schools now have departments of dental ecology covering public health, prevention, practice administration, and other subjects relating the dentist to his environment.

INDEX

Abulcasis, 44
Academy of General Dentistry, 509
Accident insurance, 479
Accident prevention, dental,
    262–264
Acquired Immune Deficiency Syn-
    drome (AIDS), control of trans-
    mission of, 265
Administration, principles of, 23,
    209–212
Adults: benefits to, from fluorida-
    tion, 409–410, 424
  health educational approaches to,
    388–390
A.F.L.–C.I.O., 484
Africa, South: caries in, 148–149,
    151
Age: dental needs by, 136–137
  as factor in disease, 117, 136–138,
    169–170
  groups, 340
  posteruptive, of teeth, 70
  as source of bias, 70
Agent: biological, 119
  chemical, 120
  microbiological, 135, 144
  physical, 120
Agent factors: in caries, 144–145
  in disease, general, 7, 119–120
  in periodontal disease, 176–177
Air pollution, 33
Alabama School of Dentistry, 439
Allowances, table of, 480
American Academy of Allergy,
    407
American Association for Health,
    Physical Education, and Recre-
    ation, 527

American Association of Orthodon-
    tists, 335
American Association of Retired
    Persons, 445
American Board of Dental Public
    Health, 224–225, 589
American Cancer Society, 261
American College Health Associa-
    tion, 564
American College of Dentists, 509
American Dental Association: ac-
    creditation work, 225, 444
  literature, 376, 377, 379, 388, 428
  policies and standards, 5, 355,
    358, 445, 484, 533, 554, 560
  recommendations, 45, 202, 233,
    235, 249, 252, 254, 265, 335,
    339, 429, 458, 461, 498,
    510–511, 632
  services, 35, 186
  study and survey work, 77, 136,
    171, 181, 190, 274, 283, 318,
    437
American Heart Association, 273
American Medical Association: code
    of ethics of, 10
  policy on industrial examinations,
    553
  recommendations of, 429
American Public Health Associa-
    tion, 21
American Typhus Commission, 11
American Waterworks Association,
    430
Analysis of variance, 79, 89
Angle's classification of malocclu-
    sion, 182, 333
Animals, caries studies in, 162, 163

Antagonism in disease, 118
Antibiotics, possible role in caries control, 164
Appointments, unimportance of, 195
Apprenticeship for dental auxiliaries, 225–226, 443
Arabs, early dental care among, 43
Areoli, G., 44
Askov, Minnesota, dental demonstrations, 549
Assistant, dental. *See* Dental assistants
Association of Latin American Dental Schools, 620
Ast, D. B., 413
Atrophy, alveolar, 168
Audio-visual aids, 374–375
Audit of dental records, 506–507
Australia, 149, 150, 154, 450–451, 464, 539
Australian (South) School Dental Service, 388, 617
Authority delegation, 211; need for, 209
Autonomy in dental public health, 212
Auxiliary dental personnel, 342, 544
Average, 60, 76

Barmes, D. E., 165, 275, 631
Barnard, C. I., 227–228
Bass toothbrushing technique, 234
Behavior, changes in, 364, 372, 391
Behavioral sciences, 17, 187
Bernard, C., 59, 60
Bill of Rights, U.S., 16
Binomial theorem, 94
Biostatistics, 59–111
    needed in epidemiology, 115
    use in public health, 8, 17, 109
Black, G. V., 49, 394
Blacks: caries among, 136–137, 160, 182
    dental needs among, 278
    periodontal disease among, 171, 178
Blue Cross-Blue Shield, 478, 480, 492, 499

Boards of health, 19
Bone loss, appraisal of, 327
Brazil: dental personnel in, 618
    training program, 618
Britain. *See* Great Britain
Brudevold, F., acid phosphate solution, 252
Budget, function and construction of, 214, 216, 313

Calcium, sources of, in diet, 246
Calculus: recognition of harm from, 44
    related to periodontal disease, 176
Cancer, oral, 182–183, 261
    and public health, 7, 27, 593
    recognition of, 260–261, 263
    surveying for, 335–336
Capitation financing, 489
Carbohydrates: in diet, related to dental disease, 49, 145, 152, 159, 164
    oral clearance, and caries, 238–239
    restriction of, 161–163, 186, 241
Caries: acute root types, 138, 143, 592
    agent factors, 144–145
    attitudes to high caries incidence, 197–198
    bilateral symmetry, 143, 144
    chemico-parasitic theory, 47, *see also* Miller
    as chronic disease, 134–135
    and civilization, 132
    and climate, 150–155
    and concomitant disease, 141–142
    decrease in recent years, 17, 39, 55, 133, 162–165, 181, 275, 281, 526, 540, 586, 631
    as deficiency disease, 135
    definition of, 323
    dietary control of, 238–247
    environmental factors, 145–165
    epidemiology, 131–165
    experience, 70–71, 83, 84, 325
    geographical variations, 145–155
    host factors, 136–143
    incidence defined, 73, 325

increases in, 165, 631
lesions of, used in surveys, 324
measures for, 60, 323–325, 348, 349
and nutrition, 50, 142
"potentiality indices," 240
and pregnancy, 140
prevalence defined, 73
prevention, 230–257
secular variations, 126, 132–133, 165
susceptibility tests for, 256–257, 357
in United States, 146–155
variations within the mouth, 142–144
Carnegie Foundation, 50
Case-finding, 38–39
in dentistry, 39
in school dental programs, 532–535
Cases, pairing of, 71, 72
Castration complex, 193
Census, Bureau of, 27
Center for Disease Control, Atlanta, Georgia, 599, 600
Certificate of need, 462, 603
Chair-time needed for dental care, 296
Children: caries-free, 163
growth and development, 24
Chinese, caries among, 136–137, 150, 279
Chi-square test, 97–101, 107
"Citizenship" concept of labor, 212, 214
Civil service systems, 220
Classrooms, open, 368
Clefts of lip or palate, 183
Climate: and dental disease, 149–155
and disease, general, 121, 194
in relation to fluoride intake, 419–420
Clinics: mobile, 460, 543
prenatal, 28, 37
well-baby, 28, 37, see also Dental clinics
Cohort study, 128
Coincidence versus causation, 64

Coinsurance, 481–482
College dental health services, 466, 563–564
Colorado brown stain, 49, 394. See also Fluorosis, dental
Commission on Chronic Illness, 407
Commission on the Survey of Dentistry in the United States, 294, 305
Committee on Costs of Medical Care, 50, 391, 557
Communication, authoritative, characteristics of, 227
Community: defined, 123
dental health council, 531
and preventive dentistry departments, 14
in public health, 9, 314–315, 390, 529–538
Community Periodontal Index of Treatment Need (CPITN), 331–332
Community-school relations, 473
Completion of treatment, interpretation of, 361
Comprehensive dental care. See Dental care, comprehensive
Comprehensive Health Planning Act, 54, 602
Computer analysis, 8, 88, 108–109
of diet, 245
programs for, 24, 109
use of, 85, 576
Conant, J. B., 61, 111
Concept, essential in research, 61, 111
Confidence interval, 79
Confidentiality in peer review, 518
Consent, informed, 66, 340
Conservation, related to ecology, 114
Consultation work, 223–224
Consumer Price Index, 283
Consumers, role in health planning, 42, 195, 307, 445, 503
Control: of disease, 14, 231
span of administrative, 209–210
Control groups: importance, 65
selection, 71

Cooperative for American Relief Everywhere (CARE), 40–41
Correlation, 100–107, 147
Correlation coefficient: calculation, 103–107
defined, 97, 102
Cost accounting, 216
Cost analysis, 519–525
Cost-benefit analysis, 217, 519–522
Cost control of care, 507, 586
Cost-effectiveness analysis, 23, 217, 303, 522
Councils, community, 41–42
Countries, developing, 12, 270–271, 275, 281, 617–620, 631
Covariance adjustment, 91–92
Cronkhite, L. W., 466
Culture: and attitudes toward health, 9
defined, 185
influence, 188–190, 631–633
Customs as factors in disease, 118
Cytology, exfoliative, in cancer detection, 261, 336

Data: actuarial, 485–486
baseline, 72
biased, 63, 67
exclusion of, 75
presentation of, 75
quality of, 62, 64
statistical, 75
Dean, H. T., 64, 70, 110, 127, 394–397
Decayed, missing, filled count. See DMF entries
Deductible amount, insurance, 481–482
"def" or "df" teeth, recording of, 324, 344, 347–348
Defluoridation, municipal, 432
Delta Dental Plans Association, 54, 495–497
Demand for dental care. See Dental care, demand for
Dental absenteeism, control of, 554–555
Dental aides, 293, 453, 618

Dental assistants, 435–438, 546
training of, 438
Dental auxiliaries: expanded function (EFDAs), 438–443, 464, 472
frontier, 454–455
utilization of, 290–291, 587
Dental care: accessibility of, 275, 318, 504
administration of, 633–635
appropriateness of, 504
attitudes toward, 190–195
auxiliary personnel in, 434–455, 634
availability of, 504
chair-time needed for, 295, 540–541
for children, 303–304
for the chronically ill, 564–567
completion, recording of, 361
comprehensive, 53, 273–274, 287, 294, 484, 607, 632–634
cost of, 290, 607
delivery of, 433–475
demand for, 281–284, 424, 472, 631–633
in developing nations, see Countries, developing
eligibility for, 584, 587
emergency, 454, 556–558
evaluation of quality, 505–514
excuse from school for, 537
geriatric, 306
for handicapped, 569–573
for home-bound, 565
for the homeless, 307
incremental, 304–306, 539–542
for industrial groups, see Industrial dentistry
initial, 295–297, 490, 497
insurance for, 479–482
maintenance, 295–297, 490
for mentally ill, 572
outcome of, 505, 506
payment for, 476–500
prepayment, see Prepayment
price-elasticity of, 282
primary, 270–271, 467, 539, 631, 635–637

private versus public, 298–301
by quadrant, 305
quality appraisal of, 450, 457
referral for, 535–538
for single-parent families, 308
in stress areas, 538–539
trends in, 633–635
Dental caries. *See* Caries
Dental clinics: attitudes toward, 189,
    301, 471
early, 44–46
functions of, 471–474
in health centers, 37, 462, 546
mobile, 388, 468–469
public relations factors, 474–475
"reasonable cost" reimbursement,
    585
school-based, 462
trends affecting, 630–631
Dental diseases, whether contagious,
    9, 164, 631
trends affecting, 630–631
See also Disease, dental
Dental equipment, portable, 468,
    567, 580
Dental examinations: classification
    by type, 339, 533–534
method for, 64
Dental examiners. *See* Examiners
Dental floss, 236
Dental health: for the aged,
    564–569
attitudes toward, 190–196
education, *see* Health education
New York State Bureau of, 24
possible future action for,
    635–637
programs, *see* Dental programs
at state level, 27
Dental Health Foundation (Austra-
    lia), 379
Dental Health Service (New York),
    295–296
Dental-hygiene teachers, 380, 463,
    471
Dental hygienists: availability of,
    318
duties of, 446–447, 472, 544, 550,
    561, 567

in home-care program, 567
originated, 47, 48
public health qualifications for,
    225
in school program, 537
in trailer program, 537
Dental inspection: classification of,
    339
reasons for, in school, 533
Dental laboratories, 444–445, 456
Dental-laboratory technicians,
    443–445
Dental "licentiates," 293, 453
Dental manpower, 284–290,
    317–318
in countries of the world, 292
new types, 293
Dental needs: of the aged, 568
classification, 357–359
frequency of treatment, 279
general, 270–281
by income, 279–281
by race, 136, 278
by regions, 280
Dental nurses, 293, 381, 447–448,
    472, 618
Dental office, hazards in, 560–561
Dental patients seen, interpretation
    of, 284, 287
Dental personnel: auxiliary, 293,
    434–455
qualifications and training of,
    224–226
Dental programs: for chronically ill,
    306
college, 563–564
industrial, 552–563
private versus public, 307–309,
    636
state, 278–293
Dental prophylaxis, function of: in
    caries prevention, 237–238,
    252, 454, 537
in periodontal disease, 258
Dental records. *See* Records
Dental rehabilitation, 231
Dental schools: educational places
    in, 289
and public health training, 589

Dental screening, 339
Dental services: "blood and
    vulcanite," 272, 282
  corporation, 492, 495–497, 499
  operative, 274–275, 277
  in order rendered, 298–299
  preliminary versus treatment,
    299–300
  scope of, 294–307, 503
  standards for, see Dental care,
    quality appraisal
  at state level, 580–586
Dental societies: cooperation with
    state dental division, 590
  function of, in disaster training,
    576
  role of, in health education, 384
Dental therapists, 293, 381, 472,
    544, 635
Dentifrices: fluoride, 235
  function of, 235
  therapeutic, 235
Dentisten (Germany), 447, 632
Dentistry: four-handed, 436
  operative, and caries control,
    248
  preventive, 230–266, 483, 485
  private practice, 4, 636
  by quadrant, 305
Dentists: advertising by, 286, 300
  attitudes toward, 197–198,
    371–372, 391
  clinic, 225, 590
  foreign-trained, in United States,
    289–290
  freedom of choice of, 484, 584
  general, 278, 287
  income of, 77, 284–285
  number of patients seen by, 284,
    287
  recruitment of, 288
  related to population, worldwide,
    284–292, 634
  role of, 202, 366, 370, 379–380,
    574–575
  specialists, 284–285, 287
Dentition, human, deemphasis of,
    630
Denturists, 445

Deviation, standard: "grand," 89
  meaning of, 78–82
  for observations of DMF teeth, 78
  use of, 358
Diabetes: causation of, 119
  as chronic disease, 134–135
  dental care problems in, 573
  Diagnosis, effect of improvement
    in, 125
Diet-history analysis, 243–245
Diets: balance in, 242
  for control of caries, 238–247
  for good general nutrition,
    242–243
  and public health, 5
Differences, significance of:
  between means, 86–89, 94
  between proportions, 94–97
Disaster programs, 574–577
Disclosing agents, for plaque, 257
Disease: agent factor in, see Agent
    factors
  attitudes toward, 190–195
  biological gradient of, 124–125
  causation factors, interplay of,
    122–123
  cardiovascular, 27, 573
  chronic, 6, 30, 31, 60, 134, 273,
    648
  communicable, 6, 24, 31–33
  concomitant, 118, 141–142, 176
  control of, in health programs,
    31–32, 528, 638
  cycles in, 126
  dental, whether contagious, 9,
    144, 164
  endemic, 113, 124
  environmental factors in, see Envi-
    ronment
  epidemic, 124
  experience defined, 70–71, 73
  host factors in, see Host factors
  mass measure, 123–124
  multifactorial, 7, 115, 132, 631
  nonoccupational, 554
  nutritional deficiency, 134
  periodontal, see Periodontal dis-
    ease
  reportable, 26

seasonal variations in, 125
secular variations, 126
transmission, 31, 32, 265
venereal, 31
DMF (decayed, missing, filled)
    count, interpretation of, 72,
    324, 336–337
DMF surfaces, use of, in surveys,
    163, 324, 337–338, 344, 350
DMF survey construction, 347–348,
    356–358
DMF teeth, 94, 146
    related to caries prevalence, 337
    related to DMF surfaces, 138, 540
    use of in surveys, 94, 163, 324,
    344, 512
Double-blind trial, 67
Down's syndrome, 404
Draker, H. L., 334

Eastern Hemisphere, dental disease
    in, 149–150
Eastman Dental Clinic (Rochester),
    5, 47
Ebersole, W. G., 46
Ecology, 113–115, 637
Economic status, related to caries,
    15, 159–160
Ecosystem, defined, 123
EDDA. See EFDA
Edentulous state, attitudes toward,
    196–197, 323, 513
Education: continuing, 509
    health, see Health education
EFDA, 438–443, 464, 472
Emotional disturbances: and caries,
    141–142
    and periodontal disease, 176
Enamel opacity, 404
Endocarditis, related to dental dis-
    ease, 273
Environment, 7, 114
    and caries, 145–162
    and disease (general), 120–122,
    315
    oral, and caries, 162, 231
    and periodontal disease, 177–179
    social, 122

Environmental Protection Agency,
    35, 419
Epidemics, defined, 113, 124–125
Epidemiologist: duties of, 31, 115,
    129–130
    qualifications of, 129–130
Epidemiology: analytic, 127
    of caries, 131–165
    defined, 7, 112–113, 116
    dental problems in, 130
    descriptive, 127
    experimental, 127
    general principles of, 112–130
    of periodontal disease, 167–182
    in public health, 7, 17, 25
    strategy of, 127–128, 587
Epilepsy, dental problems in, 572
Error, standard: of correlation coef-
    ficient, 105–106
    of difference, 86
    of mean, 85
    of proportion, 95
Eskimos, dental caries in, 158–159
Ethics in public health, 10–12, 17,
    66, 300, 474, 511, 633
Ethiopia, caries in, 150, 165
Ethnic group: as factor in caries,
    136
    as factor in disease (general),
    117
Etiology, defined, 112
Evaluation: defined, 310
    of health education, 390–392
    of quality of dental care, see Qual-
    ity
    of survey data, 359–361
Examination: dental, see Dental ex-
    amination
    physical, 6, 534
Examiners: control of, 65
    errors, 65–66
    selection, 341
Executive: characteristics of,
    226–229
    functions, 210–212
Experience, defined. See Caries, ex-
    perience
Explorer, dental, in survey work,
    341

Fatality, 72, 94
    tooth, 72
Fauchard, P., 44
Federal Emergency Relief Admin-
    istration, 51
Fédération Dentaire Internationale,
    379
Fees, 486–489
    capitation, 489
    profile of, 487
    "usual and customary," 487, 585
Field training. *See* Residency
Filled-tooth ratio, 360
Filling-extraction ratio, 360
First aid, responsibility of dentist in,
    574–575
Fisher, R. A., 89, 98
Fluoridation, 24, 34, 53, 127, 132,
    164, 591
    benefits, dental, 143, 162, 182,
        298, 393–432, 636
    and climate, 419–420
    community action upon, 206–207,
        315, 427–429
    cost, 409, 422–423
    defined, 400
    education concerning, 389
    endorsement, 429
    legal status, 424
    mechanics, 414–420
    monitoring, 420–422, 427
    opponents of, 9, 203
    and periodontal disease, 413
    religious freedom, 425
    safety of, 400–409
    of schools, 430–431, 529, 600
    as social problem, 5, 9, 202–207
    studies over 10 years, 410,
        412–413
    utilization, 5, 430–431
Fluoridator, volumetric, 416
Fluoride: accumulation in bones
        and teeth, 138
    acidulated phosphate, topical ap-
        plication, 252; gel, 252
    common sources, 415
    dietary supplementation, 164,
        254–255, 312, 431–432, 546,
        591
    epidemiology, 64, 155

gels, 252, 546
human response to, 402
ion, sources of, 415
Lukomsky topical paste, 251
measurement, electronically,
    421–422
mouth rinses, 24, 30, 252–253,
    527, 546, 591, 600
natural in United States water
    supplies, 287
as nutrient, 408
and periodontal disease, 179, 413
practicality of several preventive
    measures, 256
sodium, techniques for topical
    application, 251
stannous, 235, 251
topical application, 251–254, 409,
    546
Fluorosis, dental, 49, 394–400, 636
    epidemiology of, 399–400
    index, 396–398
Fones, A. C., 48, 235, 446
Food and Drug Administration,
    599–600
Foods: basic groups, 242–243
    detergent, 241
Food stamp programs, 122
Food supply, competition for, 114
Forsyth Dental Infirmary for Chil-
    dren (Boston), 5, 47, 344
Foundations for medical care,
    511–512
F-ratio, 89
Fraud, 502, 507
Freedom: of choice of dentist, 484,
    584
    degree of (statistical), 89, 98–100
    individual, 16, 205
    religious, 425–427
Frequency distribution: defined, 75
    examples, 81–86
Fulton, J. T., 158

Galagan, D. J., 419
Geographic variations: in caries,
    145–155
    in periodontal disease, 171, 177
Geriatric care, 27, 306, 473, 550,
    568

Germany, dental service in, 302, 615

Gibbons, R. J., 144, 164

Gies, W. J., 50

Gingiva-bone (GB) count for periodontal disease, 327, 329–330

Gingival Index of Löe, 326

Gingivitis: acute necrotizing, 177, 180
  appraisal, 326–330
  nature of, 167
  occurrence of, 172–173, 181

Gordon, J. E., 113, 114

Grand Rapids fluoridation study, 53, 410–413

Grant applications, preparation of, 215–216

Graphs, construction of, 75

Great Britain: appraisal techniques for care in, 507–508
  dental care in, 53, 613–615
  Dental Estimates Board, 518–519, 614–615
  health insurance in, 302, 478, 613–615

Greece, 132–133, 162, 302

Grenfell Mission, 271, 332, 360

Gross National Product, and health care, 195, 604, 614, 616

Group Health Association (Washington, D.C.), 53, 491

Group Health Dental Insurance (New York), 53, 491

Group practice, 455–459

Guggenheim, Murray and Leone, Clinic (New York), 47

Guidance counselor, role in health education, 383

Habits, as factors in disease, 118

Hadjimarkos, D. J., 156–157

Hagen, I. L., 404

Handicapping labiolingual deviations (Draker), 334

Handicapping Malocclusion Assessment Record, 334

Hartford (Connecticut) Health Department, preschool dental service, 548–549

Harvard Community Health Plan, 467

Head Start program, 189, 234, 548

Health: adult, 27
  defined, 5
  and the health worker, 8

Health aides, 271

Health appraisal, 528

Health care, a right, 7, 16

Health centers, 37–38, 462

Health departments: aims and organization, 18, 19, 37
  budgets, 214, 216, 313
  in health centers, 37

Health education: barriers to, 364–365
  behavior, 372
  defined, 364
  dental, 4, 283, 363–392
  evaluation of, 390–392
  fear arousal in, 370
  groups to be reached by, 367, 370, 386–390
  interdisciplinary problems, 384
  media, 373–377
  methods, 366–373
  personnel and their roles, 19–20, 379–384
  psychological principles in, 369–373
  in public health, 5, 8, 9, 17, 25, 40
  sources of dental material, 377–379

Health educators, 25, 316, 318, 383, 385

Healthful school living, 528

Health maintenance organization (HMO), 54, 461, 464–468, 500, 608

Health planning, 54

Health Systems Agency (HSA), 42, 602

Helen Hayes Hospital, N.Y. State, 23, 25

Hemophilia, dental problems in, 573

Hepatitis, transmission, control of, 265

Heredity, familial, as factors in caries, 14, 140
in disease (general), 117
Hill, A. B., 75
Hollingshead, A. B., index of social position, 199, 313
Hood Rubber Company, dental service, 557
Hospital: mental, 36
and public health, 5, 27
Host factors: in caries, 136–143
in disease, general, 7, 116–119
in periodontal disease, 169–176
Howe, P. R., 50
Human rights, 16, 66
Humidity, relative, and dental disease, 153–154
Hunter, T. A., 51
Hyatt, T. P., 49, 248
Hygienists, dental. See Dental hygienists
Hypotheses, formulation of, 127

ICNND nutrition studies, 150, 158–159, 171
Identification of dead, by teeth, 576–577
Immunity, active, 116
Immunization, 24, 29, 37, 145
Incidence, defined, 73
Incremental dental care, 304–306, 539–542
Indemnity payments, 480
India: dental hygienists in, 619
dental programs in, 619
disease in, 150, 172–173, 177, 279
WHO assistance in, 622
Indian Health Service of USPHS, 598
Indices: for dental disease, 319–336
interrelation between, 336–338
of social need, 198, 313
Indigence: estimation of, 198–201
medical, 7, 201, 306
Industrial absenteeism, 554–555
Industrial dentistry, 50, 307, 552–563
Industrial hazards, dental, 160, 559–563

Industrial health, 36
Industry, dental health education in, 389
Infection, systemic, of dental origin, 272–273
Inspection, dental, 339, 534
Insurance: accident, 479
commercial carriers of, 492
for dental care, 479–482
general principles, 477–482
health: as public health, 9, 16, 53, 302
hospital, 478
indemnity, 480
major medical, 479
service-benefit, 480
workmen's compensation, 560
International Classification of Diseases, 26
International Longshoremen's and Warehousemen's Union-Pacific Maritime Association, 54
Internship and fellowship programs, 52

Janis, I. L., 370
Japan, 292, 302
Joseph Samuels Dental Center, 571

Knutson, J. W., 96, 251, 336, 623

Laboratories, dental, 444–445, 456
Laboratory services, in public health programs, 35
Labor union dental programs, 491
Lactobacillus acidophilus, and caries, 144, 250, 258
Latitude and dental disease, 147–155
Law: and fluoridation, 424
use of, in public health, 23, 32
Leukoplakia, 184
Lewin, K., field theory in education, 371–372
Line services defined, 210
Louisville, Ky., Clinical Development Center, 439–440

McKay, F. S., 49, 127, 394
Malaysia, dental program in, 619

Malformations, epidemiology of, 182–183

Malocclusion: and loss of teeth, 306
measurement of, 333–335
occurrence of, 182–183
prevention of, 259–261
related to anxiety, 335

Management, executive, 218–223

Manpower, dental. *See* Dental manpower

Market for dental care, 275, 277

Masking of one disease by another, 170

Massachusetts Department of Public Welfare, 507, 524

Mass media in health education, 357–377

Master of Public Health degree, 224

Maternal and child health, 28, 52

Mean, arithmetic, 76, 86

Median, defined, 76, 107

Medicaid (Title XIX), 54, 301, 493–495, 499, 502, 524, 537, 538, 547, 579, 583–586, 597, 602–608
eligibility for, 504
"reasonable cost" reimbursement, 493

Medicare, 23, 54, 301, 603

Medicine: preventive and public health, 13
"socialized," 15

Mellanby, M., 50, 132

Mental health, 36, 37

Mercury, 561

Merit systems for personnel, 220

Metropolitan Life Insurance Co. (New York): dental programs for employees, 49, 297, 557–558
survey findings, 62–63, 137, 139

Military personnel, dental disease among, 146–148, 149, 180

Milk, 33–34, 246

Miller, W. D., theory of causation of caries, 45, 50, 131, 144, 232

Miswak, 233

Mode, defined, 77

Moral codes, in relation to executive work, 228

Morbidity, 26

Mortality, 26, 33, 72, 184, 403–405
maternal and infant, 28

Mosaic law, 4

Mothers: in health education, 388
in operatory, 198

Motion pictures in health education, 374

Mouthpieces for handicapped, 571–572

Mouth protectors for sports, 262–264

Muhler, J. C., 251

Multifactorial disease. *See* Disease, multifactorial

National Academy of Sciences, radiation report, 354

National Alliance Football Rules Committee, 263

National Bureau of Standards, 35

National Center for Health Statistics, 275, 516, 601

National Collegiate Athletic Association, 264

National Committee on School Health Policies, 534

National Council on Radiation Protection and Measurements, 354

National Dairy Council, 379

National Education Association, 367, 381

National Health and Nutrition Surveys (NHANES), 276

National Health Insurance:
approaches to, 630–608, 635
emergency care in, 609, 611
preventive services in, 609, 611
child dental care in, 610–611

National Health Service Corps, 598

National Institute of Dental Research, 379, 600

National Institute of Municipal Law Officers, 425–426

National Institutes of Health, 215, 600–601

National Preventive Dentistry Demonstration Program, 546

National Research Council: advisory work, 61, 408

National Research Council (*cont.*)
  recommended dietary allowances,
  245–247
Needs, dental. *See* Dental needs
Negroes. *See* Blacks
Neighborhood health centers, 462,
  546
Neuroses and periodontal disease,
  175
Newburgh-Kingston (New York),
  caries-fluorine study, 53, 403,
  410
Newspapers in health education,
  376
New York City Department of
  Health, 502
New York Naval Shipyard, dental
  conditions in, 556
New York State Department of
  Health, 21–25, 515, 591–593
New Zealand: clinics, 543, 550
  dental disease in, 150, 157, 158,
    163, 451–452
  dental nurses, 51, 293, 438
  dental program for adolescents,
    538, 542
  missing teeth among adults, 196
  School Dental Service, 51, 304,
    388, 447, 450, 464, 473, 475,
    506, 512, 617, 635
New Zealand Dental Association,
  449
Nizel, A. E., 147, 243
Normal frequency curve, 79–80,
  95
Norway, 161, 163, 302, 304, 451,
  616–618
Null hypothesis, 87, 89, 96
Nurses: dental, 51, 447–448
  public health, 29–30, 37
  school, 381–382, 536, 544–545
  visiting, 30, 37
Nursing homes, 550
  standards for, 27
  dental needs in, 565–567
Nutrient Data Bank Directory, 245
Nutrition: and caries, 49, 158–159
  in child care, 29
  in health department activity, 36
  and periodontal disease, 178

Occlusion, traumatic, related to
  periodontal disease, 175
Occupation and periodontal disease,
  175
Opacities, in enamel, 404, 406
Operations research, 222
Optical scanning systems, 344, 346
Oral hygiene, 5, 45, 46, 181,
  232–237
Oral Hygiene Committee of Na-
  tional Dental Association, 46
Oral Hygiene Index (Greene) (OHI
  and OHI-S), 332, 485
Oral Hygiene Service, London, 379
Oral rinsing: aid to hygiene,
  236–237
  with fluoride, *see* Fluoride mouth
    rinses
Orders, standing, function of, 213
Organization: administrative,
  209–212
  charts, 213
Orthodontic treatment: for the
  handicapped, 571
  in community programs, 547
Orthodontic Treatment Priority Index, 335
Osteoporosis and fluoride, 403

Pain, differing reactions to, 188,
  194
Pairing of cases, 72
Pamphlets in health education, 376
Pan-American Health Organization,
  624–626
Panels, personnel, for dental pro-
  grams, 460
Parent teacher associations, 312,
  389
Parkinson, C. N., his "law," 217
"Partnership for Health." *See* Com-
  prehensive Health Planning Act
Patients: interpretation of data on,
  361
  variations in load of, 287
Paul, B. D., 9, 187, 188, 190,
  204–205
Payment for dental care, 476–500
Pediatric care, importance of, 312
Peer review, 473, 508–514

Pennsylvania Division of Industrial Hygiene, dental program of, 563
Percentiles, defined, 77
Periodontal disease, 167–182
  agent factors in, 167, 176–177
  bacterial flora in, 176–177
  and diet, 259
  endocrine changes in, 175
  environmental factors in, 177–180
  and fluoride, 413
  geographic variations in, 172–173
  home care for, 258–259
  host factors, 169–176
  intraoral variations in, 171, 174
  measurement, 168
  metal poisoning related to, 177, 259
  prevention of, 257–259
  treatment needs, United States, 181
Periodontal Index (Russell), 179, 276, 327–328
Periodontitis, 168
Periodontosis, 168
Personnel, dental. *See also* Dental personnel
  criticism of, 227
  principles in management of, 218–222, 317
  public health types of, 20
  recruitment of, 219, 221
Philadelphia Department of Public Health, dental program, 298, 361, 473, 509, 513, 515, 635
Placebo effect, 66, 67
Plaque, bacterial, 143, 145, 176
  control of, 485
Poison: defined, 401
  in fluoride controversy, 202, 205
Polyisomerism, secondary, 630
Population: defined, 123
  elderly, 276, 277
  and public health, 12, 114
  of teeth (not persons), 142
Posters in health education, 375
Postpayment for dental care, 497–499
Poverty, "culture of," 301, 461

Practitioner, private, 15
Preferred provider organizations (PPOs), 461
Pregnancy: and caries, 140
  related to gingivitis, 175
Prepayment for dental care, 467, 482–485
  underutilization of, 483–484
Preschool dental programs, 547–549
Prevalence: defined, 73
  point versus period, 73
  use in surveys, 324, 326, 336–337, 342–343
Prevention: defined, 13
  levels of, 13, 231-232
  novelty of method in, 253–254
  of periodontal disease, 257–259
  and public health, 3, 6, 14, 265–266, 297, 636–637
Preventive dentistry, 13, 454, 581
Price elasticity of dental care, 282
Privacy, fear of, 194
Probability, interpretation of, in public health, 8, 59, 111
Procedure manuals, 213
Professional review committees, 510–511
Professional Standards Review Organizations (PSROs), 516–517, 602
Profile patterns, 507–508
Program evaluation, 222–223
Program Evaluation and Review Technique (PERT), 223
Programs, dental. *See* Dental programs
Prophylactic odontotomy, 248
Proportions, statistical appraisal of, 94–97
Public health: activities, basic, 6, 18, 21–36
  ancient examples of, 4
  characteristics of the endeavor, 6–9
  defined, 4
  laboratories, 35
  new in dentistry, 3
  and private practice, 4
  schools of, 20, 21

Public Health (*cont.*)
  techniques of, 37–41
  training and teaching at state
    level, 588–589, 593

Quality of dental care, 13, 23,
  501–525, 636
Quarantine, 6, 32
Questionnaires, value of, 65–67,
  314, 391

Race: and caries, 136
  dental needs by, 278
  and disease, general, 117
  and periodontal disease, 171, 178
Radiation, ionizing, control of, 24,
  353–356, 561
Radio in health education, 377
Rainfall and dental disease,
  154–155
Ramfjord, S., periodontal index,
  329–331
Random numbers, 70, 340
Range of variability, 78
Rates: morbidity, 26, 72
  mortality, 26, 72
  related to time, 72, 75
  tooth fatality and mortality, 72
Records, dental: function of, 213,
  217
  for identification of dead, 576
Referenda, public, in fluoridation,
  202, 205–206, 425
Refuse, removal of, 33–34
Regression, 102–106, 541
Rehabilitation, 37, 40
Research, dental, 24, 582, 619,
  637–638
Residency in dental public health,
  225, 588–589, 593
Resistance to disease, natural, 116,
  118
Rhein, M. L., 45
Rheumatic fever, 273
Russell, A. L., 122, 150, 158, 169,
  171, 178, 180, 276, 327–328,
  409, 413

Salem-Beverly, 418, 421
Salzmann, J. A., 334

Samples: size of, 69, 90–91, 339
  types of, and their function, 68, 69
Sampling, stratified, 69
Sanitation, environmental, 33–34
Saskatchewan, Canada, dental pro-
  grams of, 388, 470–471, 539,
  543, 635
Saudi Arabia, dental programs in,
  619
Scale: nominal, 107
  ordinal and ranking, 107
Scatter. *See* Variability
Schoolchildren, health-educational
  approaches to, 386–388
School curricula, types of, 367–369
School dental health programs, 50
School health, 29, 527
  education, defined, 316
  services, 316, 528–530
School lunch program, 315, 529
School medical examinations, tim-
  ing of, 534
School nurses. *See* Nurses, school
Screening, 38–39
  dental, 39, 339, 535
  multiphasic, 39
Seacoast, distance from and dental
  disease, 147–155
Sealants, pit and fissure, 24,
  248–250, 446, 449, 527, 546,
  586, 591, 609–610, 633
Selenium, and caries, 156
Semantics, 67, 373
Sewage, disposal of, 33–34
Sex: and caries, 139–140
  dental needs by, 139–140, 278
  and disease, general, 117
  and periodontal disease, 171
Significance: of difference between
  means, 78, 86–89
  of difference between propor-
  tions, 94–97
Silver nitrate in caries control, 251
Slides in health education, 375
Snyder, J. C., 11
Snyder, M. D., 257
Social classes, attitudes of, 189–192
Social factors in caries, 159–162
Social needs, measurement of,
  198–201, 313

Social science: defined, 186–188
  in dental public health, 188–190
Social scientists, and fluoridation, 203–205
Social Security Act, United States (1935), 52, 54
Social workers, function of, 201
Sognnaes, R. F., 160–162
Soils, and caries, 157
Space maintainers, 259–260
"Span of control" concept in organization, 209–210
Spearman rank correlation test, 108
Staff services, defined, 210
Staff versus line activities, 210
Standard deviation. See Deviation, standard
Standard error. See Error, standard
Standard Form No. 603, 344–345
State dental programs, 578–594
  activities of, 52, 581–582
  administration and personnel, 586–591
State Health Planning and Development Agency (SHPDA), 603
State of New York Health Department, 21–25, 210, 591–593
Statistics: defined, 60
  nonparametric, 76, 107–108
  vital, 10, 25, 26
Streptococci: in oral and systemic disease, 119, 273
  related to dental disease, 135, 144
Stress, and caries, 141–142, 308
Study: end result, 506
  epidemiological: cross-sectional or retrospective, 128, 506
  longitudinal or cohort, 128
  observational, 506
Sugar consumption and caries, 44, 161–163
Sunshine and caries, 151
Supervision, direct versus general, 448–449
Surgery, attitudes toward, 198
Surveying, 310–362
  of attitudes and resources, 311–318
  of caries, 323–325
  defined, 310

of periodontal disease, 325–333
  reversals in, 323, 341, 349
Sweden: child care, 304, 539
  dental health care, 616–617
  dental nurses, 452
  mouth rinse programs in, 452
  neighborhood clinics, 539, 543
Symmetry, bilateral, use of in surveying, 144, 338
Synergism, 118
Systems engineering, 222

Teacher, classroom, role in health education, 316, 381–382, 385, 536
TEAM programs in dental schools, 443
Teamwork, 3, 6, 436
  benefits of, 433, 442, 455
  of the future, 634
Teeth: deciduous, "def" count for, 324
  missing, appraisal of, 146, 168, 323, 326
  saving of, 181, 195, 296–297, 558
  topical protection of, 247–254
Temperature and dental disease, 152–153
Thumb sucking, control of, 259–260
Tobacco, 262
Toothbrush, 232, 233
Toothbrushing: early recommendation of, 45
  effectiveness of, 236
  for general use, 234–235
  for periodontal disease, 258–259
Tooth numbering for records, 322
Tooth resistance, developmental aids to, 254–255
Trace elements, and caries, 156–157
Tradition, importance of, 195
Trailer, dental, operation of, 537, 580
Training, in-service, 225–226
"Trench mouth," 180
t-test (statistical), 87–88
t value, 87–88, 90, 96
  test for, 89

Tuberculosis: as chronic disease, 134–135
occurrence of, 121, 125
public health problem, 31, 37–39

Underdeveloped areas. *See* Countries, developing
Unknowns, statistical treatment of, 71
United States: caries, variations within, 146–155, 163
dental care rendered by government, 596–598
United States Army Dental Corps, 47, 52
United States Department of Agriculture, 153
United States Department of Health and Human Services, 464, 599, 601–602
United States Environmental Protection Agency, 35, 419
United States Food and Drug Administration, 35
United States Naval Dental School, course in casualty handling, 575
United States Navy Dental Corps established, 47, 52
United States Peace Corps, 620
United States Public Health Service: dental department founded, 49
program activities, 597–602
educational material, 378, 428, 481
recommendations of; 202, 265, 419, 430, 547
services, 35, 432, 516
study and survey work, 34, 63, 65, 146, 148, 287, 296, 297, 431, 436
United States Supreme Court and fluoridation, 427
Universe, statistical, defined, 68, 70
Urbanization: and caries, 157, 282
and periodontal disease, 179–180

Vaccines for caries, 145
Van Burkalow, A., 155

Variability: of data, general, 74–92
measurement of, 78–92
Variables, exclusion of, 63, 64
Variance, analysis of, 79, 89
Varnishes, fluoride, 250
Vectors of disease, 33, 121
Veterans, health care for, 15, 47
Video cassettes, 374
Vietnam, 159, 165, 178, 179
Vincent's infection, 180
Vipeholm studies (Sweden), 236–237, 239
Vitamins: and caries, 50, 152, 242
and periodontal disease, 178
sources in diet, 246
Voluntary organizations: assessment of, 312
versus government, in public health, 40–41

Wallace, H. M., 198–199, 313
War, and dental caries, 160–161
Washington State Dental Service Corporation, 53
Water: consumption of, related to fluoridation, 419–420
fluoridation of, *see* Fluoridation
hardness of, and caries, 156
pipes and fluoride, 417, 418, 424
purification of, 33–34
Water Pik®, 237
Welfare funds in labor unions, 491
Williams, J. L., 45
Winslow, C. E. A., 4, 15
Woodstock, Vermont, health education conference, 283, 384–386
Women: employees, 19
and periodontal disease, 278
pregnant, 24, 140, 175
"Worker-in-his-work unit," concept of, 218
World Health Organization, 5, 21, 54, 158, 245, 430, 621–626
data bank, 55, 164
dental auxiliaries, recommendations concerning, 271, 293, 444, 453, 636
dental health programs, 623
fellowships, 624

fluoridation, policy on, 430
studies of, 435, 450–451, 512,
    623
survey methods, 319–321, 323,
    328, 331, 333, 340, 344, 362,
    624

X-rays: administrative use of, 324,
    348, 536
chest, 38–39
dental, 349–356, 534, 576

Zahnärzte, 447, 632